Lecture Notes in Computer Science 16376

The series Lecture Notes in Computer Science (LNCS), including its subseries Lecture Notes in Artificial Intelligence (LNAI) and Lecture Notes in Bioinformatics (LNBI), has established itself as a medium for the publication of new developments in computer science and information technology research, teaching, and education.

LNCS enjoys close cooperation with the computer science R & D community, the series counts many renowned academics among its volume editors and paper authors, and collaborates with prestigious societies. Its mission is to serve this international community by providing an invaluable service, mainly focused on the publication of conference and workshop proceedings and postproceedings. LNCS commenced publication in 1973.

Spyridon Bakas · Emily Dennis ·
Mehdi Astaraki · Ujjwal Baid ·
Gian Marco Conte · Martha Foltyn-Dumitru ·
Zhifan Jiang · Dominic Labella ·
Marie-Christin Metz · Udunna Anazodo ·
Maria Correia de Verdier · Florian Kofler ·
Hongwei Bran Li · Marius George Linguraru ·
Nazanin Maleki
Editors

Segmentation, Classification, and Synthesis for Brain Tumors and Traumatic Brain Injuries

MICCAI 2025 Challenges: BraTS-Lighthouse 2025 and AIMS-TBI 2025, Held in Conjunction with MICCAI 2025
Daejeon, South Korea, September 23, 2025
Proceedings, Part I

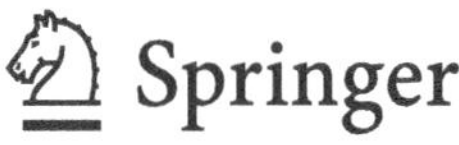

Editors
Spyridon Bakas
Indiana University School of Medicine
Indianapolis, IN, USA

Emily Dennis
University of Utah
Emerald Hills, CA, USA

Mehdi Astaraki
Karolinska Institutet
Huddinge, Sweden

Ujjwal Baid
Emory University School of Medicine
Atlanta, GA, USA

Gian Marco Conte
Mayo Clinic
Rochester, MN, USA

Martha Foltyn-Dumitru
University Hospital Bonn
Bonn, Germany

Zhifan Jiang
Children's National Hospital
Washington, D.C., USA

Dominic Labella
Duke University
Durham, NC, USA

Marie-Christin Metz
Klinikum rechts der Isar, TU Munich
Munich, Germany

Udunna Anazodo
McGill University
Montréal, QC, Canada

Maria Correia de Verdier
Uppsala University
Uppsala, Sweden

Florian Kofler
University of Tübingen
Tübingen, Germany

Hongwei Bran Li
NUS Medicine and Engineering
Singapore, Singapore

Marius George Linguraru
Children's National Hospital
Washington, D.C., USA

Nazanin Maleki
Children's Hospital of Philadelphia
Philadelphia, PA, USA

ISSN 0302-9743 ISSN 1611-3349 (electronic)
Lecture Notes in Computer Science
ISBN 978-3-032-16364-6 ISBN 978-3-032-16365-3 (eBook)
https://doi.org/10.1007/978-3-032-16365-3

This Springer imprint is published by the registered company Springer Nature Switzerland AG
The registered company address is: Gewerbestrasse 11, 6330 Cham, Switzerland

Preface

This volume contains papers accepted for the Brain TumorS (BraTS) 2025 Lighthouse Cluster of Challenges, and the Automated Identification of Moderate-Severe Traumatic Brain Injury Lesions (AIMS-TBI) 2025 Challenge. Both events were held in conjunction with the Medical Image Computing and Computer Assisted Intervention (MICCAI) conference on September 23–27, 2025 in Daejeon, Republic of Korea.

The presented manuscripts describe the latest research from computational scientists and clinical researchers working on adult and pediatric brain abnormalities, and specifically glioma, meningioma, metastases, and traumatic brain injuries. This compilation does not claim to provide a comprehensive understanding from all points of view; however, the authors present their latest advances in segmentation, detection, classification, and synthesis.

After the introductory chapter, My Model Is Better Than Yours! Statistically Aware Ranking for Fair Benchmarking of AI Models, the volume is divided into sections: The first through the seventh sections comprise a selection of accepted BraTS papers describing medical image segmentation methods for adult and pediatric brain glioblastoma, meningioma, and metastases. The eighth and ninth sections focus on accepted BraTS submissions showing advances in the field of image synthesis and inpainting for adult brain tumors. The tenth and eleventh sections focus on methods presented at the BraTS challenge, targeting the workload of classification for glioblastoma pathology sub-regions and disease progression. The twelfth section focuses on providing an overview of new medical image analysis advances from the AIMS-TBI challenge.

The focus of the first through the seventh sections is a selection of papers from the BraTS 2025 challenge participants developing the current state-of-the-art segmentation algorithms for routine, multi-institutional, clinically acquired multiparametric magnetic resonance imaging (mpMRI) scans towards addressing: Challenge 1, pre- and post-operative adult diffuse glioma (BraTS-GLI); Challenge 2, pre-treatment intracranial meningioma (BraTS-MEN); Challenge 3, pre-radiotherapy intracranial meningioma (BraTS-MEN-RT); Challenge 4, pre- and post-treatment brain metastases (BraTS-METS); Challenge 5, the underserved sub-Saharan African brain glioma patient population (BraTS-Africa); Challenge 6, pre-treatment pediatric high grade glioma patients (BraTS-PEDS); and Challenge 7, generalizability of segmentation methods across tumors (BraTS-GOAT). [Regarding the BraTS-GLI Challenge 1, Errol Colak, Adam Flanders, Felipe C. Kitamura and Luciano M. Prevedello were involved in the BraTS 2021 challenge, the data of which were used for training and validation in the 2023 and 2025 pre-treatment challenges, but they were not involved in the organization of the 2025 challenge.]

The eighth and ninth sections focus on generative artificial intelligence (AI). Challenge 8 addresses the synthesis of entire missing MRI sequences (BraTS-Synth), towards enabling the broader use of BraTS segmentation methods that mandate the availability of four structural MRI sequences (T1w, T1w with contrast, T2w, and T2-FLAIR) in clinical settings with limited imaging protocols or for the retrospective analysis of archival tumor datasets. Challenge 9 addresses the task of Local Inpainting of healthy tissue in brain tumor MRI scans (BraTS-Inpainting). Participants inpaint either brain tumor tissue or partially corrupted image regions. These forms of data corruption are often technical in nature, resulting from localized artifacts, an incomplete field of view, or missing or corrupted 2D slices. The objective is to develop algorithms that can locally synthesize missing image intensities within a predefined inpainting mask.

The tenth and eleventh sections focus on the computational workload of classification. Challenge 10 specifically includes papers representing the latest developments on AI models capable of assessing the heterogeneous histomorphologic landscape of glioblastoma by identifying nine distinct histopathologic tumor sub-regions on formalin-fixed paraffin-embedded (FFPE) H&E-stained tissue sections, acquired from standard clinical practice across 11 international sites (BraTS-Path). Challenge 11 then builds on longitudinal MRI sequences to present methods able to predict tumor progression during therapy (BraTS-PRO). Longitudinal properties are central to clinical practice, as defined by the Response Assessment in Neuro Oncology (RANO) criteria, which categorize treatment response into: complete response, partial response, stable disease, and progressive disease.

Challenge 12 focuses on the AIMS-TBI challenge, in which participants were tasked with developing new classification and segmentation algorithms for lesions due to traumatic brain injury. TBI-related lesions are highly heterogeneous and are not reliably identified by current methods focusing on other abnormalities (e.g., ischemic stroke, tumors). Our inability to accurately segment these lesions introduces significant bias in research, as lesions are either ignored, leading to methodological inaccuracies, or excluded, decreasing the generalizability of research.

Ninety papers were submitted and subsequently underwent a single-blind review process, with each receiving evaluation from a minimum of two independent reviewers. This process resulted in the acceptance of 80 papers which are presented across two volumes. We wholeheartedly hope that these two volumes will promote further exciting computational research on brain abnormalities.

October 2025

Spyridon Bakas
Emily Dennis
Mehdi Astaraki
Ujjwal Baid
Gian Marco Conte
Martha Foltyn-Dumitru
Zhifan Jiang
Dominic Labella
Marie-Christin Metz
Udunna Anazodo
Maria Correia de Verdier
Florian Kofler
Hongwei Bran Li
Marius George Linguraru
Nazanin Maleki

Organization

Challenge 1: BraTS-GLI

Leading Organizers

Spyridon Bakas	Indiana University, USA
Ujjwal Baid	Emory University, USA
Maria Correia de Verdier	University of California, San Diego, USA and Uppsala University, Sweden
Jeffrey D. Rudie	University of California, San Diego, USA and Scripps Clinic Medical Group, USA
Rachit Saluja	Cornell University, Cornell Tech, Weill Cornell Medicine, USA

Organizing Committee

Mariam Aboian	Children's Hospital of Philadelphia, USA
Mehdi Astaraki	Karolinska Institute, Sweden
Michel Bilello	University of Pennsylvania, USA
Rong Chai	Sage Bionetworks, USA
Verena Chung	Sage Bionetworks, USA
Errol Colak	University of Toronto, Canada
Gian Marco Conte	Mayo Clinic, USA
Keyvan Farahani	National Cancer Institute, USA
Nikdokht Farid	University of California, San Diego, USA
Adam Flanders	Thomas Jefferson University Hospital, USA
Louis Gagnon	University of California, San Diego, USA and University of Laval, Canada
Satyam Ghodasara	University of Pennsylvania, USA
Raymond Huang	Harvard Medical School, USA
Felipe C. Kitamura	Diagnósticos da América (DASA), Brazil
Dominic LaBella	Duke University, USA
Serghei Mangul	Sage Bionetworks, USA
Bjoern Menze	University of Zurich, Switzerland
Suyash Mohan	University of Pennsylvania, USA
Ayman Nada	University of Missouri, USA
Luciano M. Prevedello	Ohio State University, Wexner Medical Center, USA

Rachit Saluja	Cornell University, Cornell Tech, Weill Cornell Medicine, USA
Russell T. Shinohara	University of Pennsylvania, USA
Arti Singh	Sage Bionetworks, USA
Nourel Hoda Tahon	University of Missouri, USA
Philip Vollmuth	Heidelberg University, Germany

Data Contributors

Pre-treatment

Christos Davatzikos	University of Pennsylvania, USA
Spyridon Bakas	Indiana University, USA
John Mongan	University of California, San Francisco, USA
Evan Calabrese	University of California, San Francisco, USA
Jeffrey D. Rudie	University of California, San Francisco, USA
Christopher Hess	University of California, San Francisco, USA
Soonmee Cha	University of California, San Francisco, USA
Javier Villanueva-Meyer	University of California, San Francisco, USA
John B. Freymann	National Institutes of Health (NIH), USA
Justin S. Kirby	National Institutes of Health (NIH), USA
Benedikt Wiestler	Technical University of Munich, Germany
Bjoern Menze	University of Zurich, Switzerland
Errol Colak	University of Toronto, Canada
Priscila Crivellaro	University of Toronto, Canada
Rivka R. Colen	MD Anderson Cancer Center, USA
Aikaterini Kotrotsou	MD Anderson Cancer Center, USA
Daniel Marcus	Washington University in St. Louis, USA
Mikhail Milchenko	Washington University in St. Louis, USA
Arash Nazeri	Washington University in St. Louis, USA
Hassan Fathallah-Shaykh	University of Alabama at Birmingham, USA
Roland Wiest	University of Bern, Switzerland
Andras Jakab	University of Debrecen, Hungary
Marc-Andre Weber	Heidelberg University, Germany
Abhishek Mahajan	Tata Memorial Centre, Mumbai, India
Ujjwal Baid	Emory University, USA

Post-treatment

Evan Calabrese	Duke University, USA
Dominic LaBella	Duke University, USA
Jikai Zhang	Duke University, USA
Jeffrey D. Rudie	University of California, San Francisco, USA
Andreas Rauschecker	University of California, San Francisco, USA
Brandon Fields	University of California, San Francisco, USA
Javier Villanueva-Meyer	University of California, San Francisco, USA
Ayman Nada	University of Missouri, Columbia, USA
Nourel Hoda Tahon	University of Missouri, Columbia, USA
Talissa Altes	University of Missouri, Columbia, USA
Yaseen Dhemesh	University of Missouri, Columbia, USA
Filip Garrett	University of Missouri, Columbia, USA
Jaime Gass	University of Missouri, Columbia, USA
Edvin Isufi	University of Missouri, Columbia, USA
Lester J. Layfield	University of Missouri, Columbia, USA
Jason Sinclair	University of Missouri, Columbia, USA
Jonathan Thacker	University of Missouri, Columbia, USA
Jeffrey D. Rudie	University of California, San Diego, USA
Maria Correia de Verdier	University of California, San Diego, USA
Nikdokht Farid	University of California, San Diego, USA
Louis Gagnon	University of California, San Diego, USA
Jona Hattagandi Gluth	University of California, San Diego, USA
Paul Manning	University of California, San Diego, USA
Tyler Seibert	University of California, San Diego, USA
Sevcan Turk	University of Michigan, USA
Lubomir Hadjiiski	University of Michigan, USA
Sebastian Oliva	University of Michigan, USA
Patil Basavasagar	University of Michigan, USA
Ujjwal Baid	Emory University, USA
Spyridon Bakas	Indiana University, USA
Yuri S. Velichko	Northwestern University, USA

Challenge 2: BraTS-MEN

Leading Organizers

Evan Calabrese	Duke University, USA
Dominic Labella	Duke University, USA

Organizing Committee

Data Contributors

Challenge 3: BraTS-MEN-RT

Leading Organizers

Evan Calabrese	Duke University, USA
Dominic Labella	Duke University, USA

Organizing Committee

Mariam Aboian	Children's Hospital of Philadelphia, USA
Mehdi Astaraki	Karolinska Institute, Sweden
Ujjwal Baid	Emory University, USA
Spyridon Bakas	Indiana University, USA
Gian Marco Conte	Mayo Clinic, USA
Maria Correia de Verdier	University of San Diego, USA
Nourel Hoda Tahon	University of Missouri, USA
Raymond Huang	Harvard Medical School, USA
Ayman Nada	University of Missouri, USA
Andreas M. Rauschecker	University of California, San Francisco, USA
Jeffrey Rudie	University of San Diego, USA
Benedikt Wiestler	Technical University of Munich, Germany

Data Contributors

Jeffrey Rudie	University of California, San Francisco, USA
Andreas Rauschecker	University of California, San Francisco, USA
Brandon Fields	University of California, San Francisco, USA
Javier Villanueva-Meyer	University of California, San Francisco, USA
Michael Mix	SUNY Upstate, USA
Katherine Schumacher	SUNY Upstate, USA
Peter Taylor	SUNY Upstate, USA
Lia Halasz	University of Washington, USA
Justin Leu	University of Washington, USA
Ayman Nada	University of Missouri, USA
Nourel Hoda Tahon	University of Missouri, USA
Evan Calabrese	Duke University, USA
Dominic LaBella	Duke University, USA
John Kirkpatrick	Duke University, USA
Scott Floyd	Duke University, USA
Zachary Reitman	Duke University, USA
Trey Mullikin	Duke University, USA

Jonathan Shapey	King's College London, UK
Tom Vercauteren	King's College London, UK
Jeffrey D. Rudie	University of California, San Diego, USA
Maria Correia de Verdier	University of California, San Diego, USA
Nikdokht Farid	University of California, San Diego, USA
Louis Gagnon	University of California, San Diego, USA
Jona Hattagandi Gluth	University of California, San Diego, USA
Tyler Seibert	University of California, San Diego, USA

Challenge 4: BraTS-METS

Leading Organizers

Mariam Aboian	Children's Hospital of Philadelphia, USA
Nazanin Maleki	Children's Hospital of Philadelphia, USA
Ahmed Moawad	Mercy Catholic Medical Center, USA

Organizing Committee

Raisa Amiruddin	Children's Hospital of Philadelphia, USA
Nikolay Yordanov	Medical University, Sofia, Bulgaria
Crystal Chukwurah	Yale School of Medicine, USA
Pascal Fehringer	Friedrich Schiller University, Germany
Athanasios Gkampenis	University of Tübingen, Germany
Fabian Umeh	Teesside University, UK

Data Contributors

Mariam Aboian	Children's Hospital of Philadelphia, USA
Satrajit Chakrabarty	Washington University, USA
Maria Correia de Verdier	University of California, San Diego, USA
Jeffrey Rudie	University of California, San Diego, USA
Devon Godfrey	Duke University, USA
Scott Floyd	Duke University, USA
Nourel Hoda Tahon	University of Missouri, USA
Ayman Nada	University of Missouri, USA
Yuri S. Velichko	Northwestern University, USA
Ayda Youssef	National Cancer Institute, USA

Data Annotators

Fatima Memon	Medical University of South Carolina, USA
Mohanad Ghonim	University of Pennsylvania, USA
Bojan D. Petrovic	University of Chicago, USA
Mohamed Ghonim	University of Pennsylvania, USA
Justin Cramer	Mayo Clinic (Arizona), USA
Sedra Mhana	University of Pennsylvania, USA
Mark Krycia	Carolina Radiology, USA
Albara Alotaibi	Jordan University of Science and Technology, Jordan
Elizabeth Brooke Shrickel	Ohio State University, USA
Nathan Page	Friedrich Schiller University of Jena, Germany
Ichiro Ikuta	Mayo Clinic (Arizona), USA
Amirreza Manteghinejad	Children's Hospital of Philadelphia, USA
Gerard Thompson	University of Edinburgh, UK
Prisha Bhatia	Mohammed Bin Rashid University of Medicine and Health Sciences, Dubai
Lorenna Vidal	Children's Hospital of Philadelphia, USA
Yasaman Sharifi	Iran University, Iran
Vilma Kosovic	General Hospital of Dubrovnik, Croatia
Marko Jakovljevic	Children's Hospital of Philadelphia, USA
Adam Goldman-Yassen	Emory University, USA
Nikolay Yordanov	Medical University, Sofia, Bulgaria
Virginia Hill	Northwestern University, USA
Salma Abosabie	Julius-Maximilians-Universität Würzburg, Germany
Tiffany So	Chinese University of Hong Kong, China
Sara Abosabie	Charité – Universitätsmedizin Berlin, Germany
Mark Krycia	Carolina Radiology, USA
Marko Jakovljevic	Children's Hospital of Philadelphia, USA
Melisa S. Guelen	Massachusetts General Hospital, USA
Basimah Albalooshy	Children's Hospital of Philadelphia, USA
Michael Veronesi	University of Wisconsin, USA
Raisa Amiruddin	Children's Hospital of Philadelphia, USA

Challenge 5: BraTS-Africa

Leading Organizers

Udunna Anazodo	McGill University, Canada and Medical Artificial Intelligence Laboratory (MAI Lab), Nigeria
Maruf Adewole	Medical Artificial Intelligence Laboratory (MAI Lab), Nigeria

Organizing Committee

Ujjwal Baid	Emory University, USA
Spyridon Bakas	Indiana University, USA
Bjoern Menze	University of Zurich, Switzerland

Clinical Evaluators

Jeff Rudie	Scripps Health and University of California, San Diego, USA
Farouk Dako	University of Pennsylvania, USA
Abiodun Fatade	Medical Artificial Intelligence Laboratory (MAI Lab) and Crestview Radiology, Nigeria
Oluyemisi Toyobo	Medical Artificial Intelligence Laboratory (MAI Lab) and Crestview Radiology, Nigeria

Data Contributors

Kenneth Aguh	Federal Medical Centre, Umuahia, Nigeria
Rachel Akinola	Lagos State University Teaching Hospital, Lagos, Nigeria
Feyisayo Daji	National Hospital, Abuja, Nigeria
Abiodun Fatade	Medical Artificial Intelligence Laboratory (MAI Lab) and Crestview Radiology, Nigeria
Chinasa Kalaiwo	National Hospital, Nigeria
Mayomi Onuwaje	Lily Hospital, Benin, Nigeria
Olubukola Omidiji	Lagos University Teaching Hospital, Lagos, Nigeria
Mohammad Abba Suwaid	NSIA-Kano Diagnostic Center, Kano, Nigeria

Data Annotators

Adaobi Emegoakor	Nnamdi Azikiwe University Hospital, Nnewi, Nigeria
Yewande Gbadamosi	Lagos State University Teaching Hospital, Lagos, Nigeria
Chinasa Kalaiwo	National Hospital Abuja, Nigeria
Ugumba Kwikima	Muhimbili University of Health and Allied Sciences, Tanzania
Kelvin Murithi	Sonar Radiology, Kenya
Afolabi Ogunleye	Lagos State University Teaching Hospital, Lagos, Nigeria
Nancy Ojo	Federal Medical Centre, Abeokuta, Nigeria
Olubukola Omidiji	Lagos University Teaching Hospital, Lagos, Nigeria
Abbas M. Rabiu	Aminu Kano Teaching Hospital, Kano, Nigeria
Julia Rackerseder	ImFusion, Germany
Amal Saleh	Addis Ababa University, Ethiopia
Mohammad Abba Suwaid	NSIA-Kano Diagnostic Center, Kano, Nigeria
Kator Iorpagher	Benue State University, Makurdi, Nigeria

Challenge 6: BraTS-PEDS

Leading Organizers

Marius George Linguraru	Children's National Hospital and George Washington University, USA
Anahita Fathi Kazerooni	Children's Hospital of Philadelphia and University of Pennsylvania, USA

Organizing Committee

Mehdi Astaraki	Karolinska Institute, Sweden
Ujjwal Baid	Emory University, USA
Spyridon Bakas	Indiana University, USA
Verena Chung	Sage Bionetworks, USA
Keyvan Farahani	National Institutes of Health (NIH), USA
Deep Gandhi	Children's Hospital of Philadelphia, USA
Zhifan Jiang	Children's National Hospital, USA
Xinyang Liu	Children's National Hospital, USA

Data Contributors

Mariam Aboian	Children's Hospital of Philadelphia, USA
Miriam Bornhorst	Children's National Hospital, USA
Evan Calabrese	Duke University, USA
Ethan Castellino	Duke University, USA
Peter de Blank	Cincinnati Children's Hospital, USA
Michelle Deutsch	Nationwide Children's Hospital, USA
Maryam Fouladi	Nationwide Children's Hospital, USA
Lindsey Hoffman	Phoenix Children's Hospital, USA
Trent Hummel	Cincinnati Children's Hospital, USA
Benjamin Kann	Dana-Farber Brigham Cancer Center and Boston Children's Hospital, USA
Margot Lazow	Nationwide Children's Hospital, USA
Justin Low	Duke University, USA
Nazanin Maleki	Children's Hospital of Philadelphia, USA
Ali Nabavizadeh	University of Pennsylvania, USA
Avani Mangoli	Duke University, USA
Leonie Mikael	Nationwide Children's Hospital, USA
Roger Packer	Children's National Hospital, USA
Adam Resnick	Children's Hospital of Philadelphia, USA
Brian Rood	Children's National Hospital, USA
Tina Young Poussaint	FACR, Dana-Farber Brigham Cancer Center and Boston Children's Hospital, USA
Anna Zapaishchykova	Dana-Farber Brigham Cancer Center and Boston Children's Hospital, USA

Data Annotators

Debanjan Haldar	Thomas Jefferson University Hospital, USA
Shuvanjan Haldar	Children's Hospital of Philadelphia, USA
Nastaran Khalili	Children's Hospital of Philadelphia, USA
Neda Khalili	Children's Hospital of Philadelphia, USA
Hollie Lai	Children's Health Orange County, USA
Aaron McAllister	Nationwide Children's Hospital, USA
Khanak Nandolia	All India Institute of Medical Sciences, India
Sanjay Prabhu	Boston Children's Hospital, USA
Mariana Sánchez Montaño	Unidad de Patología Clínica, Mexico
Ibraheem Shaikh	Beth Israel Deaconess Medical Center, USA
Nakul Sheth	Weill Cornell Medicine and New York Presbyterian Hospital, USA
Wenxin Tu	University of Pennsylvania, USA

Bhavyasri Vunnava	Children's Hospital of Philadelphia, USA
Sanaz Varshochi	Children's Hospital of Philadelphia, USA

Data Approvers

Mariam Aboian	Children's Hospital of Philadelphia, USA
Ali Nabavizadeh	University of Pennsylvania, USA
Arastoo Vossough	Children's Hospital of Philadelphia, USA
Jeffrey B. Ware	University of Pennsylvania, USA

Challenge 7: BraTS-GOAT

Leading Organizers

Ujjwal Baid	Emory University, USA
Spyridon Bakas	Indiana University, USA
Gian Marco Conte	Mayo Clinic, USA

Data Contributors

Same data contributors as in Challenges 1, 2, 4, 5 and 6.

Challenge 8: BraTS-Synth

Leading Organizers

Hongwei Bran Li	Harvard Medical School, USA
Athinoula A. Martinos	Harvard Medical School, USA

Organizing Committee

Mariam Aboian	University of Pennsylvania, USA
Mehdi Astaraki	Karolinska Institute, Sweden
Ujjwal Baid	Emory University, USA
Spyridon Bakas	Indiana University, USA
Gian Marco Conte	Mayo Clinic, USA
Verena Chung	Sage Bionetworks, USA
Keyvan Farahani	National Institutes of Health (NIH), USA

Juan Eugenio Iglesias — Harvard Medical School, USA
Florian Kofler — Hertie AI, University of Tübingen, Germany
Marius George Linguraru — Children's National Hospital, USA
Bjoern Menze — University of Zurich, Switzerland
Matthew S. Rosen — Harvard Medical School, USA
Benedikt Wiestler — Klinikum rechts der Isar, Technical University of Munich, Germany

Data Contributors

Same data contributors as in Challenges 1, 2 and 4.

Challenge 9: BraTS-Inpainting

Leading Organizers

Florian Kofler — Hertie AI, University of Tübingen, Germany

Organizing Committee

Bjoern Menze — University of Zurich, Switzerland
Benedikt Wiestler — Klinikum rechts der Isar, Technical University of Munich, Germany
Ivan Ezhov — Technical University of Munich, Germany
Marie Piraud — Helmholtz AI, Germany

Data Contributors

Same data contributors as in Challenges 1 and 2.

Challenge 10: BraTS-Path

Leading Organizers

Spyridon Bakas — Indiana University, USA
Siddhesh Thakur — Indiana University, USA

Organizing Committee

Mehdi Astaraki	Karolinska Institute, Sweden
Ujjwal Baid	Emory University, USA
Robert Bell	Indiana University, USA
Verena Chung	Sage Bionetworks, USA
Lee A. D. Cooper	Northwestern University, USA
Jason Huse	Anderson Cancer Center, USA
Shahriar Faghani	Mayo Clinic, USA
Keyvan Farahani	National Institutes of Health (NIH), USA
Mana Moassefi	Mayo Clinic, USA

Clinical Annotators

Jose Javier Otero	Florida International University, USA
Jason Huse	Anderson Cancer Center, USA
C. J. Lucas	Johns Hopkins University, USA
Kenneth Aldape	National Cancer Institute, USA
Leo Y. Ballester	Anderson Cancer Center, USA
Aditya Raghunathan	Mayo Clinic, USA, USA
Michael L. Miller	Columbia University, USA
Valeria Barresi	University of Verona, Italy
Leonille Schweizer	University Hospital Frankfurt, Germany
Marwan M. Majeed	Indiana University, USA
Maria A. Gubbiotti	Anderson Cancer Center, USA
Michael Rodriguez	Macquarie University, Australia
Hrvoje Miletić	Haukeland University Hospital, Norway
Claire Delbridge	Technical University of Munich, Germany
Giselle Y. López	Duke University, USA
Tibor Hortobagyi	University Hospital Zurich, Switzerland
Regina Rose Reimann	University Hospital Zurich, Switzerland
Joanna J. Phillips	University of California, San Francisco, USA
MacLean P. Nasrallah	University of Pennsylvania, USA
Keith L. Ligon	Dana-Farber Cancer Institute, USA

Challenge 11: BraTS-PRO

Leading Organizers

Name	Affiliation
Yannick Kirchhoff	German Cancer Research Center (DKFZ), Germany
Philipp Vollmuth	German Cancer Research Center (DKFZ), Heidelberg and University Hospital Bonn, Germany

Organizing Committee

Name	Affiliation
Mehdi Astaraki	Karolinska Institute, Sweden
Spyridon Bakas	Indiana University, USA
Jan Egger	University Hospital Essen, Germany
André Ferreira	University of Minho, Portugal and University Hospital Essen, Germany
Martha Foltyn-Dumitru	University Hospital Bonn, Germany
Raymond Y. Huang	Mass General Brigham, USA
Balint Kovacs	German Cancer Research Center (DKFZ), Germany
Jens Kleesiek	University Hospital Essen, Germany
Klaus Maier-Hein	German Cancer Research Center (DKFZ), Germany
Mauricio Reyes	University of Bern, Switzerland
Yannick Suter	University of Bern, Switzerland
Javier Villanueva-Meyer	University of California, San Francisco, USA
Tassilo Wald	German Cancer Research Center (DKFZ), Germany
Maximilian Zenk	German Cancer Research Center (DKFZ), Germany

Challenge 12: AIMS-TBI

Leading Organizers

Name	Affiliation
Emily Dennis	University of Utah, USA
Evelyn Deutscher	Deakin University, Australia

Organizing Committee

Spyridon Bakas	Indiana University, USA
Matthew Pease	Indiana University, USA
Adrian Onicas	University of Utah, USA
Nicholas Tustison	University of Virginia, USA
Elisabeth Wilde	University of Utah, USA

Data Contributors

Robert Asarnow	University of California, Los Angeles, USA
Karen Caeyenberghs	Deakin University, Australia
Nancy Chiaravalloti	Kessler Foundation, USA
Brenda Bartnik-Olson	Loma Linda University, USA
Kristen Dams-O'Connor	Mount Sinai, USA
Ekaterina Dobryakova	Kessler Foundation, USA
Linda Ewing-Cobbs	University of Texas, Houston, USA
Helen Genova	Kessler Foundation, USA
Frank Hillary	Pennsylvania State University
Kristen Hoskinson	Nationwide Children's Hospital, USA
Nicholas Ryan	Murdoch Children's Research Institute, Australia
Stacy Suskauer	Kennedy Krieger Institute, USA
Lars Westlye	University of Oslo, Norway
Elisabeth Wilde	University of Utah, USA

Data Annotators

Emily Dennis	University of Utah, USA
Evelyn Deutscher	Deakin University, Australia
Morgan Hafen	Brigham Young University, USA
Elizabeth Hovenden	University of Utah, USA
Jamie Johnson	University of Utah, USA
Finian Keleher	University of Utah, USA
Hannah Lindsey	University of Utah, USA
Courtney McCabe	University of Utah, USA
Jake Mitchell	Monash University, Australia
Emma Read	University of Utah, USA
Madeleine Reading	Brigham Young University, USA
Emmanuella Sybrowsky	University of Utah, USA
Dayna Thayn	University of Utah, USA

Contents

Challenge 2 – BraTS-MEN

Challenge 3 – BraTS-MEN-RT

Challenge 4 – BraTS-METS

Challenge 5 – BraTS-Africa

Challenge 7 – BraTS-GOAT

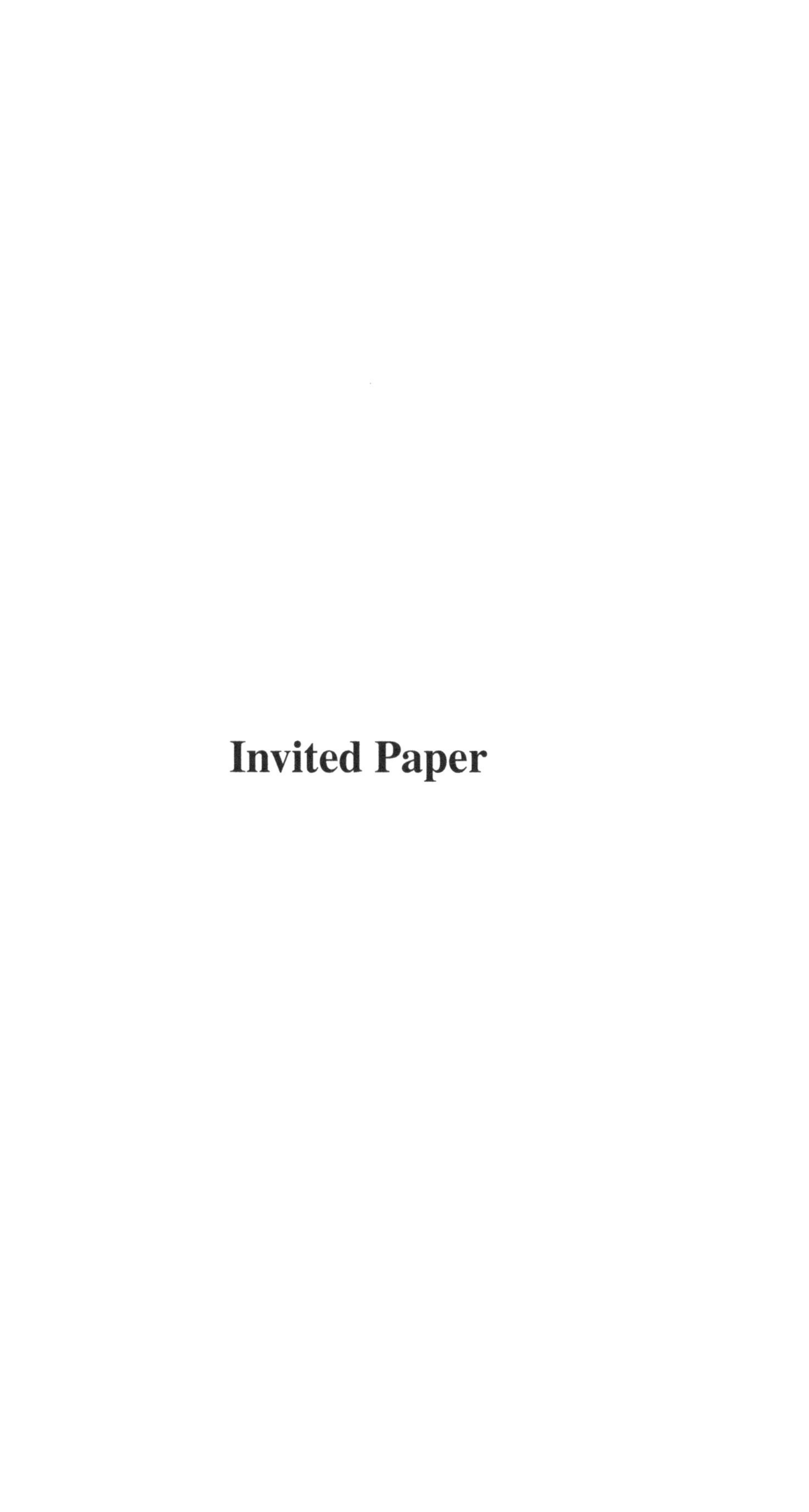

Invited Paper

My Model Is Better Than Yours! Statistically-Aware Ranking for Fair Benchmarking of AI Models

Spyridon Bakas[1,2,3,4,5(✉)], Siddhesh Thakur[1,2], Ujjwal Baid[6], Akis Linardos[1,2], Sarthak Pati[5], Jimit Doshi[7], and Russell T. Shinohara[7,8]

[1] Department of Pathology and Laboratory Medicine, Indiana University School of Medicine, Indianapolis, IN, USA
spbakas@iu.edu
[2] Indiana University Melvin and Bren Simon Comprehensive Cancer Center, Indianapolis, IN, USA
[3] Departments of Radiology and Imaging Sciences, Neurological Surgery, Biostatistics and Health Data Science, Indiana University School of Medicine, Indianapolis, IN, USA
[4] Department of Computer Science, Luddy School of Informatics, Computing, and Engineering, Indiana University, Indianapolis, IN, USA
[5] MLCommons, San Francisco, CA, USA
[6] Wallace H. Coulter Department of Biomedical Engineering at Georgia Tech and Emory University, Atlanta, GA, USA
[7] Center for Artificial Intelligence and Data Science for Integrated Diagnostics (AI2D), Perelman School of Medicine, University of Pennsylvania, Philadelphia, PA, USA
[8] Department of Biostatistics, Epidemiology, and Informatics, Perelman School of Medicine, University of Pennsylvania, Philadelphia, PA, USA

Abstract. The proliferation of artificial intelligence (AI) in healthcare has triggered the need of fair benchmarking. This, in turn, has inspired the rise of computational challenges, where participants worldwide submit models under standardized evaluation protocols. However, ranking AI models –particularly when declaring winners– raises questions about their difference from the next best (but lower-ranked) model. Here, we present a statistically-aware ranking framework, ***PermRanker***, designed to be agnostic to computational workloads (e.g., segmentation, classification, registration) and underlying data types (e.g., 2D pathology images, 3D MRI scans, or even non-imaging data). PermRanker provides fair and informative benchmarking of AI models, based on two stages: (i) a ranking score, based on case-wise cumulative rankings aggregated across multiple metrics and testing cases, and (ii) a rigorous statistical significance analysis via pairwise permutation testing across the ranked order of the AI models. This framework has served as the official ranking mechanism for over 33 international challenges between 2017 and 2025, including the BraTS, FeTS, and ISLES challenges. While mainly applied in biomedical AI challenges, PermRanker aims to address the unmet need of fair and informative benchmarking of AI models beyond this scope,

S. Bakas et al. (Eds.): MICCAI 2025, LNCS 16376, pp. 3–13, 2026.
https://doi.org/10.1007/978-3-032-16365-3_1

tackle actual real-world conditions, and hence contribute in streamlining clinical translation of AI models.

Keywords: benchmarking · ranking · statistical significance · challenges · AI

1 Introduction

Since the rapid advancement of artificial intelligence (AI) – including traditional machine learning and deep learning – and its proliferation into biomedical image analysis, there has been a rising need for fair benchmarks that adequately evaluate and compare emerging methods. This has in turn inspired the rise of multiple computational competitions (commonly known as '*challenges*'), where participants worldwide contribute innovative solutions under standardized evaluation protocols and shared datasets.

Large-scale curated datasets from such initiatives have contributed in providing fair community benchmarking environments for specific tasks (i.e., point solutions), as well as shaping the research directions of BioMedical AI. A few example of these challenges are the International Brain Tumor Segmentation (BraTS) challenges [1–7], its evolution to a MICCAI 2025 Lighthouse Cluster of Challenges covering workloads beyond segmentation and hence redefining BraTS as 'Brain TumorS' challenge [8–21], the Federated Tumor Segmentation (FeTS) challenge [22,23], the Ischemic Stroke Lesion Segmentation (ISLES) challenge [24,25], the Kidney and Kidney Tumor Segmentation (KiTS) challenge [26], the Liver Tumor Segmentation (LiTS) Benchmark [27], the QUBIQ: Uncertainty Quantification for Biomedical Image Segmentation Challenge [28], the Medical Segmentation Decathlon (MSD) [29,30], the cross-modality domain adaptation (CrossMoDA) 2021 benchmark [31], as well as a benchmark on quantifying uncertainty in brain tumor segmentation [32]. Such challenges serve as invaluable catalysts for innovation, pushing the limits of what is achievable. However, they bring to the forefront critical questions during the declaration of their "winner": Did they win by accident? Are they indeed different than the next best approach?

The conventional approach to ranking participants involves calculating a primary performance metric (e.g., Dice Similarity Coefficient (DSC) for segmentation workloads) for each test case, averaging these scores for each participating model, and then ranking the models based on this final average. This method, while widely used, has shortcomings [33]. It is susceptible to outliers, where a model might perform on a few easy cases but fail on challenging ones, yet achieve a high average score. Furthermore, it ignores the multifaceted nature of clinical tasks. For example, in tumor segmentation, delineating the enhancing tumor, the necrotic core, and the surrounding edema are all relevant, yet a single aggregated metric may obscure a model's specific strengths and weaknesses across these different subregions, and multiple metrics should be used to fairly compare 2 or more methods [34,35]. The work of Maier-Hein et al. has taken a closer look at "Why rankings of biomedical image analysis competitions should be interpreted with care", deconstructing the fragility of such simplistic leaderboards [36]: trivial perturbations, such as the choice of metric, case selection, or interpolation strategy, may alter the final rankings, suggesting that many observed performance differences are not meaningful. This echoes broader concerns in science about the reproducibility and statistical rigor of research findings [37]. Declaring a winner based on a small, and insignificant, margin in an average score does a disservice to the scientific community and can misdirect research efforts toward methods that lack true generalizability.

To address these shortcomings, here we propose ***PermRanker*** – a comprehensive statistically-informed benchmarking framework designed to be agnostic both to the computational workload (e.g., segmentation, classification, synthesis) and to the underlying data (e.g., 2D ultrasound images, 3D magnetic resonance imaging scans, or even non-imaging data). PermRanker is expected to bring substantial value to the broader biomedical AI community, since it provides a fair, transparent, and robust evaluation framework built upon two stages: ***(i)*** a ranking score generated for each evaluated model, based on case-wise cumulative rankings aggregated across pre-specified metrics and across unseen hold-out cases, and ***(ii)*** a rigorous statistical significance assessment, based on pairwise permutation testing across the ranked order of the evaluated models. Compared to a simplistic ordinal ranking, this two-staged methodology provides a more holistic assessment of model performance, identifying if performance differences between any two models are statistically significant and systematic, or the result of chance on a particular test set. While the testbed of the ranking system has so far been biomedical AI challenges, the overarching aim of PermRanker is to address the unmet need of evaluating algorithmic innovation of biomedical AI beyond this scope, tackle actual real-world conditions, and hence streamline clinical translation of AI models.

2 Methodology

2.1 Formal Problem Definition

To establish a basis for our framework, we first define the core components of a typical benchmarking of multiple models.

- $\mathcal{M} = \{M_1, M_2, \ldots, M_N\}$ is a set of N models considered for evaluation.
- $\mathcal{S} = \{S_1, S_2, \ldots, S_K\}$ is the hidden testing set, which comprises K testing cases. Note that for segmentation, registration, and synthesis tasks, a testing case represents a single subject, whereas for classification, and regression tasks a testing case describes a subset of subjects. Subsets are of equal sample size and include at least 1 case of each class.
- $\mathcal{P} = \{P_1, P_2, \ldots, P_Q\}$ is the set of Q pre-specified performance evaluation metrics. For example, in segmentation tasks, this set could include the Dice Similarity Coefficient (DSC) and the Normalized Surface Distance (NSD), whereas for classification tasks, this it might include the F1-Score and the Matthew's Correlation Coefficient (MCC).

The performance of any model $M_n \in \mathcal{M}$ on a specific testing case $S_k \in \mathcal{S}$ as measured by metric $P_q \in \mathcal{P}$ produces a scalar value, which we denote as $v(M_n, S_k, P_q)$. It is essential that the direction of optimality for each metric P_q is pre-defined, i.e., whether a higher or a lower value indicates better performance.

2.2 The Proposed Algorithmic Ranking Schema

Let the complete set of performance evaluations be represented by a three-order tensor $\mathbf{V} \in \mathbb{R}^{N \times K \times Q}$, where an element $V_{ijq} = v(M_i, S_j, P_q)$ is the scalar performance value of model M_i on case S_j using metric P_q.

Step 1: Granular Rank Transformation. For each fixed couple of (case, metric), denoted by the indices (j, q), we consider the vector of performance scores across all N models:

$$\mathbf{v}_{jq} = [v(M_1, S_j, P_q), \dots, v(M_N, S_j, P_q)]^\top \in \mathbb{R}^N \tag{1}$$

We apply a ranking operator $\mathcal{R} : \mathbb{R}^N \to \mathbb{R}^N$ to this vector to obtain a corresponding rank vector $\mathbf{r}_{jq} = \mathcal{R}(\mathbf{v}_{jq})$. The i-th component of this vector, $r(M_i, S_j, P_q)$, is the rank of model M_i.

Let σ_{jq} be a permutation of $\{1, \dots, N\}$ that sorts $\mathbf{v}_{jq}$ according to the metric's direction of optimality. Let $\delta_q \in \{-1, 1\}$ be an indicator for metric P_q, where $\delta_q = 1$ if higher is better and $\delta_q = -1$ if lower is better. Then, the sorting condition is $\delta_q \cdot v(M_{\sigma_{jq}(1)}, \dots) \geq \delta_q \cdot v(M_{\sigma_{jq}(2)}, \dots) \geq \dots$. The rank for model M_i is then defined to handle ties using the standard average rank method:

$$r(M_i, S_j, P_q) = \frac{1}{|\mathcal{A}_i|} \sum_{l \in \mathcal{A}_i} l, \tag{2}$$

where $\mathcal{A}_i = \{l \in \{1, \dots, N\} \mid v(M_i, \dots) = v(M_{\sigma_{jq}(l)}, \dots)\}$. This operation yields a rank tensor $\mathbf{R} \in \mathbb{R}^{N \times K \times Q}$.

Step 2: Case-Level Rank Aggregation. To assess the overall performance of a model on a single case, we marginalize the rank tensor $\mathbf{R}$ over the metric dimensions. This is achieved by computing the **Cumulative Rank (CR)** for model M_i on case S_j, defined as the sum of its ranks across all evaluation metrics for that case:

$$CR(M_i, S_j) = \sum_{q=1}^{Q} r(M_i, S_j, P_q). \tag{3}$$

The value $CR(M_i, S_j)$ represents an integrated performance score for model M_i on case S_j. A model that consistently ranks well across all Q evaluations for a case, will achieve a lower CR score, indicating robust performance.

Step 3: Final Model Ranking. The final ranking is determined by averaging the per-case CR scores across the entire test cohort. We define the **Final Ranking Score (FRS)** for model M_i as the empirical mean of its case-level Cumulative Ranks:

$$FRS(M_i) = \frac{1}{K} \sum_{j=1}^{K} CR(M_i, S_j). \tag{4}$$

The definitive ranking of the N models is then established by sorting them in ascending order of their FRS values. The model M^* with the lowest FRS is considered the top-performing model.

2.3 Statistical Significance of Relative Rankings via Permutation Testing

An ordinal ranking based on the FRS point estimates does not convey the statistical certainty of the observed differences. To address this, we introduce a rigorous hypothesis testing framework based on paired permutation tests to ascertain whether the performance difference between any two models is statistically significant or merely an artifact of the specific test set $\mathcal{S}$ [38,39].

Hypothesis Formulation. Consider a pair of two models M_a and M_b. For each case S_j, we have associated scalar performance summaries for each model:

$$CR(M_a, S_j) \text{ and } CR(M_b, S_j) \tag{5}$$

Let $\mathcal{D}_a$ and $\mathcal{D}_b$ be the true, unknown distributions from which these case-level CR scores are drawn. Our goal is to test for a difference in the means of these distributions, $\mu_a = \mathbb{E}[CR(M_a, S)]$ and $\mu_b = \mathbb{E}[CR(M_b, S)]$.

The null hypothesis, H_0, posits that there is no systematic difference between the two models. This implies that for any given case, the assignment of the two CR scores to either M_a or M_b is exchangeable. Formally:

$$H_0 : \mathcal{D}_a = \mathcal{D}_b. \tag{6}$$

Let us assume, without loss of generality, that $FRS(M_a) < FRS(M_b)$. The one-sided alternative hypothesis, H_1, is that model M_a is systematically superior to model M_b:

$$H_1 : \mu_a < \mu_b. \tag{7}$$

Permutation Test Algorithm. The test proceeds by constructing an empirical null distribution for a chosen test statistic.

1. **Test Statistic.** A natural test statistic is the observed difference in the FRS:

$$T_{orig} = FRS(M_a) - FRS(M_b) = \frac{1}{K} \sum_{j=1}^{K} \left(CR(M_a, S_j) - CR(M_b, S_j) \right). \tag{8}$$

2. **Null Distribution Generation.** We generate the distribution of the test statistic under the assumption that H_0 is true. This is achieved through permutations. We perform L (e.g., $L = 100,000$) simulations. In each permutation $l \in \{1, \dots, L\}$:
   (a) For each case S_j (from $j = 1, \dots, K$), we introduce a random variable $\omega_j^{(l)}$ drawn from a Rademacher distribution, i.e., $\mathbb{P}(\omega_j^{(l)} = 1) = \mathbb{P}(\omega_j^{(l)} = -1) = 0.5$.
   (b) We generate a permuted set of paired CR scores by randomly swapping the labels (M_a, M_b) for each case based on $\omega_j^{(l)}$. Let $\mathbf{d}_j = CR(M_a, S_j) - CR(M_b, S_j)$. The permuted difference for case j is $\omega_j^{(l)}\mathbf{d}_j$.
   (c) We compute the test statistic for this permutation:

$$T_{perm}^{(l)} = \frac{1}{K}\sum_{j=1}^{K} \omega_j^{(l)} \left(CR(M_a, S_j) - CR(M_b, S_j)\right). \tag{9}$$

   This procedure is equivalent to randomly swapping the CR scores for each case and recomputing the difference in means. The set $\{T_{perm}^{(l)}\}_{l=1}^{L}$ forms an empirical sample from the distribution of T under H_0.
3. **P-value Calculation.** The one-sided p-value is the probability of observing a test statistic as or more extreme as T_{orig} under the null hypothesis of no difference in performance across models. It is calculated as the proportion of permuted statistics that are less than or equal to the observed statistic:

$$p(M_a, M_b) = \frac{1 + \sum_{l=1}^{L} \mathbb{I}(T_{perm}^{(l)} \leq T_{orig})}{L + 1}, \tag{10}$$

   where $\mathbb{I}(\cdot)$ is the indicator function. The inclusion of '+1' in both the numerator and denominator accounts for the observed data itself as one possible permutation under the null hypothesis, preventing p-values of zero and yielding a more accurate estimate [38].

Interpretation and Multiple Comparisons. This pairwise test is performed for all unique pairs of models. The resulting p-values can be organized into an $N \times N$ significance matrix. For a chosen significance level α (e.g., $\alpha = 0.05$), if $p(M_a, M_b) < \alpha$, we reject H_0 and conclude that model M_a is statistically superior to M_b. If $p(M_a, M_b) \geq \alpha$, we can make no such statement. This allows for the identification of statistically indistinguishable tiers (based on the available test samples) or cliques of models. It is crucial to note that performing a large number of pairwise comparisons inflates the error rate. To maintain statistical rigor, a correction for multiple comparisons, such as the Bonferroni correction or controlling the False Discovery Rate (FDR) [40], should be applied to the p-values before interpretation.

Overall Summary of Proposed Ranking Framework: *'PermRanker'*

1: **INPUT**

a. Models considered for evaluation – *provided by the challenge participants.*
b. Evaluation metrics – *defined by the challenge organizers.*
c. Testing cases* – *provided by the challenge organizers.*

***Important**: For segmentation, registration, & synthesis tasks, a testing case is a single subject, whereas for classification & regression tasks a testing case is a subset of subjects. Subsets are of equal size & include ≥ 1 case of each class.

2: **EVALUATION MECHANISM** (per submitted model)

For each testing case

a. Evaluate the model's prediction against the target reference standard.
b. If the model prediction is missing, maximize the "penalty" for each metric, e.g., for segmentation the DSC should be zero, & for classification the prediction label should be set to the opposite of the reference standard label and calculate the metrics.

Output: A spreadsheet per evaluated model with all testing cases scored.

3: **RANKING SCHEMA** (across all evaluated models)

Input: the output spreadsheets of (2) for all submitted models:

For each testing case

- **For** each metric
  - Rank each model prediction relative to those of other models.
- Add all metrics' rankings to calculate a case-wise ranking for each model.

Output: A spreadsheet where each row describes an individual model, and each column represents the **case-wise ranking** for a specific testing case.
Averaging the case-wise rankings across columns (i.e, one average per row/model) will create the **Final Ranking Score (FRS)**.

4: **STATISTICAL SIGNIFICANCE ASSESSMENT**

Input: The spreadsheet with case-wise rankings and FRS, from (3).

- Order evaluated models & their case-wise rankings according to the FRS.
- **For** each pair of ranked participating models, e.g., M_i & M_j
  - Initialize a counter $p_{i,j} = 0$.
  - Calculate the original FRS difference: $\Delta^{orig} = |FRS_i - FRS_j|$.
  - **For** $PermNo = 100,000$ (or more)
    - * Randomly permute the case-wise rankings between M_i & M_j.
    - * Recalculate the FRS for M_i & M_j: i.e., FRS_i^{perm} & FRS_j^{perm}
    - * Calculate the FRS^{perm} difference: $\Delta^{perm} = |FRS_i^{perm} - FRS_j^{perm}|$.
    - * **If** $\Delta^{perm} \geq \Delta^{orig}$, increase the counter $p_{i,j}$ by 1.

Note: $p_{i,j}/PermNo$ represents a p-value reflecting the statistical significance of the final observed performance differences between M_i & M_j.

Output: An upper diagonal matrix of p-values for all model pairs. Example:

Models	M1	M2	M3	M4
M1	--	0.23585	0.01611	0.18780
M2		--	0.03114	0.30253
M3			--	0.79936
M4				--

3 Discussion

In this article we presented '*PermRanker*', a data-agnostic and workload-agnostic framework, to democratize the fair benchmarking of AI models, bringing them closer to clinical translation. Following the generation of a ranked order of evaluated models, PermRanker uses a permutation-based significance testing, which reduces resource bias: large academic centers or industry groups can afford to train multiple models, run extensive hyperparameter sweeps, or build ensembles to edge out a tiny performance boost (e.g., DSC of 0.851 vs 0.849), which can put their team at the top, even if the difference is within statistical noise. That discourages smaller "players", since it looks like they lost despite being essentially equivalent. The permutation-based significance testing checks whether differences between teams are statistically significant, and thus identifies when two models are indistinguishable, so instead of a single winner, we obtain a tier of top models.

PermRanker has been used since 2017 to facilitate the ranking and significance testing of hundreds of models submitted in over 33 challenges conducted in conjunction with the Annual Conferences of the Medical Image Computing and Computer Assisted Interventions (MICCAI) Society, as well as of the Radiologic Society of North America (RSNA). Specifically, between 2017 and 2025 it has facilitated the fair benchmarking of participating algorithms in more than 33 challenges including the BraTS challenges, focusing on segmentation, registration, and classification workloads [2–19], the FeTS challenges [22,23], the ISLES challenge [24,25], and the LiTS Benchmark [27]. The execution of this source code has been through the Image Processing Portal (IPP) of the Center for Biomedical Image Computing and Analytics (CBICA) at the University of Pennsylvania between 2017 and 2020, and after 2021 through the platform of Sage Bionetworks (known as synapse.org).

A key strength of the proposed framework is its inherent modularity and agnosticism to the specific clinical task or data modality. Its adaptability is conferred by the initial problem definition, where the challenge organizers (also known as the benchmark committee [41]), specify the relevant performance metrics $\mathcal{P}$ tailored to the workload at hand. For instance, a challenge on tumor volume might use metrics like volumetric difference and surface distance as its $\mathcal{P}$ set, while a classification task would use metrics like sensitivity, specificity, F1-score, and MCC. The core machinery of rank aggregation and permutation testing remains unchanged, providing a standardized, robust, and reusable tool for the broader research community (beyond the scope of challenges) to promote rigorous and fair evaluation practices.

Finally, in favor of open science, the source code of the complete package described here is available through the github repository of the Division of Computational Pathology (https://github.com/IUCompPath), following an Apache License, Version 2.0. Example files are also provided together with the source code to facilitate the seamless understanding of the implemented approach.

Acknowledgements. Research reported in this publication was partially supported by the Informatics Technology for Cancer Research (ITCR) program of the National Cancer Institute (NCI) of the National Institutes of Health (NIH), under award numbers U01CA242871 and U24CA279629. Computational resources used in this research were partially supported in part by Lilly Endowment, Inc., through its support for the Indiana University Pervasive Technology Institute. The content of this publication is solely the responsibility of the authors and does not represent the official views of the NIH or any other funding body.

U. Baid and S. Pati conducted the work reported in this manuscript while they were affiliated with the Department of Pathology and Laboratory Medicine at Indiana University School of Medicine, Indianapolis, IN, USA.

Contributions. Conceptualization: S. Bakas. **Methodology**: S. Bakas, R.T. Shinohara. **Data Curation, Formal analysis, & Validation**: S. Bakas, S. Thakur, U. Baid, A. Linardos. **Software**: S. Bakas, S. Thakur, J. Doshi, S. Pati. **Visualization**: S. Bakas, S. Thakur, U. Baid, A. Linardos. **Writing**: S. Bakas, S. Thakur, A. Linardos. **Funding acquisition, Project administration, Resources, & Supervision**: S. Bakas.

References

1. Menze, B.H., et al.: The multimodal brain tumor image segmentation benchmark (BraTS). IEEE Trans. Med. Imaging **34**(10), 1993–2024 (2015)
2. Bakas, S., et al.: Identifying the best machine learning algorithms for brain tumor segmentation, progression assessment, and overall survival prediction in the BraTS challenge. arXiv preprint arXiv:1811.02629 (2018)
3. Bakas, S., et al.: Advancing the cancer genome atlas glioma MRI collections with expert segmentation labels and radiomic features. Sci. Data **4**(1), 1–13 (2017)
4. Bakas, S., Akbari, H., Sotiras, A., et al.: Segmentation labels for the pre-operative scans of the TCGA-GBM collection. Cancer Imaging Arch. (2017)
5. Bakas, S., et al.: Segmentation labels and radiomic features for the pre-operative scans of the TCGA-LGG collection. Cancer Imaging Arch. **286** (2017)
6. Baid, U., et al.: The RSNA-ASNR-MICCAI BraTS 2021 benchmark on brain tumor segmentation and radiogenomic classification. arXiv preprint arXiv:2107.02314 (2021)
7. Adewole, M., et al.: The brain tumor segmentation (BraTS) challenge 2023: glioma segmentation in Sub-Saharan Africa patient population (BraTS-Africa). ArXiv, arXiv–2305 (2023)
8. Bakas, S., et al.: BraTS-path challenge: assessing heterogeneous histopathologic brain tumor sub-regions. arXiv preprint arXiv:2405.10871 (2024)
9. LaBella, D., et al.: Analysis of the BraTS 2023 intracranial meningioma segmentation challenge. arXiv preprint arXiv:2405.09787 (2024)
10. LaBella, D., et al.: A multi-institutional meningioma MRI dataset for automated multi-sequence image segmentation. Sci. Data **11**(1), 496 (2024)
11. LaBella, D., et al.: Brain tumor segmentation (BraTS) challenge 2024: meningioma radiotherapy planning automated segmentation. arxiv 2024. arXiv preprint arXiv:2405.18383
12. de Verdier, M.C., et al.: The 2024 brain tumor segmentation (BraTS) challenge: glioma segmentation on post-treatment MRI. arXiv preprint arXiv:2405.18368 (2024)

13. Kazerooni, A.F., et al.: The brain tumor segmentation in pediatrics (BraTS-PEDs) challenge: focus on pediatrics (CBTN-CONNECT-DIPGR-ASNR-MICCAI BRATS-PEDs). arXiv preprint arXiv:2404.15009 (2024)
14. Moawad, A.W., et al.: The brain tumor segmentation-metastases (BraTS-METS) challenge 2023: brain metastasis segmentation on pre-treatment MRI. ArXiv, arXiv–2306 (2024)
15. Li, H.B., et al.: The brain tumor segmentation (BraTS) challenge 2023: brain MR image synthesis for tumor segmentation (BraSyn). ArXiv, arXiv–2305 (2024)
16. Maleki, N., et al.: Analysis of the MICCAI brain tumor segmentation–metastases (BraTS-METS) 2025 lighthouse challenge: brain metastasis segmentation on pre- and post-treatment MRI. arXiv preprint arXiv:2504.12527 (2025)
17. Adewole, M., et al.: The BraTS-Africa dataset: expanding the brain tumor segmentation data to capture African populations. Radiol. Artif. Intell. **7**(4), e240528 (2025)
18. Amiruddin, R., et al.: Training the next generation of physicians for artificial intelligence-assisted clinical neuroradiology: ASNR MICCAI brain tumor segmentation (BraTS) 2025 lighthouse challenge education platform. arXiv preprint arXiv:2509.17281 (2025)
19. Baheti, B., et al.: The brain tumor sequence registration (BraTS-Reg) challenge: establishing correspondence between pre-operative and follow-up MRI scans of diffuse glioma patients. arXiv preprint arXiv:2112.06979 (2021)
20. Kofler, F., et al.: The brain tumor segmentation (BraTS) challenge 2023: local synthesis of healthy brain tissue via inpainting. arXiv preprint arXiv:2305.08992 (2023)
21. Kofler, F., et al.: BraTS orchestrator: democratizing and disseminating state-of-the-art brain tumor image analysis. arXiv preprint arXiv:2506.13807 (2025)
22. Zenk, M., et al.: Towards fair decentralized benchmarking of healthcare AI algorithms with the federated tumor segmentation (FeTS) challenge. Nat. Commun. **16**(1), 6274 (2025)
23. Pati, S., et al.: The federated tumor segmentation (FeTS) challenge. arXiv preprint arXiv:2105.05874 (2021)
24. Maier, O., et al.: ISLES 2015—a public evaluation benchmark for ischemic stroke lesion segmentation from multispectral MRI. Med. Image Anal. **35**, 250–269 (2017)
25. Winzeck, S., et al.: ISLES 2016 and 2017-benchmarking ischemic stroke lesion outcome prediction based on multispectral MRI. Front. Neurol. **9**, 679 (2018)
26. Heller, N., et al.: The state of the art in kidney and kidney tumor segmentation in contrast-enhanced CT imaging: the KiTS19 challenge. Med. Image Anal. **67**, 101821 (2021)
27. Bilic, P., et al.: The liver tumor segmentation benchmark (LiTS). Med. Image Anal. **84**, 102680 (2023)
28. Li, H.B., et al.: QUBIQ: uncertainty quantification for biomedical image segmentation challenge. arXiv preprint arXiv:2405.18435 (2024)
29. Antonelli, M., et al.: The medical segmentation decathlon. Nat. Commun. **13**(1), 4128 (2022)
30. Simpson, A.L., et al.: A large annotated medical image dataset for the development and evaluation of segmentation algorithms. arXiv preprint arXiv:1902.09063 (2019)
31. Dorent, R., et al.: CrossMoDA 2021 challenge: benchmark of cross-modality domain adaptation techniques for vestibular schwannoma and cochlea segmentation. Med. Image Anal. **83**, 102628 (2023)

32. Mehta, R., et al.: QU-BraTS: MICCAI BraTS 2020 challenge on quantifying uncertainty in brain tumor segmentation-analysis of ranking scores and benchmarking results. J. Mach. Learn. Biomed. Imaging (2022)
33. Kofler, F., et al.: Are we using appropriate segmentation metrics? Identifying correlates of human expert perception for CNN training beyond rolling the dice coefficient. Mach. Learn. Biomed. Imaging **2**, 27–71 (2023)
34. Reinke, A., et al.: Common limitations of image processing metrics: a picture story. arXiv preprint arXiv:2104.05642 (2021)
35. Maier-Hein, L., et al.: Metrics reloaded: recommendations for image analysis validation. Nat. Methods **21**(2), 195–212 (2024)
36. Maier-Hein, L., et al.: Why rankings of biomedical image analysis competitions should be interpreted with care. Nat. Commun. **9**(1), 1–13 (2018)
37. Ioannidis, J.P.A.: Why most published research findings are false. PLoS Med. **2**(8), e124 (2005)
38. Good, P.I.: Permutation, Parametric, and Bootstrap Tests of Hypotheses, 3rd edn. Springer Science & Business Media (2005)
39. Nichols, T.E., Holmes, A.P.: Nonparametric permutation tests for functional neuroimaging: a primer with examples. Hum. Brain Mapp. **15**(1), 1–25 (2002)
40. Benjamini, Y., Hochberg, Y.: Controlling the false discovery rate: a practical and powerful approach to multiple testing. J. Roy. Stat. Soc.: Ser. B (Methodol.) **57**(1), 289–300 (1995)
41. Karargyris, A., et al.: Federated benchmarking of medical artificial intelligence with MedPerf. Nat. Mach. Intell. **5**(7), 799–810 (2023)

Challenge 1 – BraTS-GLI

EGASegNet: An Extreme Group-Aware Segmentation Network for Glioma Segmentation

Liwei Jin and Yanjun Peng(✉)

College of Computer Science and Engineering, Shandong University of Science and Technology, Qingdao 266590, Shandong, China
yjpeng@sdust.edu.cn

Abstract. The accurate segmentation of gliomas from multi-sequence magnetic resonance imaging (MRI) remains challenging due to cross-sequence inconsistencies and boundary detection limitations. Although recent neural architectures incorporating convolutional and Transformer-based components have achieved notable advancements, many still exhibit deficiencies in modeling nonlinear inter-sequence interactions and capturing fine-grained boundaries. To address these shortcomings, we propose Extreme Group-Aware Segmentation Network (EGASegNet), a unified 3D segmentation framework that integrates edge-guided attention mechanisms with extreme group-aware transformers for enhanced boundary detection and contextual modeling. The framework introduces three core components that operate synergistically to improve segmentation accuracy. The Adaptive Edge-Guided Module (AEGM) employs boundary-aware spatial-channel joint attention to strengthen anatomically important regions through directional edge focus and adaptive channel recalibration. The Multi-Scale Directional Attention Fusion (MSDAF) module integrates multi-scale directional convolutions with cross-attention mechanisms to reduce cross-sequence misalignment while preserving detailed semantic information across different spatial orientations. The Extreme Group-Aware Attention Former (EGAF) block utilizes partition-based attention with positive-negative value handling to capture long-range dependencies and enhance feature discrimination through entropy-adjusted attention computation. These components are integrated within a hierarchical architecture that ensures coherent semantic refinement across multiple resolution levels, enabling effective fusion of global context and local boundary details for robust tumor segmentation performance. EGASegNet also demonstrates strong generalization performance on the BraTS Lighthouse Challenge testing phase. Our code is available at https://github.com/jlw9999/BraTS2025_GLI.

Keywords: Glioma segmentation · Multi-sequence MRI · Edge-guided attention · Group-aware Transformer

S. Bakas et al. (Eds.): MICCAI 2025, LNCS 16376, pp. 17–27, 2026.
https://doi.org/10.1007/978-3-032-16365-3_2

1 Introduction

Diffuse gliomas represent the most prevalent malignant primary brain tumors in adults, with their extensive infiltrative characteristics within the central nervous system rendering accurate diagnosis and treatment particularly challenging (Menze et al., 2014). Accurate and reliable segmentation of brain tumors from multi-sequence magnetic resonance imaging (MRI) is crucial for clinical diagnosis, treatment planning, and disease progression monitoring. Multi-sequence MRI typically encompasses T1, T1ce, T2, and FLAIR sequences, providing complementary anatomical and pathological information that enhances the delineation of tumor subregions (such as edema and necrotic core) and enhancing tumor components (Bakas et al., 2017). However, despite the diversity of imaging sequences, achieving precise tumor segmentation remains a significant challenge due to inter-modal heterogeneity, complex tumor morphology, and ambiguous boundary definitions (Havaei et al. 2017).

In recent years, the rapid advancement of deep learning technologies has brought revolutionary progress to medical image segmentation. Convolutional neural networks (CNNs) have achieved remarkable success in brain tumor segmentation tasks through their powerful feature extraction capabilities (Oktay et al., 2018; Isensee et al., 2021). Notably, U-Net (Ronneberger et al., 2015) and its variants have effectively integrated multi-scale feature information through encoder-decoder architectures and skip connections, establishing themselves as the canonical framework for medical image segmentation (Zhou et al., 2024).

Despite CNNs' excellence in local feature extraction, their limited receptive field characteristics constrain their ability to model long-range dependencies. To address this limitation, Transformer-based architectures have been introduced to the medical image segmentation domain (Chen et al., 2024;Wang et al., 2021). Vision Transformer (ViT) can effectively capture global contextual information through self-attention mechanisms, yet exhibits deficiencies in processing fine-grained boundaries in medical images (Hatamizadeh et al., 2022 Valanarasu et al., 2021). Recent research has attempted to fuse CNNs and Transformers to fully leverage the advantages of both approaches (Roy et al., 2023; Liu et al.,2024).

In multi-sequence medical image segmentation tasks, cross-sequence consistency and boundary precision constitute two core challenges for achieving high-quality segmentation. Although different MRI sequences (such as T1, T2, FLAIR, etc.) provide complementary structural and lesion information, registration errors, contrast variations, and nonlinear interactions between sequences often result in limited feature fusion efficiency (Dolz et al., 2019). Current fusion methods predominantly remain at the level of simple feature concatenation or weighted averaging, failing to fully exploit the potential correlations and discriminative features between sequences (Li et al., 2024). Simultaneously, brain tumor boundaries typically exhibit blurred, fragmented, or morphologically irregular characteristics, making effective identification challenging for conventional segmentation methods (Zhu et al., 2024). Although some studies have attempted to introduce edge-guided mechanisms to enhance boundary identification capabilities, fine-grained modeling of boundary information remains insufficient (Xiao et al., 2025;Lv et al., 2025). Furthermore, existing methods predominantly rely on fixed attention strategies, lacking adaptive modeling capabilities for regional heterogeneity and modal differences (Yue et al., 2025). Most multi-scale fusion mechanisms fail to adequately consider directional features, consequently demonstrating suboptimal performance when processing structurally complex or morphologically variable tumor regions (Cheng et al., 2025). Therefore, there is an urgent need for an efficient segmentation framework that can simultaneously enhance cross-modal synergistic expression, boundary awareness, and directional selectivity.

To address these problems, we propose EGASegNet, a unified 3D segmentation framework that integrates edge-guided attention mechanisms with extreme group-aware Transformers to enhance boundary detection and contextual modeling capabilities. The main contributions of this study are as follows:

- We propose the Adaptive Edge-Guided Module (AEGM), which leverages boundary-aware spatialchannel joint attention to enhance the representation of anatomically critical regions by focusing on directional edge features and adaptive channel recalibration.
- We propose the Multi-Scale Directional Attention Fusion (MSDAF) module, which integrates multi-scale directional convolutions with cross-attention mechanisms to effectively mitigate cross-sequence misalignment while preserving orientation-specific semantic details.
- We design the Extreme Group-Aware Attention Former (EGAF) block, which employs partition-based attention with positivenegative value processing to capture long-range dependencies and improve feature discrimination through entropy-adjusted attention computation.
- We construct a hierarchical architecture that ensures semantic refinement across multiple resolution levels, enabling effective fusion of global contextual information with fine-grained boundary details.

2 Methods

2.1 Overview of Network Architecture

The proposed EGASegNet employs a hierarchical encoder-decoder architecture specifically designed for volumetric brain tumor segmentation from multi-sequence MRI data, as shown in Fig. 1. The network processes 3D input volumes of dimensions W×H×D×C, where C represents the number of imaging sequences. The encoder progressively downsamples feature representations through four resolution stages via 3D convolutional blocks with strided convolution, reducing spatial dimensions by a factor of 2 at each level while systematically increasing channel dimensions from C to 2C, 4C, 8C, and 16C respectively. At the bottleneck layer, the Adaptive Edge-Guided Module (AEGM) enhances anatomical boundary representation through spatial-channel joint attention mechanisms. The decoder symmetrically reconstructs features to original resolution through multi-level skip connections that preserve spatial information.

Each upsampling stage integrates the Multi-Scale Directional Attention Fusion (MSDAF) module, which refines features using directional convolutions and cross-attention to mitigate cross-sequence misalignment. The Extreme Group-Aware Attention Former (EGAF) blocks constitute the core decoding components, implementing partition-based attention with entropy-adjusted computation to capture long-range dependencies and enhance feature discrimination. The architecture operates across multiple resolution levels (1/2, 1/4, 1/8, 1/16) with additive fusion in skip connections, ensuring progressive semantic refinement. All convolutional layers utilize 3×3×3 kernels with batch normalization and ReLU activation, while the final prediction layer employs 1×1×1 convolution for segmentation class mapping.

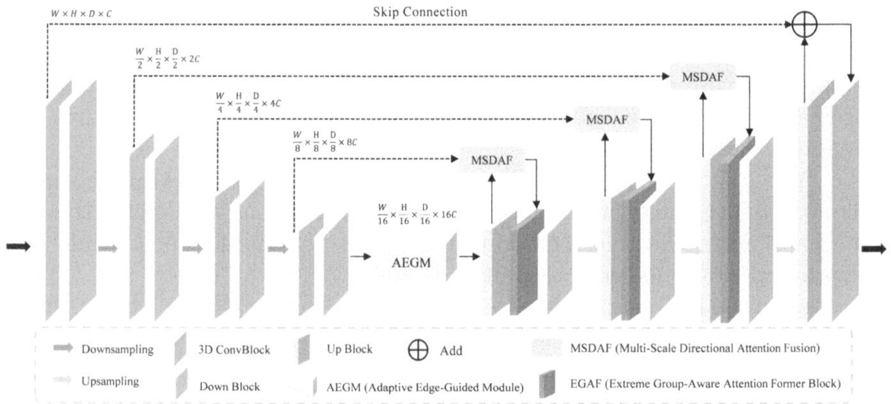

Fig. 1. The architecture of the proposed EGASegNet.

2.2 Adaptive Edge-Guided Module

The Adaptive Edge-Guided Module (AEGM) is strategically positioned at the encoder bottleneck to enhance anatomical boundary representation through sophisticated spatial-channel joint attention mechanisms. The module employs a hierarchical attention structure consisting of an EdgeAttentionUnit3D that captures fine-grained edge information via depthwise convolution operations, followed by adaptive channel recalibration through asymmetric convolutions with varying kernel sizes. The core mechanism utilizes adaptive pooling along spatial dimensions to extract global contextual information, which is subsequently processed through a dual-branch convolution pathway employing kernels of sizes (1×k×1) and (k×1×1) where k=11, enabling effective capture of cross-dimensional feature dependencies. The attention weights are computed through sigmoid activation applied to the processed global context, which are then element-wise multiplied with the edge-enhanced features to produce spatially-aware representations. The complete AEGM incorporates residual connections with learnable layer-wise scaling parameters initialized to 1×10^{-6} for training stability, complemented by a ChannelProjector3D module that performs feature transformation through point-wise convolutions with an expansion ratio of 2. The module integrates stochastic depth regularization and maintains computational efficiency through 3D operations while ensuring effective gradient propagation in deep network architectures.

2.3 Multi-scale Directional Attention Fusion

The Multi-Scale Directional Attention Fusion (MSDAF) module is designed to address cross-sequence misalignment issues prevalent in multi-sequence brain tumor segmentation by integrating features from skip connections and upsampled decoder paths. The module processes two input feature maps through independent normalization layers followed by multi-scale directional convolutions that capture spatial dependencies across different orientations and scales. The directional convolution operations employ three distinct kernel sizes (7×7×7, 11×11×11, and 21×21×21) applied separately in horizontal and vertical directions, enabling the extraction of multi-scale spatial patterns while preserving directional sensitivity. Each input feature map undergoes parallel processing through six directional convolution branches, with the resulting features aggregated through element-wise summation to form comprehensive directional representations. The module subsequently applies point-wise convolutions for feature projection, followed by a cross-attention mechanism that computes normalized query, key, and value representations for both feature branches. The attention computation utilizes L2 normalization of query and key vectors to ensure stable attention weight calculation, with the final output obtained through weighted value aggregation combined with residual connections. The MSDAF module effectively reduces feature misalignment between different sequences by leveraging directional spatial information and cross-attention mechanisms, thereby improving the quality of multi-sequence feature integration in the decoder pathway.

2.4 Extreme Group-Aware Attention Former

The Extreme Group-Aware Attention Former (EGAF) serves as the core computational block within the decoder stages, implementing partition-based attention with entropy-adjusted computation to capture long-range dependencies while maintaining computational efficiency. The module employs a Polarity-aware Perception Attention that processes input features through grouped convolutions and applies extreme perception techniques to enhance feature discrimination. The attention computation begins with the generation of query, key, and value representations through 3D convolutions:

$$Q, K, V = \text{Conv3D}_{3\times3\times3}(\text{Conv3D}_{1\times1\times1}(X)), \tag{1}$$

where the input features are processed through depthwise convolutions with dilation factor 2. The extreme perception mechanism decomposes the normalized query and key vectors into positive and negative components:

$$\begin{aligned} Q_{pos} &= \mathrm{ReLU}(Q)^{1+\alpha\cdot\sigma(s)}, \quad Q_{neg} = \mathrm{ReLU}(-Q)^{1+\alpha\cdot\sigma(s)} \\ K_{pos} &= \mathrm{ReLU}(K)^{1+\alpha\cdot\sigma(s)}, \quad K_{neg} = \mathrm{ReLU}(-K)^{1+\alpha\cdot\sigma(s)} \end{aligned} \tag{2}$$

where $\alpha = 4$ represents the power adjustment parameter and s denotes learnable scale parameters. The enhanced query and key representations are constructed as $Q_{sim} = [Q_{pos}, Q_{neg}]$ and $K_{sim} = [K_{pos}, K_{neg}]$, respectively. The attention weights are computed through temperature-scaled dot-product attention:

$$\text{Attention} = \text{softmax}\left(\frac{Q_{sim}K_{sim}^T}{\tau}\right) \tag{3}$$

where τ represents learnable temperature parameters for each attention head. The module incorporates group-aware spatial partitioning with configurable group sizes, enabling efficient processing of large volumetric data while maintaining spatial coherence, with adaptive padding to handle arbitrary input dimensions. The final output combines attention-weighted features with residual connections and multi-layer perceptron processing, ensuring effective gradient flow and feature refinement throughout the decoder pathway.

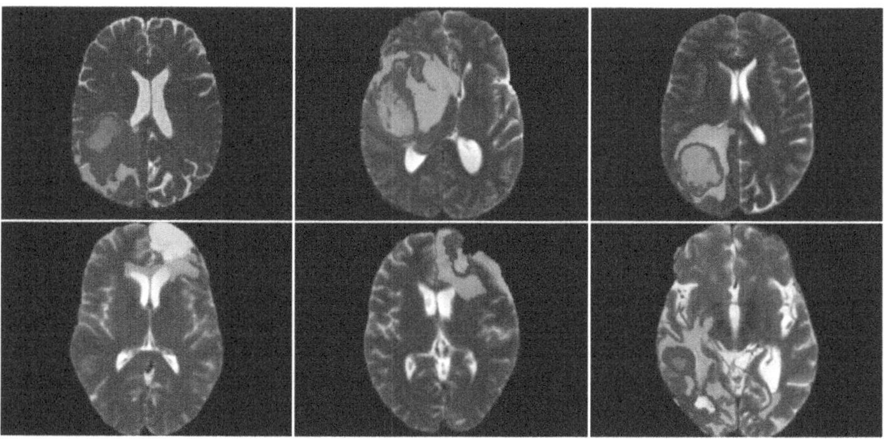

Fig. 2. Representative axial T2-FLAIR MRI slices from the BraTS2025 illustrating multi-class tumor segmentation. Pre-treatment cases are shown in the upper row, and post-treatment cases are shown in the lower row. Segmentation colors represent ET (blue), NETC (red), SNFH (green), and RC (yellow). (Color figure online)

3 Results

3.1 Datasets

This study employed multi-parametric MRI (mpMRI) scans from the BraTS-GLI challenge dataset, designed for the Pre- (Baid et al.,2021; Bakas et al., 2017) and Post-Treatment (Karargyris et al., 2023; de Verdier et al., 2024) Adult Glioma Segmentation task. The dataset includes two cohorts: the BraTS-GLI Pre-treatment dataset for pre-operative cases, and the BraTS-GLI 2024 dataset for post-treatment cases, totaling 2,872 training and 407 validation samples. Data were collected across multiple institutions using diverse clinical protocols and scanners. Each subject identifier encodes scan timepoint and treatment status, following the BraTS naming convention (e.g., 000 for pre-operative baseline, 100 for first post-treatment scan). Ground truth annotations of tumor sub-regions were created and validated by expert neuroradiologists to support quantitative evaluation, as shown in Fig. 2.

3.2 Implementation Details

All experiments were conducted using the PyTorch framework on an NVIDIA GeForce RTX 3090 GPU (24 GB). The model employed the nnU-Net preprocessing strategy, which included skull stripping, registration to a standard anatomical template, resampling to a 1 mm isotropic resolution, and data augmentation. To enhance generalization, 3D augmentation operations including random cropping, mirroring, scaling, and rotation were applied during training. The input consisted of four multi-parametric MRI sequences in NIfTI format, including native T1, T1ce, T2, and FLAIR. Manual annotations were provided by one to four expert raters and subsequently verified by experienced neuroradiologists, delineating enhancing tumor (ET), surrounding non-enhancing FLAIR hyperintensity (SNFH), non-enhancing tumor core (NETC), and resection cavity (RC). The model was optimized using AdamW optimizer with a learning rate of 1×10^{-3} and default weight decay settings. The model was trained for 1,000 epochs with a batch size of 1 to accommodate high-resolution volumetric data, using a composite loss function that combined Dice loss and cross-entropy loss to optimize segmentation accuracy. For internal validation, a 5-fold cross-validation strategy was adopted to ensure stable and reliable evaluation. Model performance was quantitatively assessed using the lesion-wise Dice Similarity Coefficient (Dice) and the Normalized Surface Distance (NSD), where the lesion-wise Dice was used to evaluate segmentation quality at the individual lesion level, reducing bias toward larger lesions and providing a more comprehensive assessment of performance in cases involving multi-focal or multi-centric tumors.

3.3 Results on the BraTS Dataset

The proposed EGASegNet demonstrates competitive performance across all evaluated tumor regions as presented in Table 1. The network achieves the high-

Table 1. LesionWise evaluation results of EGASegNet on brain tumor segmentation task. Results are reported for Dice Similarity Coefficient and Normalized Surface Distance at tolerance levels of 0.5 mm and 1.0 mm.

Region	Dice	NSD@0.5 mm	NSD@1.0 mm
ET	0.7708	0.5857	0.8133
NETC	0.7551	0.6250	0.7667
RC	0.7928	0.7145	0.7995
SNFH	0.8138	0.5461	0.8087
TC	0.7718	0.5247	0.7549
WT	0.8706	0.5450	0.8211

est Dice similarity coefficient for the whole tumor region (WT) at 0.8706, followed by surgical cavity without enhancing tumor (SNFH) at 0.8138, indicating robust performance in capturing large-scale tumor boundaries and post-surgical anatomical structures. The resection cavity (RC) and tumor core (TC) regions obtain Dice scores of 0.7928 and 0.7718 respectively, while the enhancing tumor (ET) and non-enhancing tumor core (NETC) achieve scores of 0.7708 and 0.7551, reflecting the inherent difficulty in segmenting these heterogeneous and often irregular tumor subregions. The normalized surface distance evaluation at 1.0 mm tolerance reveals consistently strong boundary localization performance, with WT achieving 0.8211, SNFH at 0.8087, and ET at 0.8133, demonstrating the effectiveness of the adaptive edge-guided module in preserving anatomical boundaries. At the more stringent 0.5 mm tolerance level, the resection cavity region shows superior performance with an NSD score of 0.7145, while other regions exhibit relatively lower scores ranging from 0.5247 to 0.6250, indicating the challenging nature of precise boundary delineation in complex brain tumor morphologies. The comprehensive evaluation across multiple tumor regions and surface distance metrics validates the robustness of the proposed architecture in handling diverse anatomical variations and pathological conditions commonly encountered in clinical brain tumor segmentation scenarios.

Following the release of the official testing phase results from the BraTS Lighthouse Challenge, EGASegNet demonstrated consistent segmentation performance on the unseen test set, achieving Dice scores of 0.8262, 0.8009, 0.7988, and 0.8649 for RC, ET, TC, and WT, respectively, with corresponding NSD@1.0 values of 0.8285, 0.8444, 0.8078, and 0.8311. These results further confirm the robustness and strong generalization capability of the proposed framework under real-world evaluation conditions. Consequently, EGASegNet ranked third in the Adult Glioma task among all participating international teams, demonstrating its competitive performance against state-of-the-art methods.

4 Discussion

The experimental results demonstrate that EGASegNet achieves robust segmentation performance across diverse brain tumor regions, with the superior performance on whole tumor (WT) segmentation highlighting the effectiveness of the hierarchical encoder-decoder architecture in capturing large-scale anatomical structures. The consistently high Dice scores for WT and SNFH regions can be attributed to the synergistic effects of the three core modules, where the Adaptive Edge-Guided Module enhances boundary representation at the bottleneck layer, the Multi-Scale Directional Attention Fusion effectively integrates multi-sequence features while reducing cross-sequence misalignment, and the Extreme Group-Aware Attention Former captures long-range dependencies through partition-based attention mechanisms. The relatively lower performance on enhancing tumor and non-enhancing tumor core regions reflects the inherent challenges in segmenting these heterogeneous subregions, which often exhibit irregular boundaries and variable intensity distributions across different MRI sequences. The normalized surface distance evaluation reveals that while the proposed method excels in overall volumetric segmentation as indicated by Dice scores, precise boundary localization remains challenging at sub-millimeter tolerance levels, particularly for complex tumor morphologies. The superior performance at 1.0 mm tolerance compared to 0.5 mm tolerance suggests that the adaptive edge-guided attention mechanism effectively captures anatomical boundaries within clinically acceptable precision ranges, which is crucial for treatment planning and surgical guidance applications. Compared to established frameworks such as nnU-Net, which relies on automated configuration and standard U-Net architectures, EGASegNet introduces specialized attention mechanisms specifically designed for multi-sequence brain MRI analysis. While nnU-Net excels through its robust preprocessing pipeline and adaptive training strategies, our approach addresses the unique challenges of brain tumor segmentation by incorporating edge-guided attention and directional fusion modules that enhance boundary delineation and cross-modal feature integration. The comprehensive evaluation across multiple tumor regions validates the generalizability of the proposed architecture, demonstrating its potential for clinical deployment in automated brain tumor segmentation workflows where accurate delineation of diverse pathological structures is essential for optimal patient care outcomes.

References

Baid, U., et al.: The rsna-asnr-miccai brats 2021 benchmark on brain tumor segmentation and radiogenomic classification. arXiv preprint arXiv:2107.02314 (v)

Bakas, S., et al.: Advancing the cancer genome atlas glioma mri collections with expert segmentation labels and radiomic features. Sci. Data **4**, 170117 (2017). https://doi.org/10.1038/sdata.2017.117

Chen, J., et al.: Transunet: rethinking the u-net architecture design for medical image segmentation through the lens of transformers. Med. Image Anal. **97**, 103280 (2024). https://doi.org/10.1016/j.media.2024.103280

Cheng, Y., Zheng, Y., Wang, J.: Cfnet: automatic multi-modal brain tumor segmentation through hierarchical coarse-to-fine fusion and feature communication. Biomed. Signal Process. Control **99**, 106876 (2025). https://doi.org/10.1016/j.bspc.2024.106876

Dolz, J., Gopinath, K., Yuan, J., Lombaert, H., Desrosiers, C., Ben Ayed, I.: Hyperdense-net: a hyper-densely connected cnn for multi-modal image segmentation. IEEE Trans. Med. Imaging **38**, 1116–1126 (2019). https://doi.org/10.1109/TMI.2018.2878669

Hatamizadeh, A., et al.: Unetr: transformers for 3d medical image segmentation. In: Proceedings of the IEEE/CVF Winter Conference on Applications of Computer Vision (WACV), pp. 574–584 (2022)

Havaei, M., et al.: Brain tumor segmentation with deep neural networks. Med. Image Anal. **35**, 18–31 (2017). https://doi.org/10.1016/j.media.2016.05.004

Isensee, F., Jaeger, P.F., Kohl, S.A.A., Petersen, J., Maier-Hein, K.H.: nnu-net: a self-configuring method for deep learning-based biomedical image segmentation. Nat. Methods **18**, 203–211 (2021). https://doi.org/10.1038/s41592-020-01008-z

Karargyris, A., et al.: Federated benchmarking of medical artificial intelligence with medperf. Nat. Mach. Intell. **5**, 799–810 (2023)

Li, Y., et al.: A review of deep learning-based information fusion techniques for multimodal medical image classification. Comput. Biol. Med. **177**, 108635 (2024). https://doi.org/10.1016/j.compbiomed.2024.108635

Liu, T., Bai, Q., Torigian, D.A., Tong, Y., Udupa, J.K.: Vsmtrans: a hybrid paradigm integrating self-attention and convolution for 3d medical image segmentation. Med. Image Anal. **98**, 103295 (2024). https://doi.org/10.1016/j.media.2024.103295

Lv, C., et al.: Cmsnet: edge-aware multimodal mri feature fusion for brain tumor segmentation. Image Vision Comput. **156**, 105481 (2025). https://www.sciencedirect.com/science/article/pii/S0262885625000691, https://doi.org/10.1016/j.imavis.2025.105481

Menze, B.H., et al.: The multimodal brain tumor image segmentation benchmark (brats). IEEE Trans. Med. Imaging **34**, 1993–2024 (2014)

Oktay, O., et al.: Attention u-net: Learning where to look for the pancreas. arXiv preprint arXiv:1804.03999 (2018)

Ronneberger, O., Fischer, P., Brox, T.: U-Net: Convolutional Networks for Biomedical Image Segmentation. In: Navab, N., Hornegger, J., Wells, W.M., Frangi, A.F. (eds.) MICCAI 2015. LNCS, vol. 9351, pp. 234–241. Springer, Cham (2015). https://doi.org/10.1007/978-3-319-24574-4_28

Roy, S., et al.: Mednext: transformer-driven scaling of convnets for medical image segmentation. In: Greenspan, H., Madabhushi, A., Mousavi, P., Salcudean, S., Duncan, J., Syeda-Mahmood, T., Taylor, R. (eds.) Medical Image Computing and Computer Assisted Intervention – MICCAI 2023, pp. 405–415. Springer Nature Switzerland, Cham (2023). https://doi.org/10.1007/978-3-031-43901-8_39

Valanarasu, J.M.J., Oza, P., Hacihaliloglu, I., Patel, V.M.: Medical transformer: gated axial-attention for medical image segmentation. In: de Bruijne, M., et al. (eds.) MICCAI 2021. LNCS, vol. 12901, pp. 36–46. Springer, Cham (2021). https://doi.org/10.1007/978-3-030-87193-2_4

de Verdier, M.C., et al.: The 2024 brain tumor segmentation (brats) challenge: Glioma segmentation on post-treatment mri. arXiv preprint arXiv:2405.18368 (2024)

Wang, W., Chen, C., Ding, M., Yu, H., Zha, S., Li, J.: TransBTS: multimodal brain tumor segmentation using transformer. In: de Bruijne, M., Cattin, P.C., Cotin, S., Padoy, N., Speidel, S., Zheng, Y., Essert, C. (eds.) MICCAI 2021. LNCS, vol. 12901, pp. 109–119. Springer, Cham (2021). https://doi.org/10.1007/978-3-030-87193-2_11

Xiao, L., Zhou, B., Fan, C.: Automatic brain mri tumors segmentation based on deep fusion of weak edge and context features. Artif. Intell. Rev. **58**, 154 (2025). https://doi.org/10.1007/s10462-025-11151-8

Yue, G., Zhuo, G., Zhou, T., Liu, W., Wang, T., Jiang, Q.: Adaptive crossfeature fusion network with inconsistency guidance for multi-modal brain tumor segmentation. IEEE J. Biomed. Health Inform. **29**, 3148–3158 (2025). https://doi.org/10.1109/JBHI.2023.3347556

Zhou, L., Jiang, Y., Li, W., Hu, J., Zheng, S.: Shape-scale co-awareness network for 3d brain tumor segmentation. IEEE Trans. Med. Imaging **43**, 2495–2508 (2024). https://doi.org/10.1109/TMI.2024.3368531

Zhu, Z., Wang, Z., Qi, G., Mazur, N., Yang, P., Liu, Y.: Brain tumor segmentation in mri with multi-modality spatial information enhancement and boundary shape correction. Pattern Recogn. **153**, 110553 (2024). https://doi.org/10.1016/j.patcog.2024.110553

Pre- and Post-Treatment Glioma Segmentation with the Medical Imaging Segmentation Toolkit

Adrian Celaya[1,2](✉), Tucker Netherton[1], Dawid Schellingerhout[1], Caroline Chung[1], Beatrice Riviere[2], and David Fuentes[1]

[1] The University of Texas MD Anderson Cancer Center, Houston, TX 77030, USA
aecelaya@rice.edu
[2] Rice University, Houston, TX 77005, USA

Abstract. Medical image segmentation continues to advance rapidly, yet rigorous comparison between methods remains challenging due to a lack of standardized and customizable tooling. In this work, we present the current state of the Medical Imaging Segmentation Toolkit (MIST), with a particular focus on its flexible and modular postprocessing framework designed for the BraTS 2025 pre- and post-treatment glioma segmentation challenge. Since its debut in the 2024 BraTS adult glioma post-treatment segmentation challenge, MIST's postprocessing module has been significantly extended to support a wide range of transforms, including removal or replacement of small objects, extraction of the largest connected components, and morphological operations such as hole filling and closing. These transforms can be composed into user-defined strategies, enabling fine-grained control over the final segmentation output. We evaluate three such strategies - ranging from simple small-object removal to more complex, class-specific pipelines - and rank their performance using the BraTS ranking protocol. Our results highlight how MIST facilitates rapid experimentation and targeted refinement, ultimately producing high-quality segmentations for the BraTS 2025 challenge. MIST remains open source and extensible, supporting reproducible and scalable research in medical image segmentation.

Keywords: Deep learning · Image segmentation · Medical imaging

1 Introduction

Medical imaging segmentation is a highly active area of research. Since its introduction in 2015, the U-Net architecture has received nearly 90,000 citations on Google Scholar [11,22]. Other architectures and frameworks like nnUNet have achieved state-of-the-art accuracy in several medical imaging benchmarks such as the Brain Tumor Segmentation (BraTS) and Medical Segmentation Decathlon (MSD) challenges [1,13,14]. Since the introduction of nnUNet in 2018, a variety of innovative segmentation methods have emerged, including transformer-based

S. Bakas et al. (Eds.): MICCAI 2025, LNCS 16376, pp. 28–37, 2026.
https://doi.org/10.1007/978-3-032-16365-3_3

architectures [24] and advanced loss functions such as boundary and generalized surface losses [8,17]. Despite these advancements, there remains a lack of standardized tools that support consistent, customizable, and reproducible comparisons across segmentation methods. Discrepancies in reported performance - where several works claim improvements over nnUNet [5,9,12,23,26] while others challenge these claims [15] - highlight the need for a common experimental framework.

To address this need, we introduced the Medical Imaging Segmentation Toolkit (MIST), a modular, end-to-end framework for training, testing, and evaluating deep learning-based segmentation methods in a standardized and reproducible manner. Using MIST, we achieved third place in the 2024 BraTS adult glioma post-treatment challenge, validating the framework's effectiveness in competitive, real-world benchmarks.

Since that submission, we have overhauled several key components of MIST to further support rapid experimentation and evaluation. These updates include a redesigned model interface supporting more flexible architecture and loss function customization, an enhanced inference engine with support for different ensembling and test-time augmentation strategies, and an entirely restructured postprocessing module that enables class-specific strategies such as morphological filtering and label reassignment. In this work, we focus on MIST's redesigned postprocessing framework and its role in producing high-quality segmentations for the BraTS 2025 pre- and post-treatment glioma segmentation challenge [2,3,3,4,16,20,25]. We present a set of postprocessing strategies composed of modular transforms, such as small object removal, hole filling, and class-specific component filtering. We also evaluate their impact on segmentation performance using the BraTS ranking protocol.

Our results show that well-designed postprocessing strategies can improve average segmentation metrics and help address specific failure modes. By enabling fine-grained control over the final segmentation output, MIST allows researchers to iterate quickly and target improvements for specific classes or failure modes. The framework remains open-source and extensible, providing a robust foundation for reproducible and scalable research in 3D medical image segmentation.

2 Methods

In this section, we begin by detailing our training protocols used to create our baseline models and results. We then describe MIST's postprocessing module, define our selected postprocessing strategies, and explain the BraTS ranking system.

2.1 BraTS 2025 Training Protocols

Our choice of architecture is the Pocket nnUNet with deep supervision (two supervision heads) and residual convolution blocks [6,13]. MIST automatically selects a patch size of $128 \times 128 \times 128$. We use two NVIDIA H100 GPUs with a batch size of four uniformly distributed across the GPUs. Additionally, we use L2 regularization with a penalty parameter equal to 1×10^{-5}. Our choice of loss function is the Dice with Cross Entropy loss. We train each model for 10,000 epochs per fold. We use a cosine learning rate schedule with an initial learning rate of 0.001 [19]. Within each fold, we set aside 2.5% of the training data as a validation set to select the best model. Once training is complete, MIST runs inference on the challenge validation data using test time augmentation (flipping along each axis and averaging each prediction) for each model. Inference uses sliding windows with an overlap of 0.5 with Gaussian blending ($\sigma = 0.125$). The predictions from all five models are averaged to produce a final prediction. All other options and hyperparameters are left at their default values. Please refer to MIST's documentation for these values.

2.2 Postprocessing Strategies

To facilitate reproducible and flexible mask refinement, we redesigned the MIST postprocessing module around a strategy-based architecture that enables users to compose class-specific transformation pipelines in a modular and declarative manner. Each strategy is defined via a JSON configuration file that specifies a sequence of transformations to apply to predicted segmentation masks. Available transformations include the removal of small objects, replacement of small components with a specified label, extraction of the top-k largest connected components, and morphological operations such as hole filling and closing. These transforms can be configured to act globally or selectively on specific segmentation labels (i.e., tumor subregions), and applied either jointly or sequentially across classes.

The user can control parameters such as size thresholds, replacement labels, and morphological operation settings directly through the strategy file, allowing for rapid experimentation without modifying code. This design separates postprocessing logic from the training pipeline, enabling efficient tuning of segmentation quality in the final prediction phase. Furthermore, the system is fully extensible—custom postprocessing transforms can be registered via a decorator-based interface within MIST's internal transform registry. Collectively, this module provides a lightweight and highly configurable framework for optimizing segmentation outputs, which is particularly beneficial in settings like BraTS, where postprocessing can have a substantial impact on both clinical relevance and leaderboard ranking.

In this submission, we compare three different postprocessing strategies:

- *Strategy 1*: Remove small objects in the RC class. We set the size threshold to 100 voxels.
- *Strategy 2*: Apply Strategy 1, retain the largest connected component in the RC class, and fill holes in the WT class with the SNFH class.
- *Strategy 3*: Replace small objects in the ET and RC classes with the SNFH class and then remove small objects from the SNFH class. The size thresholds for the RC, ET, and SNFH classes are 100, 100, and 64 voxels, respectively.

These strategies are inspired by our own experience with the BraTS challenge and existing post-processing schemes from previous BraTS challenge winners [14].

2.3 Strategy Ranking

We evaluate our baseline results alongside our three postprocessing strategies using the BraTS ranking system, which is designed to fairly assess segmentation methods across a set of test patients using multiple metrics. Specifically, we calculate the global Dice score and the 95th percentile Hausdorff distance (HD95) for the non-enhancing tumor core (NETC - label 1), surrounding non-enhancing FLAIR hyperintensity (SNFH - label 2), enhancing tissue (ET - label 3), resection cavity (RC - label 4), tumor core (TC - labels 1 and 3), and whole tumor (WT - labels 1, 2, and 3) classes for each prediction resulting from our five-fold cross-validation. For each patient, metric, and segmentation class, each strategy is ranked based on its segmentation performance. For example, for the first patient using the Dice coefficient on the NETC class, Strategy 3 might receive a rank of 1, while the baseline might receive a rank of 2, and so forth.

This ranking process is repeated across all patients, metrics, and classes, resulting in individual ranks for each strategy. We then calculate a per-patient average rank, which summarizes the overall performance of each strategy for that patient. Finally, we obtain a global rank by averaging the per-patient ranks across the entire dataset. The strategy with the lowest global average rank is considered the top performer. This rank-based evaluation emphasizes consistency and robustness across both patients and evaluation metrics, rather than relying solely on aggregated performance values (i.e., the mean of each metric).

3 Results

We use MIST and the training parameters described in Sect. 2.1 to perform a five-fold cross-validation with the BraTS Glioma Segmentation on Pre- and Post-treatment MRI challenge training dataset. Figure 1 shows an example of a baseline (i.e., no postprocessing) prediction from a pre-treatment (top) and post-treatment (bottom) case. The three postprocessing strategies described in Sect. 2.2 are applied to the predictions from the five-fold cross-validation. The accuracy of the baseline and postprocessed predictions is summarized in Table 1. Here, we see that Strategy 3 has the best average accuracy with respect to the Dice score for the SNFH, ET, TC, and WT classes, while tying Strategy 1 and the baseline for the best RC and NETC Dice scores, respectively. With respect to the Hausdorff distance, Strategy 3 achieves the best accuracy (i.e., lowest values) for the ET and TC classes, while tying the baseline and Strategy 1 for the lowest NETC and RC distances, respectively. However, Strategy 3 appears to achieve a worse average Hausdorff distance for the SNFH and WT classes compared to the baseline and Strategy 1. Strategy 2 appears to achieve the second-best performance for the average Dice and Hausdorff distance for the RC class while generally matching the baseline and Strategy 1 for the other classes.

We next apply the BraTS ranking system to our baseline and postprocessed results. Table 3a shows the average global rank across all classes and metrics. Despite Strategy 3's meaningful improvements compared to the baseline and other strategies with respect to the average metrics, it does not show an improvement when ranked against the other strategies using the BraTS ranking system. Indeed, when we compare the baseline and our postprocessing strategies using this ranking system, we see that Strategy 3 has the worst (i.e., highest) average rank.

Table 2 shows the mean and standard deviation of the global Dice, global HD95, lesion-wise (LW) Dice, and LW HD95 for the predictions on the validation set from the baseline model and postprocessed predictions from Strategies 1 and 3. Table 3b shows the average global rank of these different strategies across all classes and LW metrics for the validation set. Like with the cross-validation results, we see that Strategy 3 generally improves the overall averages of the metrics, but that this improvement in the raw averages of each metric does not translate to a high ranking under the BraTS ranking system. With the validation set, we see that the baseline predictions (i.e., no postprocessing) achieve the highest average global ranking.

Table 4 shows the mean and standard deviation of lesion-wise Dice and normalized surface Dice (1.0 mm tolerance) for the unseen test set with our baseline strategy (i.e., no post-processing). We observe that our baseline model yields results comparable to those presented in Table 2, further demonstrating that our baseline strategy effectively generalizes to unseen data.

Figure 2 shows the training and validation loss curves for a single fold. Note that the training loss is the mean of the Dice and cross-entropy loss functions, and the validation loss is the Dice loss function only with no background class. Here, we see that our model achieves a high level of convergence, with two distinct drops in each of the loss curves after about 1,000 and 6,000 epochs.

4 Discussion

Our results demonstrate that postprocessing can have a measurable impact on segmentation accuracy, particularly for challenging tumor subregions such as the ET and RC classes. Strategy 3, which combines class-specific small object replacement and targeted filtering, consistently improves the average Dice and HD95 metrics across multiple classes. These improvements suggest that thoughtful refinement of predicted masks can address common sources of segmentation error, such as small false positives. However, despite these gains in average metric values, our analysis using the BraTS ranking system reveals a more nuanced picture. While Strategy 3 generally achieves the best average metrics, these improvements do not translate into better rankings under the BraTS scoring protocol. In fact, Strategy 3 receives the worst average global rank across both cross-validation and validation set evaluations. This underperformance stems from

Table 1. Mean and standard deviation of the Dice and HD95 for each strategy and segmentation class. The best Dice (highest) and HD95 (lowest) per class are highlighted in yellow. Ties are resolved in favor of the earlier-listed strategies.

Strategy	Class	Dice	HD95 (mm)
Baseline	NETC	0.7918 (0.3058)	22.007 (75.901)
	SNFH	0.8686 (0.1380)	6.8846 (25.077)
	ET	0.8049 (0.2755)	26.069 (83.223)
	RC	0.8234 (0.3080)	31.475 (93.119)
	TC	0.8204 (0.2735)	24.252 (78.966)
	WT	0.9067 (0.1134)	6.5513 (22.732)
Strategy 1	NETC	0.7918 (0.3058)	22.007 (75.901)
	SNFH	0.8686 (0.1380)	6.8846 (25.077)
	ET	0.8049 (0.2755)	26.069 (83.223)
	RC	0.8441 (0.2867)	26.782 (86.005)
	TC	0.8204 (0.2735)	24.252 (78.966)
	WT	0.9067 (0.1134)	6.5513 (22.732)
Strategy 2	NETC	0.7918 (0.3058)	22.007 (75.901)
	SNFH	0.8686 (0.1380)	6.8846 (25.077)
	ET	0.8049 (0.2755)	26.069 (83.223)
	RC	0.8401 (0.2941)	28.780 (88.832)
	TC	0.8204 (0.2735)	24.252 (78.966)
	WT	0.9067 (0.1134)	6.5513 (22.732)
Strategy 3	NETC	0.7918 (0.3058)	22.007 (75.901)
	SNFH	0.8688 (0.1373)	7.0278 (24.403)
	ET	0.8229 (0.2596)	23.625 (78.843)
	RC	0.8441 (0.2867)	26.782 (86.005)
	TC	0.8348 (0.2606)	22.528 (75.647)
	WT	0.9071 (0.1119)	6.5872 (21.991)

the fact that while Strategy 3 improves a subset of outlier cases, it degrades performance on a larger number of patients. In other words, the strategy harms more predictions than it helps, highlighting the importance of evaluating consistency across the entire cohort rather than focusing solely on aggregate metrics.

By contrast, Strategy 1 is a more straightforward and more targeted postprocessing approach that exclusively addresses small false positives in the RC class. It achieves the best global average rank in our five-fold cross-validation because, unlike Strategy 3, it improves more cases than it degrades. Specifically, for the RC Dice coefficient, Strategy 1 improves 589 cases, leaves 2079 unchanged, and degrades 207 cases. For HD95, it improves 153 cases, leaves 2567 unchanged, and degrades 152 cases. The higher number of improvements focused on a single class, combined with no negative impact on the other five segmentation classes, explains why Strategy 1 achieves the best average rank. However, on the validation set, Strategy 1 slightly underperforms the baseline predictions.

Given this outcome and the consistent strength of the baseline across all evaluation settings, we elect to submit the baseline model with no postprocessing as our final entry. While postprocessing strategies like those tested here remain valuable in many applications [10,18,21], their effectiveness depends heavily on the model's initial performance and the broader evaluation context. In our case,

Table 2. Mean and standard deviation of the Dice, HD95, lesion-wise (LW) Dice, and LW HD95 for the baseline, Strategy 1, and Strategy 3 predictions on the validation set. The best values for each metric are highlighted in yellow. Ties are resolved in favor of the earlier-listed strategies.

Stg.	Class	Dice	HD95	LW Dice	LW HD95
Base	NETC	0.7114 (0.3556)	42.902 (105.52)	0.7450 (0.3335)	37.369 (96.851)
	SNFH	0.8608 (0.1543)	7.1704 (25.163)	0.8088 (0.2064)	24.313 (57.523)
	ET	0.7807 (0.2847)	23.670 (77.327)	0.7641 (0.2871)	35.802 (89.441)
	RC	0.8445 (0.3058)	25.010 (82.263)	0.8494 (0.2993)	29.059 (88.479)
	TC	0.7925 (0.2855)	24.582 (77.193)	0.7664 (0.2938)	38.956 (89.077)
	WT	0.9219 (0.0867)	5.9289 (18.755)	0.8663 (0.1754)	23.190 (55.493)
Stg. 1	NETC	0.7114 (0.3556)	42.902 (105.52)	0.7450 (0.3335)	37.369 (96.851)
	SNFH	0.8608 (0.1543)	7.1704 (25.163)	0.8088 (0.2064)	24.313 (57.523)
	ET	0.7807 (0.2847)	23.670 (77.327)	0.7641 (0.2871)	35.802 (89.441)
	RC	0.8484 (0.3026)	23.350 (79.303)	0.8533 (0.2959)	27.804 (86.984)
	TC	0.7925 (0.2855)	24.582 (77.193)	0.7664 (0.2938)	38.956 (89.077)
	WT	0.9219 (0.0867)	5.9289 (18.755)	0.8663 (0.1754)	23.190 (55.493)
Stg. 3	NETC	0.7114 (0.3556)	42.902 (105.52)	0.7450 (0.3335)	37.369 (96.851)
	SNFH	0.8612 (0.1556)	7.3227 (25.249)	0.8094 (0.2069)	24.533 (57.427)
	ET	0.7892 (0.2789)	23.760 (77.282)	0.7714 (0.2843)	35.365 (89.580)
	RC	0.8484 (0.3026)	23.350 (79.303)	0.8533 (0.2959)	27.804 (86.984)
	TC	0.8012 (0.2739)	23.066 (73.936)	0.7723 (0.2869)	37.949 (87.151)
	WT	0.9226 (0.0858)	5.8714 (18.738)	0.8701 (0.1718)	21.994 (53.930)

Table 3. Average global rank for each strategy. (a) Cross-validation set. (b) Validation set. Lower values indicate better performance.

Strategy	Average Rank
Strategy 1	2.470288
Strategy 2	2.474945
Base	2.491658
Strategy 3	2.563109

(a) Cross-validation.

Strategy	Average Rank
Base	1.991810
Strategy 1	1.995547
Strategy 3	2.012643

(b) Validation set.

Table 4. Mean and standard deviation of the lesion-wise Dice and normalized surface Dice (1.0 mm tolerance) on the unseen test set using our baseline strategy (i.e., no post-processing).

Class	LW Dice	LW NSD (1.0 mm)
ET	0.7875 (0.2706)	0.8340 (0.2562)
RC	0.8400 (0.3128)	0.8353 (0.3106)
TC	0.7872 (0.2911)	0.7947 (0.2760)
WT	0.8577 (0.1927)	0.8210 (0.2048)

each model was trained for 10,000 epochs using strong architectural priors (i.e., deep supervision, residual blocks), extensive data augmentation, and a conservative learning rate schedule, yielding models that are already highly optimized.

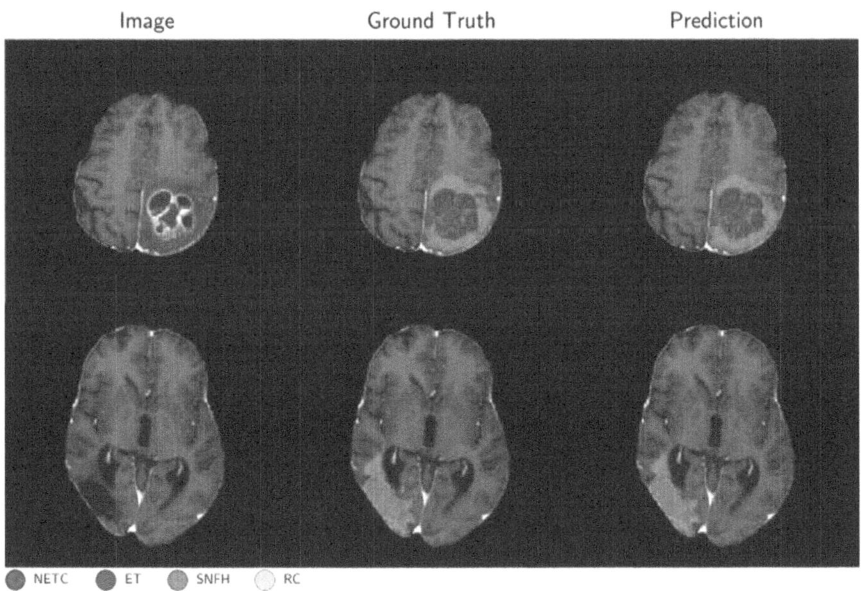

Fig. 1. From left to right, a slice of the contrast enhanced T1-weighted image, the ground truth overlaid on the image, and the baseline prediction overlaid the image for a pre-treatment case (top) and a post-treatment case (bottom).

Figure 2, which plots the training and validation loss curves for a single fold, illustrates the high level of optimization that our training scheme achieves. In this plot, we see that the model converges smoothly, with two distinct drops in the loss curves around epochs 1,000 and 6,000, followed by long plateaus. These inflection points likely mark key learning milestones, such as improved delineation of tumor subregions or the ability to distinguish between pre- and post-operative cases. The stability of the loss after these transitions suggests that the model has reached a mature optimization state, leaving

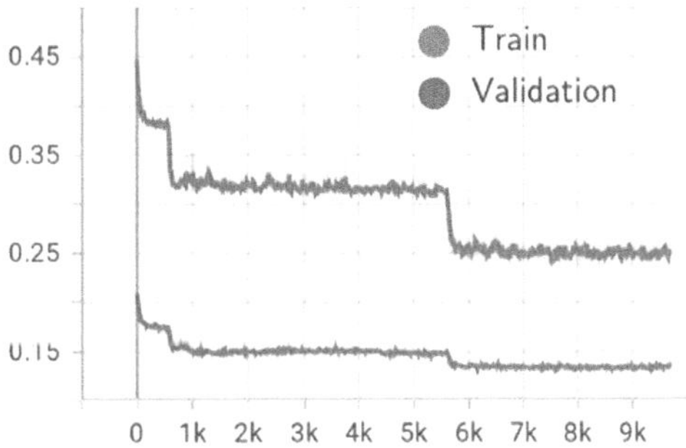

Fig. 2. Example of train (blue) and validation (red) loss curves for our model. The training loss is the mean of the Dice and cross entropy loss functions and the validation loss is the Dice loss function without the background class. (Color figure online)

limited room for additional gains through postprocessing. This observation further reinforces our decision to submit the baseline model as our final entry.

From a systems perspective, the modularity of the MIST postprocessing pipeline is crucial for facilitating this analysis. Researchers have the flexibility to experiment with a broad array of transformations without the need to retrain models or alter the underlying Python code, which accelerates experimentation and enhances reproducibility. Our strategy configuration files simplify the process of sharing and comparing various refinement approaches, ensuring that evaluations are both transparent and customizable. Collectively, our findings underscore two key considerations for future segmentation workflows: (1) postprocessing remains a valuable tool for enhancing segmentation quality but must be carefully evaluated against robust ranking systems; and (2) modular frameworks like MIST are vital for enabling flexible experimentation, especially in environments where clinical or benchmark requirements are constantly evolving. MIST is open-source (Apache 2.0 license) and is available on GitHub or PyPI. Please cite [6,7] if you use MIST for your own work.

Acknowledgments. The Department of Defense supported Adrian Celaya through the National Defense Science & Engineering Graduate Fellowship Program. This research was partially supported by the Tumor Measurement Initiative through the MD Anderson Strategic Research Initiative Development (STRIDE), NSF-2111147, NSF-2111459, and NIH R01CA195524.

References

1. Antonelli, M., et al.: The medical segmentation decathlon. Nat. Commun. **13**(1), 4128 (2022)
2. Baid, U., et al.: The RSNA-ASNR-MICCAI BRATS 2021 benchmark on brain tumor segmentation and radiogenomic classification. arXiv preprint arXiv:2107.02314 (2021)
3. Bakas, S., et al.: Segmentation labels for the pre-operative scans of the TCGA-LGG collection. The cancer imaging archive (2017)
4. Bakas, S., et al.: Advancing the cancer genome atlas glioma MRI collections with expert segmentation labels and radiomic features. Sci. Data **4**(1), 1–13 (2017)
5. Cao, H., et al.: Swin-unet: Unet-like pure transformer for medical image segmentation. In: European Conference on Computer Vision, pp. 205–218. Springer (2022)
6. Celaya, A., et al.: PocketNet: a smaller neural network for medical image analysis. IEEE Trans. Med. Imaging **42**(4), 1172–1184 (2022)
7. Celaya, A., et al.: MIST: a simple and scalable end-to-end 3d medical imaging segmentation framework. arXiv preprint arXiv:2407.21343 (2024)
8. Celaya, A., Riviere, B., Fuentes, D.: A generalized surface loss for reducing the Hausdorff distance in medical imaging segmentation. arXiv preprint arXiv:2302.03868 (2023)
9. Chen, J., et al.: TransUNet: transformers make strong encoders for medical image segmentation. arXiv preprint arXiv:2102.04306 (2021)
10. Chen, S., Gamechi, Z.S., Dubost, F., van Tulder, G., de Bruijne, M.: An end-to-end approach to segmentation in medical images with CNN and posterior-CRF. Med. Image Anal. **76**, 102311 (2022)

11. Çiçek, Ö., Abdulkadir, A., Lienkamp, S.S., Brox, T., Ronneberger, O.: 3D U-Net: learning dense volumetric segmentation from sparse annotation. In: Ourselin, S., Joskowicz, L., Sabuncu, M.R., Unal, G., Wells, W. (eds.) MICCAI 2016. LNCS, vol. 9901, pp. 424–432. Springer, Cham (2016). https://doi.org/10.1007/978-3-319-46723-8_49
12. Hatamizadeh, A., Nath, V., Tang, Y., Yang, D., Roth, H.R., Xu, D.: Swin UNETR: swin transformers for semantic segmentation of brain tumors in MRI images. In: Crimi, A., Bakas, S. (eds.) BrainLes 2021. LNCS, vol. 12962, pp. 272–284. Springer, Cham (2021). https://doi.org/10.1007/978-3-031-08999-2_22
13. Isensee, F., Jaeger, P.F., Kohl, S.A., Petersen, J., Maier-Hein, K.H.: nnU-Net: a self-configuring method for deep learning-based biomedical image segmentation. Nat. Methods **18**(2), 203–211 (2021)
14. Isensee, F., Jäger, P.F., Full, P.M., Vollmuth, P., Maier-Hein, K.H.: nnU-Net for brain tumor segmentation. In: Crimi, A., Bakas, S. (eds.) BrainLes 2020. LNCS, vol. 12659, pp. 118–132. Springer, Cham (2021). https://doi.org/10.1007/978-3-030-72087-2_11
15. Isensee, F., et al.: nnU-Net revisited: a call for rigorous validation in 3d medical image segmentation. arXiv preprint arXiv:2404.09556 (2024)
16. Karargyris, A., et al.: Federated benchmarking of medical artificial intelligence with MedPerf. Nat. Mach. Intell. **5**(7), 799–810 (2023)
17. Kervadec, H., Bouchtiba, J., Desrosiers, C., Granger, E., Dolz, J., Ayed, I.B.: Boundary loss for highly unbalanced segmentation. Med. Image Anal. **67**, 101851 (2021)
18. Kim, J., Kang, S.: Model-agnostic post-processing based on recursive feedback for medical image segmentation. IEEE Access **9**, 157035–157042 (2021)
19. Loshchilov, I., Hutter, F.: SGDR: stochastic gradient descent with warm restarts. arXiv preprint arXiv:1608.03983 (2016)
20. Menze, B.H., et al.: The multimodal brain tumor image segmentation benchmark (BRATs). IEEE Trans. Med. Imaging **34**(10), 1993–2024 (2014)
21. Patel, N., et al.: Training robust t1-weighted magnetic resonance imaging liver segmentation models using ensembles of datasets with different contrast protocols and liver disease etiologies. Sci. Rep. **14**(1), 20988 (2024)
22. Ronneberger, O., Fischer, P., Brox, T.: U-Net: convolutional networks for biomedical image segmentation. In: Navab, N., Hornegger, J., Wells, W.M., Frangi, A.F. (eds.) MICCAI 2015. LNCS, vol. 9351, pp. 234–241. Springer, Cham (2015). https://doi.org/10.1007/978-3-319-24574-4_28
23. Tang, Y., et al.: Self-supervised pre-training of swin transformers for 3D medical image analysis. In: Proceedings of the IEEE/CVF Conference on Computer Vision and Pattern Recognition, pp. 20730–20740 (2022)
24. Vaswani, A., et al.: Attention is all you need. Adv. Neural Inf. Process. Syst. **30** (2017)
25. de Verdier, M.C., et al.: The 2024 brain tumor segmentation (BraTS) challenge: Glioma segmentation on post-treatment MRI. arXiv preprint arXiv:2405.18368 (2024)
26. Zhou, H.Y., Guo, J., Zhang, Y., Yu, L., Wang, L., Yu, Y.: nnFormer: interleaved transformer for volumetric segmentation. arXiv preprint arXiv:2109.03201 (2021)

µPUA-Net: PowerMLP Model Size Shrinking Method with Accuracy Maintaining

Yu-Shan Chou[1], You-Jin Liu[2], Kai-Lun Pien[1], Tong-Hou Cheong[1], Chieh-Chen Yu[1], Ying-Hui Cheng[1], Yu-Hsuan Chiang[1], E. Ray Hsieh[3], and Chien-Chang Chen[1](✉)

[1] Department of Biomedical Sciences and Engineering, National Central University, Taoyuan, Taiwan
gettgod@ncu.edu.tw
[2] Department of Electrical Engineering, National Central University, Taoyuan, Taiwan
[3] Institute of Electronics, National Yang Ming Chiao Tung University, Hsinchu, Taiwan

Abstract. Gliomas are among the most common malignant brain tumors in adults and present significant challenges in neuro-oncology due to their heterogeneity and complex biological behavior. Accurate segmentation of gliomas using multimodal magnetic resonance imaging is essential for diagnosis and treatment planning, but it remains computationally demanding. U-Net-based models, such as Attention U-Net, UNETR, and Swin UNETR, have demonstrated strong performance in brain tumor segmentation but face inherent limitations in capturing complex nonlinear patterns. Kolmogorov-Arnold Networks (KANs) introduced learnable univariate spline functions to enhance modeling capabilities; however, their computational inefficiency poses challenges for practical deployment. In response, we propose µPUA-Net, which integrates PowerMLP layers into the UKAN-EP architecture, replacing KAN layers to improve computational efficiency while maintaining strong modeling capacity. Our approach achieves comparable accuracy to UKAN-EP with a 36.3% reduction in parameters and improves efficiency over UKAN-EP, with the lowest 3% error in accuracy compared to nn-UNet. Furthermore, our model achieves a remarkable 1/2159 reduction in inference time compared to nn-UNet, highlighting its potential as a practical and effective solution for glioma segmentation tasks.

Keywords: BraTS2025 · GLI · PowerMLP · inference time reduction

1 Introduction

Gliomas are one of the most common types of malignant brain tumors in adults and a leading cause of cancer-related mortality. Due to their complex biological behavior and significant impact on patient survival, the diagnosis and

S. Bakas et al. (Eds.): MICCAI 2025, LNCS 16376, pp. 38–47, 2026.
https://doi.org/10.1007/978-3-032-16365-3_4

treatment of gliomas pose substantial challenges in neuro-oncology. As a non-invasive assessment tool, multimodal magnetic resonance imaging (MRI) provides critical information about tumor size, location, and morphology. It serves as a primary data source for tumor segmentation tasks. Each modality has its strengths in visualizing specific tumor characteristics. For instance, enhancing tumor tissue (ET) and necrosis (non-enhancing tumor core, NETC) are most clearly observed in contrast-enhanced T1-weighted (T1Gd) mode; edema (surrounding non-enhancing FLAIR hyperintensity, SNFH) is best visualized in T2-weighted fluid-attenuated inversion recovery (FLAIR) images; resection cavity (RC) appears most prominently in T2-weighted (T2) scans. However, challenges such as intensity inconsistencies, imaging artifacts, and the requirement to process and align multimodal data significantly increase the computational burden of accurate tumor segmentation.

Over the years, U-Net-based models and their variants have demonstrated remarkable performance in brain tumor segmentation tasks. Attention U-Net [17] improves the ability to focus on relevant feature incorporation. UNETR [9] then utilizes a pure Transformer-based encoder to directly process 3D volumetric data, effectively capturing global dependencies in the input, and enabling precise segmentation by integrating global context with local spatial details. Similarly, Swin UNETR [8] employs a Swin Transformer as its encoder and combines multi-resolution representations with the decoder through skip connections. Despite their success, U-Net-based models face inherent limitations in capturing complex non-linear patterns when relying on traditional convolutional kernels, which restricts their potential for further performance improvements.

To address these issues, Kolmogorov-Arnold Networks (KANs) (Liu et al., 2024) [14] have introduced an innovative architecture, providing new possibilities for brain tumor segmentation tasks. The architecture employs learnable univariate spline functions as activation functions, replacing the fixed ones, thereby enhancing the network's capability to model complex functions. KAN improves the model interpretability and establishes a more effective connection between network structures and performance. Recently, the UKAN (Li et al., 2024) [12] model integrated KAN layers into the U-Net architecture and utilized tokenized KAN blocks to capture complex patterns better. Building upon UKAN, UKAN-EP (Chen et al., 2024) [6] was developed to address the accuracy limitations of its predecessor. Compared to other high-precision models, UKAN-EP significantly reduces the number of parameters. However, it fails to resolve the issues introduced by KAN, including high computational complexity, expensive training costs, and slow inference speed.

PowerMLP (Qiu et al., 2024) [18] was developed to conquer KAN's computational efficiency issues. This model simplifies the computation of B-splines with a basis term of powers of ReLU, avoiding the recursive calculations used in KAN, and places activation functions on edges, to achieve both higher accuracy and faster speed than KAN. Notably, PowerMLP not only reduces computational costs but also retains KAN's powerful modeling capabilities.

By synerging the advantages from PowerMLP, U-shaped architecture, and the incorporation of Attention and Aggregation mechanisms, we proposed a μPUA-Net with μ signifying the ultra-lightweight strategy. Building upon the UKAN-EP model, we replace its original KAN layers with the more computationally efficient PowerMLP layers. The study's main contributions are to validate the feasibility of architecture synergy and provide an ultra-lightweight strategy, whose accuracy is comparable to UKAN-EP with a 36.3% reduction in training parameters.

2 Related Work

2.1 UKAN

In the multilayer perceptron (MLP) architecture, weights, biases, and scaling factors collectively act on the input through linear combinations. However, MLPs typically employ nonlinear activation functions to introduce nonlinearity into the network, enhancing the model's representational capacity and fitting complex nonlinear relationships. On the other hand, KAN [14] proposes an adaptive network architecture based on the Cox-De Boor algorithm:

$$N_{i,0}(x) = \begin{cases} 1, & \text{if} \quad t_i \leq x < t_{i+1}, \\ 0, & \text{otherwise.} \end{cases} \tag{1}$$

$$N_{i,p}(x) = \frac{x - t_i}{t_{i+p} - t_i} N_{i,p-1}(x) + \frac{t_{i+p+1} - x}{t_{i+p+1} - t_{i+1}} N_{i+1,p-1}(x), \tag{2}$$

$$KAN(x) = (\Phi_{L-1} \circ \cdots \circ \Phi_1 \circ \Phi_0)(x). \tag{3}$$

KAN is designed to save resources while efficiently and rapidly approximating target functions. Compared to MLP, the KAN framework approximates target functions through a series of control points and their corresponding basis functions. The flexibility of spline functions allows them to adjust the positions and number of control points to fit the target function more accurately.

Subsequently, UKAN [12] adheres to the benchmark setup of U-Net, employing a multilayer encoder-decoder architecture with skip connections and incorporating the tokenized KAN (Tok-KAN) block. The network architecture adopts a two-phase design: the first phase involves convolution for initial feature extraction, while the second phase integrates the Tok-KAN block, where the KAN layers process tokenized features using B-spline-based activation functions. This design effectively combines the traditional U-Net architecture with the KAN framework, achieving remarkable performance in segmentation tasks. The Tok-KAN block is defined as:

$$Z_k = \text{LN}(Z_{k-1} + \text{DwConv}(\text{KAN}(Z_{k-1}))), \tag{4}$$

where Z_{k-1} represents the input feature map from the previous layer, KAN$(\cdot)$ applies the tokenized KAN transformation, DwConv$(\cdot)$ [5] denotes the depthwise convolution operation, and LN$(\cdot)$ is the layer normalization function. The Tok-KAN block enhances the feature representation by leveraging B-spline-based activation functions, enabling efficient tokenized feature processing.

2.2 UKAN-EP

Furthermore, UKAN-EP introduces ECA and PFA modules to capture information between different modalities.

Efficient Channel Attention (ECA). [6] is a lightweight and effective channel attention mechanism designed to enhance feature representation without significantly increasing computational complexity. Traditional channel attention mechanisms, such as SENet [10] and CBAM [19], rely on fully connected layers to capture cross-channel interactions. These approaches often involve dimensionality reduction of channel representations to manage computational costs, which can compromise the learning of channel-wise dependencies. In contrast, ECA avoids dimensionality reduction and efficiently learns channel attention by employing a simple 1D convolution operation to model local cross-channel interactions.

The ECA mechanism consists of three key steps:

1. **Global Feature Compression:** Global average pooling (GAP) is applied to the spatial dimensions of the input feature tensor $X = [X_{d,c,h,w}] \in \mathbb{R}^{D\times C\times H\times W}$, resulting in aggregated features $z = (z_1, \ldots, z_D) \in \mathbb{R}^D$:

$$z_c = \frac{1}{C \times H \times W} \sum_{c=1}^{C} \sum_{h=1}^{H} \sum_{w=1}^{W} X_{d,c,h,w}, \quad \text{for } d = 1, 2, \ldots, D. \tag{5}$$

   d denotes modality or feature extracted by 3D convolution. c for depth of the brain. h and w are the height and width of a 2D brain image, respectively.
2. **Local Cross-Channel Interaction Modeling:** A 1D convolution is applied to z to capture local interactions among channels, followed by a sigmoid activation function to generate channel weights:

$$(a_1, \ldots, a_C) = \text{Sigmoid}(\text{Conv1D}(z, k)). \tag{6}$$

3. **Feature Recalibration:** The channel weights $(a_1, \ldots, a_C)$ are applied to each channel of the input feature tensor $X = [X_1, \ldots, X_C]$ to produce a recalibrated feature tensor $\hat{X} = [\hat{X}_1, \ldots, \hat{X}_C]$, where informative feature channels are emphasized and less useful ones are suppressed:

$$\hat{X}_d = a_d X_d, \quad \text{for } d = 1, 2, \ldots, D. \tag{7}$$

Pyramid Feature Aggregation (PFA). Merging semantically rich deep features with spatially precise shallow features is a common strategy in hierarchical fusion frameworks [13,20,21]. Building on this principle, Pyramid Feature Aggregation (PFA) is introduced to enhance multi-scale representation by facilitating cross-scale feature continuity. Let $\{X^{(l)}\}_{l=1}^{3}$ denote the encoder feature maps, where $l = 1$ corresponds to the shallowest feature map and $l = 3$ corresponds to the deepest feature map. The PFA module aggregates features in a top-down manner, proceeding from deep to shallow layers.

At each stage $l \in \{1, 2\}$, the upsampled output from the deeper recalibrated feature $\tilde{X}^{(l+1)}$ (with $\tilde{X}^{(3)} = X^{(3)}$) is concatenated with the current encoder feature $X^{(l)}$:

$$\breve{X}^{(l)} = \text{Concat}(\text{Upsample}(\tilde{X}^{(l+1)}), X^{(l)}). \tag{8}$$

The aggregated tensor $\breve{X}^{(l)}$ is then passed through the ECA module (Sect. 2.3) to produce the recalibrated output $\tilde{X}^{(l)}$. The final outputs $\{\tilde{X}^{(l)}\}_{l=1}^{2}$ are propagated as skip connections to the decoder. This hierarchical fusion structure enhances cross-scale feature continuity and improves segmentation precision compared to conventional U-Net designs.

2.3 PowerMLP

KAN has gained significant attention due to its high accuracy in various complex tasks, such as function approximation and solving partial differential equations. However, KAN suffers from a notable drawback in computational efficiency, primarily due to the iterative computation process required by its spline functions. During training, the spline functions undergo multiple iterations for optimization to achieve optimal fitting performance, resulting in substantial time overhead and limiting KAN's applicability in large-scale tasks.

To overcome KAN's efficiency predicaments, Ruichen Qiu et al. introduced PowerMLP [18], utilizing power functions based on ReLU [16] as activation functions, simplifying the representation of non-iterative spline functions:

$$\sigma_k(x) = (\text{RELU}(x))^k = (\max(0, x))^k \quad k \in \mathbb{Z}^+. \tag{9}$$

$$\text{PowerMLP}(x) = (\Psi_{L-1} \circ \cdots \circ \Psi_1 \circ \Psi_0)(x), \quad \text{where}$$
$$\Psi_l(x_l) = \begin{cases} a_l b(x_l) + \sigma_k(w_l x_l + \gamma_l), & \text{for} \quad l < L-1, \\ w_{L-1} x_{L-1} + \gamma_{L-1}, & \text{for} \quad l = L-1. \end{cases} \tag{10}$$

This design allows the model to emulate the behavior of spline functions without iterative computation while retaining the fast training advantages of traditional MLPs. By replacing the base of the KAN algorithm with a residual activation function, PowerMLP significantly reduces computational complexity, making the training process more efficient.

3 Method

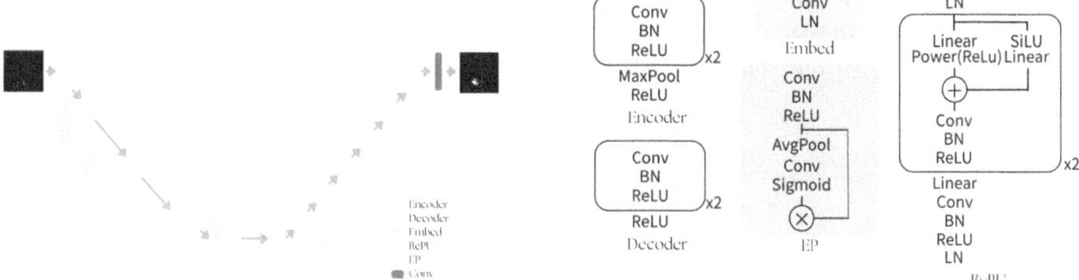

Fig. 1. µPUA-Net Architecture

Fig. 2. µPUA-Net Architecture Blocks

3.1 Dataset

Our study exclusively utilized the **training data1 v2** from the BraTS 2025 Task1.GLI Post Treatment dataset [7] is the source of training and validating data for our model. We did not utilize pre-treatment datasets [1–4,15] in our model training process. Meanwhile, we adopted AdamW with learning rate and weight decay equals to 0.01 and 0.0001, respectively.

3.2 Model Architecture

Figure 1 and Fig. 2 shows our µPUA-Net architecture, comprised of 5 major parts - Encoder, EP Block, Bottleneck, Decoder, and Skip Connection.

1. Encoder
   Each encoder block consists of two convolutional layers (Conv), each followed by a batch normalization layer (BN) and a ReLU activation function. A max-pooling layer with kernel size 2×2 is also applied to reduce the spatial dimensions. The encoder progressively extracts hierarchical features from the input image. Given an input image $X_0 = I \in \mathbb{R}^{D_0 * C_0 \times H_0 \times W_0}$, the output of the ℓ-th encoder block can be expressed as:

$$X_\ell = \text{Pool}(\text{DoubleConv}(X_{\ell-1})), \tag{11}$$

   where $X_\ell \in \mathbb{R}^{D_\ell * C_\ell \times H_\ell \times W_\ell}$ represents the feature maps at the ℓ-th layer, and Pool denotes the max-pooling operation.
2. EP Block
   The EP Block, proposed by [6], uses 3D convolution to merge brain information and effectively emphasizes informative features while suppressing less useful ones by using a 1D convolution, ensuring robust feature extraction across modalities while minimizing computational complexity.

3. Bottleneck
   The bottleneck layer serves as a compact representation of the extracted features. Inspired by [18], we employ PowerMLP within the bottleneck block to enhance computational efficiency and reduce inference time, since it integrates linear transformations, SiLU activation, and residual connections. For the bottleneck block, the transformation can be expressed as:
$$Z = \text{LayerNorm}(X_L), \tag{12}$$
$$Z = Z + \text{Linear}(\text{SiLU}(\text{Linear}(Z))), \tag{13}$$
$$Z = \text{DWConv}(Z), \tag{14}$$
   where X_L is the input from the last encoder block, and $Z \in \mathbb{R}^{H_B*W_B \times D_B*C_B}$ is the output of the bottleneck block.
4. Decoder
   The decoder reconstructs spatial dimensions and semantic information from the bottleneck features. Each decoder block consists of two Convs, each followed by a BN and a ReLU activation function. An upsampling layer (Upsample) is applied to increase the spatial resolution. Given the input from the bottleneck $Z \in \mathbb{R}^{H_B*W_B \times D_B*C_B}$, the output of the ℓ-th decoder block is computed as:
$$\hat{X}_\ell = \text{DoubleConv}(\text{Upsample}(\hat{X}_{\ell+1})), \tag{15}$$
   where $\hat{X}_\ell \in \mathbb{R}^{N_\ell*C_\ell \times H_\ell \times W_\ell}$ is the feature map at layer ℓ with N represents NumClasses, and Upsample denotes the upsampling operation.
5. Skip Connection
   Skip connections concatenate feature maps from the encoder to the corresponding decoder layers. This helps preserve spatial details and improve reconstruction quality. Let X_ℓ^{enc} denote the feature maps from the ℓ-th encoder layer, and $\hat{X}_\ell^{\text{dec}}$ denote the feature maps at the ℓ-th decoder layer. The skip connection is defined as:
$$\hat{X}_\ell^{\text{dec}} = \text{Concat}(X_\ell^{\text{enc}}, \hat{X}_\ell^{\text{dec}}), \tag{16}$$
   where Concat represents the concatenation operation along the channel dimension.

4 Result

We employed the BraTS 2025 Task1.GLI Post Treatment training data1 v2 dataset to train µPUA-Net. The µPUA-Net training tendency is presented in the Fig. 3. The loss demonstrates a rapid decline within the first 5 epochs. This is attributed to PowerMLP, which reduces the cost of model training and deployment by replacing the base functions, thereby eliminating the need for multiple iterations.

After training, we take the BraTS 2025 Task1.GLI Post Treatment training data additional dataset for inference experiments, and compare the accuracy

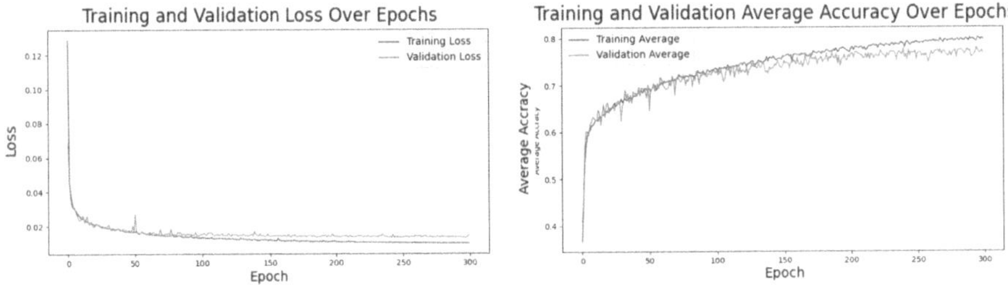

Fig. 3. Train Tendency of μPUA-Net

Table 1. Accuracy Comparison

Model	BraTs2025 Additional Dataset						Inference Time (ms)	Parameter (M)
	ET	NETC	SNFH	RC	ET+NETC	ET+SNFH+NETC		
nnUNet [11]	**0.7781**	**0.7766**	**0.8632**	**0.6596**	**0.7717**	**0.8680**	6479	88
UNETR [9]	0.6747	0.5204	0.7478	0.4102	0.6628	0.7709	522	130
SwinUNETR [8]	0.6511	0.3817	0.7468	0.4299	0.6267	0.7662	6180	62
UKAN [12]	0.2751	0.4797	0.4110	0.1823	0.2852	0.4828	20	46
UKAN-MLP	0.3439	0.4797	0.5028	0.2493	0.3565	0.5734	21	20
UKAN-EP [6]	0.6806	0.5599	0.7588	0.4800	0.6621	0.7691	5	11
μPUA-Net	0.7361	0.5630	0.8278	0.5449	0.7238	0.8383	**3**	**7**

with the contemporary models. Among them, UKAN-MLP refers to replacing the KAN layers in UKAN with PowerMLP layers. As shown in Table 1, the accuracy of the proposed μPUA-Net differs by less than 5% compared to the best-performing nnUNet in ET, SNFH, ET+NETC, and ET+SNFH+NETC. Only the differences are more pronounced for NETC and RC. However, nnUNet's inference time is 2159 times longer than that of μPUA-Net, and its parameter count is 12 times larger. Besides, Table 2 clearly presents the outstanding performance of μPUA-Net on the validation dataset.

Table 2. Validation Phrase Score

Metric	BraTs2025 Validation Dataset					
	ET	NETC	SNFH	RC	ET+NETC	ET+SNFH+NETC
Dicc	0.7148	0.5563	0.5398	0.8352	0.6777	0.8959
NSD1.0	0.7648	0.6284	0.5436	0.8194	0.6783	0.8236

Figure 4 presents the output comparison between UKAN-EP and our proposed model, as both share a similar architectural design and demonstrate comparable segmentation performance. Although our model performs better than UKAN-EP, given that much of the NETC is error annotation to RC, we speculate that the lack of comprehensive preprocessing and data augmentation causes

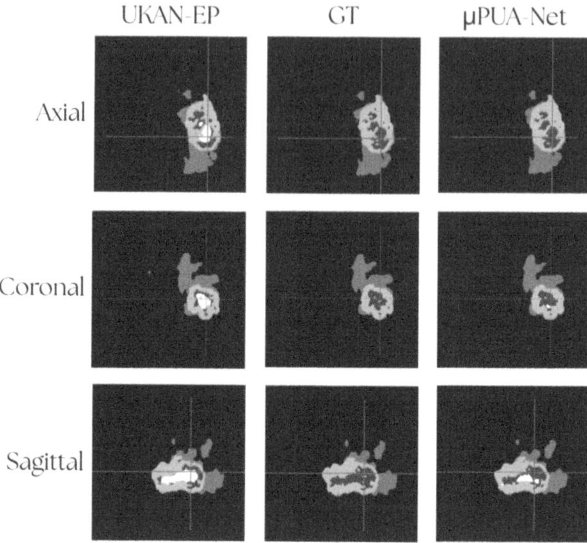

Fig. 4. Prediction Comparison between UKAN-EP and μPUA-Net

Table 3. LesionWise Score of Testing Phrase

Metric	BraTS2025 Hidden Testset			
	ET	RC	ET+NETC	ET+SNFH+NETC
Dice	0.7076	0.5874	0.6905	0.7699
NSD1.0	0.7615	0.5838	0.7045	0.7261

this. We only added noise, random rotated and random contrasted while training. Therefore, the model is unable to learn sufficient features.

Table 3 presents the quantitative performance of μPUA-Net evaluated on the hidden test set. As shown in Table 3, the majority of the scores are consistent with those in the validation set, and some even perform slightly better.

5 Discussion

While our proposed model demonstrates a slight trade-off in accuracy compared to nn-UNet, it offers significant advantages in terms of computational efficiency and deployability. Specifically, our model achieves a 12-fold reduction in parameters and an impressive 2159-time decrease in inference time, making it highly suitable for deployment on edge devices where computational resources are limited. Furthermore, despite the reduction in complexity, our model consistently outperforms previous reference works in terms of accuracy, striking a balance between performance and efficiency. These results highlight the practicality and potential of our approach for real-world applications, particularly in scenarios requiring lightweight yet practical neural networks.

References

1. Baid, U., et al.: The RSNA-ASNR-MICCAI BraTS 2021 benchmark on brain tumor segmentation and radiogenomic classification. arXiv:2107.02314 (2021)
2. Bakas, S., et al.: Segmentation labels and radiomic features for the pre-operative scans of the TCGA-GBM collection. Cancer Imaging Arch. (2017)
3. Bakas, S., et al.: Segmentation labels and radiomic features for the pre-operative scans of the TCGA-LGG collection. Cancer Imaging Arch. (2017)
4. Bakas, S., et al.: Advancing The Cancer Genome Atlas glioma MRI collections with expert segmentation labels and radiomic features. Nature Sci. Data **4**, 170117 (2017)
5. Cao, J., et al.: Do-conv: depthwise over-parameterized convolutional layer (2020)
6. Chen, Y., Tang, T., Kim, T., Shu, H.: UKAN-EP: enhancing U-KAN with efficient attention and pyramid aggregation for 3D multi-modal MRI brain tumor segmentation (2025)
7. de Verdier, M.C., et al.: The 2024 brain tumor segmentation (BraTS) challenge: Glioma segmentation on post-treatment MRI (2024)
8. Hatamizadeh, A., Nath, V., Tang, Y., Yang, D., Roth, H., Xu, D.: Swin UNETR: swin transformers for semantic segmentation of brain tumors in MRI images (2022)
9. Hatamizadeh, A., et al.: UNETR: transformers for 3d medical image segmentation (2021)
10. Hu, J., Shen, L., Albanie, S., Sun, G., Wu, E.: Squeeze-and-excitation networks (2019)
11. Isensee, F., et al.: nnU-Net: self-adapting framework for u-net-based medical image segmentation (2018)
12. Li, C., et al.: U-KAN makes strong backbone for medical image segmentation and generation. In: Proceedings of the AAAI Conference on Artificial Intelligence, vol. 39, no. 5, pp. 4652–4660 (2025). Number: 5
13. Lin, T.-Y., Dollár, P., Girshick, R., Hariharan, B., Belongie, S., He, K.: Feature pyramid networks for object detection (2017)
14. Liu, Z., et al.: KAN: Kolmogorov-Arnold networks (2025)
15. Menze, B.H., et al.: The multimodal brain tumor image segmentation benchmark (BRATS). IEEE Trans. Med. Imaging **34**(10), 1993–2024 (2015)
16. Mhaskar, H.N.: Approximation properties of a multilayered feedforward artificial neural network. Adv. Comput. Math. **1**(1), 61–80 (1993)
17. Oktay, O., et al.: Attention U-Net: learning where to look for the pancreas (2018)
18. Qiu, R., Miao, Y., Wang, S., Lijia, Yu., Zhu, Y., Gao, X.-S.: PowerMLP: an efficient version of KAN (2024)
19. Woo, S., Park, J., Lee, J.-Y., Kweon, I.S.: CBAM: convolutional block attention module (2018)
20. Zhang, Z., Sabuncu, M.R.: Generalized cross entropy loss for training deep neural networks with noisy labels (2018)
21. Zhou, Z., Siddiquee, M.M.R., Tajbakhsh, N., Liang, J.: Unet++: a nested u-net architecture for medical image segmentation (2018)

On-the-Fly Data Augmentation for Brain Tumor Segmentation

Ishika Jain[1,2(✉)], Siri Willems[1], Steven Latre[1,2], and Tom De Schepper[1]

[1] imec, Kapeldreef 75, 3001 Leuven, Belgium
kitujain15@gmail.com
[2] Department of Computer Science, UAntwerp-imec, Sint-Pietersvliet 7, 2000 Antwerp, Belgium

Abstract. Robust segmentation across both pre-treatment and post-treatment glioma scans can be helpful for consistent tumor monitoring and treatment planning. BraTS 2025 Task 1 addresses this by challenging models to generalize across varying tumor appearances throughout the treatment timeline. However, training such generalized models requires access to diverse, high-quality annotated data, which is often limited. While data augmentation can alleviate this, storing large volumes of augmented 3D data is computationally expensive. To address these challenges, we propose an on-the-fly augmentation strategy that dynamically inserts synthetic tumors using pretrained generative adversarial networks (GliGANs) during training. We evaluate three nnU-Net-based models and their ensembles: (1) a baseline without external augmentation, (2) a regular on-the-fly augmented model, and (3) a model with customized on-the-fly augmentation. Built upon the nnU-Net framework, our pipeline leverages pretrained GliGAN weights and tumor insertion methods from prior challenge-winning solutions. An ensemble of the three models achieves lesion-wise Dice scores of 0.79 (ET), 0.749 (NETC), 0.872 (RC), 0.825 (SNFH), 0.79 (TC), and 0.88 (WT) on the online BraTS 2025 validation platform. This work ranked first in the BraTS Lighthouse Challenge 2025 Task 1- Adult Glioma Segmentation.

Keywords: Generative adversarial networks · Brain tumor segmentation · nnU−Net · On−the−fly Data Augmentation · Ensemble

1 Introduction

Gliomas are the most common malignant primary brain tumors found in adults. These diffuse gliomas present significant clinical challenges due to their highly infiltrative growth into normal tissue, heterogeneous biology, and variable response to therapy. Accurate assessment of these tumors is critical for diagnosis, treatment planning, monitoring progression and predicting patient outcomes [5,11]. These assessments are performed by precise delineation, mainly performed

S. Bakas et al. (Eds.): MICCAI 2025, LNCS 16376, pp. 48–62, 2026.
https://doi.org/10.1007/978-3-032-16365-3_5

manually, of different regions of the tumor, based on information from various MRI modalities (T1, T2, FLAIR, ...). However, manual segmentation of gliomas is time-consuming, subjective and prone to human error, which motivates the need for automated and reproducible solutions.

Over the past 15 years, AI has rapidly evolved, driven by breakthroughs in neural network architectures and learning paradigms. Initially, Convolutional Neural Networks (CNNs) revolutionized image processing, including medical imaging tasks, by excelling at detecting spatial patterns [20]. Frameworks as U-Net became popular for solving unimodal and multi-modal medical imaging challenges [16]. The introduction of transformers marked a significant shift in AI, enabling models to capture long-range dependencies and contextual relationships within data [21]. Vision transformers like TransUNet [9], for example, excel at understanding spatial correlations across the entire images and have significantly improved both the accuracy and efficiency of segmentation methods, outperforming CNNs in scenarios with large, diverse datasets [22]. In general, these models leverage large-scale data, self-configuring pipelines, and attention mechanisms to better capture complex anatomical structures, reducing manual effort and accelerating clinical workflows.

To drive research further towards development of robust data-driven clinical pipelines, different challenges tackling various clinical problems are hosted at the annual Medical Image Computing and Computer Assisted Intervention (MICCAI). The Brain Tumor Segmentation (BraTS) challenge in particular provides standardized, annotated datasets and a fair, open benchmarking platform to drive research in automated brain tumor segmentation [13]. The 2025 BraTS subchallenge on pre- and post-treatment glioma [2,4,5,12] focuses on robust, automated segmentation of both pre- and post-treatment MRI images specifically, from adults diagnosed with diffuse gliomas. Hereby, aiming to create tools for objectively assessing tumor volume for treatment planning on one hand, and post surgical monitoring and outcome prediction on the other hand.

1.1 State of the Art

A well-known challenge for solving medical tasks using a data-driven approach is the scarcity of data. While there are millions of images of natural scenes, medical imaging datasets consist of only hundred or couple of thousand samples. Data augmentation strategies are key for the development of robust and strong performing models, which has been proven in previous editions of the BraTS challenge. In the BraTS 2023 **pre-treatment** adult glioma segmentation challenge, top-performing methods focused on enhancing segmentation precision through architectural innovations and advanced augmentation. The winning team "Faking It" introduced GliGAN, a GAN-based data augmentation framework that inserts realistic synthetic tumors into healthy MRIs using a Swin UNETR-based generator [1]. Other methods employed robust 3D U-Net with attention mechanism [11], and lesion-wise loss function [18] to better capture tumor boundaries and sub-regions. Some achieved competitive results by leveraging model diversity and robust post-processing [10]. The winners of the BraTS 2024 **post-treatment** glioma segmentation challenge were the same team "Faking It", continuing their success by generating massive synthetic data and ensembling diverse architectures trained across multiple folds. Other teams explored ideas, such as generating an additional input image via a linear combination of MRI sequences to emphasize contrast-enhancing tumor regions. This artificial sequence, proposed by Kim [3], improved segmentation accuracy when used alongside the original modalities in ensemble models.

While the winning methods in the BraTS 2023 and 2024 challenges achieved notably higher segmentation scores, particularly through advanced augmentation strategies, model ensembling, and synthetic data generation, several limitations remain.

- Augmentation using registration took around 2 weeks, ensembling multiple models substantially increases computational cost.
- Underrepresented subregions, remain difficult to segment accurately due to low lesion frequency and volume.
- In post-treatment gliomas, the presence of multiple small lesions, often low contrast makes accurate segmentation difficult, contributing to lower Dice scores and higher lesion-level false negatives, particularly for the tumor core.

In this work, we address these challenges by integrating on-the-fly data augmentation into the nnU-Net training pipeline. This approach not only enables the dynamic insertion of synthetic tumors during training but also allows for targeted augmentation—such as adding small lesions or omitting specific tumor classes—to address class imbalance. Furthermore, we ensemble the augmented models with a baseline model to leverage both the diversity introduced through augmentation and the stability of the original training distribution, aiming for a well-balanced and robust segmentation performance.

2 Methods

2.1 Data

The data provided by the BraTS 2025 challenge is acquired over multiple institutions and includes routine pre- and post-treatment multi-parametric MRI (mpMRI) from patients diagnosed with diffuse gliomas resulting in total in 2877 cases. Each case in the dataset has four co-registered mpMRI modalities in NIfTI format: native T1-weighted (t1n), post-contrast T1-weighted (t1ce), T2-weighted (t2w), and T2 FLAIR (t2f). All volumes are isotropically resampled to a resolution of 1 mm^3 with dimensions (182, 218, 182). Corresponding annotations (Fig. 1) consist of four tumor subregions to which we refer as 'Tumor Classes' from now on:

- Non-enhancing tumor core (NETC)- the necrosis and cysts within the tumor
- Surrounding non-enhancing FLAIR hyperintensity (SNFH)- edema, infiltrating tumor, and post-treatment changes

- Enhancing tumor (ET)- regions of active tumor
- Resection cavity (RC) -recent and chronic resection cavities (only in post-treatment scans)

For clinical decision-making, two composite regions are also of importance and are thus also considered for evaluation:

- Tumor core (TC) includes NETC and ET (labels 1 and 3), representing the lesion that is typically removed during surgical resection.
- Whole tumor (WT) includes all abnormal tissue (labels 1, 2, 3), representing the whole extent of the tumor

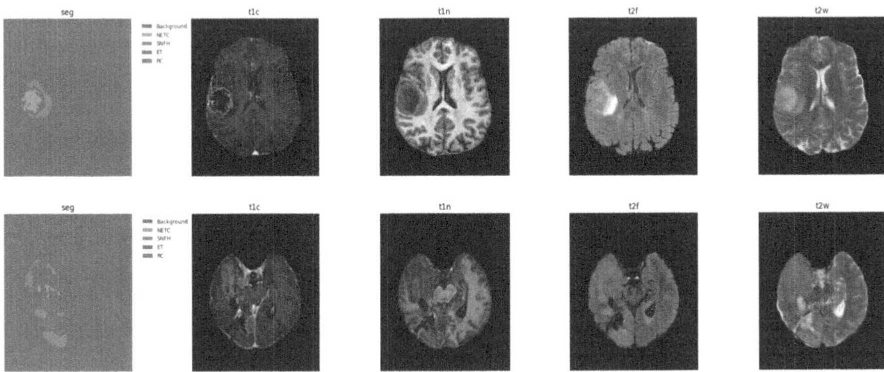

Fig. 1. Central axial slice of pre-treatment scans (upper row) and post-treatment scans (lower row)

The data is divided into a training, validation and test set. The training set includes ~2800 cases (70%), with annotations available for each case. The validation set includes ~400 cases (10%), split into 219 pre-treatment and 188 post-treatment subjects. The ground truth annotations are unavailable for the validation set. The test set comprises ~800 cases (20%), used for final evaluation is unknown.

2.2 Network Architecture

The nnU-Net framework is a self-configuring deep learning framework designed for medical image segmentation. It has been the core engine behind many winning entries in the BraTS challenges over recent years, including both baselines and customized or ensembled solutions [1]. Therefore, we also used the default fully automated nnU-Net framework [16] (3D full resolution), without any configuration changes. The input is random patches of the shape $128 \times 160 \times 112$. Batch size 2, class-based training, and deep supervised.

2.3 On-the-Fly Data Augmentation

For this work, we introduce the concept of on-the-fly data augmentation, hereby using GliGan, the GAN developed by previous winners in 2023 and 2024 [1]. The generator of the conditional GAN takes a modality with added noise in healthy areas (where the synthetic tumor has to be inserted) and a label mask as input. The generator replaces the noisy regions with a synthetic tumor that matches the shape and labels defined in the given label mask. The original work generated over 23,000 synthetic scans using this augmentation strategy applying a mix of randomly generated labels and real labels from other subjects[1].

We extend this approach by incorporating on-the-fly GAN-based data augmentation, leveraging the publicly released pre-trained weights of GliGANs for all modalities[2]. On-the-fly data augmentation refers to the process of applying data transformations dynamically during training, rather than pre-processing and storing augmented data beforehand. These augmentations are performed before the training step for each training batch. The validation data remain unaltered. The following features are added to the existing framework, see Fig. 2:

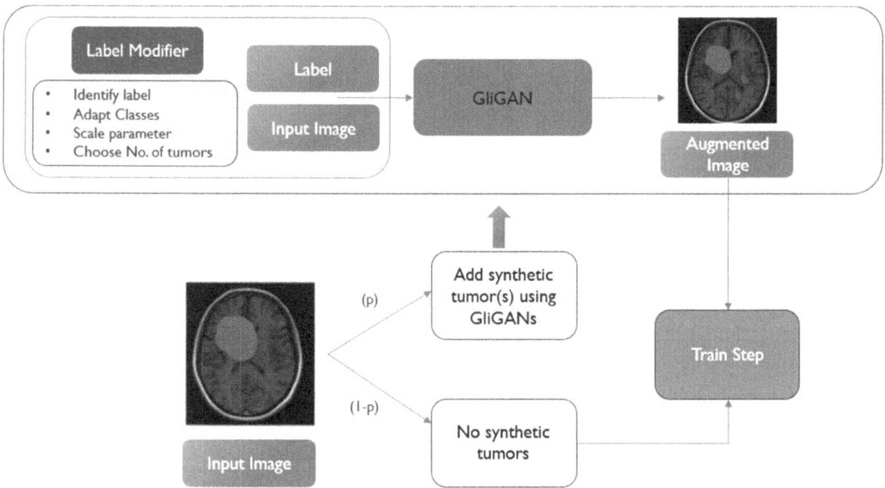

Fig. 2. On-the-fly augmentation framework: It adds synthetic tumor(s) to input image with the given probability p before proceeding to the train-step in nnU-Net training pipeline. The GliGAN uses randomly selected label from other patients and the input image to generate synthetic tumor(s) in healthy parts and returns the augmented image and label. The augmented image is now forwarded to the train step. (1-p) times input images remain unmodified.

[1] BraTS 2023-24 Challenge Winners Solution Github.
[2] GliGAN Pre-trained Weights.

- Instead of generating and storing synthetic data beforehand, our pipeline integrates GliGAN-based augmentation directly into the training loop. During each training step, the image is modified with a given probability p to insert synthetic tumor.
- Taking advantage of the conditional property of GliGAN, we direct the generator by adapting the input label mask, as illustrated in the zoomed-in view of **label modifier** in Fig. 3. First we select a label randomly from the remaining patients' labels, then we use the following parameters to modify them:
  - Adapt Tumor Classes: To handle the tumor class imbalance issue, the tumor class SNFH is replaced with ET, and ET is then replaced with NETC with a probability 0.7. This increases the number of ET and NETC tumor classes in the augmented data.
  - Scale: Since nn-UNet model uses the combination of dice scores and cross entropy loss for training, it tends to underperform on small lesions because, they contribute less to overall loss. Moreover, their features are harder to learn due to size and signal-to-noise ratio. Thus, we add the scale parameter which can be used to make the synthetic lesions smaller by simply scaling down the real label. Based on whether SNFH is present, the scale parameter randomly selects a value within a defined upper and lower bound to adapt the synthetic tumor size. If SNFH is removed, the bounds are (0.1, 0.3) and if not (0.3, 0.8). The chosen scales are less than 1 because the nnU-Net patch size is relatively small than the input image size. Augmenting smaller lesions increases their frequency, giving the model more chances to learn their patterns.
  - Choose Number of synthetic tumors to add: Unlike previous approaches that add only one synthetic tumor, our framework supports inserting up to two synthetic tumors per case. This is achieved by introducing an additional probability (0.4), if triggered, repeats the tumor insertion process. The loop continues until a maximum of two synthetic tumors have been added. Once this limit is reached, the final augmented image and corresponding label are forwarded to the training pipeline. This improves lesion-wise sensitivity and better represent multi-lesion scenarios by introducing controlled diversity, while keeping the number of synthetic tumors within a realistic range.

This allows for flexible control over augmentation parameters, such as the proportion of augmented samples(p), lesion size (through scaling), and number of synthetic tumors per image. Additionally, it significantly reduces storage requirements, as no intermediate augmented data needs to be saved.

2.4 Experiments and Evaluation

We first split the data into training (85%- 2447 cases) and test (15%- 430 cases), to have an internal test set to evaluate the performances of models with different modifications. As a **Baseline Model (1)**, the default nnU-Net framework and hyperparameters is trained using 5 fold cross-validation using the training

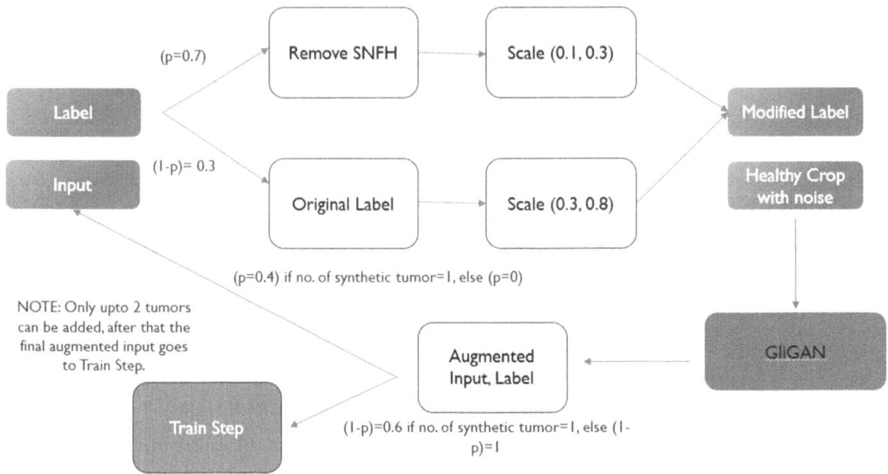

Fig. 3. Label modifier framework: if synthetic tumor probability, a randomly selected label mask is modified by probabilistically removing SNFH, scaling, and adding more synthetic tumor(s).

data without any external data augmentation using GANs. For the **On-the-fly Regular Augmentation Model (2)**, the training step of nnU-Net framework was modified to augment the input by adding synthetic tumors in a regular way with the following parameters:

- The probability to add synthetic tumor in the input image was set to 0.75. Implying 25% input images were not modified.
- If selected to augment, the synthetic tumor would be scaled down to a random value selected between (0.3, 0.8).
- The probability to add the second synthetic tumor was set to 0, implying that only one synthetic tumor is allowed per input.

A 5-fold cross-validation was performed using the training data.

For the **On-the-fly Custom Augmentation Model (3)**, the training step of nnU-Net framework was modified to augment the input by adding synthetic tumors in customized way with the following parameters:

- The probability to add synthetic tumor(s) in the input image was set to 0.6. Implying 40% input images were not modified.
- If selected to augment, the probability to remove SNFH label was set to 0.7. Thus, 70% of the augmented lesions will have only the labels ET, NETC, and RC.
- The probability to add the second synthetic tumor was set to 0.4, implying the probability of the input image to have 2 synthetic tumors is $(0.6 * 0.4 = 0.24)$ 1 synthetic tumor is $(0.6 * 0.6 = 0.36)$, and no synthetic tumor is (0.4).

Due to time constraints, the model was trained once on the full training set instead of performing a 5-fold cross validation. Last, an **Ensemble** strategy was applied to combine predictions from different models. nnU-Net performs voxel-wise averaging of the softmax outputs across all given models. The final prediction is obtained by taking the argmax over the averaged softmax map. This simple yet effective strategy helps improve segmentation performance by leveraging complementary strengths of different models. We tested all possible combinations of ensemble.

- Baseline + On-the-fly Regular Aug (1 + 2)
- Baseline + On-the-fly Custom Aug (1 + 3)
- On-the-fly Regular Aug + On-the-fly Custom Aug (2 + 3)
- Baseline + On-the-fly Regular Aug + On-the-fly Custom Aug (1 + 2 + 3)

Post Processing
Since tumor class RC (Resection Cavity) does not occur in pre-treatment cases, any predictions of RC in these cases were adjusted by setting the predicted probability of RC to zero, and then reassigning the label based on the next highest tumor class probability (i.e., using argmax after modification).

Thresholding
Lesion-wise metrics are used for evaluation, meaning the results are particularly sensitive to false positives (FP), i.e. segmentations of non-existent tumors, and false negatives (FN), i.e. missed tumors. While false negatives are difficult to correct through post-processing, false positives can be reduced by applying a threshold to remove small unusual segmentations. The threshold is defined as the minimum number of voxels a predicted lesion must have to be retained in the final segmentation. In particular, post-treatment cases often contain smaller lesions, necessitating more conservative thresholds based on the number of voxels, compared to pre-treatment cases. Even though this may lead to missing some small lesions in pre-treatment cases, it is a trade-off that significantly reduces false positives. For challenge purposes, we use higher thresholds, but in real-world clinical scenarios, thresholding should be avoided to prevent missing smaller lesions, as experts are better positioned to make informed decisions about lesion significance. The following voxel-based thresholds were tested on the best-performing model:

- **Threshold Set 1:** Common threshold for all cases: WT 200, TC 100, ET 60, RC 70
- **Threshold Set 2:** Different threshold for pre-treatment and post-treatment cases:
  - Pre-treatment threshold- WT 250, TC 150, ET 100
  - Post-treatment threshold WT 200, TC 100, ET 50, RC 80

For evaluation of the above mentioned experiments, the internal test set was used. It allows us to better understand the networks performance and perform smaller ablation studies before submitting anything to the leaderboard platform.

This means for each experiment in this study, we show results for an internal validation set first using Dice Similarity Coefficient (DSC) and lesion wise DSC. In addition, the best performing model(s) are submitted to the leaderboard and their performances on the validation and test sets provided by the challenge are used for final evaluation.
All experiments were conducted on a high-performance compute node equipped with AMD EPYC 7302 16-Core Processors, 515 GB of RAM, NVIDIA A100 GPU (PCIe, 40 GB VRAM).

3 Results

All the models explained in the above section were evaluated on the internal test set using the threshold 'set 1': WT 200, TC 100, ET 60, RC 70. Table 1 shows that the scores for all the models are very similar to each other, which makes direct comparison of models challenging. Each model excels in different tumor classes - for instance, Baseline (1) achieved top performance in RC, SNFH, and WT regions, while On-the-fly Regular (2) performed best in TC, making it difficult to identify a single "best" model through simple visual inspection. Thus, to objectively determine the most balanced and consistently performing model we use the following ranking methodology: We ranked each of the 7 models from 1 (best) to 7 (worst) across all 6 tumor classes based on their lesion dice scores, then calculated average rankings to identify overall performance as seen in Table 2. This systematic approach revealed Ensemble (1 + 3) as the top performer with the lowest average rank of 2.67, demonstrating balanced segmentation across all brain tumor classes.

Table 1. Performance on Internal Test Set Comparison: Legacy and Lesion Dice Scores (Mean ± Std)

Metric	Model	ET	NETC	RC	SNFH	TC	WT
Legacy Dice	Baseline (1)	0.829 ± 0.261	0.809 ± 0.302	0.893 ± 0.236	0.876 ± 0.156	0.843 ± 0.262	0.914 ± 0.129
	On-the-fly Regular (2)	0.829 ± 0.258	0.812 ± 0.294	0.885 ± 0.246	0.877 ± 0.145	0.844 ± 0.259	0.915 ± 0.115
	On-the-fly Custom (3)	0.828 ± 0.256	0.825 ± 0.277	0.889 ± 0.237	0.871 ± 0.147	0.842 ± 0.257	0.912 ± 0.116
	Ensemble (1 + 2)	0.829 ± 0.261	0.813 ± 0.295	0.894 ± 0.234	0.878 ± 0.149	0.845 ± 0.259	0.916 ± 0.120
	Ensemble (1 + 3)	0.833 ± 0.254	0.823 ± 0.283	0.893 ± 0.233	0.877 ± 0.148	0.847 ± 0.254	0.916 ± 0.118
	Ensemble (2 + 3)	0.832 ± 0.254	0.818 ± 0.287	0.889 ± 0.238	0.876 ± 0.146	0.846 ± 0.255	0.915 ± 0.115
	Ensemble (1 + 2 + 3)	0.829 ± 0.260	0.820 ± 0.286	0.894 ± 0.234	0.878 ± 0.147	0.843 ± 0.261	0.916 ± 0.117
Lesion Dice	Baseline (1)	0.812 ± 0.267	0.821 ± 0.288	0.894 ± 0.233	0.818 ± 0.213	0.825 ± 0.267	0.849 ± 0.205
	On-the-fly Regular (2)	0.813 ± 0.264	0.824 ± 0.281	0.883 ± 0.246	0.815 ± 0.206	0.827 ± 0.262	0.846 ± 0.202
	On-the-fly Custom (3)	0.813 ± 0.262	0.830 ± 0.271	0.888 ± 0.236	0.802 ± 0.214	0.821 ± 0.265	0.835 ± 0.208
	Ensemble (1 + 2)	0.812 ± 0.267	0.823 ± 0.283	0.893 ± 0.233	0.817 ± 0.210	0.826 ± 0.266	0.848 ± 0.204
	Ensemble (1 + 3)	0.816 ± 0.262	0.835 ± 0.268	0.892 ± 0.234	0.813 ± 0.213	0.827 ± 0.262	0.843 ± 0.207
	Ensemble (2 + 3)	0.815 ± 0.260	0.831 ± 0.272	0.889 ± 0.237	0.805 ± 0.215	0.826 ± 0.263	0.837 ± 0.209
	Ensemble (1 + 2 + 3)	0.812 ± 0.267	0.833 ± 0.271	0.893 ± 0.233	0.813 ± 0.210	0.822 ± 0.269	0.844 ± 0.204

Table 2. Lesion Dice Performance Rankings (1 = Best, 7 = Worst)

Model	ET	NETC	RC	SNFH	TC	WT	Avg Rank
Baseline (1)	5	7	1	1	5	1	3.33
On-the-fly Regular (2)	3	5	7	3	1	3	3.67
On-the-fly Custom (3)	3	4	6	7	7	7	5.67
Ensemble (1 + 2)	5	6	2	2	3	2	3.33
Ensemble (1 + 3)	**1**	**1**	4	4	**1**	5	**2.67**
Ensemble (2 + 3)	2	3	4	6	3	6	4.0
Ensemble (1 + 2 + 3)	5	2	2	4	6	4	3.83

Table 3 gives an overview of the influence of different thresholds applied to the best performing model on the internal test set, i.e. the Ensemble (1 + 3). Set 0 corresponds to No threshold and 1, 2 correspond to the respective thresholds mentioned thereafter. The performance improved after applying a thresholding step. Table 4 presents the results of paired t-tests conducted between threshold sets. The analysis reveals that both threshold sets 1 and 2 show statistically significant improvements over the no-threshold baseline (set 0), while no significant difference was observed between sets 1 and 2. Based on these findings, we choose to submit both threshold sets for evaluation on the online validation leaderboard.

Table 3. Threshold Analysis of Ensemble (1 + 3) Model on Internal Test Set: Legacy and Lesion Dice Scores

			Thresholds				Dice Scores (mean ± std)					
Metric	**Type**	**Set**	**WT**	**TC**	**ET**	**RC**	**ET**	**NETC**	**RC**	**SNFH**	**TC**	**WT**
Legacy Dice	Pre	0	0	0	0	0	0.809 ± 0.279	0.822 ± 0.283	0.868 ± 0.270	0.877 ± 0.148	0.837 ± 0.267	0.916 ± 0.118
	Post		0	0	0	0						
	Pre	1	200	100	60	70	0.833 ± 0.254	0.823 ± 0.283	0.893 ± 0.233	0.877 ± 0.148	0.847 ± 0.254	0.916 ± 0.118
	Post		200	100	60	70						
	Pre	2	250	150	100	0	0.830 ± 0.258	0.823 ± 0.281	0.892 ± 0.234	0.877 ± 0.148	0.845 ± 0.257	0.916 ± 0.119
	Post		200	100	50	80						
Lesion Dice	Pre	0	0	0	0	0	0.792 ± 0.285	0.834 ± 0.269	0.864 ± 0.273	0.806 ± 0.218	0.819 ± 0.271	0.838 ± 0.211
	Post		0	0	0	0						
	Pre	1	200	100	60	70	0.816 ± 0.262	0.835 ± 0.268	0.892 ± 0.234	0.813 ± 0.213	0.827 ± 0.262	0.843 ± 0.207
	Post		200	100	60	70						
	Pre	2	250	150	100	0	0.811 ± 0.266	0.835 ± 0.268	0.891 ± 0.235	0.813 ± 0.213	0.825 ± 0.264	0.842 ± 0.207
	Post		200	100	50	80						

Challenge Leaderboard. The validation results on the leaderboard for the above models along with the threshold applied can be seen in Table 5. This evaluation is performed online as the participants have no access to the ground-truth. The threshold set 2 performed better on validation set than the threshold set 1, thus threshold set 2, i.e. for pre-treatment cases- WT 250, TC 150, ET 100,

Table 4. Statistical Analysis of Lesion Dice Scores Across Threshold Sets (Paired t-tests)

Comparison	t-statistic	p-value	Significant ($p < 0.05$)
Threshold Set 0 vs 1	−2.6963	0.0430	**Yes**
Threshold Set 1 vs 2	1.9640	0.1067	No
Threshold Set 0 vs 2	−2.5887	0.0489	**Yes**

and for post-treatment cases WT 200, TC 100, ET 50, RC 80 has been applied to all the models. The mean value for lesion-wise metrics is best for the model Ensemble (1 + 2 + 3), although other ensembles reach a similar performance, and hence was submitted for the final test phase. The performance of the model on test set can be seen in Table 6. The submission was ranked first for the given task.

4 Discussion

The BraTS 2025 Challenge âĂŞ Glioma Segmentation on Pre- and Post-treatment MRI (Task 1) aims for multi-class segmentation of multi-modal MRI scans involving four tumor classes: ET, NETC, RC, and SNFH. The evaluation emphasizes lesion-wise performance, using Dice and normalized surface Dice (NSD) metrics.

In this work, we contribute to the challenge by proposing a segmentation pipeline that combines models trained using on-the-fly data augmentation. Our results demonstrate that ensembling models with and without augmentation— can lead to strong and robust lesion-wise performance using the strengths of each models- realism and diversity.

Both performance on internal test set and the validation leaderboard demonstrate that, overall, individual models and their ensembles produce comparable performance metrics, with each model exhibiting strengths for specific tumor classes. For instance, Baseline Model (1) achieves higher scores for the SNFH tumor class, whereas on-the-fly augmentation Models 2 and 3 show relatively better performance in the TC tumor classes. The ensemble models tend to offer intermediate performance, with a balancing and a trade-off effect: while they reduce the number of false positives by resolving spurious detections present in individual models, they can also eliminate rare true positive cases, marginally increasing false negatives. The ensemble 1 + 2 + 3 model performs the best on the lesion-wise scores on the validation platform.

Model 3 (the on-the-fly custom augmentation model) had the lowest lesion-wise Dice rankings among the evaluated models, potentially due to its lack of 5-fold cross-validation during training, which may have limited its robustness. Nevertheless, when Model 3 is combined in an ensemble with the baseline model, this pairing yields the highest overall performance, highlighting the complementary strengths of ensemble learning.

Post-processing with thresholding notably reduces false positives and enhances overall results, which is particularly beneficial in a competitive context such as the challenge; however, this approach is not typically advisable for

Table 5. Performance of Models on Online Validation Platform: Legacy and Lesion Dice Scores

Metric	Method	ET	NETC	RC	SNFH	TC	WT	Mean
Legacy Dice	Baseline(1)	0.799	0.712	0.862	0.869	0.807	0.927	0.829
	On-the-fly Regular Aug(2)	0.801	0.713	0.853	0.868	0.810	0.925	0.828
	On the fly Custom Aug(3)	0.793	0.712	0.870	0.864	0.807	0.924	0.828
	Ensemble (1 + 2)	0.802	0.715	0.862	0.870	0.813	0.927	0.832
	Ensemble (1 + 3)	0.795	0.713	0.859	0.868	0.811	0.927	0.829
	Ensemble (2 + 3)	0.795	0.710	0.866	0.867	0.810	0.926	0.829
	Ensemble (1 + 2 + 3)	0.800	0.717	0.865	0.870	0.812	0.927	0.832
Lesion Dice	Baseline(1)	0.787	0.744	0.866	0.825	0.783	0.878	0.814
	On-the-fly Regular Aug(2)	0.79	0.747	0.857	0.821	0.788	0.875	0.813
	On-the-fly Custom Aug(3)	0.783	0.745	0.878	0.814	0.784	0.871	0.812
	Ensemble (1 + 2)	0.791	0.745	0.866	0.826	0.79	0.879	0.816
	Ensemble (1 + 3)	0.787	0.746	0.867	0.820	0.791	0.875	0.814
	Ensemble (2 + 3)	0.786	0.742	0.874	0.821	0.788	0.876	0.814
	Ensemble (1 + 2 + 3)	0.790	0.749	0.872	0.825	0.790	0.880	0.818
Legacy NSD 1.0	Baseline(1)	0.835	0.733	0.867	0.86	0.784	0.871	0.825
	On-the-fly Regular Aug(2)	0.839 0.739	0.859	0.860	0.789	0.871	0.826	
	On-the-fly Custom Aug(3)	0.829	0.734	0.877	0.856	0.784	0.867	0.824
	Ensemble (1 + 2)	0.839	0.737	0.868	0.862	0.789	0.872	0.828
	Ensemble (1 + 3)	0.832	0.733	0.866	0.860	0.789	0.872	0.825
	Ensemble (2 + 3)	0.833	0.732	0.872	0.860	0.788	0.871	0.826
	Ensemble (1 + 2 + 3)	0.837	0.739	0.871	0.861	0.789	0.872	0.828
Lesion NSD 1.0	Baseline(1)	0.822	0.757	0.871	0.819	0.761	0.828	0.81
	On-the-fly Regular Aug(2)	0.828	0.763	0.861	0.817	0.769	0.827	0.811
	On-the-fly Custom Aug(3)	0.819	0.76	0.883	0.809	0.764	0.821	0.809
	Ensemble (1 + 2)	0.827	0.759	0.872	0.821	0.768	0.830	0.813
	Ensemble (1 + 3)	0.823	0.761	0.872	0.816	0.770	0.826	0.811
	Ensemble (2 + 3)	0.824	0.757	0.878	0.817	0.769	0.827	0.812
	Ensemble (1 + 2 + 3)	0.826	0.762	0.877	0.820	0.769	0.830	0.814

Table 6. Performance of Model Ensemble (1 + 2 + 3) on Test Set

Metric	ET	RC	TC	WT	Mean
Lesion Dice	0.804	0.889	0.800	0.877	0.843
Lesion NSD	0.843	0.889	0.805	0.842	0.845

clinical settings due to the potential risk of missing clinically relevant lesions. Nonetheless, for the challenge setting, thresholding results to significant score improvements.

We can conclude that on-the-fly augmentation contributes to improved robustness and stability when used together with the baseline model in an ensemble. However, the current on-the-fly augmentation pipeline is still in its early stages, and its full impact is difficult to assess due to several limitations:

- None of the models trained reached full convergence at 1000 epochs; they were still improving when training finished. This was due to time constraints of the challenge and the default nn-UNet settings which chose batch size 2, and 1000 epochs. The default nnU-Net configuration is designed to work without expecting external or custom on-the-fly augmentations—its automatic setup assumes only its built-in data augmentation strategies, which are fixed and not dynamically adapted for outside pipelines. As a result, the automatic configuration (including key parameters like patch size, batch size, and max epochs) does not account for additional, on-the-fly augmentations introduced externally. Therefore, to make the best use of our custom on-the-fly augmentation pipeline, we should have optimized these hyperparameters explicitly in the context of this added augmentation, rather than relying on defaults. Training for more epochs or increasing the batch size would allow the models to fully converge, and might better reveal the impact of on-the-fly augmentation.
- The GliGANs used for data augmentation were adopted from the BraTS 2024 winners and were trained specifically on post-treatment gliomas. Using GliGANs trained on a combined dataset—including both pre- and post-treatment cases—could provide more generalizable and effective augmentations.
- Several parts of the on-the-fly augmentation pipeline also still need tuning. For example, parameters such as the probabilities and scales for inserting synthetic tumors were selected at random, and could be optimized further for better results.
- We could add feedback mechanisms during model training, potentially generating synthetic data on the basis of feedback from the segmentation model performance.

Nevertheless, the on-the-fly augmentation approach offers the advantage of reducing both augmentation time and storage needs, while still effectively enhancing the training data with more flexibility.

Acknowledgments. This work has received funding from the Flemish Government under the "Onderzoeksprogramma Artificiele Intelligentie (AI) Vlaanderen" programme.

References

1. Ferreira, A., et al.: How we won BraTS 2023 adult glioma challenge? Just faking it! Enhanced synthetic data augmentation and model ensemble for brain tumour segmentation. arXiv preprint arXiv:2402.17317 (2024). https://github.com/ShadowTwin41/BraTS_2023_2024_solutions
2. de Verdier, M.C., et al.: The 2024 brain tumor segmentation (BraTS) challenge: glioma segmentation on post-treatment MRI, 28 May 2024. https://doi.org/10.48550/arXiv.2405.18368
3. Kim, H.: Effective segmentation of post-treatment gliomas using simple approaches: artificial sequence generation and ensemble models. In: BrainLes Workshop at MICCAI (2024)
4. Baid, U., et al.: The RSNA-ASNR-MICCAI BraTS 2021 benchmark on brain tumor segmentation and radiogenomic classification. arXiv:2107.02314 (2021)
5. Menze, B.H., et al.: The multimodal brain tumor image segmentation benchmark (BRATS). IEEE Trans. Med. Imaging **34**(10), 1993–2024 (2015). https://doi.org/10.1109/TMI.2014.2377694
6. Shorten, C., Khoshgoftaar, T.M.: A survey on image data augmentation for deep learning. J. Big Data **6**(1), 1–48 (2019)
7. Bakas, S., et al.: The BraTS 2023 challenge on brain tumor segmentation: advancing multi-institutional post-treatment glioma analysis. In: MICCAI BrainLes Workshop (2023)
8. Perez, L., Wang, J.: The effectiveness of data augmentation in image classification using deep learning. arXiv preprint arXiv:1712.04621 (2017)
9. Chen, J., et al.: TransUNet: transformers make strong encoders for medical image segmentation. In: Proceedings of MICCAI, pp. 66–76 (2021)
10. Hossain, M.S., Bhuiyan, P., Qureshi, R.U., Khan, M.A.: Advanced tumor segmentation in medical imaging: an ensemble approach for BraTS 2023 adult glioma and pediatric tumor tasks. arXiv preprint arXiv:2310.01887 (2023)
11. Cao, H., et al.: Swin-Unet: Unet-like pure transformer for medical image segmentation. Neurocomputing **522**, 58–66 (2023)
12. Bakas, S., et al.: Advancing the cancer genome atlas glioma MRI collections with expert segmentation labels and radiomic features. Nat. Sci. Data **4**, 170117 (2017). https://doi.org/10.1038/sdata.2017.117
13. Bakas, S., Reyes, M., Jakab, A., et al.: Identifying the best machine learning algorithms for brain tumor segmentation, progression assessment, and overall survival prediction in the BRATS challenge. arXiv preprint arXiv:1811.02629 (2018)
14. Isensee, F., Kickingereder, P., Wick, W., Bendszus, M., Maier-Hein, K.H.: No New-Net. arXiv preprint arXiv:1809.10486 (2018)
15. Kazerouni, A., Vaidya, A., Lin, A.A.: Diffusion models for medical image synthesis: a comprehensive survey. arXiv preprint arXiv:2210.02751 (2022)
16. Isensee, F., Jaeger, P.F., Kohl, S.A.A., Petersen, J., Maier-Hein, K.H.: nnU-Net: a self-configuring method for deep learning-based biomedical image segmentation. Nat. Methods **18**(2), 203–211 (2021). https://doi.org/10.1038/s41592-020-01008-z. https://github.com/MIC-DKFZ/nnUNet
17. Laleh, N.G., Warfield, S.O., et al.: Artificial intelligence for brain tumor segmentation: a review and contributions to BraTS. Brain Tumor Res. Treat. **11**(2), 91–104 (2023). https://doi.org/10.14791/btrt.2023.11.e14
18. Zhao, W., Xu, S., Li, H., Wang, T.: Lesion-wise loss for improving tumor subregion segmentation in MRI. In: Proceedings of MICCAI (2023)

19. LNCS Homepage. http://www.springer.com/lncs. Accessed 25 Oct 2023
20. Jia, H., et al.: Application of convolutional neural networks in medical images: a bibliometric analysis. Quant. Imaging Med. Surg. **14**(5), 3501 (2024)
21. Vaswani, A., et al.: Attention is all you need. In: Advances in Neural Information Processing Systems, vol. 30 (2017)
22. Dosovitskiy, A., et al.: An image is worth 16x16 words: transformers for image recognition at scale. arXiv preprint arXiv:2010.11929 (2020)
23. Karargyris, A., et al.: Federated benchmarking of medical artificial intelligence with MedPerf. Nat. Mach. Intell. **5**, 799–810 (2023). https://doi.org/10.1038/s42256-023-00652-2

Segmentation of Pre- and Post- Operative Glioma Tumors Using Swin UNETR and BraTS-25 Challenge Data

Mohammad Tufail Sheikh[1], Satyajit Maurya[1], and Anup Singh[1,2,3](✉)

[1] Centre for Biomedical Engineering, Indian Institute of Technology Delhi, New Delhi, India
anupsm@iitd.ac.in

[2] Department of Biomedical Engineering, All India Institute of Medical Sciences, New Delhi, India

[3] Yardi School for Artificial Intelligence, Indian Institute of Technology Delhi, New Delhi, India

Abstract. Accurate segmentation of brain tumors is critical for diagnosis, treatment planning, and post-operative assessment. In this study, we present a deep learning-based segmentation framework developed for the BraTS 2025 challenge Task-1, addressing both pre-operative and post-operative brain tumor MRI data. Due to the distinct structural and intensity variations introduced by surgical interventions, including heterogeneous resection cavities, two separate models were trained for pre-operative and post-operative cases. A patch-based training strategy with a patch size of $128 \times 128 \times 128$ was adopted using the Swin UNETR architecture, optimized for resource-constrained environments. Validation on a fixed 20% subset of the training data showed Dice Similarity Coefficients (DSC) of 0.905, 0.926, and 0.929 across enhancing tumor (ET), tumor core (TC) and whole tumor (WT) regions for the pre-operative model, and DSC of 0.764, 0.761, 0.903 and 0.761 across ET, TC, WT, and resection cavity (RC) regions, respectively for the post-operative model. The best-performing model was further evaluated on the unseen validation dataset provided via the Synapse platform, showing a combined DSC of 0.750, 0.761, 0.904, and 0.824, and lesion-wise DSC of 0.724, 0.725, 0.793 and 0.821 across ET, TC, WT, and RC regions, respectively. On the BraTS-GLI test set, the proposed model achieved lesion-wise DSC of 0.746, 0.735, 0.775 and 0.844 across the ET, TC, WT, and RC regions, respectively. Overall, the proposed methodology can automatically and accurately segment brain tumor on pre- as well as post-operative MRI images. The model provided superior performance on pre-operative compared to post-operative MRI images of Glioma patients.

Keywords: Tumor Segmentation · Deep Learning · Glioma · MRI

S. Bakas et al. (Eds.): MICCAI 2025, LNCS 16376, pp. 63–73, 2026.
https://doi.org/10.1007/978-3-032-16365-3_6

1 Introduction

The quality of human life is significantly impacted by the development of tumors, which can arise in various organs such as the lungs, liver, abdomen, and brain. The brain, a critical component of the central nervous system (CNS), is primarily composed of nerve cells (neurons) and supporting glial cells. Tumors originating in the glial cells are termed gliomas, which are among the most common primary brain tumors in adults. A subset of these, known as diffuse gliomas, is characterized by its infiltrative and invasive growth patterns. In adults, such tumors are classified as adult-type diffuse gliomas [1].

Due to the aggressive and infiltrative nature, early and accurate diagnosis of gliomas is crucial to improving treatment planning and patient outcomes. Although biopsy and immunohistochemistry remain the gold standards for definitive diagnosis, these procedures are invasive and not always feasible for repeated assessment. Therefore, non-invasive imaging methods, particularly Magnetic Resonance Imaging (MRI), play a pivotal role in the initial diagnosis, treatment planning, and monitoring of brain tumors. MRI offers excellent soft-tissue contrast and enables the visualization of tumor extent, edema, necrosis, and post-treatment changes. MRI sequences such as T1-weighted, T2-weighted, FLAIR, and contrast-enhanced T1 (T1CE) provide complementary information that aids in characterizing different tumor subregions and distinguishing between tumor progression and treatment effects.

The Brain Tumor Segmentation (BraTS) challenge [6–8] was introduced to advance the development of automated, state-of-the-art segmentation algorithms mainly for brain tumor analysis. Since its initiation, BraTS has facilitated substantial progress in automated methods for the segmentation of brain tumors. Until 2023, the challenge datasets consisted primarily of pre-operative MRI scans. However, starting from BraTS 2024 [9], the organizers have included post-operative multi-sequence MRI scans, allowing for the development of more generalized algorithms that address both pre- and post-operative clinical scenarios. This expansion enhances the potential for early diagnosis and improves treatment planning, longitudinal monitoring, and response assessment. The clinical method for delineating different regions of a brain tumor is a manual process. An experienced radiologist is responsible for segmenting the tumor regions. The accuracy of the segmentation depends heavily on the radiologist's expertise and tends to be subjective, making the process time-consuming. These segmentation masks are used to calculate the volumes of different tumor subregions in both pre-operative and post-operative scans. Moreover, analyses such as extent of resection and residual tumor volume in post-operative scans are strongly correlated with tumor recurrence. Therefore, to reduce the time required for mask generation and minimize subjectivity, there is a pressing need for accurate and automated methods for brain tumor segmentation. Notable contributions include U-Net [2], nnU-Net [3], SegResNet [14] and Swin UNETR [4], which have demonstrated high accuracy, sensitivity, and specificity across various brain tumor segmentation tasks. While these methods perform well on pre-operative MRI scans, segmentation in post-operative scenarios remains challenging, and limited literature is available on brain tumor segmentation in such cases.

Automated methods for brain tumor segmentation have become increasingly essential to support accurate and efficient clinical decision-making. Deep learning (DL) techniques have demonstrated significantly higher accuracy compared to traditional methods. However, for successful integration into clinical workflows, these DL models must be designed to perform accurately in real-time settings while addressing the inherent challenges of delineating different tumor subregions. Therefore, the objective of this study is to develop automatic segmentation methods for brain tumors using DL-based approaches, with a particular focus on post-operative cases. In this study, we develop DL based model for segmentation of both pre- and post- operative brain tumor lesions on multiparametric MRI images.

2 Methods

All training and internal validation experiments were conducted using two NVIDIA A100 GPUs, each with 40 GB of RAM. The implementation was developed using PyTorch Lightning [10] and MONAI [11], which are used in deep learning and medical imaging research. PyTorch Lightning is used to enable the Distributed Data Parallel (DDP) strategy, which facilitates efficient and synchronized multi-GPU training. The competition strategy involved decomposing the segmentation task into two subproblems: one focusing on pre-operative MRI scans and the other on post-operative scans. Accordingly, two separate models were trained independently on the respective cohorts. The methodology for the segmentation task is shown in Fig. 1. The BraTs 25 challenge data provides tags to distinguish between pre-operative and post-operative cases. Tags such as 000

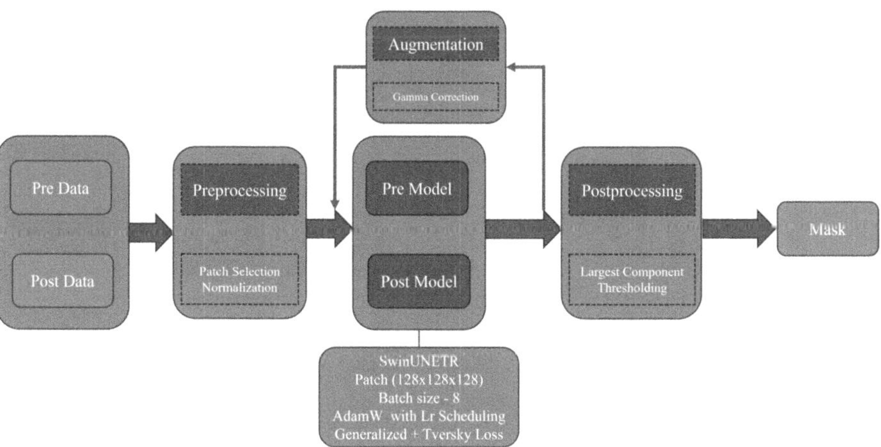

Fig. 1. Methodology

and 001 correspond to pre-operative cases, while tags in the format 10x (100 to 106) correspond to post-operative cases. DL models uses this tag to automatically identify the corresponding data for the individual models.

2.1 Datasets

The dataset is taken from the BraTs 25 competition, Task-1 Pre- and Post-Treatment Adult Glioma. It comprises 1,250 pre-operative and 1,621 post-operative brain MRI scans. Each case includes four standardized MRI sequences: T1-weighted (T1n), post-contrast T1-weighted (T1c), T2-weighted (T2w), and T2-FLAIR (T2f) (Fig. 2). The data have been collected from multiple institutions and are fully anonymized to preserve patient privacy.

The following information is provided in the BraTs challenge [9] regarding the preprocessing steps: "All scans were already preprocessed to ensure uniformity: they are skull-stripped, co-registered to a common Linear Symmetrical MNI Atlas using affine registration, and resampled to isotropic voxel dimensions of 1 mm^3". The ground truth masks are also provided in this challenge. The labels corresponding to ground truth masks are shown in Table 1.

Table 1. Different tumor regions and the corresponding label in both pre-op and post-op datasets

Tumor Region	Label	Scenario
Necrotic tumor core / Non-Enhancing Tumor Core (NETC)	1	Pre/Post
Surrounding Non-enhancing Flair Hyperintense (SNFH)	2	Pre/Post
Enhancing Tumor (ET)	3	Pre/Post
Resection cavity (RC)	4	Post

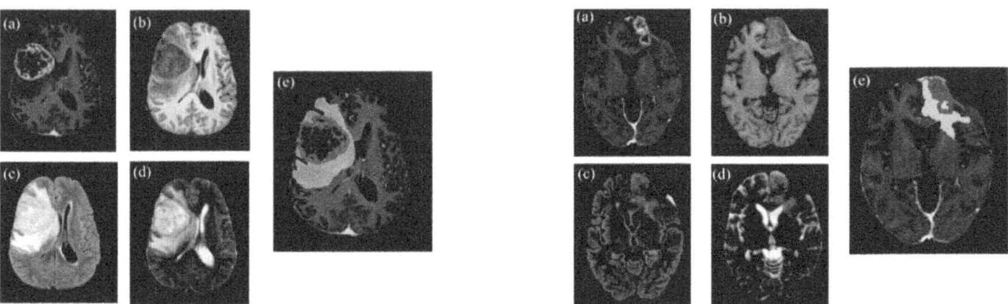

(a) Pre-operative patient (b) Post-operative patient

Fig. 2. Training dataset with given Multiparametric MRI sequences, a, b, c, d, e are T1c, T1n, T2f, T2w, and T1c + labels respectively. Labels - Necrotic region (Red), Enhancing tumor (Blue), Edema (Green), and Resection Cavity (Yellow) (Color figure online)

2.2 PreProcessing

The dataset contains scans of volumes of size $128 \times 128 \times 128$. As the size of the input volume is too large to be included in training, a patch-based approach is adopted to reduce computation. The patch-based training strategy was employed for both pre-operative and post-operative pipelines. The following patch sizes were evaluated empirically: ($64 \times 64 \times 64$, $96 \times 96 \times 96$, and $128 \times 128 \times 128$). Patches were extracted using the RandCropByPosNegLabel sampling transform from the MONAI library, configured with a positive-to-negative ratio of 1:0.2. This ensured that each sampled patch contained tumor regions with a probability of 1 out of 1.2, effectively increasing the likelihood that the network's receptive field captured relevant pathological features during training.

All image intensities were normalized using z-score normalization per volume, computed individually for each modality. This normalization ensured that intensity values had zero mean and unit variance, aiding in model convergence and stability during training. The same preprocessing pipeline was applied uniformly to both pre-operative and post-operative datasets. The z-score normalization is given by: $z = \frac{x-\mu}{\sigma}$ where μ and σ are mean and standard deviation, respectively.

2.3 Data Augmentation

To improve the model's generalization capability, gamma correction-based enhancement was applied to each of the four MRI sequences independently. For every training sample, a random gamma value between 0.8 and 1.2 was used to simulate variations in image brightness and contrast. This augmentation strategy was motivated by the observation that the dataset contained considerable intensity variability across scans.

Initially, the model was trained on the original (without augmentation) dataset. Following this, gamma-augmented versions of the dataset were used to fine-tune the model, helping it adapt to diverse intensity distributions and improving robustness to real-world imaging variability.

2.4 Deep Learning Architectures and Training Parameters

Several deep learning architectures based on the U-Net backbone were considered, like U-Net, SegResNet, and Swin UNETR. After comparative evaluation, the final model selected was Swin UNETR, a transformer-based architecture that has demonstrated superior performance over traditional convolutional neural network (CNN)-based U-Net models for medical image segmentation tasks [4].

The Swin UNETR model was configured with a feature size of 48 for both the pre-operative and post-operative segmentation pipelines. Same model parameters as given in the official Swin UNETR paper [4] were used. Each model received four input channels corresponding to the four MRI sequences (T1, T1c, T2, and FLAIR). The number of output channels was set to 3 for the pre-operative model and 4 for the post-operative model, corresponding to the annotated segmentation subregions.

The segmentation problem was formulated as a multi-label segmentation task by using a sigmoid function at the output channel to generate the likelihood probability for each pixel for the particular label, which enables the model to detect multiple overlapping regions within the tumor volume.

Training was conducted using the AdamW [12] optimizer with an initial learning rate of 1×10^{-4} with weight decay of 1×10^{-5}, and the learning rate was scheduled using a cosine annealing scheduler. The random seed of 42 was used for reproducibility. The loss function used was the Generalized Dice Focal Loss, with $\gamma = 4$, which helped address class imbalance and improved sensitivity to small structures, and the Tversky Loss [13] with $\alpha = 0.3$, $\beta = 0.7$ for penalizing the false negatives. The model was trained for 900 epochs using a batch size of 8, made feasible through DDP training across two NVIDIA A100 GPUs.

For inference, the sliding window technique (sliding_window_inference) provided by MONAI was used. A window size of $128 \times 128 \times 128$ with an overlap of 0.25 was applied. The predictions in overlapping regions were blended using 'constant' mode, ensuring smooth and stable segmentation outputs across patch boundaries.

2.5 Validation Strategy

The challenge provided an unseen validation set for final evaluation through the Synapse platform. However, during model development, a fixed internal validation split was created from the training subset to monitor training progress and guide model selection. For both the pre-operative and post-operative datasets, 80% of the training data was used for model training, and the remaining 20% was reserved for internal validation.

The model achieving the highest Dice Similarity Coefficient (DSC) on the internal validation set was selected as the best-performing model. The best model was then evaluated on the unseen validation set provided by the challenge. The performance on the unseen validation set, provided via the Synapse platform, was evaluated using the metrics, which include Lesion-wise Dice [7], standard Dice score, and Hausdorff Distance 95. These reflect generalization performance beyond the fixed validation split. The best validation scores obtained from the internal validation set and the unseen validation set are reported in the results section.

2.6 Postprocessing

Postprocessing steps were employed to improve the segmentation quality and reduce false positives. Specifically, the predicted TC and ET regions were masked by the predicted WT to ensure anatomical consistency, since both TC and ET are subregions of WT. Only the overlapping regions between TC/ET and WT were retained.

To further suppress spurious predictions, connected component analysis was performed independently on the TC, ET, and Resection RC predictions. Additionally, a voxel count threshold of 50 was applied on TC, ET and RC to remove small isolated predictions, which were likely to be false positives. This threshold was inspired by strategies adopted by top-performing teams in the BraTS 2024 challenge [5].

3 Results

The results of internal validation and unseen external validation for both pre-operative and post-operative segmentation tasks are summarized in Table 2 and Table 3, respectively. These scores represent DSC computed across relevant tumor subregions: TC, WT, ET, and RC (only in post-op). On a patch-based training strategy, the best performance was observed using $128 \times 128 \times 128$ patches, which offered a good balance between contextual information and GPU memory constraints. Table 4 shows the results of the proposed model on the BraTS-GLI test dataset. The metrics used to evaluate the submissions are Lesion-wise DSC and Lesion-wise Normalised Surface Distance (NSD).

To further analyze performance over epochs, Fig. 3 shows the Validation dice scores for individual tumor subregions and the overall mean dice score during training.

Table 2. Internal validation Dice scores for segmentation of brain tumor regions in pre-operative and post-operative MRI data of Glioma patients. ET: Enhancing Tumor; TC: Tumor Core, RC: Resection Cavity; WT: Whole Tumor.

	ET	TC	WT	RC
Pre	0.905	0.9263	0.9293	-
Post	0.764	0.761	0.9025	0.7614

Table 3. Evaluation metrics on unseen Synapse validation dataset. NETC: Non-Enhancing Tumor Core; ET: Enhancing Tumor; TC: Tumor Core, RC: Resection Cavity; SNFH: Surrounding Non-enhancing Flair Hyperintense; WT: Whole Tumor.

Metric	NETC	ET	TC	RC	SNFH	WT
Lesion-wise Dice	0.7106	0.7242	0.7253	0.8209	0.7362	0.7925
Dice	0.6776	0.7496	0.7613	0.8240	0.8349	0.9036
Hausdorff distance 95	39.4743	26.9449	21.1237	26.6858	8.6108	7.1025

Table 4. Evaluation metrics on BraTS-GLI test dataset. ET: Enhancing Tumor; TC: Tumor Core, RC: Resection Cavity; WT: Whole Tumor.

Metric	ET	TC	RC	WT
Lesion-wise Dice	0.7457 ± 0.2985	0.7351 ± 0.3218	0.8437 ± 0.2923	0.7750 ± 0.2521
Lesion-wise NSD	0.7861 ± 0.2914	0.7303 ± 0.3054	0.8333 ± 0.2895	0.7211 ± 0.2465

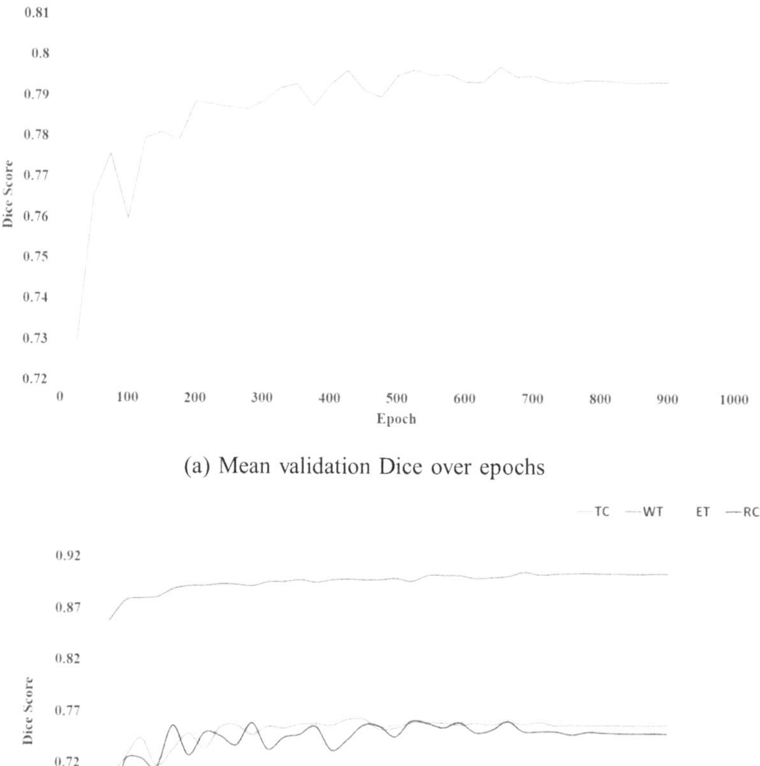

(a) Mean validation Dice over epochs

(b) Per-label Dice on validation data. ET: Enhancing Tumor; TC: Tumor Core, RC: Resection Cavity; WT: Whole Tumor.

Fig. 3. Validation performance of the model on the internal 20% validation split

4 Discussion

The DL model demonstrated promising performance in automating the segmentation of various brain tumor sub-regions in both pre-operative and post-operative scenarios. We adopted separate models for pre- and post-operative cases depending on the tag information provided with the scans. The decision was primarily motivated by the heterogeneous nature of the residual cavity, a key component in post-operative data, which can present highly variable intensity characteristics. For instance, cavities filled with air exhibit distinctly different signal properties compared to those filled with blood or other postoperative residues. These variations can visually mimic tumor regions and make segmentation more challenging.

In the current study, the training strategy followed a patch-based approach, designed to accommodate resource-constrained environments. Initially, a patch size of $64 \times 64 \times 64$ was employed; however, the accuracy was suboptimal. A larger patch size of $128 \times 128 \times 128$ provided improved contextual information and yielded better segmentation results. The model was trained for 900 epochs using sliding window inference with an overlap of 0.25 and constant padding mode, as implemented in MONAI's sliding window inference technique.

The proposed model was extensively validated on an internal validation split (from the training data) and on an unseen validation set provided by the organizers via the Synapse platform. As reported in the results, the model achieved strong internal validation metrics across tumor sub-regions. However, the unseen validation set revealed certain challenges. The performance degradation on unseen data was primarily attributed to false negatives (missed tumor regions) and some false positives, particularly in post-operative cases. In these cases, tumor regions—mainly the non-enhancing (necrotic) tumor core and resection cavity—were challenging to delineate due to their similar appearance on T2-weighted MRI scans. Conversely, cases in which the tumor regions were more distinctly visible were segmented with higher accuracy by the proposed model. On the unseen validation set, the whole tumor region achieved the highest accuracy among all subregions, with a standard Dice Similarity Coefficient (DSC) of 0.904, while the non-enhancing (necrotic) tumor core had the lowest accuracy with a DSC of 0.678. Although the standard DSC values were relatively high, lesion-wise DSC scores indicated that some smaller lesions were missed in each region, leading to lower scores. But in the necrotic subregion, the lesion-wise Dice score was higher than the standard DSC, which indicates that the model performed well on individual, isolated necrotic sub-tumor lesions.

To address the issue of false negatives, we incorporated a hybrid loss function comprising Generalized Dice Focal Loss and Tversky Loss, with the latter focusing more on penalizing false negatives. This combination was selected to improve the sensitivity of the model, especially for smaller or ambiguous tumor components. For false positive reduction, a robust post-processing pipeline was employed. This included taking only those predicted TC and ET regions that intersected with the WT, under the assumption that these sub-regions should be anatomically contained within the WT. Furthermore, a largest connected component analysis was performed independently for TC, ET, and RC predictions, followed by a size thresholding step of 50 voxels, an approach inspired by winning solutions from the previous BraTS challenge.

Although the model has automated tumor delineation and has shown reliable generalization capabilities despite computational constraints, the validation results indicate the need for further optimization to achieve greater accuracy, as the current performance is not sufficient for clinical deployment. While performance on the internal validation set was higher, the performance on the external unseen validation set highlights the inability of the model to distinguish different tumor regions from the resection cavity in complex post-operative cases. Therefore, future work will involve the application of more data augmentation techniques for better generalizability, incorporating uncertainty estimation or ensemble strategies to further enhance model reliability across diverse patient populations. Furthermore, the use of more novel and complex models, such as those based on generative modeling, is essential to better capture real-world clinical scenarios.

In conclusion, this study developed a deep learning (DL)-based framework for the automatic segmentation of brain tumors in both pre-operative and post-operative scenarios. The proposed model, Swin UNETR, demonstrated the ability to automatically delineate different tumor subregions.

Acknowledgments. The authors gratefully acknowledge the HPC facility of Indian Institute of Technology Delhi for providing the computational infrastructure and resources that supported this research. This work was supported by the Indian Council of Medical Research (ICMR) under the project Centre for Advanced Research in Quantitative Imaging and AI Modeling for Early Diagnostics and Prognostic Monitoring in Oncology (Project No. CAR-2024-01-000187). The authors also thank the organizers of the BraTS Challenge for making the dataset available to the research community.

Disclosure of Interests. The authors declare that they have no competing interests.

References

1. Louis, D.N., et al.: The 2021 WHO classification of tumors of the central nervous system: a summary. Neuro-Oncol. **23**(8), 1231–1251 (2021)
2. Ronneberger, O., Fischer, P., Brox, T.: U-Net: convolutional networks for biomedical image segmentation. In: Navab, N., Hornegger, J., Wells, W.M., Frangi, A.F. (eds.) MICCAI 2015. LNCS, vol. 9351, pp. 234–241. Springer, Cham (2015). https://doi.org/10.1007/978-3-319-24574-4_28
3. Isensee, F., Jaeger, P.F., Kohl, S.A.A., et al.: nnU-Net: a self-configuring method for deep learning-based biomedical image segmentation. Nat. Methods **18**, 203–211 (2021). https://doi.org/10.1038/s41592-020-01008-z
4. Tang, Y., et al.: Self-supervised pre-training of swin transformers for 3D medical image analysis. In: Proceedings of the IEEE/CVF Conference on Computer Vision and Pattern Recognition, pp. 20730–20740 (2022)
5. Ferreira, A., Jesus, T., Puladi, B., Kleesiek, J., Alves, V., Egger, J.: Improved multi-task brain tumour segmentation with synthetic data augmentation (2024). ArXiv. https://arxiv.org/abs/2411.04632
6. Baid, U., et al.: The RSNA-ASNR-MICCAI BraTS 2021 benchmark on brain tumor segmentation and radiogenomic classification. arXiv:2107.02314 (2021)
7. Menze, B.H., et al.: The multimodal brain tumor image segmentation benchmark (BRATS). IEEE Trans. Med. Imaging **34**(10), 1993–2024 (2015). https://doi.org/10.1109/TMI.2014.2377694
8. Bakas, S., et al.: Advancing the cancer genome atlas glioma MRI collections with expert segmentation labels and radiomic features. Nat. Sci. Data **4**, 170117 (2017). https://doi.org/10.1038/sdata.2017.117

9. De Verdier, M.C., et al.: The 2024 brain tumor segmentation (BraTS) challenge: glioma segmentation on post-treatment MRI. arXiv preprint arXiv:2405.18368 (2024)
10. Falcon, W., et al.: PyTorchLightning/pytorch-lightning: 0.7.6 Release. 0.7.6, Zenodo, 15 May 2020. https://doi.org/10.5281/zenodo.3828935
11. Cardoso, M.J., et al.: MONAI: an open-source framework for deep learning in healthcare. arXiv preprint arXiv:2211.02701 (2022)
12. Loshchilov, I., Hutter, F.: Decoupled weight decay regularization (2017). ArXiv https://arxiv.org/abs/1711.05101. Accessed 30 July 2025
13. Salehi, S.S., et al.: Tversky loss function for image segmentation using 3D fully convolutional deep networks (2017). ArXiv https://arxiv.org/abs/1706.05721. Accessed 30 July 2025
14. Myronenko, A.: 3D MRI brain tumor segmentation using autoencoder regularization (2018). ArXiv https://arxiv.org/abs/1810.11654. Accessed 31 July 2025
15. Bakas, S., et al.: Segmentation labels and radiomic features for the pre-operative scans of the TCGA-GBM collection. Cancer Imaging Arch. (2017). https://doi.org/10.7937/K9/TCIA.2017.KLXWJJ1Q
16. Bakas, S., et al.: Segmentation labels and radiomic features for the pre-operative scans of the TCGA-LGG collection. Cancer Imaging Arch. (2017). https://doi.org/10.7937/K9/TCIA.2017.GJQ7R0EF

Enhancing Tumor Subregion Segmentation Using Domain Adaptation, Pseudo-Labeling, and Post-Processing Optimization

Ajesh Saviour Paravila(✉)

National Dong Hwa University, Hualien, Taiwan
ajesh.saviour@gmail.com

Abstract. Accurate segmentation of glioma subregions in brain MRI remains a critical challenge due to high inter-subject variability and complex tumor morphology. In our submission to the BraTS 2025 challenge, we develop a pipeline based on nnU-Net, enhanced with domain adaptation, pseudo-labeling, and custom post-processing. Our method focuses on addressing distributional shifts across modalities and scanners, while improving lesion consistency through connected component filtering. The approach demonstrates moderate performance on the validation set, with strong lesion-wise Dice scores. Ongoing improvements include the integration of boundary-aware loss functions and surface-based loss functions to mitigate residual segmentation artifacts, particularly along tumor borders.

To make the process more accessible and reproducible, we focus on optimizing the pipeline for consumer-level hardware. The segmentation is performed in 2D configuration, which reduces computational overhead, making it more feasible for users with limited resources. However, while the current approach is lightweight, ongoing improvements, including the integration of boundary-aware loss functions and surface-based loss functions, are being made to address residual segmentation artifacts along tumor borders. These enhancements involve more computationally intensive tasks like Distance transform maps (DTM) calculation, which can require significant computation time, but are critical for further refinement of the segmentation accuracy and convergence.

Keywords: Brain tumor segmentation · nnU-Net · Domain adaptation · Pseudo-labeling · Distance transform maps · Boundary loss

1 Introduction

Gliomas are among the most aggressive forms of brain tumors, presenting a wide range of morphological and structural variability across patients [7]. Accurate automated segmentation of glioma subregions in multi-parametric MRI is an essential step for personalized treatment planning and longitudinal assessment [8]. The Brain Tumor Segmentation (BraTS) challenge provides a standardized platform to evaluate automated methods on multi-institutional data with annotated tumor subregions [1–6].

S. Bakas et al. (Eds.): MICCAI 2025, LNCS 16376, pp. 74–84, 2026.
https://doi.org/10.1007/978-3-032-16365-3_7

In the field of medical image segmentation, nnU-Net [9, 10] has become a widely recognized framework due to its strong performance in various segmentation challenges, including previous BraTS competitions [11]. Developed by the winners of MICCAI 2018 ISLES Challenge, nnU-Net provides an easy-to-use pipeline with powerful preprocessing tools and several configuration options such as 2D, 3D, 3D low-resolution, and 3D full-resolution architectures. This flexibility, combined with robust cross-validation capabilities (single-fold or multi-fold), makes nnU-Net an ideal choice for developing baseline models, especially when working with new and diverse datasets. Its strong out-of-the-box performance, alongside its automated preprocessing and network configuration options, make it a perfect starting point for addressing medical image segmentation tasks.

However, despite its strengths, nnU-Net is not without its challenges. While it excels in providing a solid foundation, generalizing across imaging centers and scanner protocols remains a significant hurdle due to domain shifts and intensity non-uniformity. In particular, precise delineation of tumor boundaries—especially for the enhancing tumor and tumor core—can still be inconsistent.

In our submission to BraTS 2025, we aim to address these issues by leveraging domain adaptation and pseudo-labeling [12] to improve generalization across different domains. Additionally, we introduce a robust post-processing pipeline to clean spurious predictions and small disconnected regions. Initial results indicate that the model performs well on large lesions, but boundary inconsistencies persist in smaller subregions. To tackle this, we plan to integrate boundary loss and generalized surface loss into our training framework before final submission. Our goal is to strike a balance between accuracy, robustness, and computational efficiency while addressing the challenges of domain adaptation.

2 Methods

Our approach to the BraTS 2025 Tumor Subregion Segmentation task extends the standard nnU-Net framework with domain adaptation, uncertainty-aware pseudo-labeling, and conservative post-processing optimizations. The complete pipeline is illustrated in Fig. 1.

2.1 Data and Preprocessing

We We utilized the multi-parametric MRI dataset provided by the BraTS 2025 challenge organizers, comprising both pre-treatment and post-treatment scans with four modalities (T1, T1Gd, T2, FLAIR) and corresponding expert annotations for five classes: background (0), non-enhancing tumor core/NETC (1), surrounding non-enhancing FLAIR hyperintensity/SNFH (2), enhancing tumor/ET (3), and resection cavity/RC (4). Following nnU-Net's default protocol, we employed 5-fold cross-validation at the patient level, with 80% of subjects used for training and 20% for validation in each fold.

Data Preprocessing: Standard nnU-Net preprocessing was applied including z-score normalization per modality, resampling to isotropic resolution, and data augmentation (random rotations, flips, elastic deformations, gamma transformations).

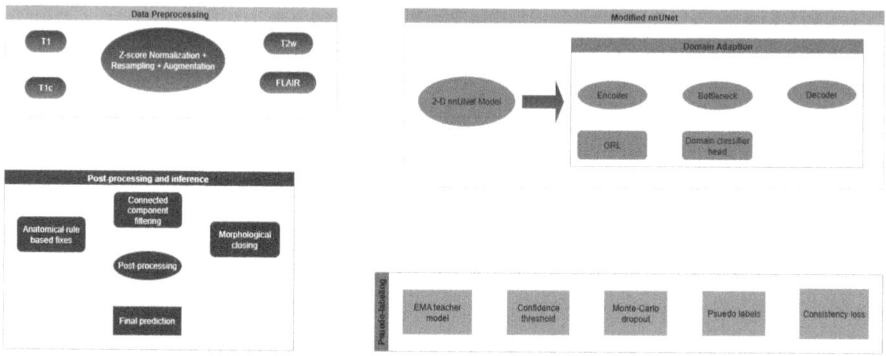

Fig. 1. Overview of the Tumor Subregion Segmentation Pipeline

2.2 Network Architecture

The nnU-Net network consists of an encoder-decoder design with skip connections, residual units, and deep supervision on intermediate decoder layers. This architecture provides a strong baseline for medical image segmentation without extensive manual tuning. No additional attention modules were added in the initial submission to ensure stable training.

2.3 Training Strategy

Domain Adaption
To address the significant domain shift between pre-treatment and post-treatment scans in the BraTS 2025 dataset due to the presence of label 4 (RC cavity), we employ a domain adversarial training approach based on gradient reversal. The approach incorporates the following components:

Architecture Modification

- **Domain Classifier Head**: A domain classifier head is added to the encoder of nnU-Net, consisting of a simple 3-layer convolutional neural network (CNN) with adaptive pooling. This classifier distinguishes between source and target domains.
- **Gradient Reversal Layer (GRL)**: The GRL applies adversarial training with coefficient λ scheduled linearly from 0 to 0.05 over the first 50 epochs, encouraging domain-invariant feature learning while maintaining segmentation performance.
- **Feature Alignment**: Feature alignment occurs at the bottleneck layer of the nnU-Net encoder with 512 channels, ensuring domain-invariant features are learned at the critical stage of the network.

Domain Labeling Strategy
In the domain adversarial setup, it is essential to differentiate between the pre-treatment and post-treatment scans. Therefore, we implement the following domain labeling strategy to facilitate supervised domain adaptation:

- **Source Domain** (pre-treatment scans) is labeled as **0**.

- **Target Domain** (post-treatment scans) is labeled as **1**.

These domain labels are automatically assigned based on the DICOM metadata and filenames, allowing the model to learn the domain-specific features that need to be adapted during training.

Training Protocol

In order to enhance model generalization across both pre-treatment and post-treatment scans, we train the baseline model on a **mixed dataset** that includes both domains simultaneously. This hybrid approach allows the model to learn from both the source and target domains concurrently, which is crucial for improving robustness to domain shifts.

- **Joint Optimization**: The model is optimized with the following losses:
  - **Segmentation Loss**: A combination of Dice and Cross-Entropy loss applied to labeled data from both the source and target domains.
  - **Domain Adversarial Loss**: A cross-entropy loss via GRL that encourages the model to learn domain-invariant features.
  - **Pseudo-Label Consistency Loss**: A regularization term based on pseudo-labels from the target domain, generated through uncertainty-aware methods.

Uncertainty-Aware Pseudo-Labeling for Target Domain

After 80 epochs of warm-up training, we activate pseudo-labeling targeting underperforming tumor classes (labels 1 and 3):

Pseudo-Label Generation.

- **Exponential Moving Average (EMA)**: An Exponential Moving Average (EMA) teacher model ($\alpha = 0.999$) generates pseudo-labels on validation data. Only voxels with prediction confidence exceeding $\tau = 0.75$ for ET and SNFH (tumor labels 1,3) are retained, as these classes showed lower baseline Dice scores.
- **Confidence Thresholding**: Pseudo-labels are generated for voxels where the model's confidence exceeds a threshold ($p > 0.85$). Specifically, we focus on tumor regions (labels 1 and 3) due to their underperformance in the baseline model, which exhibited lower Dice scores and higher variance in these areas. By concentrating on these challenging regions, we aim to improve segmentation accuracy where the model struggled in the initial training phase.
- Consistency Loss: The consistency loss between teacher pseudo-labels and student predictions is defined as:

$$L_{cons} = \frac{1}{N} \sum_{i=1}^{N} \|p_i - \tilde{p}_i\|_2^2 \tag{1}$$

where p_i represents student softmax predictions and $\tilde{p}_i$ are teacher pseudo-probabilities for confident voxels.

Uncertainty Estimation.

We use Monte Carlo dropout (5 runs) to estimate uncertainty in the pseudo-labels. Voxels with uncertainty greater than 0.1 bits are rejected, and only mutually confident regions across all runs are kept.

Curriculum Integration

A warmup period of 100 epochs is implemented before pseudo-labeling is enabled. The confidence threshold for pseudo-labeling is progressively lowered from p > 0.9 in the initial epochs to $p > 0.8$ in later epochs. A batch-wise mixing ratio of 1 labeled:1 pseudo-labeled data is used to balance the influence of labeled and pseudo-labeled data during training. To stabilize training and accelerate the convergence rate, the domain-adapted model with pseudo-labeling was initialized using the baseline nnU-Net model weights trained for 1000 epochs. This warm-start approach leveraged robust feature representations from the source domain and improved the stability of adversarial and pseudo-label loss optimization compared to training from scratch.

Loss Function Components.

The primary loss function used during training combines segmentation and domain adversarial losses:

- **Primary Loss**: The primary loss is a weighted sum of the Dice loss and Cross-Entropy loss.

$$\textit{Primary loss} = 0.5L_{DC} + 0.5L_{CE} \tag{2}$$

- **Pseudo-label Loss Weight**:

$$\lambda_{psuedo} = 0.1 * \left(\frac{currentepoch}{totalepochs}\right) \tag{3}$$

- **Domain Adversarial Loss Weight**:

$$\lambda_{domain} = \min\left(0.01, 0.05 * \left(\frac{currentepoch}{totalepochs}\right)\right) \tag{4}$$

Inference and Post-Processing

Inference is performed using nnU-Net's sliding-window approach with overlap-tile strategy to manage memory and reduce edge artifacts. Predictions from different orientations are ensembled for robustness.

Post-processing focuses on improving lesion consistency and removing spurious detections:

- **Connected component analysis (CC3D):** Conservative filtering removes isolated components smaller than label-specific thresholds: NETC < 5 voxels, SNFH < 10 voxels, ET < 3 voxels, RC < 5 voxels. These minimal thresholds preserve genuine small lesions while removing obvious artifacts.

- **Anatomical Plausibility Rules:** A rule-based system applies domain knowledge constraints. For example, if predicted enhancing tumor overlaps > 10 voxels with ventricular regions (derived from anatomical atlases), it is reclassified as edema to maintain biological plausibility.
- Gentle Morphological Operations: Optional binary closing with 3D structural elements (connectivity $= 6$, iterations $= 1$) fills small holes within tumor regions without overwriting other labels.

This step improves lesion-wise Dice scores, particularly for small and irregular tumors.

Implementation Details

Our experiments were conducted using PyTorch 2.7.1 on an NVIDIA GeForce RTX 3090 GPU (32 GB VRAM). Training was performed for 1000 epochs with a batch size of 16 and mixed precision enabled. Optimizer settings followed nnU-Net defaults with a poly learning rate schedule. Inference for a single case takes approximately 2 min, including post-processing. The full pipeline including the scripts for domain adaption and pseudo labeling is open sourced at: https://github.com/zephyr-9598/BraTS-2025.git.

3 Results

Our model was first evaluated on the BraTS 2025 training set using five-fold cross-validation and then submitted to the official validation server for blind evaluation. Performance was assessed using Dice Similarity Coefficient (DSC) and Normalized Surface Distance (NSD) at 0.5 mm and 1.0 mm tolerances, following the BraTS guidelines.

- Dice Similarity Coefficient (DSC) measures the overlap between the predicted segmentation and the ground truth, which indicates how well the model is able to capture the tumor regions.
- Normalized Surface Distance (NSD) measures the average distance between the predicted segmentation and ground truth, normalized by the surface area, giving an indication of boundary accuracy.

3.1 Internal Evaluation

During training, we monitored per-class Dice and NSD using our internal evaluation script. Table 1 and Table 2 summarizes the mean and median DSC and NSD for the training set across all tumor subregions for the baseline model and the domain-adapted model respectively.

Additionally, Figs. 2 shows the training curves for the domain-adapted models, highlighting convergence patterns and the performance gains. Representative segmentation examples are shown in Fig. 3, which illustrate both successful predictions and residual boundary inaccuracies. These challenging cases motivated the integration of boundary-aware loss functions to improve contour alignment.

These results indicate that the model performs well on the training data, with the **RC** and **SNFH** regions showing the highest Dice scores. However, the large standard deviations for NETC and ET regions suggest variability in boundary accuracy, which motivated the exploration of boundary-aware loss functions.

Table 1. Segmentation performance on training data using the baseline nnU-Net model

Label	Mean Dice	Median Dice	Mean NSD	Median NSD
NETC (1)	0.8589 (0.2554)	0.9609	0.8974 (0.2312)	0.9848
SNFH (2)	0.9130 (0.0818)	0.9352	0.9296 (0.0737)	0.9490
ET (3)	0.8616 (0.2301)	0.9398	0.9072 (0.2221)	0.9762
RC (4)	0.9307 (0.1737)	1.0000	0.9463 (0.1623)	1.000
NETC + ET	0.8836 (0.2183)	0.9581	0.9060 (0.2063)	0.9680
NETC + SNFH + ET	0.9397 (0.0589)	0.9560	0.9324 (0.0646)	09501

Table 2. Segmentation performance on training data using the complete proposed pipeline

Label	Mean Dice	Median Dice	Mean NSD	Median NSD
NETC (1)	0.8796 (0.2306)	0.9663	0.9154 (0.2084)	0.9890
SNFH (2)	0.9187 (0.0772)	0.9395	0.9374 (0.0689)	0.9459
ET (3)	0.8744 (0.2161)	0.9446	0.9198 (0.2076)	0.9808
RC (4)	0.9463 (0.1376)	1.0000	0.9625 (0.1247)	1.000
NETC + ET	0.8932 (0.2070)	0.9612	0.9168 (0.1957)	0.9730
NETC + SNFH + ET	0.9437 (0.0549)	0.9587	0.9399 (0.0581)	09561

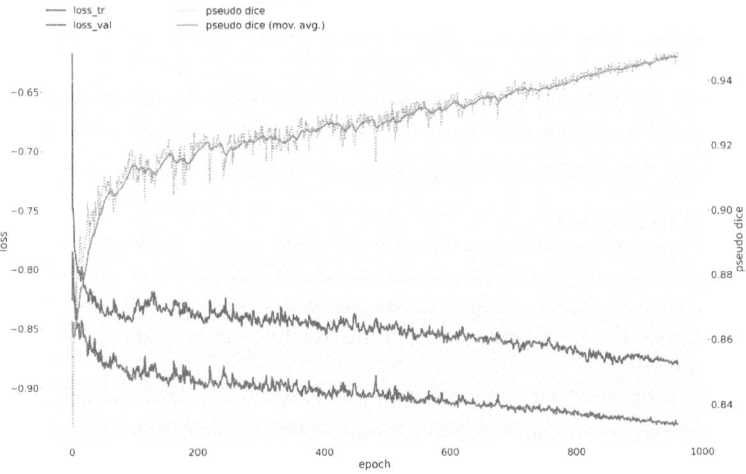

Fig. 2. The figure shows the Dice score progression over 1000 epochs for the domain adapted model.

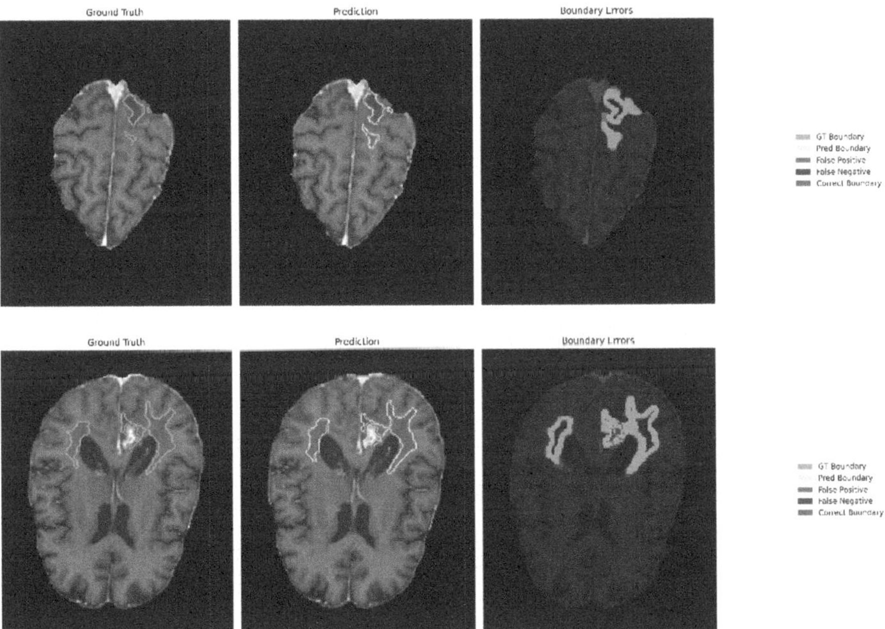

Fig. 3. The figure shows representative cases: a well-segmented example (above) and a challenging case (below) where boundary errors persist.

3.2 BraTS 2025 Evaluation Metrics

We submitted our best model with post-processing to the official BraTS 2025 submission server. Table 3 summarizes the lesion-wise Dice and NSD scores for each tumor subregion and composite labels. It is important to note that testing results for NETC and SNFH were not available as they were not officially released in the BraTS Lighthouse 2025 Challenge.

Table 3. Official BraTS 2025 validation and testing results (lesion-wise metrics).

Label	LW Dice (Validation)	LW Dice (Testing)	LW NSD@1.0 (Validation)	LW NSD@1.0 (Testing)
NETC (1)	0.7105	–	0.7216	–
SNFH (2)	0.6917	–	0.6838	–
ET (3)	0.7275	0.7349	0.7785	0.7877
RC (4)	0.7834	0.7705	0.7844	0.7651
NETC + ET	0.7275	0.7312	0.7137	0.7404
NETC + SNFH + ET	0.7271	0.7190	0.6938	0.6811

Performance was consistent across the two phases: validation and test set scores are closely matched, confirming robust generalization of the model pipeline. Notably:

- The resection cavity (RC) achieved the highest lesion-wise Dice (0.7834 on validation, 0.7705 on test), while the surrounding non-enhancing FLAIR hyperintensity (SNFH) subregion remains the most challenging (LW Dice 0.6917, LW NSD@1.0 0.6838, validation only).
- Boundary mismatches are evident from relatively lower NSD scores. Additionally, the following figure (Fig. 4) highlights boundary error maps in challenging cases, supporting our decision to introduce **Boundary Loss** [13] and **Generalized Surface Loss** [14] for the final containerized submission.

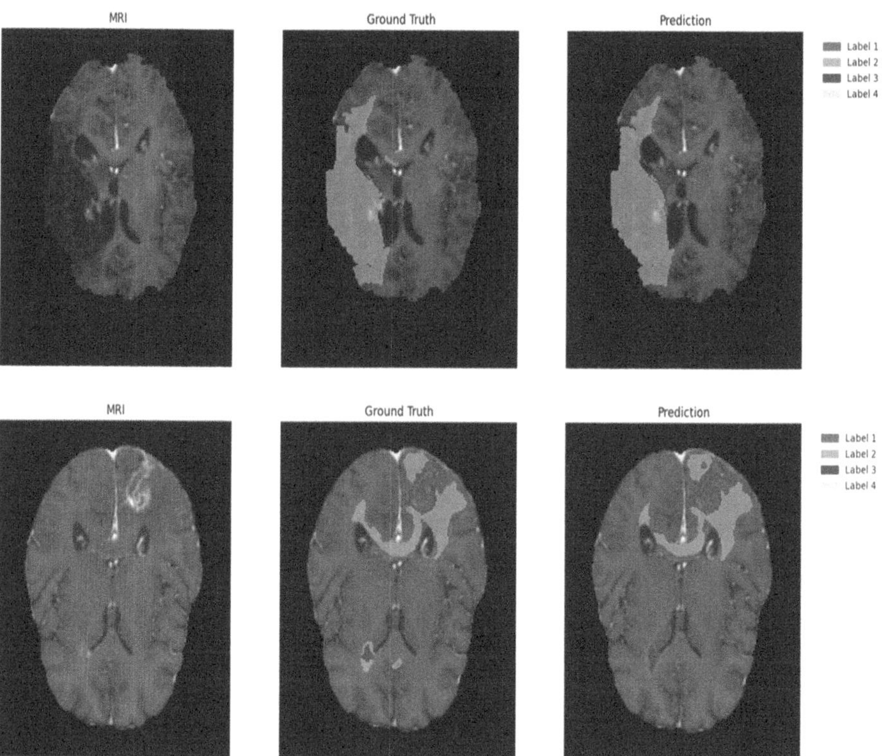

Fig. 4. Boundary errors (red) in a difficult case, motivating the planned integration of boundary loss and generalized surface loss.

4 Discussion

Our domain-adapted nnU-Net, with pseudo-labeling and post-processing, achieved moderate and consistent tumor subregion segmentation performance on two distinct, organizer-held datasets. RC and SNFH regions showed the strongest results; however, the SNFH and enhancing tumor (ET) classes continue to pose challenges, as reflected in both validation and test results. These findings are consistent with challenges commonly reported in brain tumor segmentation:

- **Domain shift sensitivity**, where scanner-specific intensity distributions reduce generalization;
- **Boundary ambiguity**, particularly in regions with low contrast or infiltrative tumor growth;
- **Class imbalance**, which causes smaller enhancing regions to be underrepresented during training.

Our combined use of domain adaptation and pseudo-labeling enhanced generalization across data centers and imaging protocols, yet some boundary sensitive gaps remain between subregional classes. Overall, the model demonstrates strong stability across independent unseen datasets, establishing a solid basis for further improvements in clinical segmentation reliability.

Acknowledgements. We thank God for His continuous guidance and blessings throughout this work. We also gratefully acknowledge the **National Health Research Institutes (NHRI), Taiwan**, and **Dr. Maxim Solovchuk** for providing the computational resources and support that made this research possible.

References

1. Baid, U., et al.: The RSNA-ASNR-MICCAI BraTS 2021 Benchmark on Brain Tumor Segmentation and Radiogenomic Classification. arXiv preprint arXiv:2107.02314 (2021)
2. Menze, B.H., Jakab, A., Bauer, S., Kalpathy-Cramer, J., Farahani, K., Kirby, J., et al.: The multimodal brain tumor image segmentation benchmark (BRATS). IEEE Trans. Med. Imaging **34**(10), 1993–2024 (2015). https://doi.org/10.1109/TMI.2014.2377694
3. Bakas, S., Akbari, H., Sotiras, A., Bilello, M., Rozycki, M., Kirby, J.S., et al.: Advancing the cancer genome atlas glioma mri collections with expert segmentation labels and radiomic features. Sci. Data **4**, 170117 (2017). https://doi.org/10.1038/sdata.2017.117
4. Bakas, S., Akbari, H., Sotiras, A., Bilello, M., Rozycki, M., Kirby, J.S., et al.: Segmentation labels and radiomic features for the pre-operative scans of the TCGA-GBM collection. Cancer Imaging Archive (2017). https://doi.org/10.7937/K9/TCIA.2017.KLXWJJ1Q
5. Bakas, S., Akbari, H., Sotiras, A., Bilello, M., Rozycki, M., Kirby, J.S., et al.: Segmentation labels and radiomic features for the pre-operative scans of the TCGA-LGG collection. Cancer Imaging Archive (2017). https://doi.org/10.7937/K9/TCIA.2017.GJQ7R0EF
6. Baid, U., et al.: The RSNA-ASNR-MICCAI BraTS 2024 Challenge on Brain Tumor Segmentation and Outcome Prediction. arXiv preprint arXiv:2405.18368 (2024). https://doi.org/10.48550/arXiv.2405.18368
7. Karargyris, A., et al.: Federated benchmarking of medical artificial intelligence with MedPerf. Nat. Mach. Intell.. **5**, 799–810 (2023)
8. Guadagno, E., et al.: Anti-apoptotic and anti-oxidant proteins in glioblastomas: immunohistochemical expression of beclin and DJ-1 and its correlation with prognosis. Int. J. Mol. Sci. **20**(16), 4066 (2019). https://doi.org/10.3390/ijms20164066
9. Kazerooni, A., et al.: Automated tumor segmentation and brain tissue extraction from multiparametric MRI of pediatric brain tumors: a multi-institutional study. medRxiv preprint (2023). https://doi.org/10.1101/2023.01.02.22284037

10. Isensee, F., Jaeger, P.F., Kohl, S.A.A., Petersen, J., Maier-Hein, K.H.: NnU-Net: a self-configuring method for deep learning-based biomedical image segmentation. Nat. Methods **18**(2), 203–211 (2021). https://doi.org/10.1038/s41592-020-01008-z
11. Isensee, F., Jaeger, P., Full, P., Kickingereder, P., Maier-Hein, K.: nnU-Net for brain tumor segmentation. arXiv preprint arXiv:2011.00848 (2020). https://doi.org/10.48550/arXiv.2011.00848
12. Gunawardhana, M., Xu, F., Zhao, J.: How good is nnU-Net for segmenting cardiac MRI: a comprehensive evaluation. Research Square preprint (2024). https://doi.org/10.21203/rs.3.rs-4786465/v1
13. Yao, H., Hu, X., Li, X.: Enhancing pseudo label quality for semi-supervised domain-generalized medical image segmentation. arXiv preprint arXiv:2201.08657 (2022). https://doi.org/10.48550/arXiv.2201.08657
14. Kervadec, H., Bouchtiba, J., Desrosiers, C., Granger, E., Dolz, J., Ben Ayed, I.: Boundary loss for highly unbalanced segmentation. In: Proceedings of the Medical Imaging with Deep Learning (MIDL 2019), PMLR, vol. 102, pp. 285–296 (2019). Also published in Med. Image Anal. **67**, 101851 (2021). https://doi.org/10.1016/j.media.2020.101851
15. Celaya, A., Riviere, B., Fuentes, D.: A generalized surface loss for reducing the Hausdorff distance in medical imaging segmentation. arXiv preprint arXiv:2302.03868v3 (2024). https://doi.org/10.48550/arXiv.2302.03868

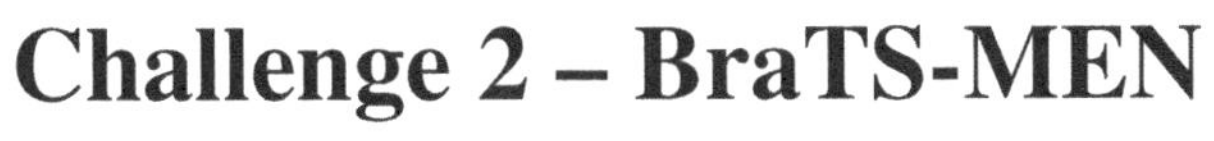

Challenge 2 – BraTS-MEN

PTransBTS: A Hybrid Transformer Integrating Priors for Brain Tumor Segmentation

Haitao Yu and Yanjun Peng(✉)

College of Computer Science and Engineering, Shandong University of Science and Technology, Qingdao 266590, Shandong, China
pengyanjuncn@163.com

Abstract. Brain tumor segmentation (BTS) using magnetic resonance imaging (MRI) plays a crucial role in the diagnosis, treatment, and research of brain tumors. With advancements in computer vision technology, numerous effective BTS models have been developed to tackle various challenges. However, most existing models overlook the incorporation of medical prior knowledge to guide the learning of intrinsic features beyond the label data. In this paper, we present PTransBTS, a prior-integrated brain tumor segmentation model that effectively leverages both the relationships between imaging modalities and lesion regions, as well as tumor shape priors. To address two key challenges in brain tumor segmentation—localization and precise delineation of fuzzy tumor boundaries—we introduce a Conv-head Global Attention (CHGA) block that combines parallel convolutional and Transformer-based architectures. Instead of directly merging all modalities, we propose a universal Brain Tumor Segmentation Stem (BTSS), which individually extracts features from each modality and applies weights for transmission to distinct decoder branches for segmenting different tumor subregions. To incorporate shape priors, we design a Learnable Dynamic Prior (LDP) block utilizing cross-attention mechanisms.

Keywords: Brain tumor segmentation · medical prior knowledge · multimodal fusion

1 Introduction

Magnetic resonance imaging (MRI) is a routine modality for brain tumor diagnosis. Radiologists assess brain tumors by integrating multiple imaging modalities and focusing on enhanced regions, tumor necrosis, and peritumoral edema. These features—greater enhancement, necrosis, and edema—often indicate high-grade brain tumors with a poor prognosis. As such, precise and automated segmentation of lesions is crucial for neuro-precision medicine, influencing areas such as treatment planning and quantitative analysis.

S. Bakas et al. (Eds.): MICCAI 2025, LNCS 16376, pp. 87–98, 2026.
https://doi.org/10.1007/978-3-032-16365-3_8

Over the past decades, convolutional neural networks (CNNs) have been widely applied to medical image segmentation tasks, including brain tumor segmentation (BTS), owing to their strong feature representation capability [10]. However, the limited receptive field of convolution kernels constrains their ability to model global context. Recently, self-attention mechanisms have shown great success in natural language processing and have subsequently been introduced into computer vision and medical imaging [3,27]. These methods have demonstrated impressive performance in BTS [7,8], leading to a variety of Transformer-based variants [5,6,33]. Given the complementary strengths of CNNs and self-attention mechanisms, researchers have explored hybrid models that integrate the two architectures. For example, CKDTransBTS [15] and SlimUNETR [23] adopt a serial integration of convolution and attention, but are prone to the semantic gap between CNN and Transformer features. In contrast, other studies have explored parallel architectures, resulting in several promising BTS models [18,19]

Moreover, current brain tumor segmentation methods often overlook the integration of medical prior knowledge. We contend that designing architectures that allow models to autonomously learn parameters for medical prior knowledge is highly effective, as it aids the model in learning intrinsic features beyond labels and improves interpretability. In clinical practice, different MRI modalities have varying relevance for segmenting distinct lesion regions. However, existing methods that focus on modality fusion typically process and combine modalities only at the encoder stage [15] [32], often neglecting the associations between modalities and lesion regions.

To address these challenges, we propose PTransBTS, a prior-integrated hybrid brain tumor segmentation network. Our model incorporates a Brain Tumor Segmentation Stem (BTSS) that leverages clinical prior knowledge, using convolutions for independent feature computation in the top layers of the encoder and decoder. Multi-layer perceptrons (MLPs) in skip connections weight and transmit information from different modalities to the segmentation heads for distinct lesion regions. For deep feature encoding and decoding, inspired by recent studies [2,22], we develop a Conv-head Global Attention (CHGA) module. By treating convolution as a head within the attention mechanism, CHGA bridges the semantic gap between CNNs and Transformers. Additionally, upsampling and downsampling are performed before and after attention computation to reduce computational overhead and accelerate receptive field expansion. Finally, a Learnable Dynamic Prior (LDP) module is integrated into skip connections. Using spatial and channel cross-attention, LDP injects self-learned shape priors into relevant channels, enabling faster lesion localization.

2 Related Work

2.1 CNN and Transformer Based Segmentation

Transformers excel at capturing global representations, while CNNs possess strong inherent local inductive biases. To combine these complementary capabilities, various methods have been proposed to integrate Transformers and CNNs.

TransUNet [1] was the first to apply Transformers to medical image segmentation, using a CNN encoder to extract slice-level features and introducing a Transformer at the bottleneck to capture long-range dependencies between features. nnFormer [33] adopts a serial backbone that combines both architectures, while PHtrans [19] utilizes a parallel backbone to alleviate the semantic gap between CNN and Transformer features. VSmTrans [18] introduces a lightweight parallel convolutional branch to a Transformer backbone, thereby incorporating inductive biases.

2.2 Multi-modal Fusion Models

Early brain tumor segmentation (BTS) models often ignored the multi-modal fusion problem by simply concatenating different modalities as input channels. More recent studies have proposed network architectures that more effectively fuse multi-modal information. Zhang et al. [31] introduced learnable weights to estimate the contribution of each modality, inspired by clinical diagnostic reasoning. Zhou et al. [34] designed four independent encoders for four modalities, fusing features in latent space. CKD-TransBTS [15] created two branch encoders to separately extract features from two related modality pairs: T1, T1Gd and T2, FLAIR. AAHN [32] adopted a dual-branch encoder where all modalities were input into the Transformer branch, while a single primary modality was processed by the CNN branch. These methods achieved effective fusion at the encoder stage by exploring relationships among MRI modalities.

2.3 Prior Embedding Methods

Early approaches primarily employed explicit statistical shape models [9] to embed priors. However, these methods are sensitive to noise and dynamic backgrounds and are difficult to embed within deep learning architectures. To implicitly introduce anatomical priors into U-shaped segmentation networks, some methods leverage convolutional attention mechanisms. BB-UNet [4] enhances skip connections using pre-defined bounding box (BB) filters during training, providing organ-specific shape cues. However, generating BB filters requires manual annotation. Attention U-Net [25] incorporates attention gates (AGs) to amplify task-relevant features while suppressing redundant activations from irrelevant regions, effectively capturing shape priors to a limited extent. Nevertheless, due to the limited receptive field of CNNs, such methods struggle to model long-range dependencies.

3 Methods

The architecture of the proposed PTransBTS model is shown in Fig. 1. We designed the Brain Tumor Segmentation Stem (BTSS), which are applied both at the modality input stage in the encoder and at the final segmentation stage in the decoder.

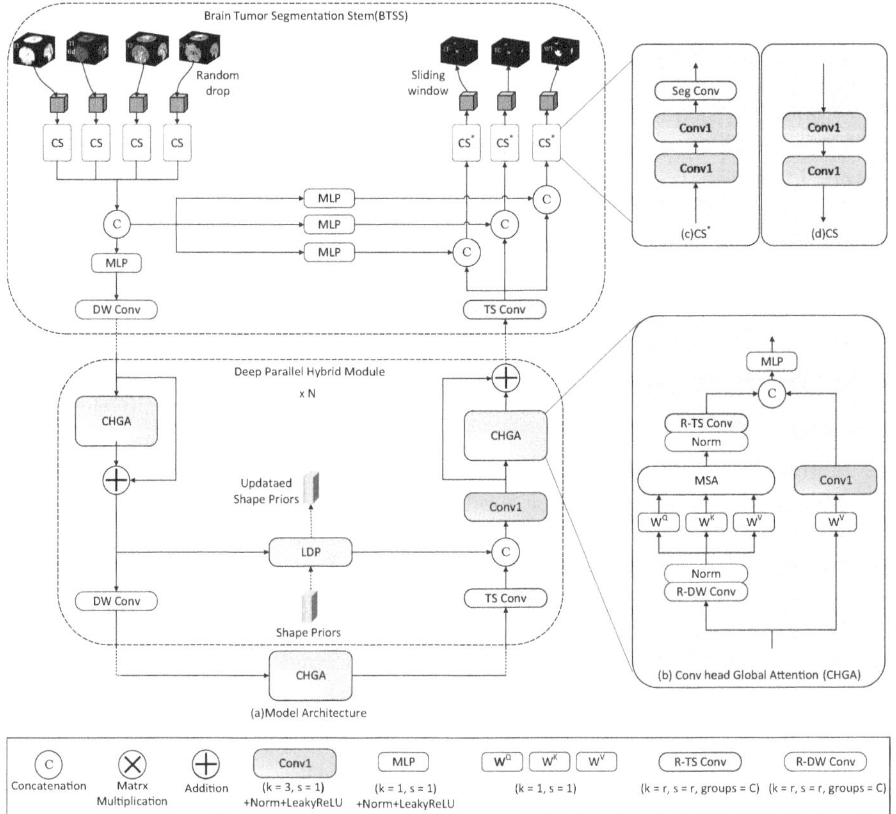

Fig. 1. The architecture of the proposed PTransBTS. (a) This model is a U-Net-like structure that processes features using multiple parallel convolutional Brain Tumor Segmentation Stems (BTSS) in the shallow layers, and employs N layers of hybrid Transformer feature extraction blocks in the deeper layers. (b) Conv-head Global Attention (CHGA), which embeds convolution as one head into the attention mechanism. (c) Convolutional Stem (CS*) to use in the decoder. (d) Convolutional Stem (CS) to use in the encoder.

In the deeper layers of the model, we incorporate N-layer Conv-head Global Attention (CHGA) modules, where convolution and Transformer processes operate in parallel to refine feature representations progressively. Additionally, a Learnable Dynamic Prior (LDP) block is integrated into the skip connections to inject dynamic shape prior.

3.1 Brain Tumor Segmentation Stem

As illustrated in Fig. 1, at the input stage, we employ convolutional operations to stabilize the optimization of subsequent Transformer layers [30]. Specifically, we design a convolutional stem (CS) composed of several serially connected convolutions. Four independent stems are used to extract features from the four MRI modalities $T1, T1ce, T2, FLAIR$:

$$\bar{X}m = \mathrm{CS}(Xm), \quad m \in T1, T1ce, T2, FLAIR \tag{1}$$

The extracted features are concatenated as:

$$X^* = \mathrm{Concat}(\bar{X}_{t1}, \bar{X}_{t1Gd}, \bar{X}_{t2}, \bar{X}_{flair}) \tag{2}$$

Subsequently, deeper feature representations are obtained by applying a $1 \times 1 \times 1$ convolution (MLP) followed by the deep module (DeepM):

$$X_{\text{mainstream}} = \mathrm{DeepM}\left(\mathrm{MLP}(X^*)\right) \tag{3}$$

At the decoding stage, three additional convolutional stems (CS*) are introduced to independently predict the tumor subregions ET, TC, WT. To enhance modality-region correspondence, MLP blocks in skip connections learn modality-specific weights for each subregion, enabling weighted transmission of encoder features. The segmentation process is formulated as:

$$Y_r = CS^* \left(\mathrm{Concat}\big(\mathrm{MLP}(X^*), X_{\text{mainstream}}\big)\right), \quad r \in ET, TC, WT \tag{4}$$

where Y_{ET}, Y_{TC}, and Y_{WT} denote the final predictions for the three tumor regions.

3.2 Conv-Head Global Attention

The Conv-head Global Attention (CHGA) module, illustrated in Fig. 1, combines convolutional and attention-based operations to jointly capture local and global features. It consists of two branches: a convolutional branch focusing on high-frequency edge features and a Transformer branch capturing low-frequency global features.

In the Transformer branch, depthwise separable convolutions (DWconv) are used for spatial downsampling before attention computation, reducing the computational load:

$$F_{\text{trans}} = R\text{-DWconv}(F), \quad F_{\text{trans}} \in \mathbb{R}^{C \times \frac{H}{r} \times \frac{W}{r} \times \frac{L}{r}} \tag{5}$$

Here, R-DWconv() denotes a depthwise separable convolution with stride r, used for spatial downsampling.

The Query and Key tensors for attention are computed as:

$$\begin{cases} Q = W^Q(F_{\text{trans}}), & Q \in \mathbb{R}^{(1-\alpha)C \times \frac{H}{r} \times \frac{W}{r} \times \frac{L}{r}} \\ K = W^K(F_{\text{trans}}), & K \in \mathbb{R}^{(1-\alpha)C \times \frac{H}{r} \times \frac{W}{r} \times \frac{L}{r}} \end{cases} \tag{6}$$

The attention matrix is computed as:

$$Att = \mathrm{Softmax}\left(\frac{QK^T}{\sqrt{d}}\right) \tag{7}$$

Att is the attention matrix calculated by the Transformer branch. In parallel, the Value tensors from both branches are defined as:

$$\begin{cases} V_{\text{conv}} = W^V(F), & V_{\text{conv}} \in \mathbb{R}^{\alpha C \times H \times W \times L} \\ V_{\text{trans}} = W^V(F_{\text{trans}}), & V_{\text{trans}} \in \mathbb{R}^{(1-\alpha)C \times \frac{H}{r} \times \frac{W}{r} \times \frac{L}{r}} \end{cases} \tag{8}$$

Note that V_{conv} is computed from the original feature map without an explicit attention mechanism. Instead, convolution itself serves as an inductive bias, functioning as a form of localized "natural attention". The parameter α is the proportion of channels occupied by the convolution head.

The outputs from both branches are computed as:

$$\begin{cases} F_{\text{attn}} = R\text{-TSconv}(Att \cdot V_{\text{trans}}) \\ F_{\text{conv}} = \text{Conv}(V_{\text{conv}}) \end{cases} \tag{9}$$

Here, F_{attn} represents the global feature extracted from the Transformer branch, and F_{conv} represents the local feature extracted by the convolutional branch.

Finally, the two branches are concatenated and fused through an MLP layer to produce the final output:

$$F_{\text{out}} = \text{MLP}(\text{concat}(F_{\text{attn}}, F_{\text{conv}})) \tag{10}$$

3.3 Learnable Dynamic Prior

As shown in Fig. 1, the LDP is integrated into the skip connection of the model. It utilizes shape priors and decoder features to extract relevant shape information, which is then embedded into the features at the skip connection. These shape priors are updated with each layer, allowing the LDP block to refine the shape knowledge at each stage. Initially, the shape priors are represented as a learnable tensor.

The structural details of the LDP block are shown in Fig. 2. Part (b) of Fig. 2 illustrates the spatial cross-attention mechanism used for extracting relevant priors. In this mechanism, the shape priors are projected into Value and Key matrices, while the downsampled decoder features are projected into the Query matrix. After the cross-attention operation, an upsampling step is applied to restore the feature size.

Part (a) of Fig. 2 employs a channel cross-attention mechanism, which injects the relevant features into the skip connection features. In this case, the skip connection features are reshaped into Key, and the relevant shape prior features are reshaped into Query and Value. After the channel cross-attention calculation, the skip connection features are enhanced with the relevant shape priors. Finally, the features are compressed using a convolution operation, and the updated shape prior is concatenated with the extracted relevant prior to form the new shape prior.

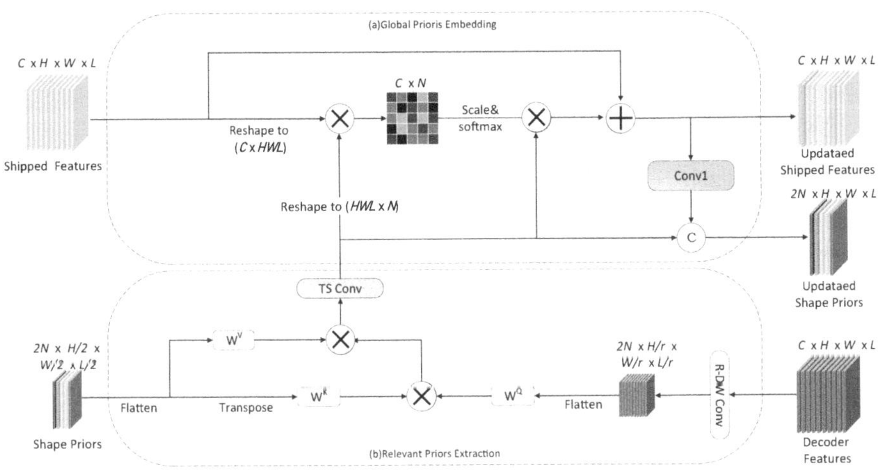

Fig. 2. Illustration of the Learnable Dynamic Prior (LDP). DLP consists of the Relevant Priors Extraction and Global priors Embedding.

3.4 Loss Function

To train the segmentation model, we adopt a combination of soft Dice loss [21] and focal loss [16]. Finally, the total loss function used for training is the sum of the Dice and focal losses:

$$L_{\text{total}} = L_{\text{focal}} + L_{\text{dice}} \tag{11}$$

4 Experimental Setup

In this section, we describe the experimental setup for 3D brain tumor segmentation, including the datasets used, evaluation metrics, and implementation details.

4.1 Datasets

We evaluated PTransBTS on the BraTS2023-MEN [14] and BraTS2024-PED [12,13] datasets. Since their validation and test sets are private, we used the publicly available training sets for experiments. Following prior works, the BraTS2023-MEN dataset (1,000 cases) was split into 80% training, 15% validation, and 5% testing, while the BraTS2024-PED dataset (261 cases) was divided into 80% training and 20% validation.

4.2 Evaluation Metrics

In our experiments, we use the Dice score, 95% Hausdorff distance (HD95).

Table 1. Comparison of Segmentation Performance in BRATS 2023-Men Dataset. The Top-3 Results are in Red, Blue and Green

Method	Dice				HD95			
	ET	TC	WT	Mean	ET	TC	WT	Mean
TransBTS[29]	0.8910	0.8715	0.8798	0.8808	12.27	12.16	11.79	12.07
nnUNet[11]		0.8894				9.36	9.24	9.47
3D ResUNet[24]	0.9068	0.8964	0.8970	0.9001	14.62	14.10	13.93	14.22
UNETR[7]	0.8460	0.8205	0.8318	0.8327	25.79	24.31	24.26	24.78
Swin UNETR[6]	0.8891	0.8789	0.8813	0.8831	20.93	20.93	20.61	20.82
PHtrans[19]	0.8383	0.8077	0.8240	0.8233	24.17	21.49	21.20	22.28
CKD-TransBTS[15]	0.8772	0.8554	0.8644	0.8657	21.36	21.30	21.32	21.33
SlimUNETR[23]	0.8451	0.8267	0.8365	0.8361	18.01	17.36	16.93	17.43
VSmTrans[18]	0.8914	0.8786	0.8848	0.8849	16.89	16.64	16.05	16.53
UNETR++[26]	0.8215	0.8055	0.7969	0.8080	41.83	42.32	42.14	42.10
PHNet[17]	0.9098		0.9025	0.9017	8.06	8.40	8.07	8.18
HMCG[28]	0.9022	0.8910	0.8959	0.8964	10.30			
ours	0.9225	0.9082	0.9172	0.9160	6.12	7.18	6.69	6.66

4.3 Implementation Details

We implement all experiments using PyTorch and MONAI, training models on a workstation equipped with an NVIDIA 4090D GPU. The learning rate is set to 3e-4 and adjusted via the cosine annealing algorithm [20]. The model is trained for 400 epochs with a weight decay of 1e-5. The number of layers in the deep model, denoted as N, is set to 4, and the channel split ratio α in CHGA is fixed at 0.8. Identical preprocessing and postprocessing steps are applied to all datasets. Identical preprocessing and postprocessing steps are applied to all datasets.

During training, we first compute the minimum bounding box of the volume and then randomly partition it into 128×128x128 volumes. To enrich data distribution and mitigate overfitting, we employ multiple data augmentation techniques: random zooming, three-directional random flipping, Gaussian noise, Gaussian blur, and random contrast adjustment. These augmentations are applied to all four modalities with consistent configurations. For testing, the sliding window method is used with a 0.6 overlap rate.

After obtaining the model performance, we adopted an 80:20 five-fold cross-validation scheme. We did not use any additional data. The final result is an ensemble of five PTransBTS models to enhance performance.

5 Experimental Results

5.1 Comparison With the State-of-The-Art Methods

We evaluated PTransBTS on the BraTS2023-MEN and BraTS2024-PED datasets against twelve state-of-the-art models. The results are summarized in Table 1 and Table 2, with the top-3 methods highlighted in red, blue, and green.

On BraTS2023-MEN, PTransBTS consistently surpasses competing methods, achieving the best Dice and HD95 scores across ET, TC, and WT regions.

On BraTS2024-PED, PTransBTS attains the highest mean Dice score while maintaining moderate computational cost (891.28 GFLOPs, 44.65M parameters). It outperforms strong baselines such as PHNet and HMCG, demonstrating both accuracy and efficiency.

Table 2. Comparison of Segmentation Performance, Model Parameter Size and Computational Complexity In BRATS 2024-Ped Dataset. The Top-3 Results are in Red, Blue and Green

method	Dice				GFLOPs	MParams
	ET	TC	WT	Mean		
TransBTS[29]	0.4932	0.8332	0.8582	0.7282	263.67	30.62
nnUNet[11]	0.5818	0.8699	0.8812	0.7777	539.56	31.20
3D ResUNet[24]	0.5330	0.8268	0.8416	0.7338	437.68	9.50
UNETR[7]	0.4509	0.7889	0.8158	0.6852	179.92	101.72
Swin UNETR[6]	0.5557	0.8298	0.8470	0.7442	793.92	61.99
PHtrans[19]	0.5342	0.8597	0.8792	0.7577	1349.63	71.49
CKD-TransBTS[15]	0.4730	0.8217	0.8449	0.7132	459.98	81.42
SlimUNETR[23]	0.2115	0.7976	0.8149	0.6080	12.39	1.77
VSmTrans[18]	0.5089	0.8173	0.8312	0.7191	857.99	49.87
UNETR++[26]	0.4945	0.7827	0.8084	0.6952	139.35	19.98
PHNet[17]	0.4630	0.9063		0.7627	1027.11	24.91
HMCG[28]	0.4707		0.9202		1674.24	87.42
ours		0.9081	0.9352	0.7942	891.28	44.65

Table 3. Quantified Metrics in the Testing Phase for the Multi-Consortium International Pediatric Brain Tumor Segmentation Challenges

Metric	statistic	ET	TC	WT
Dice	Mean	0.8769	0.8699	0.8492
	std	0.2249	0.2325	0.2387
NSD(1mm)	Mean	0.8803	0.8718	0.8413
	std	0.2244	0.2323	0.2394

Table 4. Quantified Metrics in the Testing Phase for the Meningioma Radiotherapy Segmentation Challenges

Metric	statistic	CC	ED	ET	NETC	TC	WT
Dice	Mean	0.6757	0.8919	0.6822	0.8397	0.8953	0.9016
	std	0.4702	0.3119	0.3333	0.2108	0.1572	0.1529
NSD(1mm)	Mean	0.6757	0.8919	0.7350	0.7948	0.7989	0.8076
	std	0.4702	0.3119	0.3271	0.2057	0.2284	0.2176

5.2 Performance in the Testing Phase

Our proposed method continues to demonstrate excellent performance in the testing phase, where we achieved first place in the Preoperative Meningioma Tumor task and third place in the Multi-Consortium International Pediatric Brain Tumor task. The specific metrics are shown in Tables 3 and 4.

6 Discussion and Conclusion

In this paper, we present a novel brain tumor segmentation model, PTransBTS, which integrates medical prior knowledge to enhance segmentation accuracy. The model learns the relationships between imaging modalities and lesion subregions, utilizing both convolutional and Transformer-based feature extraction in parallel. We argue that designing an architecture that allows the model to autonomously learn parameters that incorporate medical prior knowledge is an effective approach.

From a technical standpoint, we introduce three innovative modules. First, recognizing that different tumor subregions often require distinct modality combinations for effective segmentation in clinical brain tumor diagnosis, we designed the Brain Tumor Segmentation Stem (BTSS). This module allows the model to autonomously assign weights to modalities based on their relevance to different tumor subregions, thereby mitigating interference from irrelevant modalities and enhancing the representation of the most relevant features. Second, acknowledging the shape regularities of brain tumors despite their variable locations, we developed the Learnable Dynamic Prior (LDP) module. The LDP enables the model to autonomously learn tumor shape patterns, embedding relevant shape priors into the encoder features at skip connections through high-level decoder features via cross-attention mechanisms. Finally, brain tumor segmentation poses two critical challenges: tumor localization and precise delineation of fuzzy tumor boundaries. To address these, we proposed the Convolutional Head Global Attention (CHGA) module. This hybrid feature extraction block combines the global attention mechanism for rapid tumor localization with the convolutional inductive bias for accurate segmentation of indistinct tumor boundaries.

Evaluated on two datasets, PTransBTS demonstrates superior overall performance, outperforming state-of-the-art models.

References

1. Chen, J., et al.: Transunet: transformers make strong encoders for medical image segmentation. arXiv preprint arXiv:2102.04306 (2021)
2. Cordonnier, J.B., Loukas, A., Jaggi, M.: On the relationship between self-attention and convolutional layers. arXiv preprint arXiv:1911.03584 (2019)
3. Dosovitskiy, A., et al.: An image is worth 16x16 words: Transformers for image recognition at scale. arXiv preprint arXiv:2010.11929 (2020)
4. El Jurdi, R., Petitjean, C., Honeine, P., Abdallah, F.: Bb-unet: U-net with bounding box prior. IEEE J. Selected Topics Signal Process. **14**(6), 1189–1198 (2020)
5. Gao, Y., Zhou, M., Metaxas, D.N.: UTNet: a hybrid transformer architecture for medical image segmentation. In: de Bruijne, M., et al. (eds.) MICCAI 2021. LNCS, vol. 12903, pp. 61–71. Springer, Cham (2021). https://doi.org/10.1007/978-3-030-87199-4_6
6. Hatamizadeh, A., Nath, V., Tang, Y., Yang, D., Roth, H.R., Xu, D.: Swin unetr: swin transformers for semantic segmentation of brain tumors in mri images. In: International MICCAI Brainlesion Workshop, pp. 272–284. Springer (2021). https://doi.org/10.1007/978-3-031-08999-2_22
7. Hatamizadeh, A., et al.: Unetr: transformers for 3d medical image segmentation. In: Proceedings of the IEEE/CVF winter Conference on Applications of Computer Vision, pp. 574–584 (2022)
8. Hatamizadeh, A., Xu, Z., Yang, D., Li, W., Roth, H., Xu, D.: Unetformer: A unified vision transformer model and pre-training framework for 3d medical image segmentation. arXiv preprint arXiv:2204.00631 (2022)
9. Heimann, T., Meinzer, H.P.: Statistical shape models for 3d medical image segmentation: a review. Med. Image Anal. **13**(4), 543–563 (2009)
10. Hesamian, M.H., Jia, W., He, X., Kennedy, P.: Deep learning techniques for medical image segmentation: achievements and challenges. J. Digit. Imaging **32**, 582–596 (2019)
11. Isensee, F., Jaeger, P.F., Kohl, S.A., Petersen, J., Maier-Hein, K.H.: nnu-net: a self-configuring method for deep learning-based biomedical image segmentation. Nat. Methods **18**(2), 203–211 (2021)
12. Kazerooni, A.Fet al.: The brain tumor segmentation in pediatrics (brats-peds) challenge: Focus on pediatrics (cbtn-connect-dipgr-asnr-miccai brats-peds). arXiv preprint arXiv:2404.15009 (2024)
13. Kazerooni, A.F., et al.: The brain tumor segmentation (brats) challenge 2023: Focus on pediatrics (cbtn-connect-dipgr-asnr-miccai brats-peds). ArXiv pp. arXiv–2305 (2024)
14. LaBella, D., et al.: The asnr-miccai brain tumor segmentation (brats) challenge 2023: Intracranial meningioma. arXiv preprint arXiv:2305.07642 (2023)
15. Lin, J., et al.: Ckd-transbts: clinical knowledge-driven hybrid transformer with modality-correlated cross-attention for brain tumor segmentation. IEEE Trans. Med. Imaging **42**(8), 2451–2461 (2023)
16. Lin, T.Y., Goyal, P., Girshick, R., He, K., Dollár, P.: Focal loss for dense object detection. In: Proceedings of the IEEE International Conference on Computer Vision, pp. 2980–2988 (2017)
17. Lin, Y., Fang, X., Zhang, D., Cheng, K.T., Chen, H.: Boosting convolution with efficient mlp-permutation for volumetric medical image segmentation. IEEE Trans. Med. Imaging (2025)

18. Liu, T., Bai, Q., Torigian, D.A., Tong, Y., Udupa, J.K.: Vsmtrans: a hybrid paradigm integrating self-attention and convolution for 3d medical image segmentation. Med. Image Anal. **98**, 103295 (2024)
19. Liu, W., et al.: Phtrans: parallelly aggregating global and local representations for medical image segmentation. In: International Conference on Medical Image Computing and Computer-Assisted Intervention, pp. 235–244. Springer (2022). https://doi.org/10.1007/978-3-031-16443-9_23
20. Loshchilov, I., Hutter, F.: Sgdr: Stochastic gradient descent with warm restarts. arXiv preprint arXiv:1608.03983 (2016)
21. Milletari, F., Navab, N., Ahmadi, S.A.: V-net: fully convolutional neural networks for volumetric medical image segmentation. In: 2016 Fourth International Conference on 3D Vision (3DV), pp. 565–571. IEEE (2016)
22. Pan, X., et al.: On the integration of self-attention and convolution. In: Proceedings of the IEEE/CVF Conference on Computer Vision and Pattern Recognition, pp. 815–825 (2022)
23. Pang, Y., et al.: Slim unetr: scale hybrid transformers to efficient 3d medical image segmentation under limited computational resources. IEEE Trans. Med. Imaging **43**(3), 994–1005 (2023)
24. Pei, L., Liu, Y.: Multimodal brain tumor segmentation using a 3d resunet in brats 2021. In: International MICCAI Brainlesion Workshop, pp. 315–323. Springer (2021). https://doi.org/10.1007/978-3-031-08999-2_26
25. Schlemper, J., et al.: Attention gated networks: learning to leverage salient regions in medical images. Med. Image Anal. **53**, 197–207 (2019)
26. Shaker, A., Maaz, M., Rasheed, H., Khan, S., Yang, M.H., Khan, F.S.: Unetr++: delving into efficient and accurate 3d medical image segmentation. IEEE Trans. Med. Imaging **43**(9), 3377–3390 (2024)
27. Shamshad, F., et al.: Transformers in medical imaging: a survey. Med. Image Anal. **88**, 102802 (2023)
28. Wang, Z., Cheng, Y., Zhou, X., Yu, P., Wang, G., Tamura, S.: Hierarchical multi-class group correlation learning network for medical image segmentation. IEEE J. Biomed. Health Inform. (2025)
29. Wang, W., Chen, C., Ding, M., Yu, H., Zha, S., Li, J.: TransBTS: multimodal brain tumor segmentation using transformer. In: de Bruijne, M., et al. (eds.) MICCAI 2021. LNCS, vol. 12901, pp. 109–119. Springer, Cham (2021). https://doi.org/10.1007/978-3-030-87193-2_11
30. Xiao, T., Singh, M., Mintun, E., Darrell, T., Dollár, P., Girshick, R.: Early convolutions help transformers see better. Adv. Neural. Inf. Process. Syst. **34**, 30392–30400 (2021)
31. Zhang, D., et al.: Exploring task structure for brain tumor segmentation from multi-modality mr images. IEEE Trans. Image Process. **29**, 9032–9043 (2020)
32. Zheng, S., et al.: Asymmetric adaptive heterogeneous network for multi-modality medical image segmentation. IEEE Trans. Med. Imaging (2025)
33. Zhou, H.Y., Guo, J., Zhang, Y., Yu, L., Wang, L., Yu, Y.: nnformer: Interleaved transformer for volumetric segmentation. arXiv preprint arXiv:2109.03201 (2021)
34. Zhou, T., Ruan, S., Guo, Y., Canu, S.: A multi-modality fusion network based on attention mechanism for brain tumor segmentation. In: 2020 IEEE 17th international symposium on biomedical imaging (ISBI), pp. 377–380. IEEE (2020)

Efficient Meningioma Tumor Segmentation Using Ensemble Learning

Mohammad Mahdi Danesh Pajouh(✉) and Sara Saeedi

University of Calgary, Calgary, Canada
mohammadmahdi.danesh@ucalgary.ca

Abstract. Meningiomas represent the most prevalent form of primary brain tumors, comprising nearly one-third of all diagnosed cases. Accurate delineation of these tumors from MRI scans is crucial for guiding treatment strategies, yet remains a challenging and time-consuming task in clinical practice. Recent developments in deep learning have accelerated progress in automated tumor segmentation; however, many advanced techniques are hindered by heavy computational demands and long training schedules, making them less accessible for researchers and clinicians working with limited hardware.

In this work, we propose a novel ensemble-based segmentation approach that combines three distinct architectures: (1) a baseline SegResNet model, (2) an attention-augmented SegResNet with concatenative skip connections, and (3) a dual-decoder U-Net enhanced with attention-gated skip connections (DDUNet). The ensemble aims to leverage architectural diversity to improve robustness and accuracy while significantly reducing training demands. Each baseline model was trained for only 20 epochs and Evaluated on the BraTS-MEN 2025 dataset. The proposed ensemble model achieved competitive performance, with average Lesion-Wise Dice scores of 77.30%, 76.37% and 73.9% on test dataset for Enhancing Tumor (ET), Tumor Core (TC) and Whole Tumor (WT) respectively. These results highlight the effectiveness of ensemble learning for brain tumor segmentation, even under limited hardware constraints. Our proposed method provides a practical and accessible tool for aiding the diagnosis of meningioma, with potential impact in both clinical and research settings.

Keywords: Meningioma · Tumor Segmentation · Ensemble Learning

1 Introduction

1.1 Clinical Introduction

A meningioma is a tumor that forms in the meninges, which are three layers of tissue that cover and protect the brain and spinal cord. Meningiomas originate specifically from arachnoid cells, which are found in the thin, spiderweb-like membrane surrounding the brain and spinal cord. This membrane is one of the three layers that make up the meninges shown in Fig. 1.

S. Bakas et al. (Eds.): MICCAI 2025, LNCS 16376, pp. 99–111, 2026.
https://doi.org/10.1007/978-3-032-16365-3_9

Most meningiomas are not cancerous (benign), although they can sometimes be malignant (cancerous). In general, if a tumor is cancerous, it means it is aggressive, can invade other tissues, and potentially spread to other parts of the body. A benign tumor, on the other hand, does not spread.

Meningiomas are most often found near the top and outer curve of the brain. They may also form at the base of the skull. Spinal meningiomas are rare. Meningiomas tend to grow slowly and inward. Often, they have grown quite large before being diagnosed. Even benign meningiomas can become life-threatening if they compress or affect nearby areas of the brain. There are three types of meningioma based on grade:

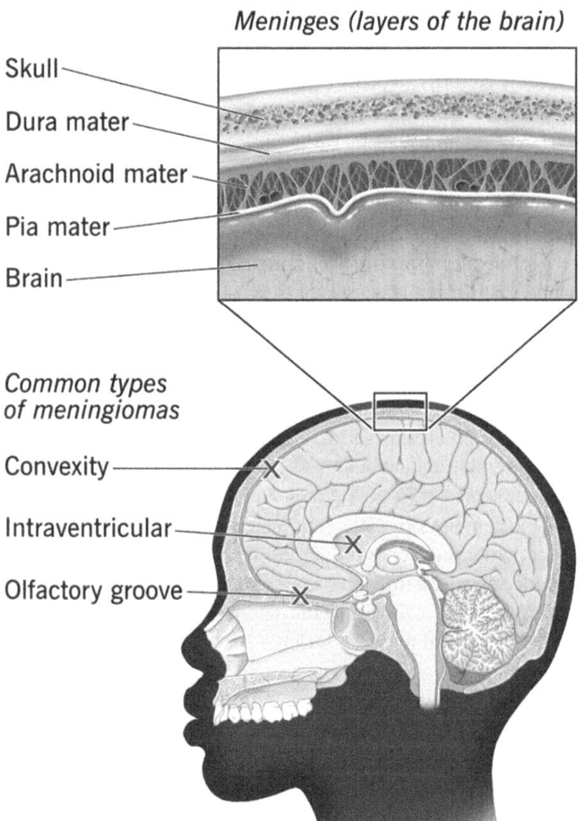

Fig. 1. Visualization of Meninges layers and its common types. Image is from Cleveland Clinic [1]

- **Grade I (typical):** A benign meningioma that grows slowly. These tumors represent approximately 80% of cases.
- **Grade II (atypical):** A noncancerous meningioma that grows more quickly and can be more resistant to treatment. These account for about 17% of cases.

- **Grade III (anaplastic):** A malignant (cancerous) meningioma that grows and spreads quickly. These represent approximately 1.7% of cases [1].

Accurate and early segmentation of meningiomas from MRI is essential for diagnosis, treatment planning (e.g., surgical resection or radiation therapy), and longitudinal monitoring. However, their variable location and morphology make automated segmentation a challenging task.

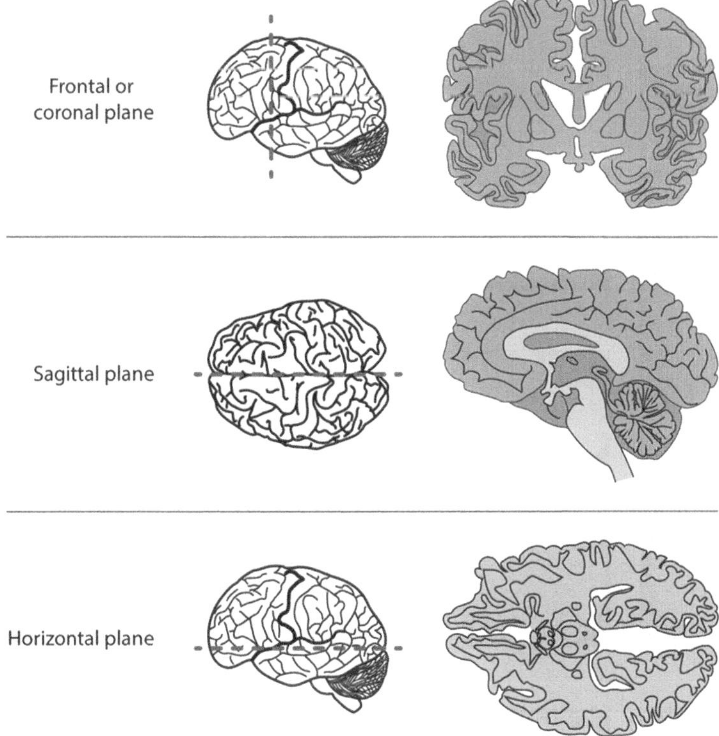

Fig. 2. Representation of the three principal orientations commonly employed in MRI. The upper row illustrates the coronal (frontal) view, which sections the brain from side to side, separating anterior from posterior regions. The middle row displays the sagittal perspective, slicing the brain lengthwise to distinguish the left and right hemispheres. The lower row shows the axial (horizontal) orientation, which produces top-to-bottom slices spanning superior to inferior aspects. Taken together, these planes provide complementary insights into brain anatomy and are widely utilized in both diagnostic practice and neuroscientific research. Image adapted from Foundations of Neuroscience by Casey Henley (2021), licensed under CC BY-NC-SA 4.0.

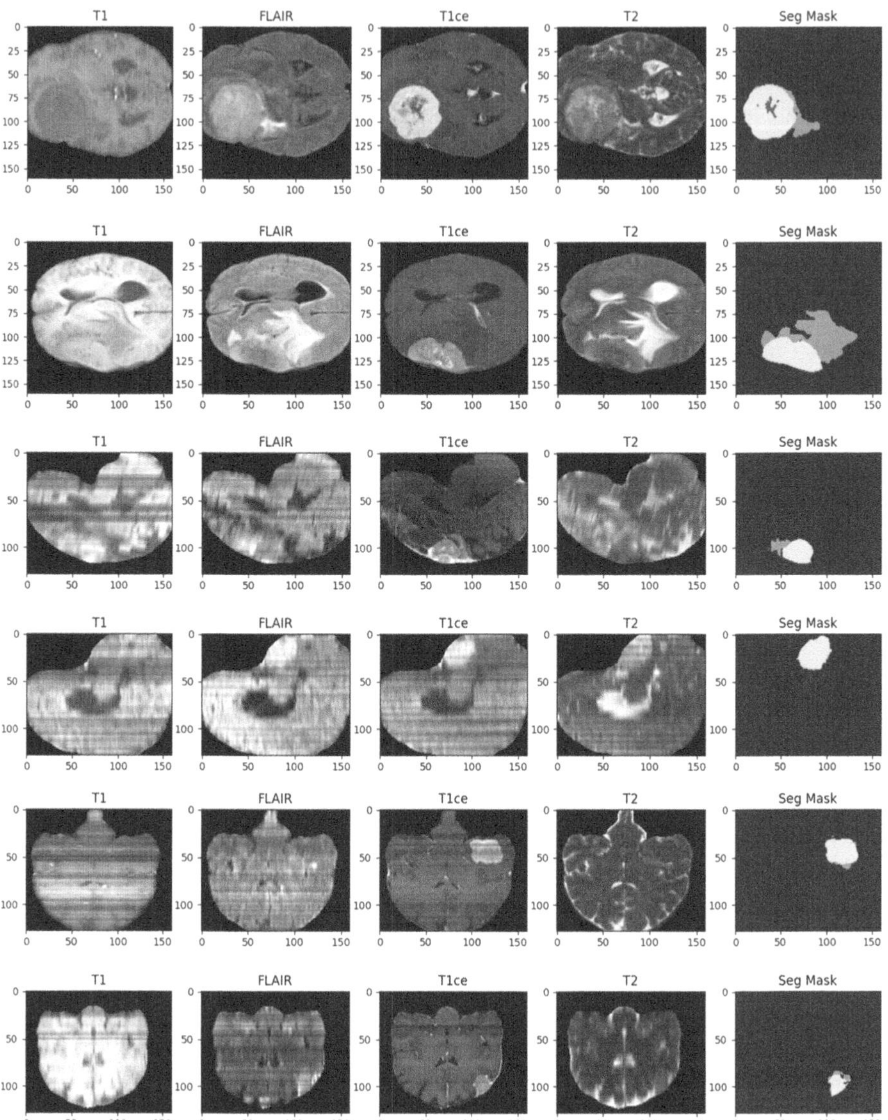

Fig. 3. Illustration of multi-modal MRI scans from the BraTS-MEN 2025 dataset. For each patient, representative horizontal, sagittal, and axial views are shown across four imaging sequences: T1-weighted (T1), Fluid-Attenuated Inversion Recovery (FLAIR), contrast-enhanced T1-weighted (T1ce), and T2-weighted (T2). The final column illustrates the corresponding ground-truth segmentation. Together, these modalities highlight complementary structural and contrast patterns that are essential for reliable identification of tumor regions.

1.2 Magnetic Resonance Imaging

Magnetic Resonance Imaging (MRI) is a powerful, non-invasive diagnostic tool used extensively in clinical and research settings to obtain high-resolution anatomical images.

By detecting variations in the alignment of hydrogen nuclei in response to magnetic fields and radiofrequency pulses, MRI enables visualization of internal tissues, particularly those with high water content [2]. In the context of brain tumors, clinicians typically rely on a combination of MRI sequences, each tailored to highlight different tissue properties.

The most frequently used MRI modalities in brain tumor evaluation include:

- **T1-weighted (T1):** Provides clear anatomical structure and is useful for visualizing normal brain anatomy.
- **T1-weighted post-contrast (T1ce):** Acquired after the administration of a gadolinium-based contrast agent, this sequence enhances visualization of vascularized regions, such as tumor tissue or inflammation.
- **T2-weighted (T2):** Highlights fluid-rich areas, making it ideal for detecting edema and cystic regions.
- **FLAIR (Fluid-Attenuated Inversion Recovery):** Suppresses the signal from cerebrospinal fluid, thereby enhancing the visibility of lesions adjacent to ventricles and sulci.

These modalities work synergistically to offer a multi-faceted view of tumor characteristics, aiding in diagnosis, treatment planning, and monitoring of progression.

MRI data is acquired as volumetric 3D scans, consisting of stacked 2D slices. For interpretation and analysis, images are typically viewed in three standard anatomical planes depicted in Fig. 2:

- **Axial View:** Horizontal slices from top to bottom of the brain.
- **Coronal View:** Vertical slices dividing the brain into anterior (front) and posterior (back) halves.
- **Sagittal View:** Vertical slices that split the brain into left and right sections.

This multi-planar approach provides essential spatial context for accurately assessing tumor size, location, and interaction with surrounding brain structures, which is critical for segmentation tasks.

1.3 Dataset

The BraTS-MEN 2025 dataset visualized in Fig. 3, which is the same as the 2023 version, is a widely recognized benchmark in brain tumor segmentation research. It provides multi-modal MRI scans accompanied by detailed manual annotations that delineate key tumor subregions.

These annotations distinguish tissue characteristics critical for clinical interpretation. Specifically:

- **Label 0** represents background,
- **Label 1** denotes non-enhancing tumor core, including necrotic regions and cystic changes or calcifications,
- **Label 2** corresponds to the surrounding FLAIR hyperintensity, capturing the full extent of abnormal FLAIR signal not part of the core,
- **Label 3** indicates enhancing tumor, reflecting actively growing or vascularized tumor tissue.

Researchers often aggregate these labels into clinically meaningful regions:

- **Whole Tumor (WT):** Union of labels 1, 2, and 3,
- **Tumor Core (TC):** Union of labels 1 and 3,
- **Enhancing Tumor (ET):** Label 3 only.

By offering comprehensive and standardized annotations, the BraTS dataset supports consistent evaluation across segmentation models and facilitates the development of algorithms capable of accurately distinguishing between tumor components [3, 4].

1.4 Proposed Model

As a result of thorough experimentation with various architectures and approaches, we found that the best performance was achieved through an ensemble of models. For this task, the ensemble includes the following components:

- **MONAI's SegResNet** [5], which is essentially a U-Net variant with residual connections,
- A **modified SegResNet** with attention gates in the skip connections and concatenation instead of summation,
- A modified version of **attention-based dual-decoder U-Net (DDUNet)** previously introduced in [6].

All models in the ensemble are evaluated on validation set by BraTS challenge using lesion-wise dice score and hausdorff95.

The rationale for proposing this method is twofold, reflecting both performance-oriented and practical objectives:

1. **Achieving Accurate Segmentation**

The proposed ensemble was achieved through experimenting with different architectural designs, hyperparameters, and training strategies. The aim was to identify a solution that provides robust segmentation performance while keeping computational demands low. Among all tested configurations, the ensemble approach consistently outperformed individual models on the validation set.

1. **Promoting Accessibility and Hardware Efficiency**

A primary motivation behind this work is to develop a model that is accessible to users with limited computational resources. Many high-performing models in the literature require GPUs with large memory and long training times, making them impractical for many researchers and clinicians. In contrast, our ensemble was trained and tested on modest hardware (e.g., a standard home PC), for a few epochs, yet still delivered strong results. This makes it feasible for others to reproduce, fine-tune, or deploy the model without requiring high-end infrastructure.

2 Methodology

2.1 Overview

To address the task of meningioma segmentation, we adopt an ensemble-based strategy that integrates MONAI's implementation of SegResNet, an attention residual UNet which is different from SegResNet due to addition of attention gate modules in skip connections and using concatenation of encoder features (through skip connections) and decoder features, unlike SegResNet that uses summation. Lastly a modified version of attention dual-decoder UNet (DDUNet) [6] was used. The DDUNet in this work differs from original by incorporating channel-wise attention (squeeze-and-excitation) and adding residual connections. Adding this attention module empirically improved the performance. The attention gate module was used in the last two models, allowing the networks to prioritize tumor-relevant regions while suppressing irrelevant background information. The models were trained using a combination of dice loss and focal loss which helps mitigate class imbalance in the dataset. To further promote generalization, we incorporated 3D dropout and weight decay during optimization. We utilize the BraTS-MEN 2025 dataset with four MRI modalities.

2.2 Preprocessing

Each subject in the BraTS-MEN 2025 dataset is provided with four volumetric MRI sequences, together with a segmentation mask annotated across four categories (labels 0–3). Raw volumes are stored in 3D format and were converted into NumPy arrays for efficient processing. The modalities were concatenated along the channel dimension to form a unified input tensor.

Because the original scans are large ($240 \times 240 \times 155$ voxels), we applied center cropping to reduce input size and computational cost while preserving anatomical fidelity. This yielded a final crop of $160 \times 160 \times 128$ voxels, which was used across all experiments. Segmentation masks were transformed into one-hot encodings to represent the four target classes. The training dataset contains 1000 subjects, while the validation set contains 141 subjects.

Intensity normalization was performed on each subject individually using z-score standardization, ensuring consistent intensity distributions across patients. To improve generalization and reduce overfitting chance, several random augmentations are applied to each training sample for the first epochs of DDUNet model such as: random affine scaling and rotation, random Gaussian noise, blurring and scaling intensities. This was done only on DDUNet because it has more parameters compared to the other two models. Adding augmentation to the other two, did not improve performance.

2.3 Model Architectures

The ensemble is designed to take advantage of several models' strength. It uses three lightweight models that grow in complexity, simple SegResNet which is quite light, a more complex version of residual UNet with attention and the highest number of parameters belongs to residual DDUNet with channel-wise attention. We will discuss each one in more detail.

SegResNet

We employ the MONAI's implementation of SegResNet (without variational autoencoder regularization) as our first model. There are four encoder layers with 1, 2, 2 and 4 residual blocks per each level respectively. The decoder has three levels each containing 1 residual block. The dropout probability is set to 0.2 and the initial number of filters is 16.

Attention Residual UNet (Modified SegResNet)

We implemented this model by overriding MONAI's SegResNet class and adding attention gate mechanisms at each skip connection (explained in detail later in this subsection). Unlike SegResNet, we decided to concatenate the features coming from encoder through skip connections and decoder features. This provides the model with more flexibility to choose from the features. Number of blocks in encoder and decoder, dropout rate and initial filters is the same as our SegResNet model.

Modified DDUNet

DDUNet is the result of our previous work, in which more than 100 training strategies and architectures were tested for the task of glioma brain tumor segmentation. The model was modified and tailored to the new task of meningioma tumor segmentation. We found that adding channel-wise attention modules improve the performance. In addition, the convolution blocks in DDUNet were replaced by residual blocks. A short summary of the modified DDUNet is presented below:

Encoder.

The encoder portion adopts a five-stage hierarchical design similar to U-Net, where each level consists of a residual block containing between two and four 3D convolutions (depending on depth). Every convolution is followed by Group Normalization and a ReLU activation. Group Normalization [7] was selected in place of the more common Batch Normalization [8] because training is performed with a batch size of one, where group-based statistics provide greater stability. Feature channel dimensions expand gradually across layers as follows:

$$\text{Input} = 4 \rightarrow 16 \rightarrow 32 \rightarrow 64 \rightarrow 128 \rightarrow 256$$

Dual Decoders.

Instead of a single decoding path, the network uses two separate decoder streams. Each branch performs upsampling and merges its activations with the attention-weighted skip features from the encoder. The merged tensors are then refined with a residual block.

- Decoder 1 is composed of four, four, three, and two convolutional blocks across its levels.
- Decoder 2 includes three, three, two, and two convolutional blocks.

Both branches produce independent segmentation outputs. These predictions are concatenated along the channel dimension and passed through a concluding $1 \times 1 \times 1$

convolution to yield the final voxel-level segmentation map. This late fusion step enables the model to exploit complementary feature representations learned by the two decoders.

Normalization and Regularization.

All residual units utilize Group Normalization, which is well-suited for very small batch sizes (in our case, one). To encourage robustness, 3D dropout with probability 0.1 is applied after each residual block. Unlike standard dropout, Dropout3D discards entire feature maps rather than individual activations, which helps maintain structural consistency, an advantage when segmenting tumors that may be spatially small. Weight decay regularization with weight 0.001 is also applied.

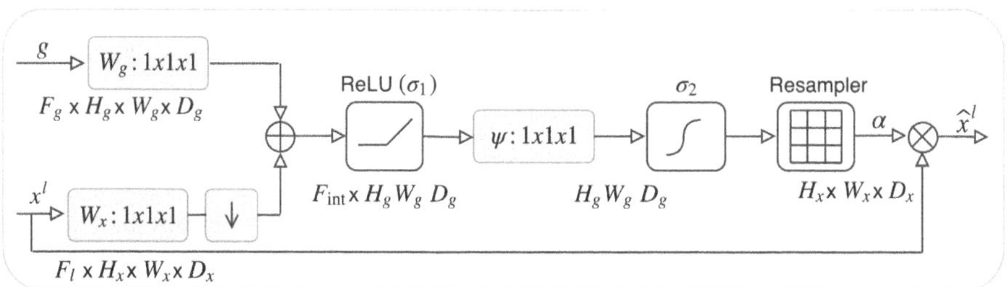

Fig. 4. Illustration of the Attention Gate (AG) as introduced by Oktay et al. in the Attention U-Net [9]. Each gate receives two inputs: a gating signal g from a deeper decoder layer and a skip connection x^l from the encoder. Both inputs are first projected via $1 \times 1 \times 1$ convolutions to reduce channel dimensions. The resulting feature maps are combined through element-wise addition, passed through a ReLU, and then processed with another $1 \times 1 \times 1$ convolution followed by a sigmoid activation to generate attention coefficients α. These coefficients modulate the encoder features, emphasizing relevant spatial regions.

In the original Attention U-Net, a resampling step aligns the spatial dimensions of the gating signal and encoder features. In contrast, our adaptation operates at the same spatial resolution for both inputs, eliminating the need for resampling while retaining fine-grained spatial details.

To improve the effectiveness of skip connections, attention gate modules are integrated independently into each decoder of the DDUNet as well as into the modified SegResNet models. These gates calculate attention weights for encoder features based on the activations of the corresponding decoder stage. The mechanism follows an additive attention formulation.

In the original Attention U-Net (Oktay et al., 2018) [9] shown in Fig. 4, the gating signal is obtained from a deeper, lower-resolution decoder layer, which modulates the encoder features prior to fusion. While this helps suppress irrelevant background signals, it may also compromise the preservation of fine spatial details.

Our DDUNet variant employs same-level gating, where the gating signal is derived from decoder features at the same spatial resolution as the encoder skip connections. The encoder features (X) and decoder signal (G) are first projected into a shared feature space through $1 \times 1 \times 1$ convolutions. Their combination is passed through a ReLU activation, followed by another $1 \times 1 \times 1$ convolution with a sigmoid function to produce the attention map. This map is then applied to reweight the encoder features before they are concatenated with the decoder outputs. By aligning gating and encoder features at the same resolution, the network preserves more local detail, which improves segmentation of small or complex tumor structures.

Loss Function

To handle the inherent class imbalance and enhance segmentation accuracy across tumor subregions, we employ a hybrid loss that integrates multi-class Dice Loss with multi-class Focal Loss. Dice Loss encourages high overall overlap with ground truth masks, while Focal Loss emphasizes voxels that are more difficult to classify, effectively guiding the model to focus on challenging regions. The combination ensures robust performance across all tumor classes by balancing global structure alignment with fine-grained voxel-level attention.

Multi-Class Dice Loss.

The Dice similarity coefficient is a widely used metric for evaluating segmentation performance, particularly in cases where class imbalance is prevalent. In multi-class segmentation, the Dice score is calculated separately for each class, and the overall loss is derived by averaging the class-wise scores. This approach helps ensure that smaller tumor subregions receive sufficient gradient contribution during training. The Dice loss is expressed as:

$$L_{Dice} = 1 - 2 \times \frac{P \cap T}{P + T}$$

where P is the predicted set and T is the ground truth.

Multi-Class Focal Loss.

Focal loss extends the conventional cross-entropy loss by assigning reduced weights to well-classified voxels and amplifying the impact of harder, misclassified examples. This re-weighting mechanism is especially beneficial in medical segmentation tasks where easily classified background voxels can dominate the loss. The focal loss is defined as:

$$L_{Focal} = -\sum_{n=1}^{N} -\alpha(1 - p_t)^{\gamma}\log(p_t)$$

If ground truth is 1, then $p_t = p$, otherwise $p_t = 1 - p$. γ is called the focusing parameter and in our setup it is 2. Additionally, $\alpha = 0.25$ is the parameter for class-balancing.

Final Loss.

The two loss terms are combined to form the final loss function:

$$L_{total} = \lambda_1 \times L_{Dice} + \lambda_2 \times L_{Focal}$$

In our experiments, we use $\lambda_1 = 0.75, \lambda_2 = 0.25$ as they demonstrated superior performance.

2.4 Post-Processing

After the segmentation masks are created for validation set by getting the majority vote of the result of each model, the images are padded with label 0 to match their original shape. An affine transform is applied to position the masks according to the challenge guidelines.

2.5 Training Procedure

We trained our models using the AdamW optimizer with AMSGrad and learning rate of 5×10^{-5}. A combination of dice loss and focal loss were used to address the class imbalance issue.

Training was carried out with batch size one, using a GTX1080 GPU with 8GB vram.

3 Experiments and Results

On validation set, for each subresion namely enhancing tumor (ET), tumor core (TC) and whole tumor (WT), the average and median results of each baseline model and the ensemble is presented in Table 1 and Table 2 respectively. Throughout our experiments, the ensemble constantly outperformed single models.

Table 1. Average results of the three baseline and the ensemble models on validation set

Model	Lesion-wise Dice ET (%)	Lesion-wise Dice TC (%)	Lesion-wise Dice WT (%)	Lesion-wise hausdorff95 ET	Lesion-wise hausdorff95 TC	Lesion-wise hausdorff 95 WT
SegResNet	73.9	74	72.4	63.29	60.2	62.6
Modified SegResNet	73.3	75.7	67.8	73.3	63.5	92.4
Modified DDUNet	62.6	63	61.5	109	107.1	110.8
Ensemble	76.7	76.2	73.8	56.5	55.9	63.1

Table 2. Median results of the three baseline and the ensemble models on validation set

Model	Lesion-wise Dice ET (%)	Lesion-wise Dice TC (%)	Lesion-wise Dice WT (%)	Lesion-wise hausdorff95 ET	Lesion-wise hausdorff95 TC	Lesion-wise hausdorff95 WT
SegResNet	89.6	88.2	87.3	1.9	2	2.4
Modified SegResNet	92.4	93.3	87.6	1.4	1.6	3.6
Modified DDUNet	79.4	79.7	77.7	5	5	5.7
Ensemble	91.8	91	88.2	1.4	1.4	2.2

On the test set, the lesion-wise dice is reported as 77.30%, 76.37% and 73.92% with standard deviations of 0.29, 0.30 and 0.28 for enhancing tumor (ET), tumor core (TC) and whole tumor (WT) respectively.

Through experimentation, we realized that these models complement each other in various samples. For example DDUNet, would usually overestimate tumor regions leading to more false positives. However, adding it to the ensemble improved performance as SegResNet models were too conservative when used alone.

We also observed that sometimes improving the performance of a model causes the performance of the ensemble to deteriorate, which shows there is no guarantee that improving overall performance of a model would improve its contribution to ensemble per sample.

Additionally, there were 9 samples in validation set that all the tested models predicted wrongly. These samples could correspond to cases in which the model has not been trained on.

Another notable aspect of this work is that each baseline model was trained for only 20 epochs, which further highlights a good choice of architecture could result in competitive results in one to two days.

4 Conclusion

Meningioma is a very common primary brain tumor. In recent years, AI has proved to be a great tool to diagnose and detect diseases. In the case of brain tumors however, due to the abnormal morphology of tumors, the development of accurate, efficient, and generalizable segmentation models continues to pose significant challenges, particularly in settings with limited computational resources. In this study, we introduced a novel ensemble-based approach composed of three lightweight models: a baseline SegResNet, an attention-augmented SegResNet with concatenative skip connections, and a modified attention dual-decoder U-Net with added channel-wise attention and residual blocks (DDUNet). Each baseline model used in the ensemble was trained for only 20 epochs.

Our ensemble was evaluated on the BraTS-MEN 2025 dataset and achieved competitive performance on unseen test set, with average Lesion-Wise Dice scores of 77.30%, 76.37% and 73.92% for Enhancing Tumor (ET), Tumor Core (TC) and Whole Tumor (WT) respectively. These results demonstrate that it is possible to achieve great segmentation accuracy without relying on large-scale hardware or extensive training schedules.

Beyond accuracy, the strength of our approach lies in its accessibility and practical applicability. By leveraging architectural diversity and attention mechanisms, our method balances performance and efficiency, making it an ideal solution for deployment in clinical or research settings with limited resources.

Acknowledgment. This research was supported by University of Calgary. The authors would like to thank Hossein Danesh Pajouh for his encouragement and providing the computer used in this research.

References

1. Johns Hopkins Medicine. (n.d.). Brain tumor. https://www.hopkinsmedicine.org/health/conditions-and-diseases/brain-tumor
2. Cleveland Clinic. (n.d.). Meningioma. https://my.clevelandclinic.org/health/diseases/17858-meningioma
3. National Institute of Biomedical Imaging and Bioengineering. (n.d.). Magnetic resonance imaging (MRI). U.S. Department of Health & Human Services. https://www.nibib.nih.gov/science-education/science-topics/magnetic-resonance-imaging-mri
4. Karargyris, A., et al.: Federated benchmarking of medical artificial intelligence with MedPerf. Nat. Mach. Intell. **5**, 799–810 (2023). https://doi.org/10.1038/s42256-023-00652-2
5. LaBella, D., et al.: The asnr-miccai brain tumor segmentation (brats) challenge 2023: Intracranial meningioma. arXiv preprint arXiv.2305.07642. (2023)
6. Myronenko, A.: 3D MRI brain tumor segmentation using autoencoder regularization. In: International MICCAI brainlesion workshop, pp. 311–320. Springer International Publishing, Cham (September 2018)
7. Danesh Pajouh, M.M.:Efficient Brain Tumor Segmentation Using a Dual-Decoder 3D U-Net with Attention Gates (DDUNet). arXiv preprint arXiv:2504.13200. (2025)
8. Wu, Y., He, K.: Group normalization. In: Proceedings of the European Conference on computer vision (ECCV), pp. 3–19 (2018). https://doi.org/10.1007/978-3-030-01261-8_1
9. Ioffe, S., Szegedy, C.: Batch normalization: accelerating deep network training by reducing internal covariate shift. In: International Conference on Machine Learning, pp. 448–456. PMLR (June 2015)
10. Oktay, O., et al.: Attention U-Net: Learning Where to Look for the Pancreas (2018). arXiv preprint arXiv:1804.03999

Brain Tissue Context for Enhancing Brain Tumor Segmentation: A Contribution to BraTS 2025

Mehdi Astaraki[1,2,3](✉), Farangis Sajadi Moghadam[4], and Iuliana Toma-Dasu[1,2]

[1] Department of Medical Radiation Physics, Stockholm University, Solna, Sweden
[2] Department of Oncology-Pathology, Karolinska Institutet, Solna, Sweden
[3] Department of Clinical Science, Intervention and Technology, Karolinska Institutet, Huddinge, Sweden
[4] Department of Biomedical Engineering, Amirkabir University of Technology, Tehran, Iran

Abstract. The development of deep learning methodologies has significantly impacted medical image segmentation, leading to highly accurate models for critical applications such as brain tumor delineation in MRI volumes. Precise tumor segmentation is indispensable for quantitative analysis, surgical planning, radiation treatment delivery, and disease monitoring. This paper presents a novel context-aware segmentation pipeline, conceptually rooted in anomaly detection, by integrating brain tissues as an auxiliary segmentation class. This inclusion enhances the discriminability between pathological and healthy tissues. To mitigate the class imbalance inherent in this added segmentation scheme, we incorporated a class-adaptive loss function within the nnU-Net and MedNeXt frameworks. The efficacy of this approach was rigorously evaluated on five tasks within the Brain Tumor Segmentation (*BraTS*) 2025 MICCAI Lighthouse challenge: adult glioma (*GLI*), pediatric glioma (*PED*), brain metastasis (*MET*), meningioma in pre-operative (*MENpre*), and meningioma in treatment planning (*MENrt*) segmentation. Our method demonstrated promising overall whole tumor segmentation performance on the validation set, yielding lesion-wise Dice scores of 0.873 (*GLI*), 0.945 (*PED*), 0.861 (*MENpre*), 0.845 (*MENrt*), and 0.679 (*MET*). The final phase of testing demonstrated that the proposed solutions performed among the top-ranked algorithms for the *MET*, *MENpre*, *MENrt*, and *GLI* challenges.

Keywords: brain tumor · MRI · segmentation · brats challenge

1 Introduction

Brain tumors, though constituting a relatively infrequent oncological diagnosis, impose a substantial burden of morbidity and mortality across the demographic spectrum. These heterogeneous neoplasms are broadly categorized into primary brain tumors, originating within the *central nervous system (CNS)* parenchyma,

S. Bakas et al. (Eds.): MICCAI 2025, LNCS 16376, pp. 112–126, 2026.
https://doi.org/10.1007/978-3-032-16365-3_10

and secondary or metastatic tumors, which represent extracranial malignancies that have disseminated to the brain [30]. This inherent diversity manifests deeply in their genetic, histological, and ultimately, their characteristic imaging signatures [11]. Their imaging pattern is notably inhomogeneous, frequently comprising extensive necrotic regions, vigorously enhancing vital tumor components, and substantial peritumoral edema.

Magnetic Resonance Imaging (MRI) serves as the indispensable imaging modality for brain tumor screening, owing to its unparalleled capacity to generate high-resolution images of cerebral soft tissues [25]. These images are critically important for accurate diagnostic assessment, *radiotherapy (RT)* planning, and disease monitoring. In clinical practice, *multi-parametric MRI (mpMRI)* sequences are routinely employed to characterize the heterogeneous subregions of brain tumors, each exhibiting distinct signal intensities across various *MRI* pulse sequences. The intrinsic variability and complex morphology of these tumors render their manual assessment and delineation a technically demanding and exceedingly time-consuming endeavor. Accurate and consistent delineation of brain tumors is paramount for precise diagnosis and *RT* planning; however, this task is widely recognized as labor-intensive and susceptible to both inter-observer and intra-observer variability [9]. Hence, the development of automated tumor segmentation algorithms in *MRI* emerges as a clinically transformative tool capable of supporting surgical planning, optimizing *RT* dosimetry, and facilitating objective and quantitative assessment of treatment response.

Advances in *Deep Learning (DL)* methodologies resulted in the emergence of numerous computational models for brain tumor segmentation, predominantly utilizing institutional datasets. Nevertheless, the systematic benchmarking and comparative performance analysis of these diverse strategies have historically been impeded by several confounding factors. These include variations in the specific imaging modalities employed (e.g., structural *MRI* vs. multi-modal CT-*MRI* combinations), differences in the investigated brain tumor types (e.g., high-grade vs. low-grade gliomas), and inconsistencies in the evaluation criteria applied (e.g., subject-wise overlapping metrics vs. lesion-wise distance metrics).

To overcome these significant limitations, the *Brain Tumor Segmentation (BraTS)* challenge was established in the Medical Image Computing and Computer Assisted Intervention (MICCAI) 2012 conference. The primary objective of *BraTS* was to facilitate the objective and standardized evaluation of state-of-the-art algorithms for automated brain tumor segmentation in *MRI*. Specifically, for each annual MICCAI conference, *BraTS* organizers have consistently provided a carefully examined collection of structural *MRI* scans, *native T1-weighted (T1n)*, *contrast enhanced T1-weighted (T1c)*, *T2-weighted (T2w)*, and *T2-weighted fluid-attenuated inversion recovery (T2f)* images, accompanied by corresponding expert-generated segmentation masks [3,16,26].

Initially centered on segmenting *glioma (GLI)* in pre-operative *MRI*, the *BraTS* challenge has significantly broadened its scope. It now includes a wider array of segmentation tasks, such as post-treatment *GLI*, *meningioma (MEN)* (pre- and post-*RT*), *pediatric (PED)* brain tumors, brain *metastasis (MET)*, and gliomas in *Sub-Saharan African populations (SSA)*.

The remarkable advancements in *DL* techniques have deeply facilitated the development of robust algorithms for automated brain tumor segmentation. Inspired by groundbreaking architectures such as the U-Net [32] and V-Net [27], a multitude of encoder-decoder models have been subsequently developed for diverse segmentation tasks. These models primarily introduce innovations through architectural modifications and/or refined optimization procedures. Several *Convolutional Neural Network (CNN)*, transformer-based models, and recently State Space Sequence Models including U-Mamba [23], STU-Net [12], U-Net++ [38], SegResNet [29], nn-UNet [14], MedNeXt [34], Swin UNetR [10], have recently demonstrated superior performance in the challenging domain of brain tumor segmentation.

Previous years' top-performing algorithms in brain tumor segmentation have consistently utilized a diverse array of methodologies, encompassing sophisticated preprocessing techniques, various segmentation network architectures, and refined post-processing strategies. For example, the winning solution for BraTS GLI in both 2023 and 2024 leveraged a generative model in conjunction with image registration techniques [7]. This approach significantly augmented the volume of training data, which was then used to train nnU-Net and Swin UNETR models. Subsequent stages involved thresholding and model ensemble methods to refine the segmentation output. Similarly, the winner of BraTS GLI 2022 developed an ensemble of three distinct segmentation models: DeepSeg, DeeoSCAN, and a modified nnU-Net, with the final segmentation generated using the STAPLE algorithm [37]. The BraTS GLI 2021 winner, in contrast, focused on architectural modifications to the nnU-Net model, specifically by increasing the number of filters within its encoder and bottleneck sections while retaining the original decoder structure [22].

Our proposed approach for segmenting various brain tumor entities in the BraTS 2025 cluster of challenges integrates healthy brain tissue as an additional segmentation label. This inclusion aims to enrich the learning process by providing crucial anatomical context. Hence, we have expanded the number of segmentation classes to incorporate healthy brain tissues and employ several robust segmentation pipelines, including nnU-Net, and MedNeXt for the *GLI*, *PED*, *MET*, and *MEN* tasks.

2 Materials and Methods

This study utilized annotated multi-modal *MRI* datasets provided through the MICCAI *BraTS* 2025 Lighthouse Challenge, comprising five segmentation tasks: adult *GLI*, pre-operative *MEN*, *MEN* radiotherapy, brain *MET*, and *PED* tumors. All datasets were distributed in Neuroimaging Informatics Technology Initiative (NIfTI) via the Synapse platform.

2.1 Studied Dataset

Task 1: Adult Glioma (GLI) – This dataset consists of pre- and post-treatment scans from 2601 training, and 407 validation subjects [1,2,5]. Each case includes four *mpMRI* sequences: *T1n*, *T1c*, *T2w*, and *T2f*. Segmentation annotations covered four tumor subregions: *Enhancing tumor (ET)*, *non-enhancing tumor core (NETC)*, *surrounding non-enhancing FLAIR hyperintensity (SNFH)*, and *resection cavity (RC)*. Combined regions including *tumor core (TC)* and *Whole tumor (WT)* are defined, respectively, *ET* plus *NETC* and the union of *ET*, *NETC*, and *SNFH*. The provided dataset underwent rigorous preprocessing, including coregistration of all sequences, skull stripping for non-brain tissue removal, and rigid registration to the Montreal Neurological Institute (MNI) atlas space [8].

Task 2: Pre-operative Meningioma (MEN-pre) – This dataset comprises 1000 training, and 141 validation of *mpMRI*s including *T1n*, *T1c*, *T2w*, and *T2f* [20]. Tumor annotations delineate the following constituent subregions: *ET*, *NETC*, and *SNFH*. The dataset was released after applying several preprocessing steps, including coregistration of all sequences, skull stripping, and rigid registration to the SRI24 atlas space [31].

Task 3: Meningioma Radiotherapy (MEN-rt) – Designed for *RT* planning, this task contains 500 training, and 70 validation [21]. Each subject is provided with a single 3D *T1c* sequence alongside a binary mask representing the *gross tumor volume (GTV)*. Crucially, each *MRI* scan is provided in its native anatomical space, without prior image preprocessing steps such as normalization to an atlas space.

Task 4: Brain Metastases (MET) – This dataset includes 1296 labeled training, and 179 validation subjects [24,28]. Each subject contains four *MRI* sequences (*T1n*, *T1c*, *T2w*, *T2f*) with segmentation labels of *ET*. *NETC*, *RC*, and *SNFH*. The majority of the data underwent preprocessing, which included coregistration of all sequences, skull-stripping, and registration to the SRI24 atlas space. However, a subset of the data was provided with coregistration and skull-stripping but remained in its native anatomical space.

Task 6: Pediatric Tumors (PED) – This dataset provides 261 training, and 91 validation cases [18,19]. Similar to other tasks with *mpMRI* scans, each subject includes the four standard sequences. Segmentation labels consist of *ET*, *NETC*, *Cystic component (CC)*, and *edema (ED)*. The preprocessing step of this dataset includes the coregistration of sequences, registration to SRI24 atlas space, and defacing.

2.2 Methods

Preprocessing: Prior to model training, image preprocessing was executed in two distinct stages. The initial stage focused on optimizing patch extraction for subsequent network input. This involved cropping MRI volumes to maximally exclude background regions. A series of thresholding and connected component analysis steps were employed to segment the volumes into foreground (body) and background, with the body's skin serving as the anatomical boundary. Following this procedure, a bounding box was generated to encompass the widest portion of the volume. This cropping approach facilitated the optimal loading of relevant brain tissues within each patch, thereby effectively eliminating extraneous background information.

The second preprocessing stage addressed the critical issue of intensity normalization. Recognizing the substantial variability in maximum intensity values across different MRI volumes, a normalization scheme was implemented. Specifically, for sequences exhibiting peak intensities exceeding 800, values above the 99th percentile were clipped. The final preprocessing operation involved channel-wise Z-score standardization, ensuring consistent intensity distributions across the dataset.

nnU-Net ResENC Model: nnU-Net is a self-configuring and self-adapting deep learning framework for biomedical image segmentation [14]. It systematically optimizes preprocessing, network architecture, and training, achieving state-of-the-art performance across diverse datasets without manual tuning.

The fist segmentation pipeline implemented was based on the nnU-Net V2 framework, specifically employing a ResNet-enhanced U-Net architecture – nnU-Net ResENCM – with its default configurations [15]. For the *GLI*, *PED*, *MEN*pre, and *MET* tasks, the model processed four channel input data, comprising *T1n*, *T1c*, *T2w*, and *T2f* sequences. On the other hand, the *MEN*rt task utilized a single-channel *T1c* input. Model training was conducted over 1500 epochs, employing a 5-fold cross-validation strategy. Each epoch consisted of 250 training iterations and 50 validation iterations. The optimization process was initiated with a learning rate of 10e-2, a batch size of 3, and incorporated deep supervision.

The input patch dimensions were $128 \times 160 \times 112$ voxels for the *GLI* and *MEN*pre tasks, $112 \times 160 \times 128$ for *MET* and *PED*, and $96 \times 160 \times 160$ for *MEN*rt task. All models in this pipeline featured six encoder stages, except for the *MEN*rt which included seven states of encoder blocks, initiating from 32 feature maps in the first block to 512 in the latent space. This pipeline was trained with both label-based and region-based optimization approaches.

MedNeXt Model: The second segmentation pipeline is MedNeXt [33] which leverages an architecture composed exclusively of ConvNeXt blocks [35] to capitalize on their design advantages. To maintain contextual information during upsampling and downsampling operations, the network replaces standard up-down/sample blocks with Residual Inverted Bottlenecks. Furthermore, to mitigate performance saturation commonly associated with large kernel sizes, training can be initiated with smaller kernels, which can then be progressively increased using the UpKern technique. Overall, MedNeXt functions as a scalable encoder-decoder framework optimized for 3D segmentation tasks, designed to maximize the potential of ConvNeXt architectures even when faced with the constraints of limited datasets.

In this study, we explored MedNeXt's functionality for the label-based and region-based segmentation of all the studied tumor types. Both models were trained using large-scale network architectures with a kernel size of $3 \times 3 \times 3$, a batch size of 2, isotropic spacing of 1mm, and a patch size of $128 \times 128 \times 128$, adhering to the nnU-Net training protocol.

Context-Aware Tumor Segmentation: In recent years, numerous studies have demonstrated that the integration of contextual information into the learning process significantly enhances model learning capacity and, therefore, improves overall performance. Within the domain of deep learning for medical imaging, contextual information can be incorporated through various mechanisms, including modifications to network architecture, optimization procedures, or the explicit inclusion of relevant anatomical data [6,36].

Concurrently, in anomaly detection applications, the primary objective is to identify deviations from learned representations of healthy anatomical structures. This implicitly categorizes image content as either healthy or abnormal [4].

Inspired by these principles, this paper proposes a segmentation strategy that includes brain tissues as an additional class, alongside tumoral regions, within the segmentation labels. The underlying hypothesis is that this approach will enable the model to not only directly segment tumoral regions but also to effectively differentiate between healthy tissues and pathological areas. This strategy can enhance the model's learning capacity by simultaneously leveraging information from both target tumors and their surrounding healthy tissues. To implement this concept, we utilized HD-BET, a rigorously validated algorithm known for its robust segmentation of brain tissues even in the presence of pathologies such as tumors [13]. By excluding the tumoral regions from the binary segmentation output of HD-BET, a new mask representing healthy brain tissue was generated. This new mask was then integrated as an additional label into the tumor label mask. Therefore, for each task, a new label was appended to the segmentation target. For example, the *MEN*rt segmentation masks were transformed from a binary to a two-class segmentation scheme. Figure 1 provides illustrative examples of the implemented strategy.

As expected, the inclusion of brain tissues as a new class introduces a highly imbalanced segmentation problem, wherein the volume of healthy tissues significantly exceeds that of the target tumoral regions. The use of conventional segmentation loss functions in such scenarios typically results in lower *Dice similarity coefficient (DSC)* values for classes with smaller regions compared to those with larger ones. To mitigate this imbalance, Kato and Hotta proposed the Adaptive t-vMF *DSC* loss [17]. Their work re-evaluated the standard *DSC* loss and demonstrated its reformulability using cosine similarity. Building upon this, their novel t-vMF *DSC* loss leverages t-vMF similarity, an extension of cosine similarity, to construct a more compact similarity loss function. The Adaptive

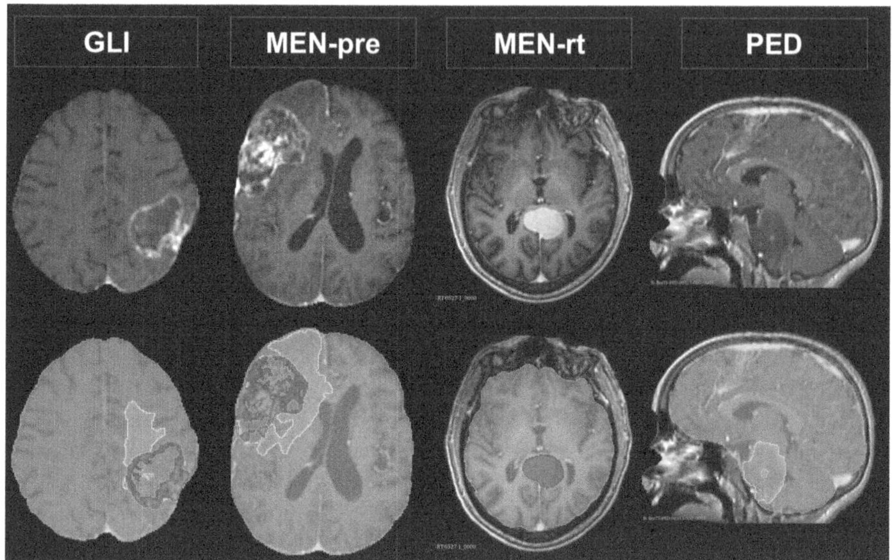

Fig. 1. Segmentation labels including healthy brain tissues alongside *GLI*, *MEN*-pre, *MEN*-rt, and *PED* samples. Tumor subregions are represented by green, blue, yellow, and red, with healthy brain tissue shown in thistle. (Color figure online)

t-vMF *DSC* loss further incorporates an algorithm that dynamically adjusts a parameter for the t-vMF similarity based on validation accuracy. This adaptability enables the model to apply more compact similarities for easily discriminable classes and broader similarities for challenging classes, thereby facilitating adaptive training based on class accuracy and ultimately improving *DSC* for imbalanced segmentation tasks. This loss function was integrated into the nnU-Net pipeline for the optimization of the ResENC-M and MedNeXt models across the evaluated datasets.

3 Results

The segmentation models were developed using a 5-fold cross-validation methodology on the training dataset. For simplicity and clarity, this paper only presents the quantitative subject-wise *DSC* for training data and lesion-wise *DSC* for the validation set. The following abbreviations will be used to denote our proposed solutions:

- B: Baseline – corresponds to segmentation models utilizing original data.
- P: Preprocessed – refers to segmentation models trained with preprocessed data.
- ML: Modified Loss – indicates segmentation models incorporating the modified loss function.

- Br: Brain tissue – denotes segmentation models leveraging brain tissue labels as contextual information.

Tables 1 through 5 present the subject-wise *DSC* metrics, showcasing the segmentation performance of the optimal results obtained across all conducted experiments. While various permutations of preprocessed datasets, the inclusion or exclusion of contextual information, diverse network architectures, and different loss functions were independently investigated and evaluated, this section only presents the highest performing configurations. Furthermore, it is noteworthy that two independent models were developed for the *GLI* task, addressing pre- and post-treatment datasets, separately (Tables 2 and 3).

Table 1. Quantified subject-wise *DSC* metrics for *GLI* task on the training set.

Entity	Data/Model	Architecture	Task ID	DSC ($\mu \pm \sigma$)					
				ET	NETC	RC	SNFH	TC	WT
Pre	B	ResENC-M	GLIpre1	0.866 ± 0.190	0.767 ± 0.271	–	0.860 ± 0.173	0.921 ± 0.136	0.929 ± 0.072
	P	ResENC-M	GLIpre2	0.877 ± 0.187	0.775 ± 0.284	–	0.870 ± 0.139	0.929 ± 0.141	0.933 ± 0.073
	P-ML	ResENC-M	GLIpre3	0.881 ± 0.169	0.781 ± 0.269	–	0.898 ± 0.170	0.929 ± 0.158	0.933 ± 0.068
	P-ML-Br	MedNeXt-L	GLIpre4	0.889 ± 0.171	0.793 ± 0.252	–	0.889 ± 0.162	0.931 ± 0.122	0.941 ± 0.065
Post	B	ResENC-M	GLIpost1	0.758 ± 0.283	0.611 ± 0.361	0.736 ± 0.272	0.907 ± 0.079	0.751 ± 0.314	0.902 ± 0.086
	P	ResENC-M	GLIpost2	0.762 ± 0.292	0.607 ± 0.354	0.758 ± 0.313	0.919 ± 0.091	0.755 ± 0.298	0.916 ± 0.090
	P-ML	ResENC-M	GLIpost3	0.749 ± 0.339	0.633 ± 0.388	0.718 ± 0.368	0.913 ± 0.083	0.706 ± 0.339	0.922 ± 0.078
	P-ML-Br	MedNeXt-L	GLIpost4	0.751 ± 0.299	0.643 ± 0.347	0.768 ± 0.298	0.911 ± 0.085	0.756 ± 0.257	0.920 ± 0.081

Table 2. Quantified subject-wise *DSC* metrics for *PED* task on the training set.

Data/Model	Architecture	Task ID	DSC ($\mu \pm \sigma$)					
			ET	NETC	CC	SNFH	TC	WT
B	ResENC-M	PED1	0.558 ± 0.366	0.794 ± 0.230	0.240 ± 0.347	0.160 ± 0.284	0.865 ± 0.170	0.887 ± 0.149
P	ResENC-M	PED2	0.571 ± 0.282	0.830 ± 0.218	0.310 ± 0.301	0.230 ± 0.284	0.881 ± 0.183	0.898 ± 0.135
P-ML	ResENC-M	PED3	0.601 ± 0.219	0.810 ± 0.307	0.298 ± 0.252	0.281 ± 0.158	0.879 ± 0.195	0.908 ± 0.120
P-ML-Br	MedNeXt-L	PED4	0.592 ± 0.307	0.819 ± 0.272	0.339 ± 0.287	0.268 ± 0.184	0.884 ± 0.173	0.904 ± 0.142

Table 3. Quantified subject-wise *DSC* metrics for *MET* task on the training set.

Data/Model	Architecture	Task ID	DSC ($\mu \pm \sigma$)			
			ET	RC	TC	WT
B	ResENC-M	MET1	0.721 ± 0.268	0.447 ± 0.402	0.751 ± 0.259	0.754 ± 0.281
P	ResENC-M	MET2	0.740 ± 0.244	0.469 ± 0.332	0.765 ± 0.255	0.774 ± 0.247
P-ML	ResENC-M	MET3	0.711 ± 0.244	0.416 ± 0.398	0.754 ± 0.282	0.750 ± 0.278
P-ML-Br	MedNeXt-L	MET4	0.732 ± 0.219	0.431 ± 0.284	0.737 ± 0.318	0.748 ± 0.321
P-ML cascade	MedNeXt-L/ResENC-M	MET5	0.692 ± 0.320	0.399 ± 0.379	0.707 ± 0.346	0.715 ± 0.254

For the *MET* task, the inclusion of brain tissue as an additional label was deemed impractical due to the often tiny size of the lesions. This disparity in class sizes led to significant imbalance, causing segmentation results to be consistently skewed towards the brain tissue, even with the application of class-adaptive loss functions. To address this challenge, a cascaded model approach was implemented. Initially, a two-class segmentation model was trained to differentiate between the union of all tumor subregions and the surrounding brain tissue. The output of this initial model underwent post-processing to generate a binary segmentation mask specifically for the metastatic regions. This mask was then incorporated as an additional input channel for a second network, which was directly optimized for the segmentation of metastases subregions.

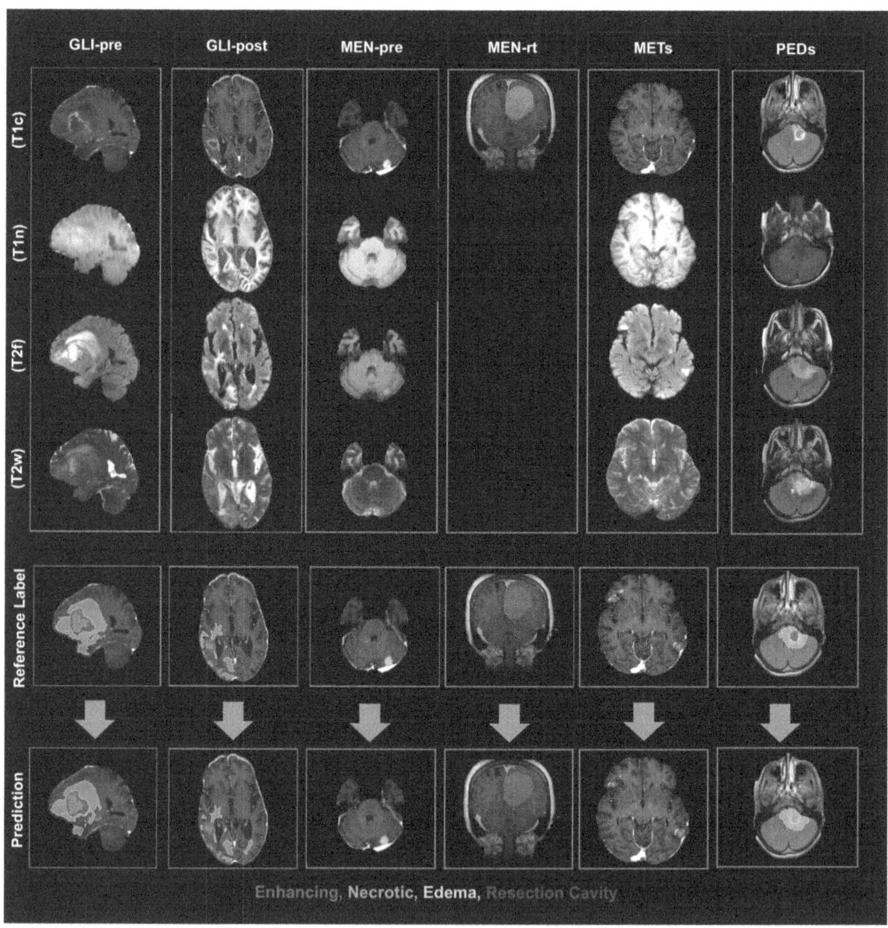

Fig. 2. Overview of studied segmentation tasks. Each column delineates a specific segmentation task, while the upper four rows indicate the corresponding MRI modalities required. Tumor subregions, including *ET*, *NETC*, *SNFH*, *RC*, *CC* and *GTV*, are depicted with distinct color-coded segmentation labels superimposed on representative 2D slices.

Figure 2 details the segmentation tasks by illustrating the studied *MRI* sequences, segmentation labels, and the corresponding predicted labels for each task (Tables 4 and 5).

Table 4. Quantified subject-wise *DSC* metrics for *MEN*pre task on the training set.

Data/Model	Architecture	Task ID	DSC ($\mu \pm \sigma$)		
			ET	TC	WT
B	ResENC-M	MENpre1	0.931 ± 0.146	0.929 ± 0.147	0.919 ± 0.151
P	ResENC-M	MENpre2	0.934 ± 0.131	0.932 ± 0.138	0.919 ± 0.146
P-ML	ResENC-M	MENpre3	0.937 ± 0.134	0.935 ± 0.140	0.926 ± 0.143
P-ML-Br	ResENC-M	MENpre4	0.939 ± 0.131	0.936 ± 0.138	0.928 ± 0.142

Table 5. Quantified subject-wise *DSC* metrics for *MEN*rt task on the training set.

Data/Model	Architecture	Task ID	DSC ($\mu \pm \sigma$)
			GTV
B	ResENC-M	MENrt1	0.781 ± 0.250
P	ResENC-M	MENrt2	0.792 ± 0.241
P-ML	ResENC-M	MENrt3	0.788 ± 0.239
P-ML-Br	MedNeXt-L	MENrt4	0.795 ± 0.238

The reported metrics clearly demonstrate that including brain tissue as an additional label consistently improved segmentation accuracy across various tumor entities and their subregionse except for the *MET* task.

Quantified metrics indicate that no single configuration consistently achieved optimal accuracy across all examined regions. For instance, for the *GLI*pre task, configuration *GLIpre4* demonstrated superior performance for the *ET* and *NETC* regions, whereas configuration *GLIpre3* yielded more accurate segmentations for the *SNFH* region. Therefore, an ensemble approach, aggregating these two models, was employed for the final *GLI*pre task.

This strategy was similarly applied to other tasks where feasible. Thus, the various Task IDs presented in Table 6 denote the instances of model aggregation employed. This table further details the optimal performance achieved from the submitted masks on the Synapse platform's validation datasets. It is important to note that the models with the configurations outlined in Table 6 were subsequently utilized as containerized algorithms for the final submission during the testing phase, under the Synapse username **Astaraki** and Synapse project ID **syn67269876**.

The proposed algorithms were containerized and subsequently submitted to the Synapse platform for evaluation against unseen testing datasets. A summary of the quantitative metrics, as provided by the challenge organizers, is presented in Table 7. The results indicate that the proposed solutions performed among the top-ranked algorithms for the *MET*, *MEN*-pre, *MEN*-rt, and *GLI* challenges. However, for reasons of transparency, these results were excluded from the official ranking, as the primary author of this paper was a member of the organizing committee.

Table 6. Quantified lesion-wise *DSC* metrics for all the studied tasks on the **validation** set.

Entity	Task IDs	DSC ($\mu \pm \sigma$)					
		ET	NECT	RC/CC	SNFH/ED	TC	WT
GLI-pre	GLIpre3 GLIpre4	0.827 ± 0.230	0.748 ± 0.282	–	0.788 ± 0.203	0.840 ± 0.231	0.884 ± 0.146
GLI-post	GLIpost2 GLIpost3 GLIpost4	0.739 ± 0.305	0.797 ± 0.352	0.710 ± 0.365	0.846 ± 0.200	0.717 ± 0.305	0.861 ± 0.201
GLI-all	GLIpre3 GLIpre4 GLIpost2 GLIpost3 GLIpost4	0.786 ± 0.270	0.770 ± 0.317	0.866 ± 0.286	0.822 ± 0.204	0.783 ± 0.274	0.873 ± 0.173
PED	PED2 PED3 PED4	0.630 ± 0.427	0.917 ± 0.123	0.752 ± 0.415	0.967 ± 0.179	0.945 ± 0.107	0.945 ± 0.108
MET	MET2	0.678 ± 0.276	–	0.930 ± 0.224	–	0.695 ± 0.279	0.679 ± 0.272
MEN-pre	MENpre4	0.873 ± 0.223	–	–	–	0.886 ± 0.200	0.861 ± 0.213
MEN-rt	MENrt2 MENrt4	GTV 0.845 ± 0.165					

4 Discussion

The *BraTS* 2025 MICCAI Lighthouse challenge comprises eleven tasks, encompassing the segmentation of various brain pathologies in MRI volume which includes adult *GLI* (pre- and post-operative), *PED* glioma (pre-operative), *MEN* (pre-operative and RT planning), and *MET*.

In the last few years, while a body of literature has proposed robust solutions for medical image segmentation, including brain tumors for the *BraTS* challenge, the specific strategy of incorporating brain tissues as an additional segmentation class to enhance the distinction between normal brain tissues and tumoral regions has not been previously explored, at least to the best knowledge of the authors.

Table 7. Quantified lesion-wise *DSC* metrics for all the studied tasks on the **testing** set.

Entity	DSC ($\mu \pm \sigma$)			
	ET	RC/CC	TC	WT
GLI	0.805 ± 0.262	0.886 ± 0.254	0.800 ± 0.286	0.872 ± 0.182
PED	0.725 ± 0.305	0.603 ± 0.468	0.898 ± 0.156	0.904 ± 0.153
MET	0.595 ± 0.287	–	0.607 ± 0.292	0.604 ± 0.292
MEN-pre	0.880 ± 0.213	–	0.875 ± 0.215	0.853 ± 0.226
MEN-rt	0.829 ± 0.173			

In this study, we investigated the efficacy of this novel approach when integrated into state-of-the-art models for segmenting different brain tumor entities. Our method involved simultaneously segmenting both tumoral regions and brain tissues, which necessitated modifying the loss function to accommodate the inherent imbalance in the size of these structures. The proposed pipeline incorporated a simple yet effective image preprocessing sequence, including brain tissue cropping and intensity normalization. For the segmentation models, we selected nnU-Net ResENC-M and MedNeXt due to their demonstrated superior performance in various segmentation applications. Finally, an aggregation of top-performing models from the training phase was utilized for the ultimate submission across the validation and testing phases of the challenge.

Our experiments generally demonstrate the efficacy of the proposed approach for all tasks investigated, with the exception of the *MET* task. Specifically, the inclusion of brain tissues during the training of both nnU-Net and MedNeXt models, when optimized with the modified loss function, led to improved segmentation accuracy across different tumor subregions. However, the significantly smaller size of *MET* lesions compared to the large size of brain tissue resulted in a substantial imbalance ratio, leading to poor performance for the MET task despite the modified loss function's attempt to balance this ratio during optimization.

While both ResENC and MedNeXt baseline models exhibited robust segmentation performance when applied directly to raw datasets, our findings indicate that preprocessing the datasets, providing additional contextual information during the training procedure, and subtle optimizations to the training protocols can further enhance the segmentation accuracy of these models. Post-processing methods that utilize size and intensity thresholds have been demonstrated in other studies to be effective in reducing false positive segmentation errors; therefore, we plan to integrate such methods into our proposed pipeline in our future research.

In summary, our contributions to the *BraTS* 2025 challenge culminated in robust segmentation models for each of the five tasks investigated, yielding competitive results on the validation sets, which were subsequently evaluated and reported on the unranked Synapse leaderboards.

Acknowledgmenet. This research was supported by the Cancer Research Funds of Radiumhemmet. The Swedish Cancer Society and The Swedish Research Council (grant number 2020-04618) are gratefully acknowledged for their support. The authors also extend their appreciation to Stockholm Medical Artificial Intelligence and Learning Environments (SMAILE) for providing access to their computational resources.

Disclosure of Interests. The authors have no competing interests to declare that are relevant to the content of this article.

References

1. Baid, U., Ghodasara, S., et al.: The RSNA-ASNR-MICCAI BraTS 2021 benchmark on brain tumor segmentation and radiogenomic classification (2021). https://arxiv.org/abs/2107.02314
2. Bakas, S., et al.: Advancing the cancer genome atlas glioma MRI collections with expert segmentation labels and radiomic features. Sci. Data **4**(1), 170117 (2017). https://doi.org/10.1038/sdata.2017.117
3. Bakas, S., Reyes, M., Jakab, A., Bauer, S., Rempfler, M., et al.: Alessandro Crimi. Identifying the best machine learning algorithms for brain tumor segmentation, progression assessment, and overall survival prediction in the BraTS challenge (2019). https://arxiv.org/abs/1811.02629
4. Baur, C., Denner, S., Wiestler, B., Navab, N., Albarqouni, S.: Autoencoders for unsupervised anomaly segmentation in brain MR images: a comparative study. Med. Image Anal. **69**, 101952 (2021). ISSN 1361-8415. https://doi.org/10.1016/j.media.2020.101952. https://www.sciencedirect.com/science/article/pii/S1361841520303169
5. de Verdier, M.C., Saluja, R., et al.: The 2024 brain tumor segmentation (BraTS) challenge: glioma segmentation on post-treatment MRI (2024). https://arxiv.org/abs/2405.18368
6. Feng, S., et al.: CPFNet: context pyramid fusion network for medical image segmentation. IEEE Trans. Med. Imaging **39**(10), 3008–3018 (2020). https://doi.org/10.1109/TMI.2020.2983721
7. Ferreira, A., et al.: How we won BraTS 2023 adult glioma challenge? Just faking it! Enhanced synthetic data augmentation and model ensemble for brain tumour segmentation (2024). https://arxiv.org/abs/2402.17317
8. Fonov, V.S., Evans, A.C., McKinstry, R.C., Almli, C.R., Collins, D.L.: Unbiased nonlinear average age-appropriate brain templates from birth to adulthood. NeuroImage **47**, S102 (2009). ISSN 1053-8119. https://doi.org/10.1016/S1053-8119(09)70884-5. https://www.sciencedirect.com/science/article/pii/S1053811909708845. Organization for Human Brain Mapping 2009 Annual Meeting
9. Growcott, S., Dembrey, T., Patel, R., Eaton, D., Cameron, A.: Inter-observer variability in target volume delineations of benign and metastatic brain tumours for stereotactic radiosurgery: results of a national quality assurance programme. Clin. Oncol. **32**(1), 13–25 (2020). ISSN 0936-6555. https://doi.org/10.1016/j.clon.2019.06.015. https://www.sciencedirect.com/science/article/pii/S0936655519302766
10. Hatamizadeh, A., Nath, V., Tang, Y., Yang, D., Roth, H.R., Xu, D.: Swin UNETR: swin transformers for semantic segmentation of brain tumors in MRI images. In: Crimi, A., Bakas, S. (eds.) Brainlesion: Glioma, Multiple Sclerosis, Stroke and Traumatic Brain Injuries, pp. 272–284. Springer, Cham (2022)

11. Hu, L.S., Hawkins-Daarud, A., Wang, L., Li, J., Swanson, K.R.: Imaging of intratumoral heterogeneity in high-grade glioma. Cancer Lett. **477**, 97–106 (2020)
12. Huang, Z., et al.: STU-Net: scalable and transferable medical image segmentation models empowered by large-scale supervised pre-training (2023). https://arxiv.org/abs/2304.06716
13. Isensee, F., et al.: Automated brain extraction of multisequence MRI using artificial neural networks. Hum. Brain Mapp. **40**(17), 4952–4964 (2019). https://doi.org/10.1002/hbm.24750
14. Isensee, F., Jaeger, P.F., Kohl, S.A.A., Petersen, J., Maier-Hein, K.H.: nnU-Net: a self-configuring method for deep learning-based biomedical image segmentation. Nat. Methods **18**(2), 203–211 (2021). ISSN 1548-7105. https://doi.org/10.1038/s41592-020-01008-z
15. Isensee, F., et al.: nnU-Net revisited: a call for rigorous validation in 3D medical image segmentation (2024). https://arxiv.org/abs/2404.09556
16. Karargyris, A., Umeton, R., Sheller, M.J., et al.: Federated benchmarking of medical artificial intelligence with MedPerf. Nat. Mach. Intell. **5**(7), 799–810 (2023). https://doi.org/10.1038/s42256-023-00652-2
17. Kato, S., Hotta, K.: Adaptive t-vMF dice loss: an effective expansion of dice loss for medical image segmentation. Comput. Biol. Med. **168**, 107695 (2024). ISSN 0010-4825. https://doi.org/10.1016/j.compbiomed.2023.107695. https://www.sciencedirect.com/science/article/pii/S0010482523011605
18. Kazerooni, A.F., Khalili, N., et al.: The brain tumor segmentation (BraTS) challenge 2023: focus on pediatrics (CBTN-CONNECT-DIPGR-ASNR-MICCAI BraTS-PEDs) (2024). https://arxiv.org/abs/2305.17033
19. Kazerooni, A.F., Khalili, N., et al.: The brain tumor segmentation in pediatrics (BraTS-PEDs) challenge: focus on pediatrics (CBTN-CONNECT-DIPGR-ASNR-MICCAI BraTS-PEDs) (2024). https://arxiv.org/abs/2404.15009
20. LaBella, D., Adewole, M., et al.: The ASNR-MICCAI brain tumor segmentation (BraTS) challenge 2023: intracranial meningioma (2023). https://arxiv.org/abs/2305.07642
21. LaBella, D., Abramova, V., Astaraki, M., et al.: Analysis of the 2024 BraTS meningioma radiotherapy planning automated segmentation challenge (2025). https://arxiv.org/abs/2405.18383
22. Luu, H.M., Park, S.-H.: Extending nn-UNet for brain tumor segmentation. In: Crimi, A., Bakas, S. (eds.) Brainlesion: Glioma, Multiple Sclerosis, Stroke and Traumatic Brain Injuries, pp. 173–186. Springer, Cham (2022)
23. Ma, J., Li, F., Wang, B.: U-Mamba: enhancing long-range dependency for biomedical image segmentation (2024). https://arxiv.org/abs/2401.04722
24. Maleki, N., Amiruddin, R., et al.: Analysis of the MICCAI brain tumor segmentation – metastases (BraTS-METs) 2025 lighthouse challenge: brain metastasis segmentation on pre- and post-treatment MRI (2025). https://arxiv.org/abs/2504.12527
25. Menze, B., et al.: Analyzing magnetic resonance imaging data from glioma patients using deep learning. Comput. Med. Imaging Graph. **88**, 101828 (2021). ISSN 0895-6111. https://doi.org/10.1016/j.compmedimag.2020.101828. https://www.sciencedirect.com/science/article/pii/S0895611120301233
26. Menze, B.H., Jakab, A., Bauer, S., et al.: The multimodal brain tumor image segmentation benchmark (BraTS). IEEE Trans. Med. Imaging **34**(10), 1993–2024 (2015). https://doi.org/10.1109/TMI.2014.2377694

27. Milletari, F., Navab, N., Ahmadi, S.-A.: V-Net: fully convolutional neural networks for volumetric medical image segmentation. In: 2016 Fourth International Conference on 3D Vision (3DV), pp. 565–571 (2016). https://doi.org/10.1109/3DV.2016.79
28. Moawad, A.W., Janas, A., et al.: The brain tumor segmentation (BraTS-METs) challenge 2023: brain metastasis segmentation on pre-treatment MRI (2024). https://arxiv.org/abs/2306.00838
29. Myronenko, A.: 3D MRI brain tumor segmentation using autoencoder regularization. In: Crimi, A., et al. (eds.) BrainLes 2018. LNCS, vol. 11384, pp. 311–320. Springer, Cham (2019). https://doi.org/10.1007/978-3-030-11726-9_28
30. Ostrom, Q.T., Francis, S.S., Barnholtz-Sloan, J.S.: Epidemiology of brain and other CNS tumors. Current Neurol. Neurosci. Rep. **21**(12), 68 (2021). ISSN 1534-6293. https://doi.org/10.1007/s11910-021-01152-9
31. Rohlfing, T., Zahr, N.M., Sullivan, E.V., Pfefferbaum, A.: The SRI24 multichannel atlas of normal adult human brain structure. Hum. Brain Mapp. **31**(5), 798–819 (2010)
32. Ronneberger, O., Fischer, P., Brox, T.: U-Net: convolutional networks for biomedical image segmentation. In: Navab, N., Hornegger, J., Wells, W.M., Frangi, A.F. (eds.) MICCAI 2015. LNCS, vol. 9351, pp. 234–241. Springer, Cham (2015). https://doi.org/10.1007/978-3-319-24574-4_28
33. Roy, S., et al.: MedNext: transformer-driven scaling of convnets for medical image segmentation. In: Greenspan, H., et al. (eds.) Medical Image Computing and Computer Assisted Intervention – MICCAI 2023, pp. 405–415. Springer, Cham (2023)
34. Roy, S., et al.: MedNext: transformer-driven scaling of convnets for medical image segmentation (2024). https://arxiv.org/abs/2303.09975
35. Woo, S., et al.: ConvNeXt V2: co-designing and scaling convnets with masked autoencoders (2023). https://arxiv.org/abs/2301.00808
36. Xie, X., et al.: CANet: context aware network with dual-stream pyramid for medical image segmentation. Biomed. Sig. Process. Control **81**, 104437 (2023). ISSN 1746-8094. https://doi.org/10.1016/j.bspc.2022.104437. https://www.sciencedirect.com/science/article/pii/S1746809422008916
37. Zeineldin, R.A., Karar, M.E. Burgert, O., Mathis-Ullrich, F.: Multimodal CNN networks for brain tumor segmentation in MRI: a BraTS 2022 challenge solution. In: Bakas, S., et al. (eds.) Brainlesion: Glioma, Multiple Sclerosis, Stroke and Traumatic Brain Injuries, pp. 127–137. Springer, Cham (2023)
38. Zhou, Z., Siddiquee, M.M.R., Tajbakhsh, N., Liang, J.: UNet++: redesigning skip connections to exploit multiscale features in image segmentation (2020). https://arxiv.org/abs/1912.05074

Challenge 3 – BraTS-MEN-RT

DeSURVAE: A Dual-Encoder Dual-Decoder Neural Network for GTV Semantic Segmentation of Meningioma Brain Tumor in Radiotherapy Planning

Nima Sadeghzadeh[1], Jason A. Correia[2], Samantha J. Holdsworth[3,4,5], Poul M. F. Nielsen[1], Michael Dragunow[3,6], Richard L. M. Faull[3,5], and Hamid Abbasi[1,3](✉)

[1] Auckland Bioengineering Institute, The University of Auckland, Auckland, New Zealand
{nima.sadeghzadeh,p.nielsen,h.abbasi}@auckland.ac.nz
[2] Department of Neurosurgery, Auckland City and Starship Hospitals, Auckland, New Zealand
[3] Centre for Brain Research, The University of Auckland, Auckland, New Zealand
{s.holdsworth,m.dragunow,rlm.faull}@auckland.ac.nz
[4] Mātai Medical Research Institute, Gisborne, New Zealand
[5] Department of Anatomy with Radiology, University of Auckland, Auckland, New Zealand
[6] Departments of Pharmacology and Clinical Pharmacology, The University of Auckland, Auckland, New Zealand

Abstract. Meningiomas are the most common primary central nervous system (CNS) tumors in adults, typically arising from arachnoid cells in the meninges. While often benign, their recurrence and treatment planning, particularly following surgical resection, require precise volumetric delineation. Accurate segmentation of postoperative gross tumor volume (GTV) in meningioma remains a largely unaddressed challenge in automated medical image analysis. This study proposes a novel hybrid architecture, DeSURVAE (Dual-encoder Swin UNETR VAE), designed to improve segmentation performance in this setting. DeSURVAE integrates a dual-encoder framework that combines convolutional and transformer-based encoders to jointly capture local and global contextual features. A variational autoencoder (VAE) branch is incorporated to regularize the latent space and improve generalization. The model was trained on a combination of the BraTS'24 meningioma radiotherapy dataset with 500 postoperative contrast-enhanced T1-weighted (T1W + C) MRIs, and the BraTS'23 meningioma dataset with 1,000 preoperative T1W + C MRIs with consistent single-label tumor delineations. DeSURVAE achieved an average lesion-wise Dice score of 0.779 ± 0.011 and a 95th percentile Hausdorff Distance (HD95) of 21.6 ± 2.51 mm. These results represent an improvement over baseline architectures, including SegResNet with 0.696 ± 0.012 Dice and 64.2 ± 2.70 mm HD95, as well as Swin UNETR with 0.711 ± 0.018 Dice and 57.3 ± 3.74 mm HD95. Stratified analysis across tumor sizes indicated consistent performance, with poor segmentation observed in only 8% of test cases. The results suggest that hybrid encoder designs combining convolutional and transformer-based representations, along with latent space regularization (VAE branch), can effectively address the variability inherent in postoperative imaging.

S. Bakas et al. (Eds.): MICCAI 2025, LNCS 16376, pp. 129–138, 2026.
https://doi.org/10.1007/978-3-032-16365-3_12

Keywords: Hybrid Neural Network · Transformer · BraTS · Variational Auto-Encoder · Dual Decoder

1 Introduction

Meningiomas are the most common CNS tumors in adults, especially among women [1–5]. They arise from arachnoid cells in the meninges, the protective layers surrounding the brain and spinal cord [1, 2]. World Health Organization classifies meningiomas into three grades: Grade I (least aggressive), Grade II (higher risk of recurrence), and Grade III (most aggressive, associated with poor clinical outcomes) [1, 2]. Tumors are commonly analyzed via magnetic resonance imaging (MRI) or computed tomography scans [1–3].

Gross tumor volume (GTV) represents the tumor area visible on post-contrast MRI scans, and its segmentation has a crucial role in radiation therapy planning [6–9]. Manual segmentation, however, is time-consuming, labor-intensive, and prone to inter-observer variability, often resulting in incomplete resection or suboptimal surgical planning that can exacerbate the situation, especially for small tumors (e.g., smaller than 3 ml) that are difficult to delineate manually [10–12]. On the other hand, an accurate automatic segmentation system addresses these challenges by providing consistent, reproducible, and rapid tumor delineation, reducing the dependency on human expertise and minimizing errors.

To date, automated segmentation techniques from medical images have proven effective in delivering consistent and precise delineations of brain tumors [13, 14]. In recent years, deep learning approaches have demonstrated state-of-the-art performance of more than 0.90 Dice score for pretreatment meningioma tumor segmentation, largely driven by the strong representational capacity of convolutional neural networks (CNNs) and transformers [15–17]. However, to the best of our knowledge, no study has specifically focused on postoperative meningioma GTV segmentation [9, 18], except for one nnU-Net, reporting 0.67 Dice score on BraTS'24 dataset [19]. To bridge this gap, we propose an approach for GTV segmentation in postoperative cranial/facial meningioma radiotherapy planning to support improved clinical outcomes.

2 Methods

2.1 Architecture Inspiration

Our architecture is a dual-encoder framework that integrates convolutional and transformer-based encoders to jointly capture local and global contextual features. Transformers are provenly great choices for segmentation due to their exceptional long-range feature extraction capabilities, drawing inspiration from the Swin UNETR [20], the winner of BraTS'21 with 0.889 Dice score. The task was to receive a 3D MRI with four channels of T1-weighed (T1W), contrast-enhanced T1W (T1W + C), T2-weighed (T2W), and fluid attenuation inversion recover (FLAIR) to segment three classes of the enhancing tumor (ET), tumor core (TC), and whole tumor (WT) [21]. Moreover, SegResNet architecture, the winner of BraTS'18 with 0.866 Dice on a similar task [22], combines a fully-convolutional encoder-decoder with a variational autoencoder (VAE) branch for bottleneck regularization. This branch encourages a structured latent space and helps the network to learn more robust feature representations for segmentation.

2.2 Dataset

We use BraTS'24 meningioma radiotherapy planning dataset which contains 500 T1W + C MRI scans showing intact or postoperative meningioma that underwent either conventional external beam radiotherapy or stereotactic radiosurgery [9]. Segmentations include a single-label target volume representing the GTV and any at-risk postoperative regions. For preoperative meningiomas, the target volume encompasses the entire GTV and associated nodular dural tail, while for postoperative cases, it includes at-risk resection cavity margins as determined by the corresponding treating institution.

To improve performance, we also include BraTS'23 pre-operative meningioma dataset for training, which contains 1,000 multimodal (T1W, T1W + C, T2W, and T2W-FLAIR) meningioma MRIs, with corresponding segmentations, including enhancing tumor (ET), non-enhancing tumor core (NETC), and surrounding non-enhancing FLAIR hyperintensity (SNFH) [3]. Fig. 1 shows three examples of each dataset. Images in the BraTS'24 dataset are defaced and in native acquisition space, while those in the BraTS'23 dataset are skull stripped and co-registered to the SRI24 atlas space.

2.3 Pre-processing

Before training, isotropic voxel resampling was implemented for BraTS'24 dataset to standardize the MRI resolutions to $1 \times 1 \times 1$ mm; however, BraTS'23 dataset was standardized by default and did not require this step. Moreover, we utilize only the T1W + C modality from the BraTS'23 dataset and merge the ET and NETC regions, excluding SNFH, to generate TC masks. This reformulation enables binary segmentation (i.e., tumor versus background) consistent with the characteristics of the BraTS'24 dataset. All MRIs were subsequently normalized using z-score normalization.

During training, the input 3D MRIs were randomly cropped to a $192 \times 192 \times 192$ region of interest. The average height, width, and depth that a tumor can have in the dataset is respectively $36.8 \times 41.6 \times 19.7$ (SD $23.8 \times 27.3 \times 14.4$) mm (each mm^3 corresponds to one $pixel^3$) with the largest being $140 \times 170 \times 105$ mm; therefore, a $192 \times 192 \times 192$ voxel patch sufficiently covers the entire tumor and most of the brain tissue without significant loss in data. The data was augmented through random intensity shifts, scaling, skew, rotation, and flipping.

2.4 Network Architecture

Inspired by the architectural designs of Swin UNETR and SegResNet, we combined key elements from both to develop a novel hybrid model. Our architecture follows a U-Net structure, incorporating both residual convolutional and transformer-based encoders, along with a decoder and a VAE branch. We named the architecture DeSURVAE (Dual-encoder Swin UNETR VAE) for convenience and presented it in Fig. 2.

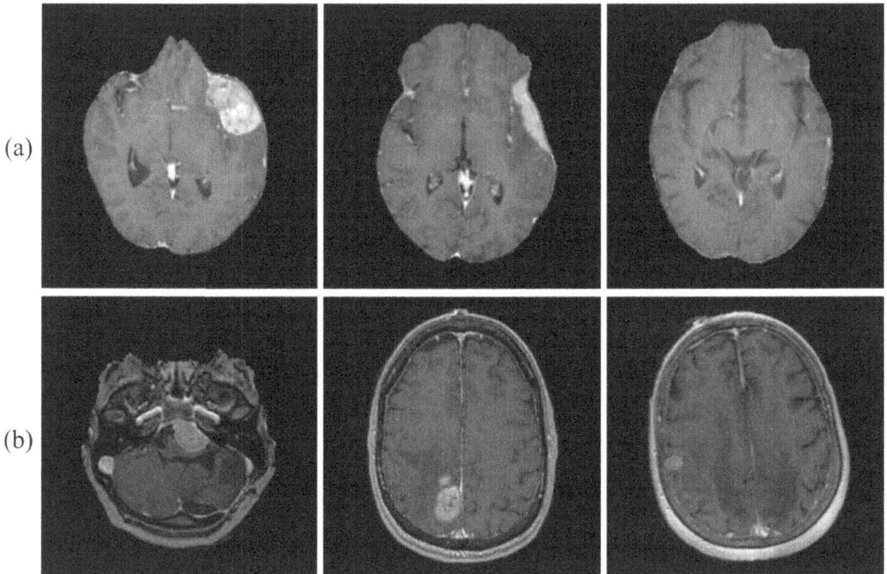

Fig. 1. Examples of the (a) BraTS'23 and (b) BraTS'24 datasets. Tumors are indicated with red outline for a better visualizations, generated using Matplotlib from the masks provided by BraTS.

Specifically, in the transformer encoder, a 3D 1-channel input volume with dimensions H × W × D × 1 (where H, W, and D are all set to 192) is linearly embedded and passed through four hierarchical Swin layer blocks [23]. Each block progressively reduces the spatial dimensions while increasing feature channel depth, yielding feature maps of size $\frac{H}{2^i} \times \frac{W}{2^i} \times \frac{D}{2^i} \times 2^{i-1}F$ (adapted from Swin UNETR [20]), where F is a constant control variable and is set to 48 (maximum possible value due to the GPU constraints), while i is the block index and is used in this paper to refer to the feature map dimension configuration. The bottleneck block of the encoder ($i = 5$) is a convolutional block and is to capture high-level abstract representations. On the other hand, the convolutional encoder receives the same input in parallel and passes through four convolutional blocks with an identical feature map setting culminating in the bottleneck at $i = 5$.

In the decoder, feature maps from each encoder blocks are fed via skip connections into additional dedicated convolutional blocks, concatenated with the output of a previous block, and then upsampled using a deconvolution block. The decoder blocks mirror the encoder in reverse order, processing each level from $i = 4$ down to $i = 1$. The final feature maps are then passed through an additional deconvolution block with the $i = 1$ configuration, followed by a convolution block to restore the feature map size to its original input dimensions.

Simultaneously, an additional decoder branch (i.e., VAE) is introduced to reconstruct the original input image. This branch receives the bottleneck feature maps (at $i = 5$) and passes to a convolution block ($i = 4$ configuration), from which a Gaussian distribution $\mathcal{N}(\mu, \sigma^2)$ is estimated (i.e., in variational bottleneck) and forwarded into four upstream blocks, culminating in a convolution block with $i = 1$ configuration. This branch encourages a structured latent space in the bottleneck and helps the network to learn more robust feature representations for segmentation.

Lastly, the models, including the baselines (i.e., Swin UNETR and SegResNet), were trained for 500 epochs via Dice loss, Adam optimizer with 10^{-4} learning rate, 10^{-5} weight decay, cosine annealing scheduler, and using three-fold cross-validation. BraTS'24 dataset was split to a 67:33, with the 67% sets combined with the entire BraTS'23 for training, and the 33% sets for testing. After training, the VAE branch was discarded as it only served to tune learnable parameters while training. Training was conducted on NVIDIA A100 82GB GPUs, using Python 3.9 and PyTorch 2.5 via Cuda 12.6. Lastly, lesion-wise Dice and 95th percentile Hausdorff Distance (HD95) scores were used to evaluate the models and enable consistent comparison with future studies. For testing, normalized surface distance (NSD) is reported per evaluation by BraTS.

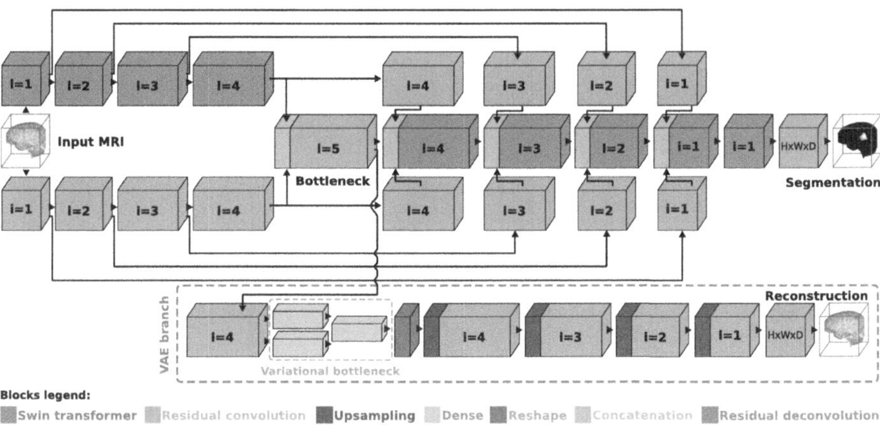

Fig. 2. DeSURVAE architecture. Residual blocks consist of two consecutive convolution or deconvolution layers (as needed), each preceded by group normalization and ReLU activation. A skip connection adds the input directly to the output of the second layer, for residual learning.

3 Results

The evaluation results (Table 1) show that DeSURVAE achieved a lesion-wise Dice score of 0.779 ± 0.011 [24] which is 6.8–8.3% improvement from the baselines; and an average of 21.6 ± 2.51 mm HD95 which is 35–42 mm lower than the baselines. Figure 3 shows lesion-wise Dice and HD95 scores for different tumor volumes, indicating that only 8% of the test data have lower than 1% Dice, while the majority fall in the 80th accuracy percentile. Accurate and inaccurate segmentation examples are also available in Fig. 4 with top rows showing successful segmentations (> 0.8 Dice), while bottom rows show challenging cases (< 0.5 Dice), while Fig. 5 compares the three models side-by-side. Results do not show any specific patterns, such as strength in a particular tumor location or size. Challenges in both figures could be associated with motion artifacts.

DeSURVAE generally showed better alignment with ground truth, particularly around complex boundaries and resection margins. However, BraTS reported 0.63 ± 0.30 Dice and 0.42 ± 0.27 NSD_1 for DeSURVAE on the official test set, presumably marking the lower bound of its performance across unseen data.

Table 1. Evaluation results for three-fold cross-validation.

Architecture	Lesion-wise Dice	Lesion-wise HD95
DeSURVAE	**0.779 ± 0.011**	**21.6 ± 2.51**
Swin UNETR	0.711 ± 0.018	57.3 ± 3.74
SegResNet	0.696 ± 0.012	64.2 ± 2.70

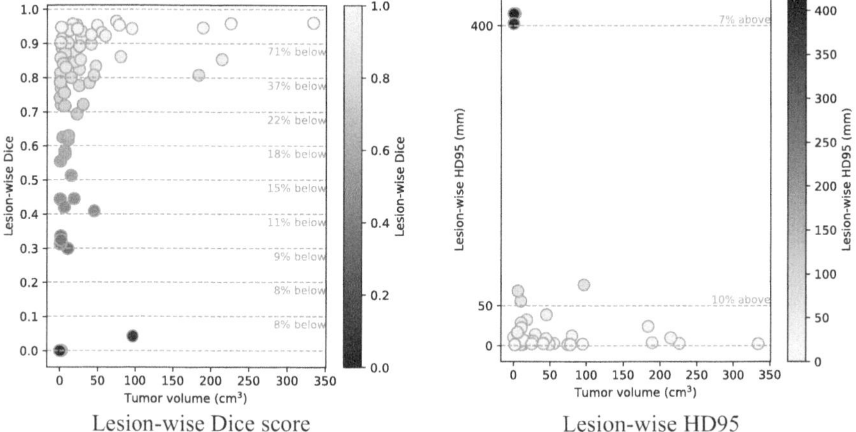

Fig. 3. Quantitative evaluation of DeSURVAE performance across test cases. The horizontal dashed lines indicate what percentage of the test data falls below or above the line.

4 Discussion and Conclusion

We proposed the DeSURVAE architecture, which utilizes a dual-encoder framework combining the long-range feature extraction of Swin transformers with the local feature capture of residual convolutional blocks, alongside a VAE branch for latent space regularization. DeSURVAE demonstrates significant advancements in postoperative meningioma GTV segmentation, achieving high lesion-wise Dice and low HD95, outperforming baseline models of Swin UNETR, SegResNet, and nnU-Net [19], achieving substantial training performance gains. The model's ability to segment most of the test cases effectively, as shown in Fig. 3, highlights its potential to enhance radiotherapy planning by providing consistent, reproducible, and accurate tumor delineations, thereby reducing inter-observer variability and improving clinical outcomes.

The results indicate that a hybrid architecture more effectively captures both local and global context via multiple branches, as the baseline single-branch models achieved lower Dice scores and higher HD95. Future work should also explore the model's applicability to other CNS tumors and validate its performance in prospective clinical settings to ensure robustness and scalability.

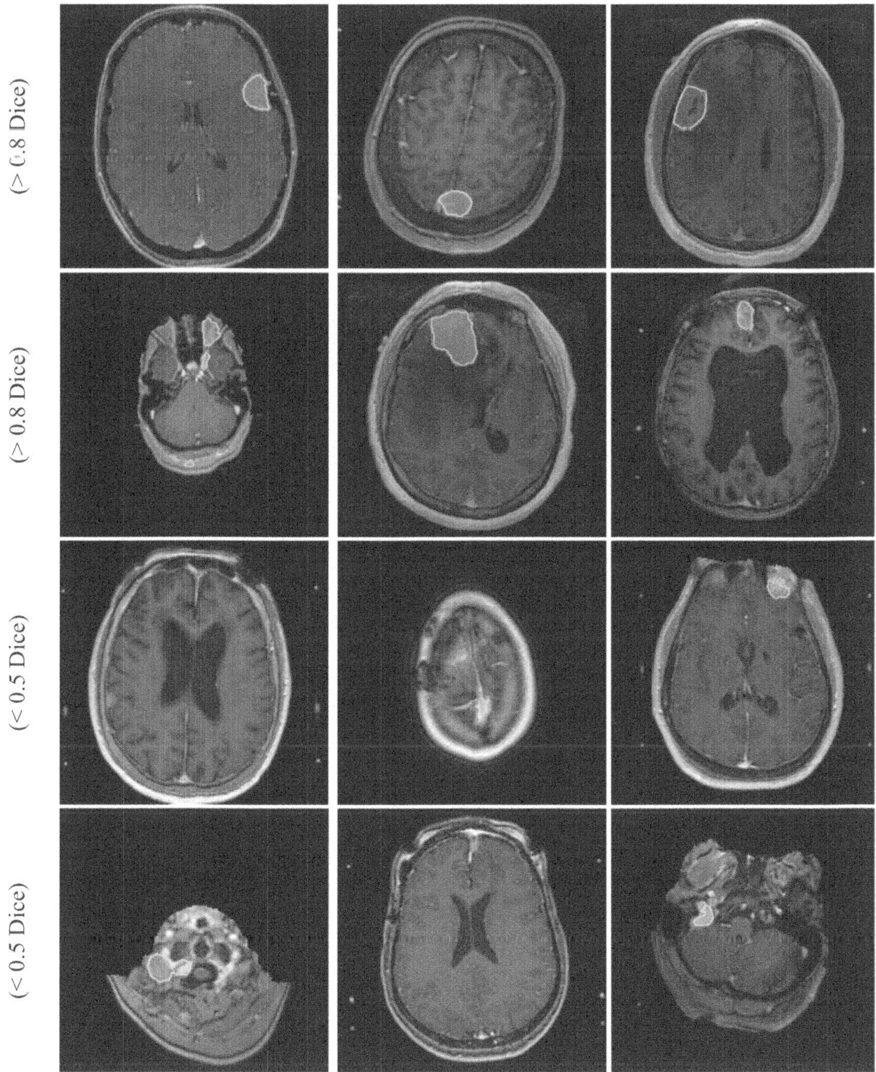

Fig. 4. Accurate and inaccurate segmentations. Red: ground truth, Green: segmentation. Brains were not aligned to conform with BraTS'25 evaluation criteria [9].

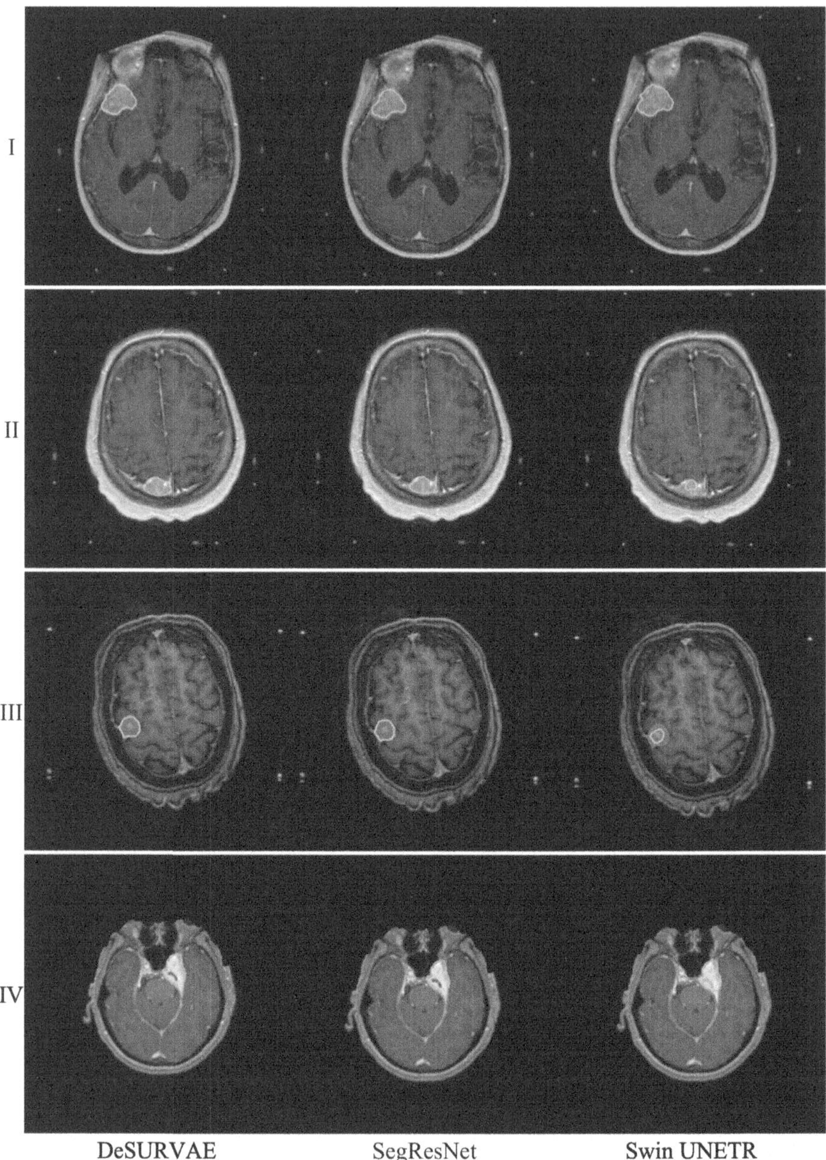

Fig. 5. Model comparisons for samples I-IV across the three models. Brains were not aligned to conform with BraTS'25 evaluation criteria [9].

Acknowledgements. We acknowledge the financial support provided by the Freemasons Neurosurgery Research Unit at the Centre for Brain Research, University of Auckland, for this study.

Disclosure of Interests. The authors have no competing interests to declare that are relevant to the content of this article.

References

1. Yang, L., Wang, T., Zhang, J., Kang, S., Xu, S., Wang, K.: Deep learning–based automatic segmentation of meningioma from T1-weighted contrast-enhanced MRI for preoperative meningioma differentiation using radiomic features. BMC Med. Imaging. **24**, 56 (2024)
2. Mostafa, H., Haddad, N., Mohamed, H., Taha, Z.A.E.H., Classification, B.M.R.I.: Segmentation of Glioma, Pituitary and Meningioma Tumors Using Deep Learning Approaches. In: 2024 Intelligent Methods, Systems, And Applications (IMSA), vol. 2024, pp. 482–488. IEEE, Giza, Egypt
3. LaBella, D., et al.: The ASNR-MICCAI Brain Tumor Segmentation (BraTS) Challenge 2023: Intracranial Meningioma, (2023)
4. Sadeghzadeh, N., et al.: Deterministic Value of Neurosurgeon-Assessed Meningioma Features in MRI and CT Scans for Predicting Tumor Growth Risk and Volumetric Progression, in: IEEE. Christchurch, New Zealand (2025)
5. Sadeghzadeh, N., et al.: Single-scan machine learning prediction of meningioma tumor growth risk and progression using neurosurgeon-evaluated MRI and CT scan features, IEEE, Copenhagen, Denmark (2025)
6. Hanna, C., et al.: Review of meningioma diagnosis and management. Egypt. J. Neurosurg. **38**, 16 (2023)
7. Wang, J.Z., et al.: International consortium on Meningiomas consensus review on scientific advances and treatment paradigms for clinicians, researchers, and patients. Neuro-Oncology. (2024)
8. Farajzadeh, N., Sadeghzadeh, N., Hashemzadeh, M.: A fully-convolutional residual encoder-decoder neural network to localize breast cancer on histopathology images. Comput. Biol. Med. **147**, 105698 (2022)
9. LaBella, D., et al.: brain tumor segmentation (brats) challenge 2024: meningioma radiotherapy planning automated segmentation (2024)
10. Bouget, D., Pedersen, A., Hosainey, S.A.M., Solheim, O., Reinertsen, I.: Meningioma segmentation in T1-weighted MRI leveraging global context and attention mechanisms. Front. Radiol. **1** (2021)
11. Maniar, K.M., et al.: Traditional machine learning methods versus deep learning for meningioma Classification, grading, outcome prediction, and segmentation: a systematic review and meta-analysis. World Neurosurg. **179**, e119–e134 (2023)
12. Farajzadeh, N., Sadeghzadeh, N., Hashemzadeh, M.: Brain tumor segmentation and classification on MRI via deep hybrid representation learning. Expert Syst. Appl. **224**, 119963 (2023)
13. Saifullah, S., Dreżewski, R.: Brain tumor segmentation using ensemble CNN-transfer learning models: DeepLabV3plus and ResNet50 approach. In: Franco, L., de Mulatier, C., Paszynski, M., Krzhizhanovskaya, V.V., Dongarra, J.J., Sloot, P.M.A. (eds.) Computational Science – ICCS 2024, pp. 340–354. Springer Nature Switzerland, Cham (2024)
14. Lv, C., et al.: MamTrans: magnetic resonance imaging segmentation algorithm for high-grade gliomas and brain meningiomas integrating attention mechanisms and state-space models. Quant. Imaging Med. Surg. **15**, 5796–5810 (2025)
15. Bai, H., et al.: Meningioma segmentation with GV-UNet: a hybrid model using a ghost module and vision transformer. SIViP. **18**, 2377–2390 (2024)
16. Huang, H., Liu, P., Liu, J.: TAGU-net: transformer convolution hybrid-based U-net with attention gate for atypical meningioma segmentation. IEEE Access. **11**, 53207–53223 (2023)
17. Rai, H.M., Yoo, J., Dashkevych, S.: Two-headed UNetEfficientNets for parallel execution of segmentation and classification of brain tumors: incorporating postprocessing techniques with connected component labelling. J. Cancer Res. Clin. Oncol. **150**, 220 (2024)

18. Bianconi, A., et al.: Deep learning-based algorithm for postoperative glioblastoma MRI segmentation: a promising new tool for tumor burden assessment. Brain Inf. **10**, 26 (2023)
19. Hazaimeh, H., Nemma, R., Al-Ajarmeh, A., Alkasabrah, A.R.: Automated segmentation of meningioma gross tumor volume (GTV) in radiotherapy planning using deep learning (nnU-net) (P9-6.008). Neurology. **104**, 1640 (2025)
20. Hatamizadeh, A., Nath, V., Tang, Y., Yang, D., Rothm, H., Xu, D.: Swin UNETR: Swin Transformers for Semantic Segmentation of Brain Tumors in MRI Images (2022)
21. Baid, U., et al.: The RSNA-ASNR-MICCAI BraTS 2021 benchmark on brain tumor segmentation and radiogenomic classification, (2021)
22. Myronenko, A.: 3D MRI Brain Tumor Segmentation Using Autoencoder Regularization (2018).
23. Liu, Z., et al.: Swin Transformer: Hierarchical Vision Transformer Using Shifted Windows, pp. 10012–10022 (2021)
24. Karargyris, A., et al.: Mattson, federated benchmarking of medical artificial intelligence with MedPerf. Nat. Mach. Intell. **5**, 799–810 (2023)

Boundary-Aware Approach for Meningioma Segmentation in Radiotherapy Planning MRI

Valeriia Abramova(✉), Agustin Cartaya Lathulerie, Uma M. Lal-Trehan Estrada, Cansu Yalçın, Rachika E. Hamadache, Clara Lisazo, Micaela Rivas Díaz, Adrià Casamitjana, Arnau Oliver, and Xavier Lladó

Computer Vision and Robotics Institute, University of Girona, Girona, Spain
valeriia.abramova@udg.edu

Abstract. Meningiomas are the most prevalent type of primary intracranial tumor, with radiotherapy commonly used for treating high-grade cases. Precise identification and delineation of tumor boundaries on magnetic resonance imaging (MRI) are essential for effective radiotherapy planning. However, this task is both time-consuming and labor-intensive, highlighting the need for automated segmentation solutions in clinical practice. To support progress in this area, the BraTS-MEN-RT challenge was launched in 2024, and continued in 2025, aiming to benchmark automated meningioma segmentation on MRI. In this paper, we describe our submission to the 2025 edition of the challenge, which utilizes the widely adopted nnU-Net framework. Our approach specifically focuses on improving the pre-processing steps and the delineation of tumor borders. It ranked first during the testing stage of the challenge, achieving the average Dice score of 0.816.

Keywords: Meningioma · nnU-Net · Brain tumor segmentation

1 Introduction

Meningiomas are the most prevalent intracranial tumors and can be characterized with high mortality and morbidity rates [1]. Radiotherapy is a common treatment solution, and all World Health Organization (WHO) grade 2 and 3 meningiomas go through radiotherapy, while WHO grade 1 meningiomas can also be eligible for radiotherapy in some cases [2]. Accurate segmentation of the preoperative meningioma gross tumor volume (GTV) is essential for radiotherapy planning, and for this purpose magnetic resonance imaging (MRI), especially post-contrast T1-weighted sequence (T1c) is used in clinical settings. However, GTV segmentation is a complex and time-consuming task, which requires certain level of expertise [2]. Therefore, there is a need in reliable automatic meningioma segmentation methods that can assist clinicians in defining the GTV necessary for radiotherapy planning.

S. Bakas et al. (Eds.): MICCAI 2025, LNCS 16376, pp. 139–147, 2026.
https://doi.org/10.1007/978-3-032-16365-3_13

Currently, there is a limited research on automated meningioma GTV segmentation [2]. Since the works of previous Brain Tumor Segmentation (BraTS) challenges mainly focused on preoperative tumors and the images were preprocessed in a certain way, the clinical utility of those results remained limited. Therefore, in 2024, the Brain Tumor Segmentation Meningioma Radiotherapy (BraTS-MEN-RT) challenge was organized to create a benchmark for automated segmentation of meningioma GTV based on pre-radiotherapy planning brain MRI exams. The results of this challenge identified the state-of-the-art methods for meningioma segmentation, and in 2025 the challenge was opened for submissions again.

In this work, we present our proposal for meningioma GTV segmentation from T1c brain MRI scans based on nnU-Net framework [3]. nnU-Net is based on U-Net architecture [4,5] which is currently a state-of-the-art in many biomedical segmentation tasks. We studied the impact of performing additional preprocessing of the training images such as bias field correction inside the brain area. Moreover, we introduced a two class segmentation inside nnU-Net (the inner part of the tumor and boundary region) to improve overall segmentation accuracy.

2 Methods

2.1 Data

The BraTS-MEN-RT 2025 challenge dataset is the same as the previous year edition, and consists of 750 brain MRI post-contrast T1-weighted scans (T1c) from 7 different clinical sites across United States. Notice that the scans from one of the institutions are not included in neither training nor validation sets, and are reserved exclusively for testing stage [2]. The main difference of 2025 edition of the challenge compared to the previous year BraTS-MEN-RT challenge is that a subset of a testing cohort will include annotations from multiple annotators. This is done to compare the results of submitted algorithms against a variety of human experts to discover the role of intra-observer and inter-observer variability for meningioma segmentation.

The dataset is made publicly available by the challenge organizers[1]. They released 500 images with ground truth masks available for the training stage, and 70 images without masks for the validation stage. The private test set consisting of 180 cases will be used to evaluate the participants algorithms to determine the final ranking.

Compared to other subtasks of the BraTS-Lighthouse 2025 Challenge, the pre-processing done in the BraTS-MEN-RT challenge tried to mimic the data available for most radiotherapy planning scenarios. Firstly, the images were converted from DICOM and DICOM-RT to NIfTI format. The MRI scans were presented in their native acquisition space and an automated defacing was performed to keep patient anonymity while preserving intracranial tissues other

[1] https://www.synapse.org/Synapse:syn64153130/wiki/631057.

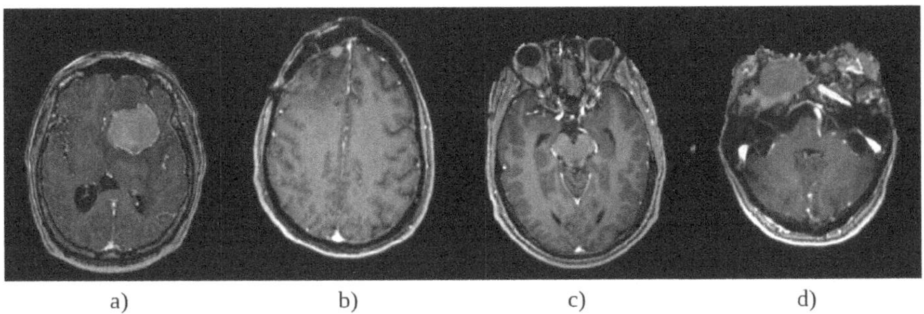

Fig. 1. Different examples of the provided training set. There is a high variability in the sizes of meningiomas (a, b). The scans are not skull stripped and some parts of meningiomas can be located outside of the brain in the intracranial area (c, d).

than brain which can also include meningiomas. Since the scans can be in both preoperative and postoperative settings, the target ground truth volume (GTV) was defined as either the portion of the tumor visible on the T1c MRI for the preoperative protocol or post-op resection bed and any residual enhancing tumor visible on the T1c MRI for postoperative protocol. Some examples of the images together with the corresponding ground truth masks available in BraTS-MEN-RT are shown in the Fig. 1.

We also performed an additional pre-processing as part of our approach. Firstly, since the provided images were not skull-stripped, we extracted the brain mask using TotalSegmentator toolbox [6]. We used this brain mask as an additional input for N4 bias field correction algorithm from SimpleITK [7], so that only voxels of the brain were used to estimate the bias field. In Sect. 3, we will analyze the influence of this pre-processing step on the final segmentation results.

2.2 Model

We based our approach on the standard 3D configuration of the nnU-Net [3] with the resolution of $1.1 \times 0.9375 \times 0.9375$ mm^3, the patch size of $96 \times 160 \times 160$ and batch size of 2. The architecture we used was a plain convolutional U-Net trained for 1000 epochs using as a loss function the combination of Dice and binary cross-entropy losses and a stochastic gradient descent optimizer [3].

For the training of our approach, we employ the two-class region-based training strategy introduced in the nnU-Net framework, initially proposed for gliomas segmentation in the BraTS challenge [8]. In that case, the target areas that were used to compute the metrics were combined from the individual classes represented in the dataset. In contrast, in our case in the BraTS-MEN-RT 2025 challenge, in order to improve segmentation of the boundaries of the tumors, we used the multi-class training of nnU-Net model to be able to train at the same time a model that can predict the full tumor segmentation and also a good contour segmentation. To perform this multi-class segmentation, we have to define the ground truth label for the tumor border, which was computed as the difference between the original ground truth mask and an eroded version of the same ground truth mask using a square structure element of size $3 \times 3 \times 3$. Therefore, the regions provided for the nnU-Net training were: (*i*) the foreground, consisting of the inner part of the tumor, and (*ii*) the specific region, representing only the tumor boundary. Note that our proposed boundary region consists only of the pixels existing in the original ground truth label.

We trained our model in a 5-fold cross validation manner on the training set (N = 450), splitting it into 5 folds following a proportion of 80% of the images for training and 20% for validation per fold. Notice that we separated 50 scans from the provided training set to internally evaluate our approach and the proposed modifications prior to opening of the validation stage. A weighted average ensemble of the 5 models provided by the cross validation strategy was computed inside nnU-Net framework when performing inference in the validation set and the internal testing subset. Since the proposed model predicts 2 class labels, the inner part of the tumor and its boundary, in inference we combined both classes to produce a single segmentation label.

All approaches were implemented using PyTorch 2.2.1 and experiments were run on an NVIDIA TITAN V with 12 GB RAM with nnU-Net 2.5.1. The erosion operation was performed using scipy library of the version 1.11.3.

3 Experimental Results

3.1 Metrics

The BraTS-MEN-RT challenge utilizes two metrics to evaluate the performance of submitted methods: lesion-wise Dice score and normalized surface distance (NSD), which measures the boundary overlap between the predicted and ground truth segmentations. NSD is computed at two tolerance values (0.5 and 1.0). This is different from the previous editions of BraTS challenge, where the lesion-wise Hausdorff distance-95 was used instead of NSD.

3.2 Quantitative and Qualitative Results

In this section, we describe the different experiments performed to choose the best model configuration for the final approach to be used for the testing phase of BraTS-MEN-RT challenge.

Firstly, we carried an experiment to analyze the influence of our additional pre-processing of the training images on the final results. We trained two models in a 5-fold cross validation manner with exactly the same hyperparameters and train/val splits, but in the first case we used the original training images, and in the second case we used pre-processed images. After evaluating this experiments, we also analyzed the effect of adding the tumor boundary information as an additional label when performing the region-based training of nnU-Net. We tested all these configurations on our internal test set, separated from the initial training dataset. From the results, we noticed that training with pre-processed images improved all the metrics of interest, e.g. the mean Dice score improved from 0.625 to 0.676, and the mean NSD at tolerance of 1.0 improved from 0.518 to 0.564. Moreover, we observed that performing the two class region-based training on the original images instead of a standard single-class segmentation enhanced the segmentation results, improving the mean Dice score from 0.625 to 0.677. We also ran inference of all the mentioned cross validation ensembles on the validation set and submitted the resulting masks for an online evaluation. The inference results on the official challenge validation set are presented in the Table 1.

Table 1. Results of ensembles of nnU-Net models from 5-fold cross validation trained on either the original or pre-processed images with and without incorporation of tumor border as an additional class. The results are presented for the validation dataset (N=70, results obtained after submission)

	Lesion-wise Dice score ↑	Lesion-wise NSD@0.5 ↑	Lesion-wise NSD@1.0 ↑
	Inference on 70 validation cases (ensemble of cross validation models)		
Original images	0.768 ± 0.290	0.500 ± 0.254	0.636 ± 0.294
Pre-processed images	0.826 ± 0.200	0.541 ± 0.225	0.694 ± 0.250
Original images + border	0.827 ± 0.196	0.533 ± 0.209	0.703 ± 0.237
Pre-processed images + border	0.843 ± 0.160	0.547 ± 0.214	0.707 ± 0.238

From these online validation results, we noticed that similarly to our internal test subset, the segmentation results on the validation images improved when images were initially pre-processed. Analyzing the validation results case by case, we observed that the effect of pre-processing was not so significant for big and well defined lesions since they were initially segmented very well (Fig. 2a,b); but we noticed significantly improved results for cases where meningiomas were smaller and/or located outside of the brain in intracranial structures. For example, for one case with small meningioma located outside of the brain tissues, using pre-processed images improved the Dice score from 0 to 0.932 (Fig. 2c and d). We noticed a similar behavior when analyzing the results on the internal test subset within our cross validation.

Moreover, from Table 1 we observed an improvement of the results when performing two class region-based training when training with either original or pre-processed images in comparison to the same input images but a single-class training. In addition, in this case we also observed that region-based training with pre-processed images surpassed the same with original images. Since in this setting we provided two ground truth regions for training, the inner part of

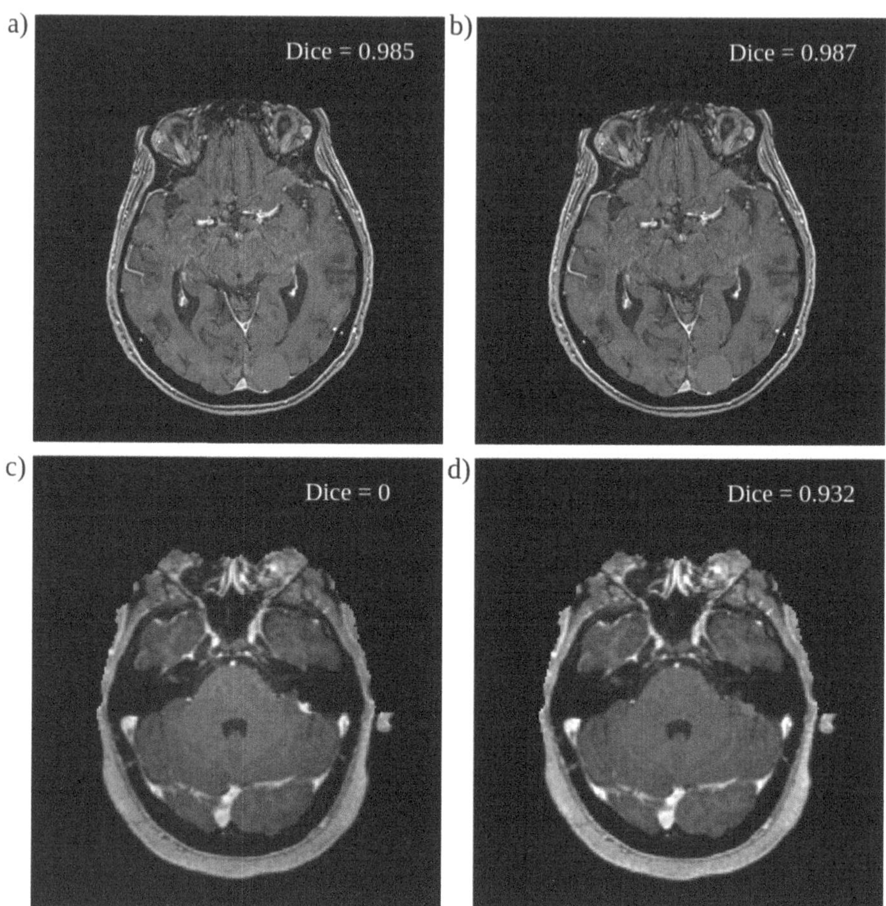

Fig. 2. Example of segmentations obtained when the training was done on original images (a, c) and on pre-processed images (b, d). We noticed that for some tumors of larger size and round shape the results did not improve significantly since cases already had high Dice score (>0.98) after initial training. However, for small lesions located outside of the brain, training with pre-processed images could significantly improve segmentation metrics (c, d), improving the Dice score from 0 to 0.932.

the tumor, and only the lesion boundary, nnU-Net oversampled this region, generating more training patches with meningiomas. We also observed that one case had an empty prediction when tested with the model trained on original images with a binary segmentation model, however we obtained a Dice score of 0.528 for this case when using the model trained with pre-processed in a two class region-based setting. Individually analyzing the results obtained in the online validation stage, we noticed that for some cases even when overall volumetric Dice score was not improved with the region-based training, the normalized surface distance, which specifically focuses on the boundary overlap, increased, therefore, showing the effect of the inclusion of the boundary information within the model. Qualitative results obtained with two class region-based training compared to a standard single-class training are shown on Fig. 3. From the figure we can say that two class region-based training helped to segment more true positive voxels without significantly oversegmenting the lesion. Despite the fact that in the challenge the Hausdorff distance metric was not tracked, we also computed it in all our experiments, and it showed the lowest results for region-based training with pre-processed images (average HD95 of 13.02 mm vs. 50.47 mm for the model trained on original images in a binary segmentation setting), meaning that in this case we achieve a better segmentation and specially the better delineation of the boundaries.

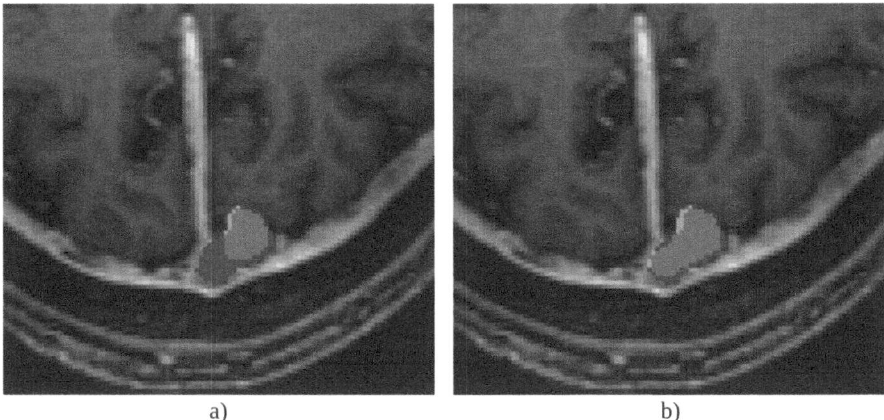

Fig. 3. Example of segmentations obtained with the ensemble of models trained using the original truth lesion mask (a) and ensemble of models trained in a two class region-based manner with tumor boundary as an additional region (b). The colors of the segmentation mask represent: true positive pixels (red), false positive pixels ( ), false negative pixels (blue). Oversampling patches containing ground truth voxels helps the model to segments more true positive voxels without significantly increasing false positives. (Color figure online)

Considering all the performed experiments, for our final submission to the testing stage of the challenge [9] we chose the following configuration of nnU-Net: an ensemble of 5 models trained within a cross validation framework using the provided training images after additional pre-processing. The models were trained using a two class region-based training with full tumor and its boundary as separate classes. At inference time, the obtained segmentation mask was binarized to coincide with the initial binary segmentation task. During testing stage, this approach achieved the average Dice score of 0.816 ± 0.193 and the average NSD at 1.0 tolerance of 0.699 ± 0.239, ranking first among other submitted approaches.

4 Discussion

In this work, we described our approach used for the BraTS-MEN-RT challenge. Similarly to our submission for the last year's edition of the challenge, we focused on improving tumor boundary segmentation. Moreover, since initial pre-processing of the dataset is limited to defacing only, we applied bias field correction inside the brain area of the provided images.

As nnU-Net is widely used for biomedical segmentation tasks, being a winner in different challenges, we used it as our baseline model in its automatically configured setting. However, in our proposal we focused the training on both the tumor region and also tumor boundaries, providing this way an overall better segmentation results (both in terms of volumetric Dice and boundary specific NSD). We compared the results of the trainings performed on the original images and on the pre-processed ones, using either a single label or two labels with the boundary included. The best results on both internal test set and validation set were achieved with pre-processed images and with addition of tumor boundary as another class. Our final approach produced robust results in the online validation stage with the average Dice score of 0.843 as well as in the testing stage with the average Dice score of 0.816.

Acknowledgments. Valeriia Abramova and Agustin Cartaya Lathulerie hold FPI grants from the Ministerio de Ciencia, Innovación y Universidades with reference numbers PRE2021-099121 and PREP2023-001473, respectively. Uma M. Lal-Trehan Estrada and Rachika E. Hamadache hold an IFUdG2022 and IFUdG2024 grants from Universitat de Girona, respectively. Cansu Yalçın and Clara Lisazo hold FI grants from the Catalan Government with reference numbers 2023 FI-1 00096 and 2024 FI-1 00103, respectively. Micaela Rivas Díaz holds a DEXCOM Chair grant (TSI-100932-2023-1) from the Spanish Ministry for Digital Transformation and Public Service, co-funded by the European Union NextGenerationEU. Adrià Casamitjana holds a POSTDOC-UdG2023 grant from Universitat de Girona. This work has been supported by PID2023-146187OB-I00 from the Ministerio de Ciencia, Innovación y Universidades and also by the ICREA Academia program.

References

1. LaBella, D., et al.: The ASNR-MICCAI brain tumor segmentation (BRATS) challenge 2023: intracranial meningioma (2023). https://doi.org/10.48550/ARXIV.2305.07642, https://arxiv.org/abs/2305.07642
2. LaBella, D., et al.: Analysis of the 2024 BRATS meningioma radiotherapy planning automated segmentation challenge (2024). https://doi.org/10.48550/ARXIV.2405.18383, https://arxiv.org/abs/2405.18383
3. Isensee, F., Jaeger, P.F., Kohl, S.A.A., Petersen, J., Maier-Hein, K.H.: nnU-net: a self-configuring method for deep learning-based biomedical image segmentation. Nat. Methods **18**(2), 203–211 (2020)
4. Ronneberger, O., Fischer, P., Brox, T.: U-net: convolutional networks for biomedical image segmentation (2015). https://doi.org/10.48550/ARXIV.1505.04597, https://arxiv.org/abs/1505.04597

5. Çiçek, O., Abdulkadir, A., Lienkamp, S.S., Brox, T., Ronneberger, O.: 3d u-net: learning dense volumetric segmentation from sparse annotation (2016). https://doi.org/10.48550/ARXIV.1606.06650, https://arxiv.org/abs/1606.06650
6. Akinci D'Antonoli, T., et al.: Totalsegmentator MRI: robust sequence-independent segmentation of multiple anatomic structures in MRI. Radiology **314**(2) (2025). https://doi.org/10.1148/radiol.241613, http://dx.doi.org/10.1148/radiol.241613
7. Tustison, N.J., Gee, J.: N4itk: Nick's n3 itk implementation for MRI bias field correction. Insight J. (2010). https://doi.org/10.54294/jculxw, http://dx.doi.org/10.54294/jculxw
8. Isensee, F., Jäger, P.F., Full, P.M., Vollmuth, P., Maier-Hein, K.H.: nnu-net for brain tumor segmentation. In: Crimi, A., Bakas, S. (eds.) Brainlesion: Glioma, Multiple Sclerosis, Stroke and Traumatic Brain Injuries, pp. 118–132. Springer, Cham (2021)
9. Karargyris, A., et al.: Federated benchmarking of medical artificial intelligence with medperf. Nat. Mach. Intell. **5**(7), 799–810 (2023). https://doi.org/10.1038/s42256-023-00652-2, http://dx.doi.org/10.1038/s42256-023-00652-2

Condition-Based Ensemble Modelling of Swin UNETR and 3D U-Net for Meningioma Segmentation in Radiotherapy Planning

Sanskriti Srivastava[1], Kuldeep Raghuwanshi[1], and Anup Singh[1,2,3](✉)

[1] Centre for Biomedical Engineering, Indian Institute of Technology Delhi, Delhi, India
anupsm@iitd.ac.in

[2] Department of Biomedical Engineering, All India Institute of Medical Sciences, Delhi, India

[3] Yardi School of Artificial Intelligence, Indian Institute of Technology Delhi, Delhi, India

Abstract. Segmentation of meningioma tumors is important for effective radiotherapy planning. Despite recent advances in medical image segmentation, automatic and accurate segmentation of meningioma tumors on T1-contrast-enhanced (T1CE) MRI sequences remains a challenge, particularly across varied tumor shapes and sizes.

This study proposed an automatic segmentation of meningioma on T1CE MRI, as a part of the BraTS-Lighthouse 2025 Meningioma Radiotherapy Segmentation Task, by leveraging state-of-the-art deep learning architectures. In the current study, two deep learning 3D segmentation networks, 3D U-Net and Swin UNETR, were trained on T1CE brain MRI volumes of 500 patients provided by BraTS-Lighthouse 2025, followed by fine-tuning of models. Further, a condition-based ensemble strategy is implemented for combining Swin UNETR and 3D U-Net to achieve an optimum Dice Similarity Coefficient (DSC).

Individual model evaluation showed that Swin UNETR outperformed the 3D U-Net. On the local training dataset comprising 50 patients, the optimized Swin UNETR achieved a lesion-wise DSC of 0.81 ± 0.18, compared to 0.74 ± 0.23 for the optimized 3D U-Net. Similarly, on the external validation dataset of 70 patients, Swin UNETR achieved a DSC of 0.65 ± 0.29, while 3D U-Net obtained 0.61 ± 0.33.

Furthermore, both models are condition-based ensembled for the final predictions, the ensemble model provides a lesion-wise DSC of 0.83 ± 0.13 on local training dataset of 50 patients and lesion-wise DSC of 0.70 ± 0.28 for the external validation dataset of 70 patients.

Our study describes the effectiveness of condition-based ensemble using a transformer-based (Swin UNETR) and convolutional neural network-based (3D U-Net) models for Gross Tumor Volume (GTV) segmentation of meningioma tumors in MRI scans.

Keywords: Meningioma segmentation · MRI · Radiotherapy planning · Swin UNETR · Ensemble learning · 3D U-Net

S. Srivastava and K. Raghuwanshi—(Share equal Authorship)

S. Bakas et al. (Eds.): MICCAI 2025, LNCS 16376, pp. 148–158, 2026.
https://doi.org/10.1007/978-3-032-16365-3_14

1 Introduction

The most prevalent primary brain tumors of the central nervous system are meningiomas, which account for 37% [1, 2] across all brain tumors in adults. According to the World Health Organization (WHO), meningioma tumors are classified into three grades i.e. Grade 1 (Benign), Grade 2 (Atypical), and Grade 3 (Anaplastic) based on tumor morphology, tumor aggressiveness, mitotic activity, and infiltration of meningioma tissue in the brain. These grades are further classified into 15 subtypes [3, 4]. The incidence rate and the prognosis of meningioma tumors depend on the grade of the tumor. Magnetic Resonance Imaging (MRI) is the routinely used for the pre-operative characterization and treatment planning of meningiomas. The T1-contrast-enhanced (T1CE) MR sequence is primarily used to provide information about the tumor morphology, tumor heterogeneity, dura tail enhancement, and leakage of contrast in the tumor tissue [5]. These features are important imaging features for preoperative treatment planning and radiotherapy.

The treatment planning of meningioma tumor patients requires a balance between definitive treatment of the tumor and the avoidance of iatrogenic neurologic damage [6]. The surgical intervention and radiotherapy are the first-line treatment methods for meningiomas. The different methods of radiotherapy are the external beam radiotherapy (EBRT), stereotactic radiosurgery (SRS), intensity-modulated radiotherapy (IMRT), fractionated stereotactic radiotherapy (FSRT), and Proton radiotherapy [6, 7]. Radiotherapy serves as an important adjuvant treatment in meningiomas for improving local control and reducing the risk of recurrence. In radiotherapy, the accurate prediction of Gross Tumor Volume (GTV) will help in reducing the risk of recurrence and improving the prognosis-free survival.

Meningioma tumors are heterogeneous, multifocal, and have different imaging features depending upon the grade of the tumor, so the automatic segmentation of GTV is a challenging task. In the literature, there are several studies on the segmentation of meningioma tumors. Bouget et al. 2021 [8] trained two Deep Learning (DL) models, 3D U-Net and PLS-Net, on 698 T1CE scans, with PLS-Net excelling in speed and large tumor segmentation, and achieved Dice scores of ~70%. In their another study of Bouget D et al. [9] they introduced attention-based models AGUNet and DAUNet, and they are able to get the DSC of 81.6% particularly effective for tumors >3 ml. Laukamp et al. [10] used a pretrained 3D U-Net on 10,000 healthy MRIs and fine-tuned it on 806 meningioma cases and achieving a median DSC of 88.2%. These studies have several limitations. Firstly, they are evaluating their models on the larger tumor regions; also, the segmentation of the tumors based on tumor enhancement, and challenges remain in the segmentation of GTV for radiotherapy planning.

Therefore, the purpose of this study was to investigate the ability of 3D DL models and their condition-based ensemble approach for the accurate segmentation of GTV of the pre-operative meningioma tumors in the T1CE MRI sequence, which will be useful for radiotherapy planning.

2 Methods

2.1 Dataset Description

In this study, the dataset used was obtained from the BraTS 2025 Meningioma Radiotherapy Segmentation Challenge [11]. During the training phase, T1CE MRI sequence dataset of 500 patients is provided with its corresponding GTV masks. An additional 70 patient dataset is provided in the validation phase, where masks were not present. As mentioned in the challenge, the dataset was collected from different centers across the world and was specifically curated to support automated segmentation of the GTV in meningiomas.

2.2 Preprocessing

The dataset has varying pixel dimensions and volumetric shapes, which are due to different imaging protocols, acquisition parameters, and scanner types, so the dataset requires standardized preprocessing to train the DL model. So, a structured preprocessing pipeline was implemented using the Medical Open Network for AI (MONAI) framework [12]. Fig. 1 shows the pipeline of the proposed methodology.

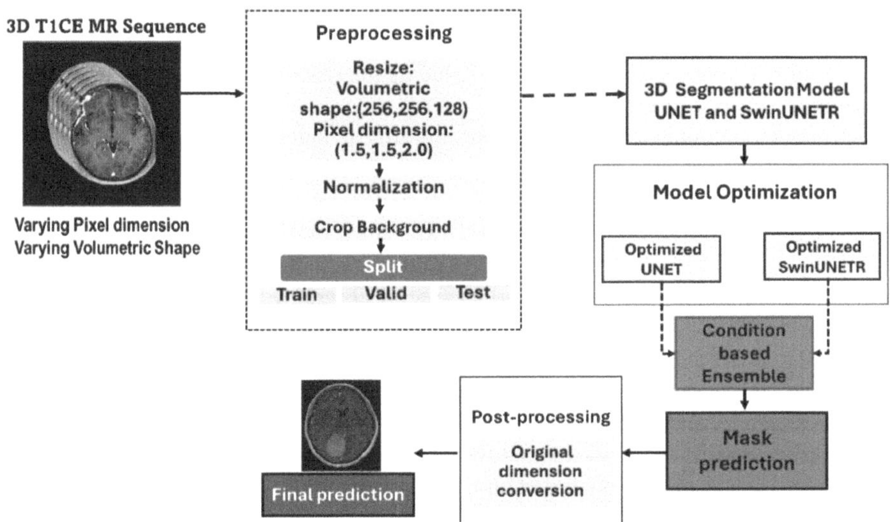

Fig. 1. Proposed pipeline for segmentation of meningioma tumors for radiotherapy planning.

The preprocessing involves the loading of image-label pairs, followed by reformatting to a channel-first layout for PyTorch compatibility. Intensity values of all volumes were normalized to the [0, 1] range to mitigate inter-patient brightness variations. Non-informative background regions were also removed to focus on relevant anatomy.

To ensure spatial and anatomical consistency, all volumes were reoriented to the RAS coordinate system and resampled to a uniform voxel spacing of $1.5 \times 1.5 \times 2.0$ mm using bilinear interpolation for images and nearest-neighbor for labels. Each volume was then resized or padded to (256, 256, 128) for compatibility with the networks input size.

Before the preprocessing, the training dataset (local dataset) was randomly divided into three subsets: Training Set: 400 volumes (80%), Validation Set: 50 volumes (10%), and Testing Set: 50 volumes (10%). For training the model, the volumes of training dataset were divided into patches of size ($96 \times 96 \times 96$). The approach extracts four random sub-volume patches per image. This strategy helps the model to learn effectively despite class imbalance. In contrast, a sliding window inference of size ($96 \times 96 \times 96$) is used on the validation volumes to provide a stable and consistent reference for evaluating model performance.

2.3 Deep Learning Algorithm and Training

This study was conducted on a high-performance computing system with dual NVIDIA A100 (40GB) and 2x Intel Xeon Platinum 8358 (32 cores, 2.6 GHz) connected to 200G HDR InfiniBand. The models were implemented in PyTorch 2.6.0 with MONAI 1.5.0. with cuDNN enabled. Also, parallel computing was enabled using PyTorch's DataParallel module, which allowed the simultaneous use of multiple GPUs. We implemented two 3D image segmentation architectures: 3D U-Net [13] and Swin UNETR [14]. The training configuration for both models were trained using Dice Loss including the AdamW optimizer with a starting learning rate of 1e-4, a batch size of 8, and 200 epochs, followed by fine-tuning of the model. Further, we implemented a condition-based ensemble modeling strategy for optimum results.

2.4 Fine-Tuning via Learning Rate

In this step, we fine-tuned both 3D U-Net and Swin UNETR models, by applying a staged decay in learning rate. The weights of trained 3D U-NET and 3D Swin UNETR models were loaded, and optimization continued by gradually reducing the learning rate across multiple stages. We began with a learning rate of 0.0001, which was then decreased to 0.00001 and subsequently to 0.000001, with validation performance closely monitored at each stage. This fine-tuning strategy allowed the models to refine their parameters more precisely.

2.5 Condition-Based Ensemble Model

Using the above-mentioned training strategies, we obtained two optimized and well-performing models, 3D U-Net and Swin UNETR. Further, in the detailed evaluation, it was observed that each model had its own limitations. In some cases, either model failed to accurately segment regions with intensity values similar to surrounding bone structures, particularly near the basal ganglia, medulla oblongata, and skull base. However, there were also instances where Swin UNETR missed tumor regions, but the U-Net was able to detect them.

To leverage the complementary strengths of both models, we implemented a condition-based ensemble modeling strategy. This involved a pixel-wise fusion of the predicted masks. If Swin UNETR(M1) predicted a pixel as a tumor (value = 1), it was accepted as the final prediction. If Swin UNETR predicted 0, we checked the 3D U-Net(M2) prediction. If the U-Net predicts the pixel as a tumor (value = 1), we analyzed the intensity value of its 8-connected neighborhood if the sum of the neighborhood intensity values is more than five, then the U-Net prediction is the final prediction. Fig. 2 illustrates the flowchart of this decision process.

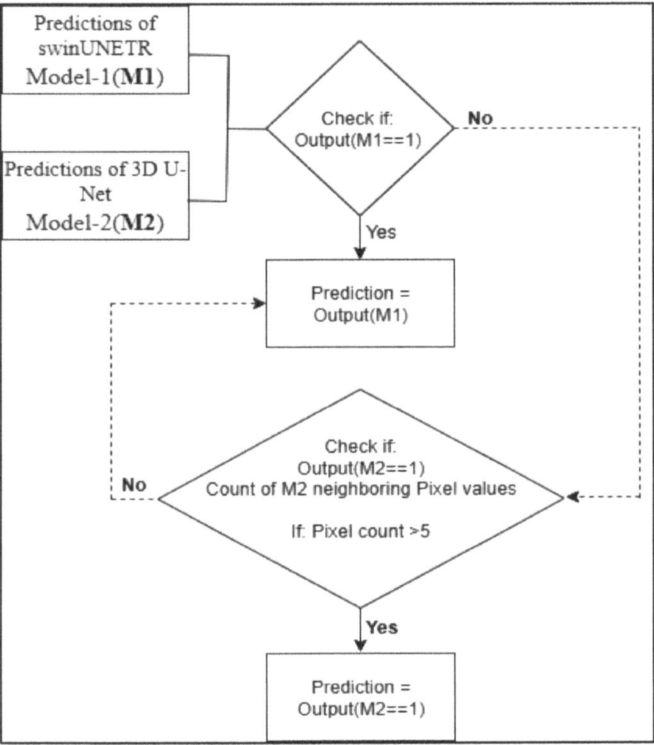

Fig. 2. Condition-based ensemble model for segmentation of meningioma tumors.

2.6 Prediction and Post-Processing

For the prediction of the mask, the preprocessing steps involve cropping the background and resizing the volume to a model-compatible size, which is mentioned above, and intensity normalization is done. Further, the post-processing is done by MONAI, inverted to save the mask in the same orientation, volumetric size, and pixel spacing.

3 Performance Evaluation

To evaluate the model performance, the mean of lesion-wise DSC [16–17], median of lesion-wise DSC and 75th percentile of lesion-wise DSC was used. These matrices provide a more clinical meaning to access the GTV for radiotherapy.

4 Results

We trained and evaluated two deep learning-based segmentation models: 3D U-Net and Swin UNETR. Model performance was primarily assessed using lesion-wise DSC, Median, and 75th percentile matrices for both local test data and the external validation dataset of 70 patients. Table 1 shows the performance evaluation of all trained models.

Table 1. Segmentation performance of all DL models tested on local data (train data) and external validation data.

Evaluation on test data extracted from training dataset (50 cases)			
Models	**Lesion-Wise DSC (MEAN ± SD)**	**Lesion-Wise DSC Median**	**Lesion-Wise DSC 75TH percentile**
3D U-Net	0.65 ± 0.29	0.78	0.88
3D U-Net optimized	0.74 ± 0.23	0.82	0.88
3D Swin UNETR	0.76 ± 0.25	0.87	0.91
3D Swin UNETR optimized	0.81 ± 0.18	0.87	0.90
Ensemble(U-Net + Swin UNETR)	**0.83 ± 0.13**	**0.87**	**0.90**
Evaluation on separate validation data provided by BraTS-Lighthouse 2025 Challenge (70 cases)			
Models	**Lesion-Wise DSC (MEAN ± SD)**	**Lesion-Wise DSC Median**	**Lesion-Wise DSC 75TH percentile**
3D U-Net	0.58 ± 0.36	0.75	0.89
3D U-Net optimized	0.61 ± 0.33	0.78	0.86
3D Swin UNETR	0.64 ± 0.32	0.78	0.88
3D Swin UNETR optimized	0.67 ± 0.29	0.80	0.89
Ensemble(U-Net + Swin UNETR)	**0.70 ± 0.28**	**0.82**	**0.90**

In the initial training, the Swin UNETR performs better than the 3D U-Net; the mean lesion-wise DSC for 3D UNET and Swin UNETR were 0.65 ± 0.29 and 0.76 ± 0.25, on local test data and 0.58 ± 0.36 and 0.64 ± 0.32 on external validation data, respectively. The models get improved by fine-tuning; the mean lesion-wise DSC for 3D UNET and Swin UNETR was 0.74 ± 0.23 and 0.81 ± 0.18 on local test data, respectively, and 0.61 ± 0.33 and 0.67 ± 0.29 on external validation data, respectively. The final condition-based ensemble model achieved a lesion-wise DSC of 0.70 ± 0.28 on the external validation data and 0.83 ± 0.13 on local test data. On the final test dataset condition-based ensemble model achieved the mean DSC of 0.68 ± 0.30. A comparative analysis of optimized 3D U-Net, Swin UNETR, and condition-based ensemble model, shown in Fig. 3, shows that the ensemble model provides better results among all models. Fig. 4 represents the best-performing and underperforming cases.

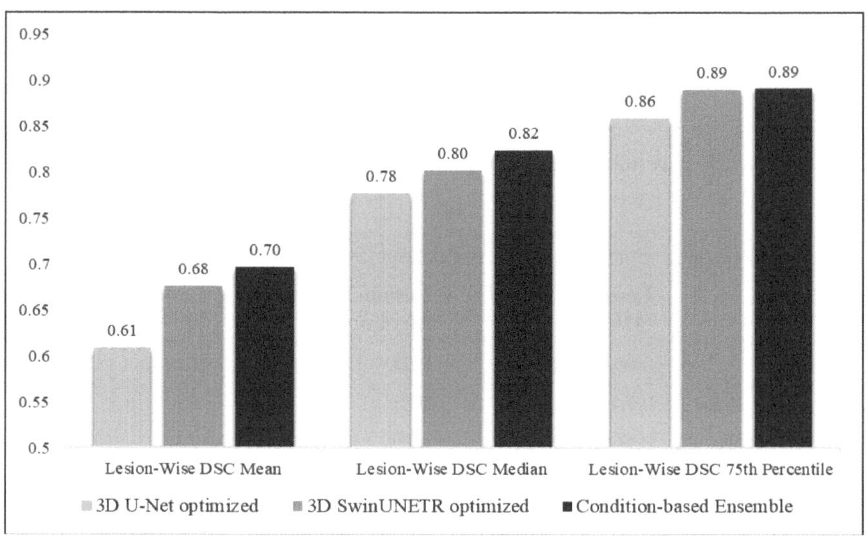

Fig. 3. Comparison of lesion-wise DSC metrics using Mean, Median, and 75th Percentile across 3D U-Net, Swin UNETR, and Condition-based ensemble models.

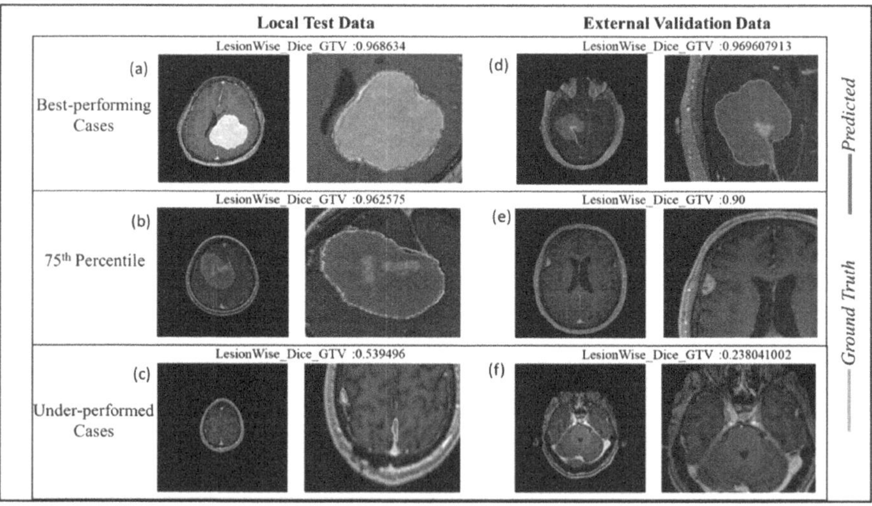

Fig. 4. Examples illustrate both accurate and inaccurate lesion predictions by the condition-based ensemble model. The green boundary represents the ground truth, while the red boundary denotes the predicted segmentation mask. Subfigures (a), (b), and (c) correspond to predictions on the local test dataset, whereas (d), (e), and (f) show results on the external validation dataset.

5 Discussion

This study aims to develop and evaluate DL-based models for accurate segmentation of meningioma lesions on T1CE MRI sequence, which is generally required for radiotherapy planning. For this task, we implemented, optimized, and evaluated two state-of-the-art architectures, 3D U-Net and Swin UNETR, both trained with identical preprocessing and training pipelines. While Swin UNETR demonstrated superior performance in most cases, in some cases, 3D U-Net consistently outperformed where Swin UNETR was unable to predict. Recognizing the complementary strengths of these models, we proposed to integrate them through an ensemble-based decision strategy.

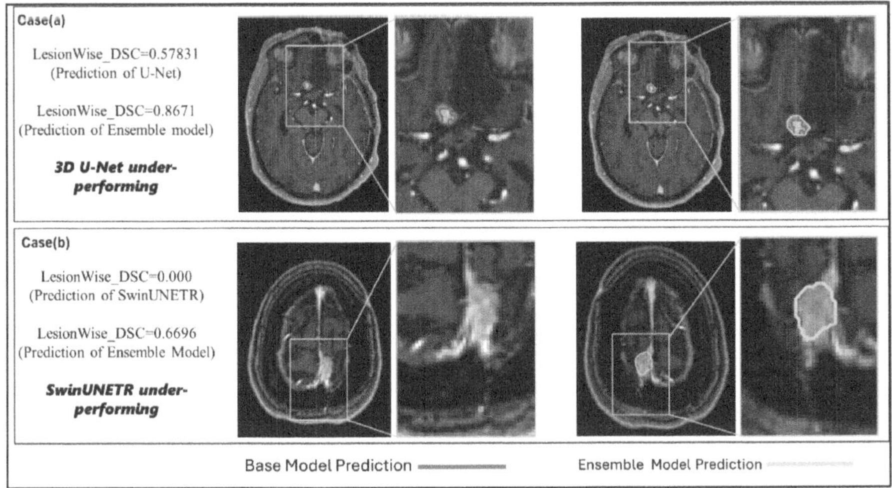

Fig. 5. (a) Case where 3D U-Net provided underestimates prediction of tumor mask, whereas condition-based ensemble model is able to predict the lesion with substantially high accuracy. (b) Case where Swin UNETR is unable to predict the lesion whereas condition-based ensemble model is able to predict the lesion with a high accuracy. The mask predicted by the 3D U-Net is represented by magenta, whereas the mask predicted by the condition-based ensemble is represented as cyan.

The Swin UNETR attention-based transformer architecture has the ability to capture global contextual information and long-range dependencies than traditional CNN-based architectures. Its hierarchical structure and shifted window attention mechanism enabled better modeling of tumor boundaries in complex anatomical regions. On the other hand, the 3D U-Net, with its residual connections and spatial skip pathways, proved effective at preserving fine details, particularly in high-resolution superficial areas. While each model had its individual strengths and limitations. To address these limitations and to enhance the segmentation accuracy, we implemented a condition-based ensemble strategy. Visual representation of cases where the 3D U-Net and Swin UNETR are underperforming, and the condition-based ensemble model is able to predict the lesion, is shown in Fig. 5.

Recent studies have shown that T1CE MRI alone is often sufficient for accurate brain tumor segmentation, particularly in enhancing regions. A study done by Chan. C. et al.

[18] in which they segment the tumor for the grading of meningiomas, they have used 2D U-NET and 3D U-NET for the segmentation of tumor and got the accuracy of 0.92 DSC on validation data. V.K. et al. [19] has implemented an adapted DeepMedic and achieved a 0.78 Dice, detecting 55 of 56 tumors despite scan variability. Another study done by Kang. et al. [20] They implemented the 2D nnU-NET for the segmentation of meningioma tumors and achieved a median DSC of 0.89 on external validation data for tumor size >1 cm^3. In the literature, it was found that there are some limitations in their studies, as the reported model performance on median DSC does not provide the overall performance of the model, and is tested on validation data from a single centre. Also, in some studies, they are testing their model for larger lesions. These findings highlight the need for efficient deep learning models to segment the tumor region for radiotherapy planning. To the best of our knowledge, no ensemble-based deep learning model is trained on radiotherapy planning, utilizing multicentric data with high lesion-wise DSC. So, in the current study, we are dealing with multicentric MRI Scans and achieved commendable accuracy by utilizing ensemble-based modelling.

There are some limitations in this study. First, the increased complexity from combining two models raises computational demands; moreover, the condition-based ensemble modelling may also create some false predictions in the segmentation of GTV. Further testing on a large multicentric dataset is required.

6 Conclusion

The current study proposed presented a deep learning ensemble-based model for accurate meningioma segmentation utilizing the T1CE MR Sequence. Among the architectures evaluated, 3D U-Net and Swin UNETR, the transformer-based Swin UNETR demonstrated superior performance across multiple metrics, particularly in the mean, median, and 75th percentile of lesion-wise Dice scores. The proposed condition-based ensemble approach improved generalization and robustness, especially in cases with smaller tumor lesions and intensity similarity between bone and tumor. Overall, our findings underscore the importance of transformer-based architecture, convolution-based architecture, fine-tuning, and ensemble strategies in achieving accurate and robust segmentation of contrast-enhancing meningioma lesions for radiotherapy planning.

Acknowledgments. The authors thanks for the funding support from Indian Council of Medical Research, India (Project No. CAR-2024-01-000187), IIT Delhi HPC facility for computational resources and also would like to thank all MedImg lab members for their guidance and support.

Disclosure of Interests

The authors declare that they have no conflict of interest.

References

1. McNeill, K.A.: Epidemiology of brain tumors. Neurol. Clin. **34**(4), 981–998 (Nov. 2016). https://doi.org/10.1016/J.NCL.2016.06.014

2. Park, Y.W., et al.: Radiomics and machine learning may accurately predict the grade and histological subtype in meningiomas using conventional and diffusion tensor imaging. Eur. Radiol. **29**(8), 4068–4076 (Aug. 2019). https://doi.org/10.1007/s00330-018-5830-3
3. Nasrallah, M.L.P., Aldape, K.D.: Molecular classification and grading of meningioma. Springer, (01 Jan 2023). doi:https://doi.org/10.1007/s11060-022-04228-9.
4. Louis, D.N., et al.: The 2021 WHO classification of tumors of the central nervous system: a summary. Neuro-Oncology. **23**(8), 1231–1251 (2021). https://doi.org/10.1093/NEUONC/NOAB106
5. Kim, H., Kim, H.G., Oh, J.H., Lee, K.M.: Deep-learning model for diagnostic clue: detecting the dural tail sign for meningiomas on contrast-enhanced T1 weighted images. Quant. Imaging Med. Surg. **13**(12), 8132–8143 (2023). https://doi.org/10.21037/qims-23-114
6. Hartrampf, P.E., et al.: Long-term results of multimodal peptide receptor radionuclide therapy and fractionated external beam radiotherapy for treatment of advanced symptomatic meningioma. Clin. Trans. Radiat. Oncol. **22**, 29–32 (2020). https://doi.org/10.1016/j.ctro.2020.03.002
7. Hwang, K.L., Hwang, W.L., Bussière, M.R., Shih, H.A.: The role of radiotherapy in the management of high-grade meningiomas. AME Publishing Company, (Jul 01 2017). doi:https://doi.org/10.21037/cco.2017.06.09.
8. Bouget, D., Pedersen, A., Hosainey, S.A.M., Vanel, J., Solheim, O., Reinertsen, I.: Fast meningioma segmentation in T1-weighted magnetic resonance imaging volumes using a lightweight 3D deep learning architecture. J. Med. Imaging. **8**(02) (Mar. 2021). https://doi.org/10.1117/1.JMI.8.2.024002
9. Bouget, D., Pedersen, A., Hosainey, S.A.M., Solheim, O., Reinertsen, I.: Meningioma segmentation in T1-weighted MRI leveraging global context and attention mechanisms. Front. Radiol. **1** (2021). https://doi.org/10.3389/FRADI.2021.711514
10. Laukamp, K.R., et al.: Fully automated detection and segmentation of meningiomas using deep learning on routine multiparametric MRI. Eur. Radiol. **29**(1), 124–132 (2019). https://doi.org/10.1007/S00330-018-5595-8
11. LaBella, D. et al.: Analysis of the 2024 BraTS Meningioma Radiotherapy Planning Automated Segmentation Challenge. vol. 45, p. 70, (May 2024). Available: https://arxiv.org/pdf/2405.18383
12. MONAI: Medical Open Network for AI. Accessed 29 Jul (2025). [Online]. Available: https://monai.io/
13. Çiçek, Ö., Abdulkadir, A., Lienkamp, S.S., Brox, T., Ronneberger, O.: 3D U-net: learning dense volumetric segmentation from sparse annotation. In: Lecture Notes in Computer Science (Including Subseries Lecture Notes in Artificial Intelligence and Lecture Notes in Bioinformatics), vol. 9901, pp. 424–432. LNCS (Jun. 2016). https://doi.org/10.1007/978-3-319-46723-8_49
14. Hatamizadeh, A., Nath, V., Tang, Y., Yang, D., Roth, H.R., Xu, D.: Swin UNETR: swin transformers for semantic segmentation of brain tumors in MRI images. In: Lecture Notes in Computer Science (including subseries Lecture Notes in Artificial Intelligence and Lecture Notes in Bioinformatics), vol. 12962, pp. 272–284. LNCS (Jan. 2022). https://doi.org/10.1007/978-3-031-08999-2_22
15. Moore, C., Bell, D.: Dice similarity coefficient. Radiopaedia.org. (Mar 2020). doi:https://doi.org/10.53347/RID-75056.
16. Nawaz, M., et al.: Unraveling the complexity of optical coherence tomography image segmentation using machine and deep learning techniques: a review. Comput. Med. Imaging Graph. **108** (2023). https://doi.org/10.1016/j.compmedimag.2023.102269
17. Ren, T., Honey, E., Rebala, H., Sharma, A., Chopra, A., Kurt, M.: An optimization framework for processing and transfer learning for the brain tumor segmentation. In: Lecture Notes in

Computer Science (Including Subseries Lecture Notes in Artificial Intelligence and Lecture Notes in Bioinformatics), vol. 14669, pp. 165–176. LNCS (2024). https://doi.org/10.1007/978-3-031-76163-8_15
18. Chen, C., et al.: Automatic meningioma segmentation and grading prediction: a hybrid deep-learning method. J. Pers. Med. **11**(8), 786 (2021). https://doi.org/10.3390/JPM11080786/S1
19. Boaro, A., et al.: Deep neural networks allow expert-level brain meningioma segmentation and present potential for improvement of clinical practice. Sci. Rep. **12**(1) (2022). https://doi.org/10.1038/S41598-022-19356-5
20. Kang, H., et al.: Fully automated MRI segmentation and volumetric measurement of intracranial meningioma using deep learning. J. Magn. Reson. Imaging. **57**(3), 871–881 (2023). https://doi.org/10.1002/JMRI.28332;SUBPAGE:STRING:FULL

Challenge 4 – BraTS-METS

Segmentation of Pre and Post-treatment Brain Metastases Using nnU-Nets

Maria Bancerek[1], Piotr Rudzki[1], and Jakub Nalepa[1,2](✉)

[1] Graylight Imaging, Gliwice, Poland
{mbancerek,prudzki}@graylight-imaging.com
[2] Silesian University of Technology, Gliwice, Poland
jnalepa@graylight-imaging.com, Jakub.Nalepa@polsl.pl

Abstract. Monitoring brain metastases is a time-consuming process, especially when relying on manual analysis of multiple small lesions. While Response Assessment in Neuro-Oncology Brain Metastases (RANO-BM) guidelines recommend unidimensional measurements, volumetric assessment of tumors and surrounding edema is critical for informed clinical decisions. Manual methods, however, are often error-prone and subjective, motivating the development of automated, reproducible artificial intelligence-powered solutions for monitoring the progress of the disease. In this work, we address the problem of automated brain metastasis detection and multi-class segmentation using the nnU-Net framework—a self-configuring deep learning model for medical image analysis. We evaluate different configurations of nnU-Net, including changes to loss functions, model size, training duration, and post-processing routines. Our experiments (GLI-team) on the BraTS-METS 2025 dataset demonstrate robust performance of nnU-Nets across diverse MRI scanners and clinical protocols (exceeding the Dice score of 0.78 for the enhancing part of the tumor). This heterogeneity makes BraTS-METS a crucial benchmark for assessing model generalizability. Our results highlight the promise of automated, objective tools in supporting more consistent and scalable clinical workflows for managing patients with brain metastases. Finally, our approach outperformed all other techniques and was the winning solution in the BraTS-METS 2025 Challenge.

Keywords: Brain metastasis · Detection · Segmentation · nnU-Net

1 Introduction

Monitoring metastatic brain disease is a labor-intensive and time-consuming process, particularly when multiple metastases are present, and assessments rely on manual techniques. According to the Response Assessment in Neuro-Oncology Brain Metastases (RANO-BM) guidelines, brain metastases are typically evaluated by measuring their largest unidimensional diameter. However, accurate volumetric estimates of both the lesions and the surrounding edema are crucial

M. Bancerek and P. Rudzki—Joint first author with equal contribution.

S. Bakas et al. (Eds.): MICCAI 2025, LNCS 16376, pp. 161–172, 2026.
https://doi.org/10.1007/978-3-032-16365-3_15

for informed clinical decision-making, and for improving predictions of treatment outcomes. This task is, unfortunately, further complicated by the fact that brain metastases are commonly small, making the detection and segmentation of lesions especially challenging. Of note, manual analysis of (virtually any) medical images may be human-biased and prone to a variety of errors, thus building reproducible, unbiased and objective (deep) machine learning techniques for medical image analysis tasks is an important focus of the community nowadays.

The algorithms for brain metastasis detection can be broadly categorized into (*i*) classic and (*ii*) deep learning (CML and DL, respectively) approaches. A systematic review by Cho et al.[4] of recent studies highlights a shift from CML to DL after 2018, driven by access to larger, and substantially more heterogeneous datasets [18]. Early CML methods include Ambrosini et al.'s [1] 3D spherical tumor models for detecting lesions in single-modal magnetic resonance images (MRIs), which may miss tumors with atypical shapes or intensity profiles. Similarly, Farjam et al. [5] used optimized 3D spherical shell templates tailored for small lesions, while Pérez-Ramírez et al. [19] proposed a template-matching method for this task. These approaches are often combined with ML techniques, such as unsupervised clustering, for candidate detection and classification for reducing false positive detections [20]. Notably, many of these studies were single-center and lacked pathological confirmation of metastases, limiting their generalizability [20]. Therefore, building large-scale, objective and multi-center benchmarks, such as BraTS-METS [16], developed within the framework of the famous Brain Tumor Segmentation (BraTS) family of challenges, is of paramount importance to verify (and quantify) the generalization capabilities of the emerging algorithms for brain metastasis detection and segmentation.

In this paper, we tackle the problem of automated brain metastasis detection and multi-class segmentation, and propose an automatically-optimized deep learning method for this task. We build on the nnU-Net framework, which is a self-configuring method originally developed for medical image analysis. We explore several nnU-Net variants differing in loss functions, parameter settings (e.g., number of training epochs), model sizes, and post-processing strategies (Sect. 3). Our experimental validation, performed over the BraTS-METS 2025 dataset shows strong generalization capabilities of our approach (Sect. 4). This is worth emphasizing, as the released dataset is heterogeneous in terms of the MRI scanners that were used for acquiring the image data, as well as in terms of the protocols followed in a variety of clinical sites. We believe that our efforts may become an important step toward building generalizable methods that could help improve the way patients with brain metastases are managed and treated, through making it more objective, reproducible, and free from human bias.

This article is structured as follows. The dataset used in this study and released within the BraTS MICCAI 2025 Lighthouse Challenge is discussed in Sect. 2. The deep learning algorithms used for brain metastasis detection and multi-class segmentation are presented in Sect. 3. The experimental results are discussed in Sect. 4, whereas Sect. 5 concludes the paper.

2 Data

In this study, we exploit the dataset which was made available through the BraTS MICCAI 2025 Lighthouse Challenge (*Task 4: Pre- and Post-Treatment Brain Metastases*) [16]. The dataset contains retrospective pre- and post-treatment brain metastases multiparametric (mpMRI) scans obtained from various institutions, and acquired standard clinical conditions, using different imaging protocols and scanners. Therefore, it presents a high level of data-level heterogeneity (in terms of image quality and characteristics), hence may be used to verify the clinical utility of the developed brain metastasis detection and segmentation techniques that are to be ultimately deployed in clinical practice. For each study, the following MRI sequences are available: pre-contrast T1-weighted (T1W), post-contrast T1-weighted (T1C), T2-weighted (T2W), and T2-weighted Fluid Attenuated Inversion Recovery (FLAIR). The images are accompanied by the ground-truth segmentation masks, containing the following classes of interest:

- **Nonenhancing tumor core (NETC)**, being all portions of the tumor core without contrast enhancement that are enclosed by enhancing tumor (ET). It represents the bulk of the tumor—this part is typically considered for surgical excision in clinical settings.
- **Surrounding non-enhancing FLAIR hyperintensity (SNFH)**, being the peritumoral edematous and infiltrated tissue, defined by the abnormal hyperintense signal envelope on the T2 FLAIR volumes, which includes the infiltrative non enhancing tumor, together with the vasogenic edema in the peritumoral region. The authors of the dataset emphasized that the non tumor related FLAIR signal abnormality, such as prior infarcts or microvascular ischemic white matter changes, are not included in this class.
- **Enhancing Tumor (ET)**, being all tumor areas with noticeable contrast enhancement on postcontrast T1-weighted images. Similarly, the adjacent blood vessels, bleeding or intrinsic T1 hyperintensity are not included here.
- **Resection Cavity (RC)**, being the resection of region within the brain tissue in the post-treatment cases.

Overall, the training part ($\boldsymbol{T}$) of the dataset includes 1296 multiparametric MRI scans (obtained for 890 patients), whereas the validation set ($\boldsymbol{V}$), for which the ground-truth labels have not been released, encompasses 179 such scans (for 166 patients). Indeed, the training set manifests significant diversity of the imaged brain metastases, also in terms of their number and specific regions in the $\boldsymbol{T}$ patients. In Fig. 1, we can appreciate that the majority of patients have a relatively small number of brain metastatic lesions. However, there are cases in which the number of tumorous regions reach 50. It is of paramount importance to precisely detect and segment such lesions, as it would allow for a reproducible and objective monitoring of the disease progression (or regression), and for designing an appropriate treatment pathway which is more patient-specific.

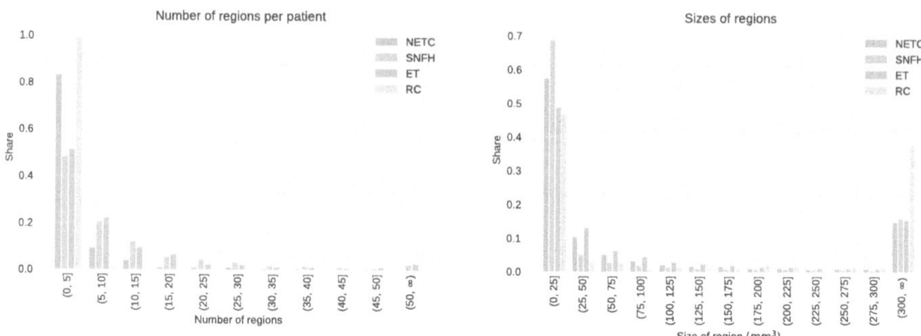

Fig. 1. The distribution of the number of brain metastatic-related regions in all training set ($\boldsymbol{T}$) patients (left panel, *Share* ranges from 0–1, and sums up to 1 across all regions), together with the distribution of sizes of these regions in all $\boldsymbol{T}$ scans (right panel).

3 Methods

In this section, we discuss the nnU-Nets, a self-configuring deep learning method for segmenting (not only [7]) medical images [6,8], originally introduced by Isensee et al. [10,12], which we utilized to detect and segment brain metastatic lesions (Sect. 3.1). Afterwards, we present the quality metrics that are used within the challenge to assess the quality of the algorithms (Sect. 3.2).

3.1 Detecting and Segmenting Brain Metastases Using nnU-Nets

In this study, we build upon the nnU-Net framework, being a self-configuring method designed for the analysis of medical image data (of note, it was further adopted to a variety of other domains and data modalities [7,13,14], proving its inherent generalizability). This approach is built upon fully-convolutional neural networks, and it has already established the state of the art in an array of medical image segmentation tasks in various organs, lesions and modalities [9,11,17,21]. Also, it was exploited in our recent work which introduced deep learning ensembles for detecting brain metastases in longitudinal multi-modal MRI studies [15]. In this paper, we investigated several versions of the nnU-Net, with different loss functions, parameterizations (concerning e.g., the maximum number of epochs), size of the model, and post-processing routines. These versions, together with their identifiers extracted from the submission system, are presented in Table 1.

3.2 Quality Metrics and Classes of Interest

To quantify the quality of predictions generated using the developed brain metastasis detection and segmentation methods, the following metrics are exploited, and both of them are calculated *subject-wise*:

- **Dice Similarity Coefficient (DSC)**, being the overlap metric calculated for the predicted and ground-truth region (ranges from zero to one, with one indicating the perfect score, i.e., the full agreement with the ground truth).

Table 1. The nnU-Net variants, with different loss functions, hyperparameters and post-processing routines, investigated in this study. For each variant, we report its identifier (as extracted from the submission system), and the submission name.

ID (brats id)	Submission name	Description
1 (9754176)	baseline	Settings: – baseline nnU-Net trained on all available data: 1000 epochs, – initial learning rate 0.01, – learning rate with the polynomial decay: $lr_{epoch} = lr_{init} \cdot (1 - epoch/N_{epochs})^{0.9}$, – loss function: cross-entropy (CE) + Dice, – planner: `nUNetPlannerResEncXL`, configuration: `3d_fullres`
2 (9754396)	baseline, finetuned	Settings: – baseline nnU-Net model fine-tuned on the TopK ($k = 10\%$) loss function [2]: 400 epochs, – initial learning rate: $5 \cdot 10^{-3}$ (together with the default decay), – loss function: the TopK loss weighting CE (without Dice)
3 (9754611)	baseline, postprocessed	Settings: – baseline nnU-Net model post-processed by removing all blobs below $5\,\text{mm}^3$ from predictions
4 (9755836)	smaller model, modified loss	Settings: – smaller nnU-Net (L) model trained on all available data: 1000 epochs, – initial learning rate: 0.01, – learning rate polynomial decay: $lr_{epoch} = lr_{init} \cdot (1 - epoch/N_{epochs})^{0.9}$, – loss function: Top10 CE + Dice, – planner: `nUNetPlannerResEncL`, config: `3d_fullres`

– **Normalized Surface Distance (NSD)**, being the overlap metric calculated for two boundaries (predicted and ground truth) of a given lesion part (the higher, the better, with one indicating the perfect score).

While calculating the quality metrics, the following equally-important classes of interest are considered (the metrics are calculated for each class separately): (*i*) tumor core, (*ii*) enhancing tumor, and the (*iii*) whole tumor. The definitions of (*i*) and (*ii*) were given in Sect. 2, and (*iii*) includes all tumor sub-regions.

4 Experiments and Discussion

In this section, we present our experimental study, starting with the experimental setup detailed in Sect. 4.1. The results obtained using the investigated models are gathered and discussed in Sect. 4.2.

4.1 Experimental Setup

All the experiments were executed using a computational server equipped with an NVIDIA A100-PCIE-40GB Graphics Processing Unit (GPU). All nnU-Net hyperparameters were kept as suggested in their default values[1]. Training the model selected for evaluation took approx. 177 h, whereas its inference was approx. 5.5 s per one multi-modal MRI scan on average. To ensure reproducibility and traceability of the experimentation, we exploited MLFlow [3]. Our team identifier on the Synapse platform is **GLI-team**.

4.2 Results and Discussion

The experimental results, obtained for all investigated nnU-Net models over the validation set ($\boldsymbol{V}$), as returned by the evaluation server, are gathered in Table 2 (as our final model, we selected and dockerized the *baseline* configuration, as presented in Table 1). We can observe that all models were consistent, leading to very similar quality scores. Additionally, applying post-processing (to remove small detections, that might be considered false-positive candidates; the threshold of 5 mm^3 was selected experimentally over the training set) in the third model gave only marginal alterations of the quantity measures, e.g., the Normalized Surface Distances for ET and TC. However, at the same time, the post-processing led to the minimal drop in the Dice score for the clinically-important enhancing tumor subregion. The experiments show that indeed the automatically optimized fully-convolutional networks offer high-quality delineation of all classes of interest in segmenting brain metastases from multi-modal MRI scans, and they are robust against different characteristics of the acquired image data (the MRI scans were captured using different equipment and acquisition procedures). The relationships between the prediction metrics and ground truth characteristics are visualized in Fig. 2. These visualizations show that larger metastatic brain lesions might be easier to automatically delineate.

In Figs. 3 and 4, we render example nnU-Net predictions for selected MRI scans, in which small and large metastases are respectively visible (additionally, we report the corresponding metrics, as the ground-truth segmentation masks are publicly available for the training set; the LW metrics indicate the lesion-wise scores). Although the quantitative metrics are slightly better for larger metastases, nnU-Nets delivered precise delineation of all classes in both cases.

[1] The nnU-Net parameterization used in our study can be found in the nnU-Net original repository available at: https://github.com/MIC-DKFZ/nnUNet/blob/master/nnunetv2/training/nnUNetTrainer/nnUNetTrainer.py (last access: July 28, 2025).

Table 2. The results obtained over the validation set $\boldsymbol{V}$, as returned by the evaluation server for all investigated nnU-Net models. We report the Dice score (dsc), and the Normalized Surface Distance (nsd) for all classes: ET (enhancing tumor), RC (resection cavity), TC (tumor core), and WT (whole tumor). Both metrics should be maximized ($\uparrow$), and the best results for each metric are **boldfaced**.

ID (brats id)	ET_{dsc}	ET_{nsd}	RC_{dsc}	RC_{nsd}	TC_{dsc}	TC_{nsd}	WT_{dsc}	WT_{nsd}
1 (9754176)	**0.781**	0.615	0.921	0.880	**0.800**	0.623	**0.797**	**0.518**
2 (9754396)	0.772	0.599	0.918	0.876	**0.800**	0.609	0.794	0.507
3 (9754611)	0.780	**0.616**	0.921	0.880	**0.800**	**0.624**	**0.797**	**0.518**
4 (9755836)	0.763	0.591	**0.937**	**0.895**	0.791	0.604	0.795	0.503

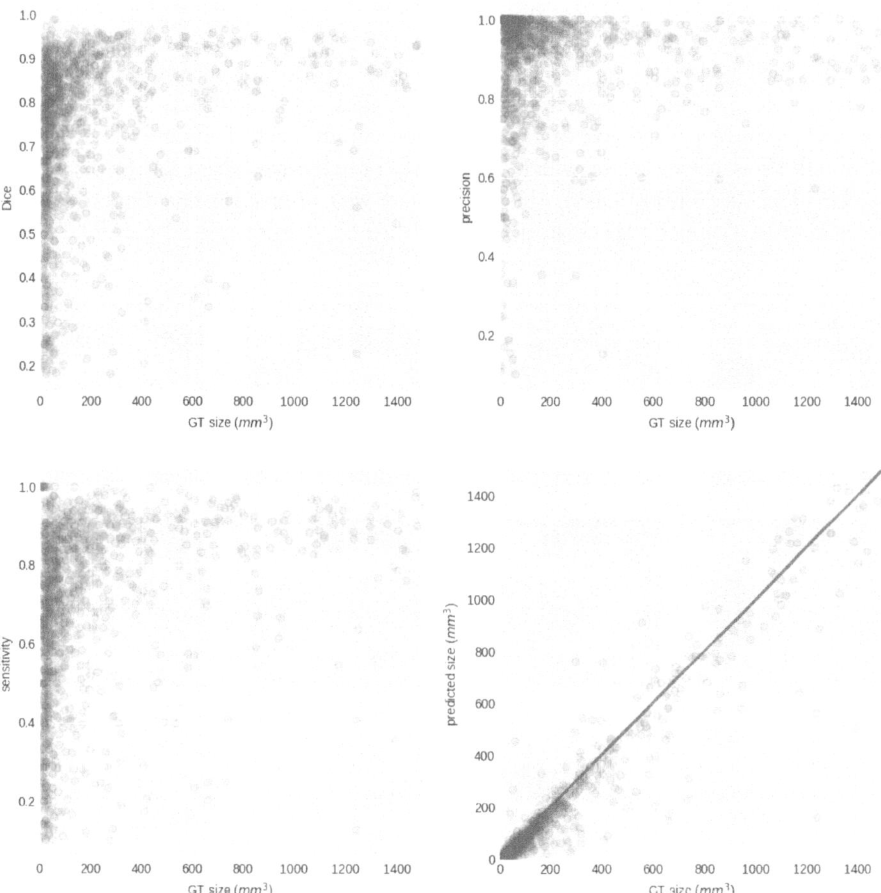

Fig. 2. Overlap metrics for the matched pairs of predictions and ground-truth segmentations for the training set. Each point corresponds to one of such pairs.

Table 3. The results obtained over the test set Ψ, as returned by the evaluation server for the final submission. We report the Dice score (*dsc*), and the Normalized Surface Distance (*nsd*) for all classes: ET (enhancing tumor), RC (resection cavity), TC (tumor core), and WT (whole tumor). Both metrics should be maximized (↑).

metric	ET_{dsc}	ET_{nsd}	RC_{dsc}	RC_{nsd}	TC_{dsc}	TC_{nsd}	WT_{dsc}	WT_{nsd}
mean	0.578	0.664	0.906	0.905	0.590	0.666	0.586	0.633
std dev.	0.292	0.310	0.261	0.262	0.295	0.310	0.292	0.291

Automatically detecting and segmenting small metastases is of paramount clinical importance, as these steps allow us to effectively quantify the progress of the disease in an unbiased and fully reproducible way. Finally, in Fig. 5, we render the predicted segmentation masks for the validation cases, for which the ground truth has not been released (therefore, we do not present the ground-truth masks). However, the validation quality metrics (calculated by the evaluation server) indicate the strong generalization capabilities of the nnU-Net model. Although there are cases for which the quality metrics are rather low (see e.g., the BraTS-MET 00844-000 case), the metastasis was appropriately detected here, and therefore could be tracked in the longitudinal studies of this patient [15].

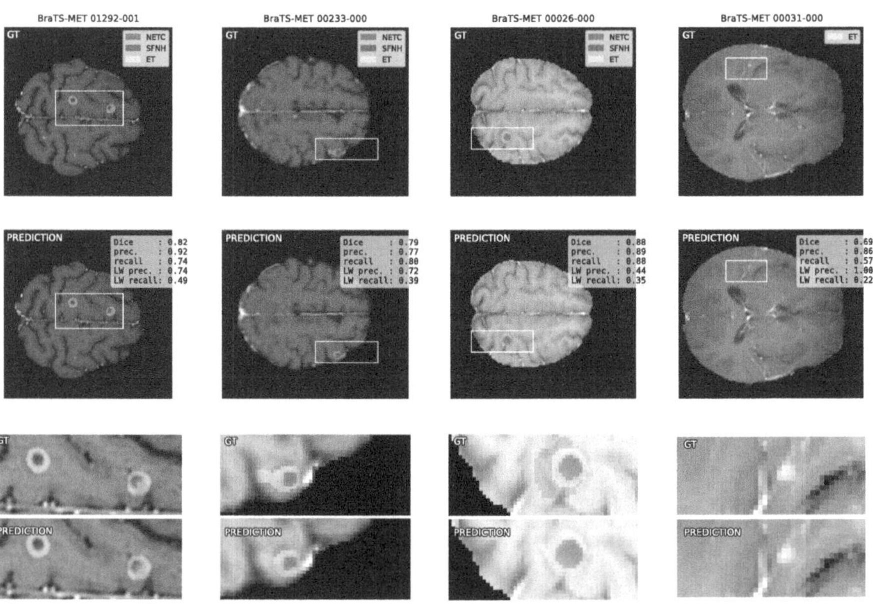

Fig. 3. Example predictions obtained for the *small* metastases for the training set ($\boldsymbol{T}$) multiparametric MRI scans, along with ground truth segmentations. The bottom row displays zoomed-in fragments corresponding to the areas marked with white boxes.

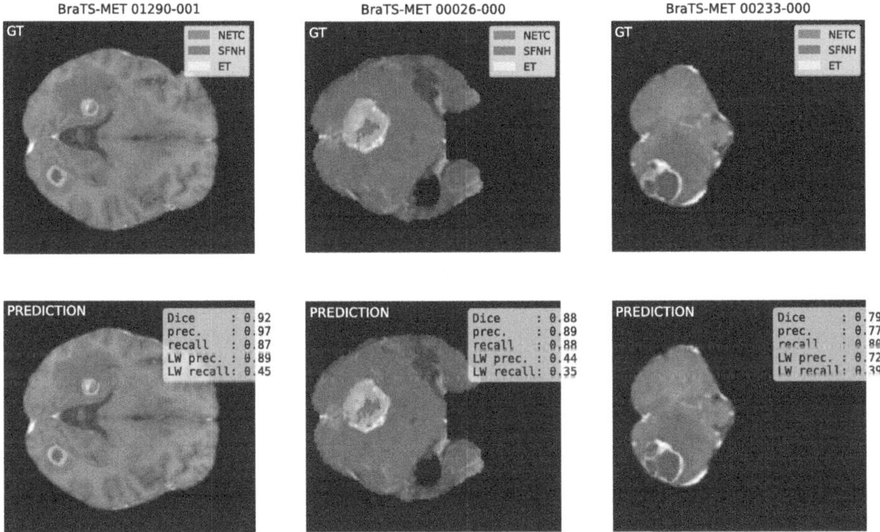

Fig. 4. Example predictions obtained for the *large* metastases for the training set ($\boldsymbol{T}$) multiparametric MRI scans.

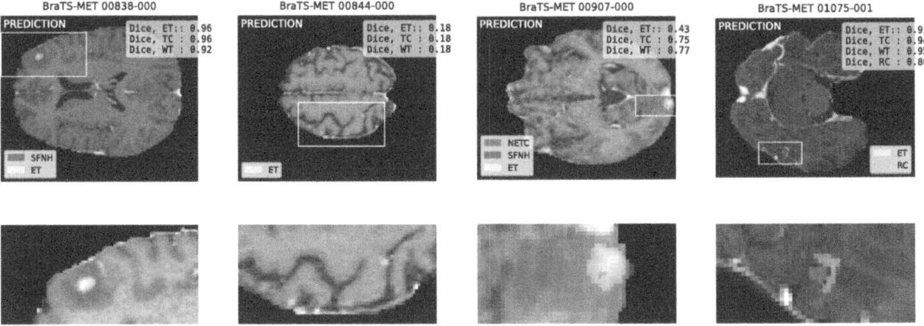

Fig. 5. Example predictions obtained using the nnU-Net model for the metastases for the validation set ($\boldsymbol{V}$) multiparametric MRI scans. The bottom row displays zoomed-in fragments corresponding to the areas marked with white boxes.

The results obtained over the unseen test set are gathered in Table 3. They highlight the generalizability of our model—it outperformed all other techniques in the BraTS-METS 2025 Challenge and was the winning solution.

5 Conclusion

Detecting and segmenting brain metastases have become extremely important in clinical practice, in order to effectively track the disease progress. Since the manual annotation of such lesions is troublesome, prone to human errors and bias, and it is time-consuming (thus not scalable), developing objective, automatic, and fully-reproducible techniques for this task has been blooming in the field of medical image analysis. In this work, we followed this research pathway, and introduced nnU-Nets for automatic brain metastasis detection and multi-class segmentation. The experiments, performed on a large-scale and heterogeneous (in terms of scanners and acquisition protocols) dataset showed that the automatically optimized fully-convolutional neural networks offer high-quality brain metastasis delineation, exceeding the Dice score of 0.78 for the enhancing part of the tumor (being clinically extremely important) in the unseen validation set. Finally, the results obtained over the test set and calculated by the evaluation server further confirmed the capabilities of our technique—it was the winning solution of the BraTS-METS 2025 Challenge.

Acknowledgments. JN was supported by the Silesian University of Technology grant for maintaining and developing research potential. The authors would like to thank Daria Bernys (Graylight Imaging) for her valuable help in managing this study.

This paper is in memory of Dr. Grzegorz Nalepa, an extraordinary scientist, pediatric hematologist/oncologist, and a compassionate champion for kids at Riley Hospital for Children, Indianapolis, USA, who helped countless patients and their families through some of the most challenging moments of their lives.

References

1. Ambrosini, R.D., Wang, P., O'Dell, W.G.: Computer-aided detection of metastatic brain tumors using automated three-dimensional template matching. J. Magn. Reson. Imaging **31**(1), 85–93 (2010). https://doi.org/10.1002/jmri.22009
2. Berrada, L., Zisserman, A., Kumar, M.P.: Smooth loss functions for deep top-k classification. In: International Conference on Learning Representations (2018)
3. Chen, A., et al.: Developments in MLflow: a system to accelerate the machine learning lifecycle. In: Proceedings of the Fourth International Workshop on Data Management for End-to-End Machine Learning. DEEM '20. Association for Computing Machinery, New York, NY, USA (2020). https://doi.org/10.1145/3399579.3399867
4. Cho, S.J., Sunwoo, L., Baik, S.H., Bae, Y.J., Choi, B.S., Kim, J.H.: Brain metastasis detection using machine learning: a systematic review and meta-analysis. Neuro-Oncology **23**(2), 214–225 (2020). https://doi.org/10.1093/neuonc/noaa232
5. Farjam, R., Parmar, H.A., Noll, D.C., Tsien, C.I., Cao, Y.: An approach for computer-aided detection of brain metastases in post-Gd T1-W MRI. Magn. Reson. Imaging **30**(6), 824–836 (2012). https://doi.org/10.1016/j.mri.2012.02.024
6. González, C., Ranem, A., Pinto dos Santos, D., Othman, A., Mukhopadhyay, A.: Lifelong nnU-net: a framework for standardized medical continual learning. Sci. Rep. **13**(1), 9381 (2023). https://doi.org/10.1038/s41598-023-34484-2

7. Grabowski, B., et al.: Squeezing adaptive deep learning methods with knowledge distillation for on-board cloud detection. Eng. Appl. Artif. Intell. **132**, 107835 (2024). https://doi.org/10.1016/j.engappai.2023.107835, https://www.sciencedirect.com/science/article/pii/S0952197623020195
8. Heidenreich, J.F., Gassenmaier, T., Ankenbrand, M.J., Bley, T.A., Wech, T.: Self-configuring nnU-net pipeline enables fully automatic infarct segmentation in late enhancement MRI after myocardial infarction. Eur. J. Radiol. **141**, 109817 (2021). https://doi.org/10.1016/j.ejrad.2021.109817, https://www.sciencedirect.com/science/article/pii/S0720048X21002989
9. Huang, X., Chen, W., Liu, X., Wu, H., Wen, Z., Shen, L.: Left and right ventricular segmentation based on 3D region-aware U-net. In: 2022 IEEE 35th International Symposium on Computer-Based Medical Systems (CBMS), pp. 137–142 (2022). https://doi.org/10.1109/CBMS55023.2022.00031
10. Isensee, F., Jaeger, P.F., Kohl, S.A.A., Petersen, J., Maier-Hein, K.H.: nnU-Net: a self-configuring method for deep learning-based biomedical image segmentation. Nat. Methods **18**(2), 203–211 (2021). https://doi.org/10.1038/s41592-020-01008-z
11. Isensee, F., Ulrich, C., Wald, T., Maier-Hein, K.H.: Extending nnU-net is all you need. In: Deserno, T.M., Handels, H., Maier, A., Maier-Hein, K., Palm, C., Tolxdorff, T. (eds.) BVM 2023, pp. 12–17. Springer, Wiesbaden (2023). https://doi.org/10.1007/978-3-658-41657-7_7
12. Isensee, F., et al.: nnU-net revisited: a call for rigorous validation in 3D medical image segmentation. In: Linguraru, M.G., et al. (eds.) MICCAI 2024. LNCS, vol. 15009, pp. 488–498. Springer, Cham (2024). https://doi.org/10.1007/978-3-031-72114-4_47
13. Justo, J.A., et al.: Semantic segmentation in satellite hyperspectral imagery by deep learning. IEEE J. Sel. Top. Appl. Earth Observ. Remote Sens. **18**, 273–293 (2025). https://doi.org/10.1109/JSTARS.2024.3487360
14. Kovac, D., et al.: Deep learning for in-orbit cloud segmentation and classification in hyperspectral satellite data. In: 2024 9th International Conference on Frontiers of Signal Processing (ICFSP), pp. 68–72 (2024). https://doi.org/10.1109/ICFSP62546.2024.10785468
15. Machura, B., et al.: Deep learning ensembles for detecting brain metastases in longitudinal multi-modal MRI studies. Comput. Med. Imaging Graph. **116**, 102401 (2024). https://doi.org/10.1016/j.compmedimag.2024.102401, https://www.sciencedirect.com/science/article/pii/S0895611124000788
16. Moawad, A.W., et al.: The Brain Tumor Segmentation (BraTS-METS) Challenge 2023: Brain Metastasis Segmentation on Pre-treatment MRI (2024). https://arxiv.org/abs/2306.00838
17. Nalepa, J., et al.: Deep learning automates bidimensional and volumetric tumor burden measurement from MRI in pre- and post-operative glioblastoma patients. Comput. Biol. Med. **154**, 106603 (2023). https://doi.org/10.1016/j.compbiomed.2023.106603
18. Park, Y.W., Lee, N., Ahn, S.S., Chang, J.H., Lee, S.K.: Radiomics and deep learning in brain metastases: current trends and roadmap to future applications. Investig. Magn. Reson. Imaging **25**(4), 266–280 (2021). https://doi.org/10.13104/imri.2021.25.4.266
19. Perez-Ramírez, U., Arana, E., Moratal, D.: Brain metastases detection on MR by means of three-dimensional tumor-appearance template matching. J. Magn. Reson. Imaging **44**(3), 642–652 (2016). https://doi.org/10.1002/jmri.25207

20. Sunwoo, L., et al.: Computer-aided detection of brain metastasis on 3D MR imaging: observer performance study. PLOS ONE **12**(6), 1–18 (2017). https://doi.org/10.1371/journal.pone.0178265
21. Zhang, G., Yang, Z., Huo, B., Chai, S., Jiang, S.: Automatic segmentation of organs at risk and tumors in CT images of lung cancer from partially labelled datasets with a semi-supervised conditional nnU-Net. Comput. Methods Programs Biomed. **211**, 106419 (2021). https://doi.org/10.1016/j.cmpb.2021.106419

Automated Segmentation for the Brain Tumor Segmentation (BraTS) Metastases 2025 Challenge Using Multi-Architectural Deep Learning

Wes Krikorian[1](✉) and Ananya Purwar[2]

[1] Horace Mann School, Bronx, NY, USA
wnkrikorian@gmail.com
[2] Harvey Mudd College, Claremont, CA, USA

Abstract. Brain metastases are the most frequently diagnosed brain tumors and are associated with significant clinical and economic burdens. Accurate segmentation of metastases is essential for minimally invasive treatment but remains a time-consuming and labor-intensive process. This work presents a machine learning-based segmentation pipeline to compete in the Brain Tumor Segmentation (BraTS) Metastases 2025 Challenge, using the MONAI Auto3DSeg framework with three neural network architectures: SegResNet, DiNTS, and Swin-UNETR. The model was trained on 1,296 cases, each including four sequences (T1, T1-post contrast, T2, and FLAIR), with an NVIDIA ADA 6000 GPU. Training was done with two-fold cross-validation on 100 epochs with early stopping after 5 epochs. Once training was completed, the models each made predictions on 179 unlabeled cases, which were then post-processed by removing noise, enforcing a label hierarchy, and filling in holes. Then, the final predictions were submitted to the BraTS Synapse page for model evaluation. The final predictions achieved Dice Similarity Coefficients (DSC) of 0.87 for the resection cavity, 0.69 for the tumor core, 0.68 for the whole tumor, and 0.66 for the enhancing tumor. These results highlight the combination of multiple architectures and a robust post-processing pipeline to improve segmentation accuracy. Future work will focus on using more cross-validation folds, optimizing model architectures through neural architecture search, and expanding training data to improve the detection of smaller tumor regions.

Keywords: Brain Metastases · Neural Network · Transformer · Autosegmentation · Ensemble

1 Introduction

Brain metastases are the most diagnosed brain neoplastic lesions and occur as a complication in patients with primary solid tumors in the lung, breast, colon, etc. [1, 2]. In some studies, the percentage of patients with primary cancer who develop brain metastatic disease can be as high as 30% with correspondingly significant morbidity,

S. Bakas et al. (Eds.): MICCAI 2025, LNCS 16376, pp. 173–181, 2026.
https://doi.org/10.1007/978-3-032-16365-3_16

mortality, and cost [3]. In one study, synchronous brain metastases, which are present at the time of initial primary cancer diagnosis, are associated with a median survival of less than 5 months [4–6]. Treatment options for these patients are generally limited to systemic chemotherapy and radiation therapy. Surgery is generally not an option due to location and risk of injury to adjacent critical intracranial structures [7, 8]. As such, any technology to improve outcomes for these patients is desperately needed.

Accurate segmentation of brain metastases is crucial for diagnosis, treatment planning, and monitoring. However, this requires extensive manual effort by radiologists to ensure adequate precision. This is particularly important for prognostication and for therapies such as stereotactic radiosurgery, where just a few millimeters can make a difference in clinical outcome. The ability to precisely delineate tumor boundaries enables clinicians to deliver targeted radiation doses while minimizing damage to healthy brain tissue [9–11]. In the United States, there remains a shortage of radiologists due to rising imaging volumes and training bottlenecks, such that in 2024, 45% of hospitals report being understaffed in radiology [12]. This scenario presents a significant opportunity for AI innovation.

One effort to address this clinical and research need is the Brain Tumor Segmentation Challenge (BraTS), an international competition that provides a standardized dataset and evaluation framework for developing automated brain tumor segmentation algorithms using multimodal MRI scans. The brain metastases segmentation model presented in this scientific work was created using MonAI's Auto3dSeg, an open-source framework for medical image segmentation. It simplifies the complex process of setting up, training, and implementing AI models for medical image analysis. The framework has proven effective in various medical applications, particularly in identifying and outlining anatomical structures like aortas, kidneys, and tumors in CT scans. Deep learning architectures used in this training include: SegResNet, Swin-UNETR, and DiNTS architectures, discussed in greater detail below. [13–15].

2 Methodology

2.1 Dataset

The BraTS-METs 2025 challenge includes two unique datasets [16]: 1296 labeled cases and a 176-unlabeled dataset. The larger, labeled dataset was used for training, while the smaller, unlabeled dataset was used for validation.

The dataset includes pre-contrast T1-weighted (T1W), post-contrast T1-weighted (T1C), T2-weighted (T2W), and T2-weighted Fluid Attenuated Inversion Recovery (FLAIR) sequences. Each scan is annotated for four key tumor subregions: the tumor core (TC), the whole tumor (WT), the enhancing tumor (ET), and the resection cavity (RC). The dataset used to train the model represents a large-scale, multi-institutional collection of brain MRI scans for metastasis segmentation. Ultimately, the trained model generates the predictions that would be subsequently uploaded to the BraTS Synapse page for evaluation. Please note that the first paragraph of a section or subsection is not indented. The first paragraphs that follows a table, figure, equation etc. does not have an indent, either.

2.2 Annotation Protocol

Annotations were generated using a multi-step pipeline to address the size of the data and ensure clinical accuracy. An automated metastasis segmentation tool first produced initial labels, which were then manually refined by trained medical students. These refined labels were subsequently reviewed and verified by neuroradiologists. This approach ensures high-quality ground truth to train accurate models.

2.3 Architecture

To enhance the robustness of final predictions and leverage the complementary strengths of different architectures, we trained the models using SegResNet, base-level DiNTS, and Swin-UNETR. This multi-architecture approach allowed certain models to compensate for the weaknesses of others, improving overall segmentation performance. SegResNet, base DiNTS, and Swin-UNETR represent three neural network architectures commonly used in medical image segmentation, each suited to different use cases.

SegResNet, a convolutional residual network, is known for its efficiency and strong performance on standard segmentation tasks, making it ideal for quick experimentation and deployment in resource-limited environments. The base DiNTS model serves as the starting point for neural architecture search (NAS), offering a generic UNet-style structure that can be optimized to fit the characteristics of a specific dataset better. While its baseline performance is modest, it lays the groundwork for more powerful custom models. Swin-UNETR, a transformer-based architecture, excels in capturing long-range spatial dependencies and is particularly well-suited for complex, multimodal imaging tasks such as brain tumor segmentation. Although computationally intensive, it often delivers state-of-the-art results when sufficient data and GPU resources are available. Together, these models cover a wide spectrum of segmentation needs, from baseline efficiency to maximum accuracy [17–21].

2.4 Pre-Processing

All cases in the BraTS-METs 2025 dataset underwent pre-processing by the BraTS organizers. The pipeline started with a format conversion where the original Digital Imaging and Communication in Medicine (DICOM) files were converted into the Neuroimaging Informatics Technology Initiative (NIfTI) format. During this step, all private patient information was removed. Next, spatial registration was conducted: all sequences were aligned so the tumors would be in the same spot for each sequence. Then the images were resampled to an isotropic resolution of 1 mm^3. Lastly, a final anonymization was done by using a deep learning model to skull-strip the image for further patient privacy.

Then, when training the model, MONAI's Autorunner pre-processed the data so it would be compatible with the SegResNet architecture. It changed the input dimensions from 3D to 5D; a channel dimension of four was added (one for each MRI modality), and a batch dimension of one was added. The Autorunner's pre-processing pipeline also resampled voxel spacing and voxel intensity. Lastly, it cropped the image to the annotated portions to remove unnecessary background.

The final step of pre-processing involved assembling all the data into a metadata.json file, allowing the model to easily access the dataset. This metadata file included three keys: training, validation (which was unused), and testing. All 1,296 labeled cases were assigned to the training key, which was then randomly split into five folds. The 176 unlabeled cases were placed under the testing key.

2.5 Training

Model training was performed using an NVIDIA Ada 6000 GPU, chosen for its high memory capacity suitable for large 3D medical imaging workloads. Although the dataset was split into five folds for cross-validation, only models for folds 0 and 1 were trained due to time and computational resource constraints. Each model was trained for up to 100 epochs, with early stopping applied after five consecutive epochs without improvement in validation performance to prevent overfitting and reduce training time. A patch size of $160 \times 160 \times 160$ and a batch size of 1 were used to fit the models within GPU memory limits. Additionally, a low cache rate was configured in the Auto3DSeg training pipeline to manage system memory during data loading. Lastly, the learning rate was set to 1e-4 with a warmup cosine scheduler to avoid large early updates, which could potentially harm the model. This setup balanced performance, resource usage, and time constraints while still allowing for meaningful model evaluation.

2.6 Ensembling and Post-psrocessing

Building on the multi-architecture training approach, the post-processing pipeline further refines segmentation predictions to enhance accuracy and clinical relevance. First, ensembling combines outputs from the SegResNet, base DiNTS, and Swin-UNETR models to leverage their complementary strengths, producing more robust and stable segmentations. Using the MONAI Auto3DSeg Autorunner, the ensemble method was set to select the top-performing algorithm from each fold based on validation performance and combined them using the majority voting scheme that was configured for this implementation. The models were equally weighted in our approach.

Next, hierarchy enforcement ensures that the segmented regions respect anatomical relationships, such as containment or exclusion rules, which is critical in complex structures like brain tumors. Small, isolated clusters (five voxels or fewer), often representing noise or false positives, are then removed to clean the segmentation maps. Finally, any holes or gaps within segmented regions are filled to generate smooth, continuous structures. This carefully designed post-processing pipeline transforms the combined raw model outputs into precise and reliable segmentations (Fig. 1).

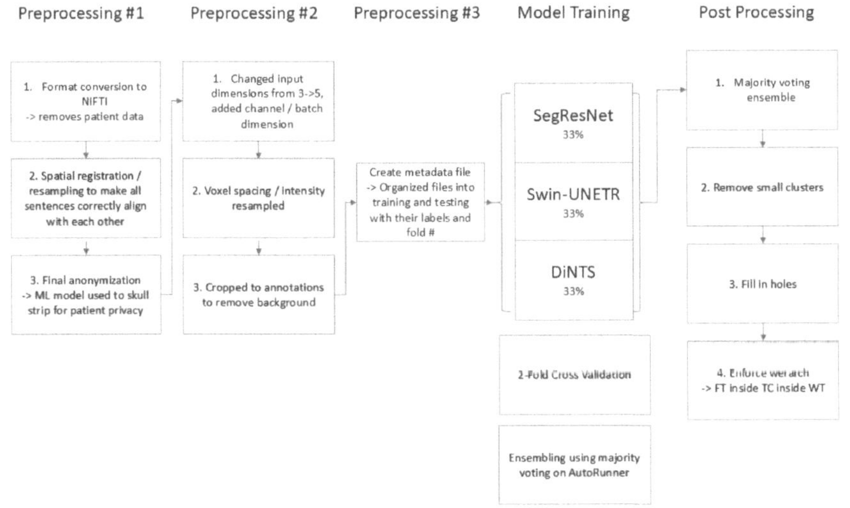

Fig. 1. Schematic of preprocessing, training, and post processing pipeline for automated segmentation for the BraTS Metastases 2025 Challenge using multi-architectural deep learning

2.7 Evaluation Metrics

For the validation and testing phases of the BraTS challenge, the model would be evaluated by the Dice Similarity Coefficient (DSC) and Normalized Surface Distance (NSD) on the tumor core, whole tumor, enhancing tumor, and the resection cavity.

3 Results

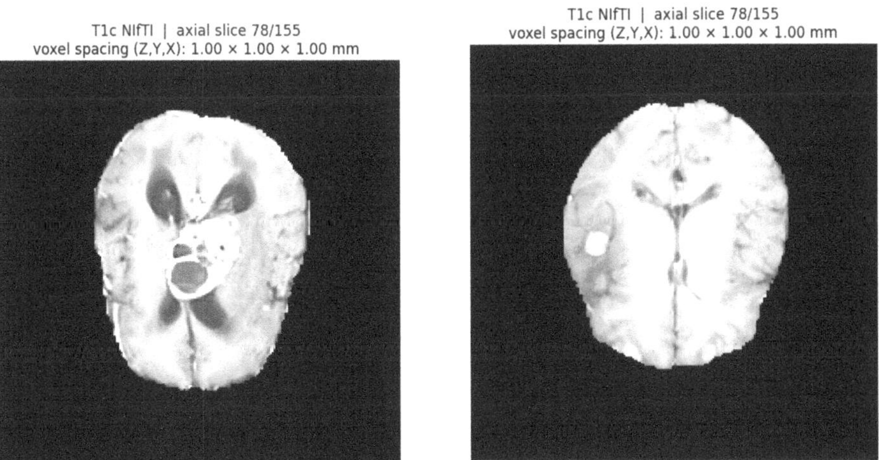

Fig. 2. Examples of axial T1 post contrast images demonstrating enhancing brain metastases.

During model training, the SegResNet model performed a validation epoch every three training epochs (the Swin-UNETR and DiNTS models did not perform any validation due to time constraints). The SegResNet model peaked at an average DSC of 0.64 across all classes. The fully ensembled model demonstrated improvement in performance: from the validation phase, the enhancing tumor had a DSC of 0.66 and an NSD of 0.47; the resection cavity had a DSC and NSD of 0.87; the tumor core had a DSC of 0.69 and an NSD of 0.47; the whole tumor had a DSC of 0.68 and an NSD of 0.35Please note that the first paragraph of a section or subsection is not indented. During the testing phase, the ensemble saw lower dice scores but higher normalized surface distances. The enhancing tumor had a DSC of 0.52 ± 0.29 with an NSD of 0.59 ± 0.30; the resection cavity had a DSC and NSD of about 0.85 ± 0.36; the tumor core had a DSC of 0.53 ± 0.30 and an NSD of about 0.60 ± 0.31; lastly, the whole tumor had a DSC of 0.52 ± 0.29 and an NSD of about 0.56 ± 0.29 (Fig. 2, 3 and 4).

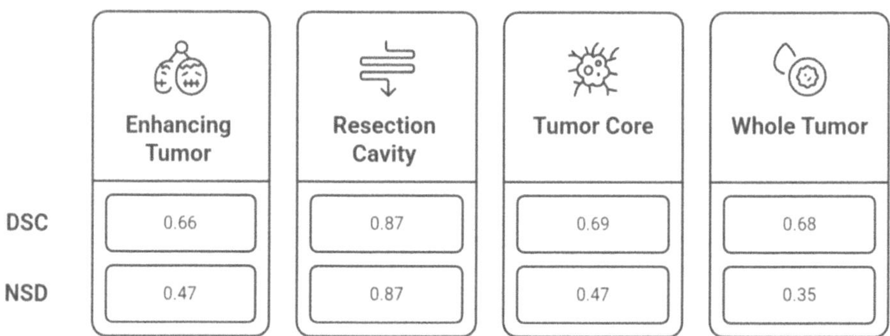

Fig. 3. The final ensemble model's dice similarity coefficient and normalized surface distance for each of the tumor classes during validation.

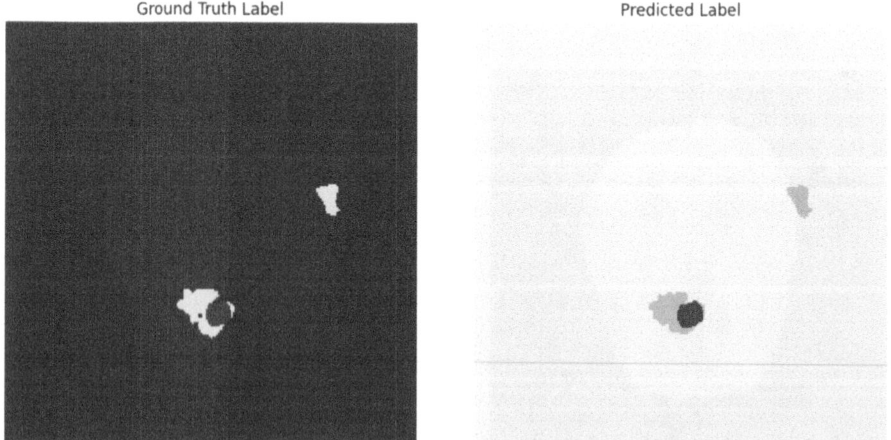

Fig. 4. Visual representation of one example of a pair of the ground truth lable and the final ensemble model's predicted segmentation

4 Discussion

Despite evolving treatment, brain metastatic disease is associated with substantial morbidity and mortality [1, 5]. The Graded Prognostic Assessment (GPA) varies depending on the primary cancer site and the selected treatment approach and strategy [4]. In a recent Norwegian study of 912 patients with first-time brain metastasis, the mean overall survival for the entire cohort was 5.9 months, with 50% of the patients succumbing to their disease within 6 months after the diagnosis had been established [5]. In addition to the unfavorable prognosis, brain metastases incur a significant economic burden. A recent nationwide study conducted in the US found that patients with lung cancer with central nervous system (CNS) spread incurred healthcare costs that were approximately $13,000 higher than those with lung cancer but no brain metastases [3].

According to the Congress of Neurological Surgeons guidelines on brain metastases treatment, surgery plus whole-brain radiotherapy (WBRT) is the recommended initial approach for patients with first-time diagnosed brain metastatic disease [9]. However, WBRT is associated with significant side effects such as, but not limited to, fatigue, nausea, anorexia, cognitive dysfunction, and hearing loss [7]. In contrast to WBRT, stereotactic radiosurgery (SRS) has a less negative effect on neurocognition and quality of life [11]. In addition, Level 3 evidence exists that stereotactic radiosurgery alone can be considered as an alternative treatment to surgery plus WBRT, with the caveat that the patient has oligometastatic disease, i.e., 1 to 4 lesions [11].

For the radiation delivered by SRS to be highly focused, precise contouring of the lesions is performed by radiation oncologists using a radiotherapy planning software. This approach is tedious and time-consuming [15]. Deep Learning (DL) models for brain metastases segmentation, such as the MetNet developed by Zhou et al. [15], have been proposed as a tool to mitigate the challenges with manual lesion delineation. However, to our knowledge, there is no widely distributed tool that is routinely used in clinical practice to autosegment and quantify the volume of intracranial lesions.

The ensemble model achieved the highest segmentation accuracy on the resection cavity (DSC of 0.87), while performance on the enhancing tumor was more modest (DSC of 0.66). These results highlight the effectiveness of both the post-processing pipeline and the ensembling strategy in improving segmentation quality. The strong performance on the resection cavity is likely due to its well-defined and consistent appearance across patients. In contrast, the lower Dice score for the enhancing tumor may stem from its smaller size, variability in appearance, and lower prevalence within the dataset.

In a clinical setting, this model has the potential to significantly reduce the time burden associated with manual segmentation. Rather than delineating lesions from scratch, radiologists could use the model's outputs as a baseline and make minor adjustments as needed, streamlining the workflow and increasing efficiency.

A major limitation of this study was time. Due to computational and scheduling constraints, only two out of the five cross-validation folds were trained. This limitation would likely reduce model performance and reduce generalizability. Additionally, the DiNTS model was used in its unoptimized, base form, without applying neural architecture search (NAS) to tailor it to the dataset. Model parameters were also adjusted for faster training rather than optimal performance. For example, training was capped at 100 epochs with an aggressive early stopping criterion, which may have limited the model's learning capacity.

Future work will address these limitations by completing training on all five folds, conducting a full architecture search for DiNTS, and tuning hyperparameters for performance rather than speed. Moreover, we plan on expanding the training dataset with more cases containing smaller, less common labels, such as enhancing tumors, which may improve sensitivity and segmentation accuracy for underrepresented regions.

References

1. Sharma, P., et al.: Trends in survival in solid malignancies with synchronous brain metastases: a population-based study. JCO **42**, e23299–e23299 (2024)
2. Lamba, N., Wen, P.Y., Aizer, A.A.: Epidemiology of brain metastases and leptomeningeal disease. Neuro Oncol. **23**(9), 1447–1456 (2021). https://doi.org/10.1093/neuonc/noab101
3. Shim, Y.-B., Byun, J.-Y., Lee, J.-Y., Lee, E.-K., Park, M.-H.: Economic burden of brain metastases in non-small cell lung cancer patients in South Korea: a retrospective cohort study using nationwide claims data. PLoS ONE **17**(9), e0274876 (2022). https://doi.org/10.1371/journal.pone.0274876
4. Sperduto, P.W., et al.: Survival in patients with brain metastases: summary report on the updated diagnosis-specific graded prognostic assessment and definition of the eligibility quotient. J. Clin. Oncol. **38**(32), 3773–3784 (2020). https://doi.org/10.1200/JCO.20.01255
5. Yri, O.E., et al.: Survival and quality of life after first-time diagnosis of brain metastases: a multicenter, prospective, observational study. Lancet Reg. Health - Europe **49**, 101181 (2025). https://doi.org/10.1016/j.lanepe.2024.101181
6. Ostrom, Q. T., Wright, C. H., Barnholtz-Sloan, J.S.: Brain metastases: epidemiology. In Handbook of Clinical Neurology, vol. 149, pp. 27–42. Elsevier (2018). https://doi.org/10.1016/B978-0-12-811161-1.00002-5
7. Aizer, A.A., et al.: Brain metastases: a society for Neuro-Oncology (SNO) consensus review on current management and future directions. Neuro Oncol. **24**(10), 1613–1646 (2022). https://doi.org/10.1093/neuonc/noac118
8. Nahed, B.V., et al.: Congress of neurological surgeons systematic review and evidence-based guidelines on the role of surgery in the management of adults with metastatic brain tumors. Neurosurgery **84**(3), E152–E155 (2019). https://doi.org/10.1093/neuros/nyy542
9. Brown, P.D., Ahluwalia, M.S., Khan, O.H., Asher, A.L., Wefel, J.S., Gondi, V.: Whole-brain radiotherapy for brain metastases: evolution or revolution? J. Clin. Oncol. **36**(5), 483–491 (2018). https://doi.org/10.1200/JCO.2017.75.9589
10. Brown, P.D., et al.: Hippocampal avoidance during whole-brain radiotherapy plus memantine for patients with brain metastases: phase III trial NRG oncology CC001. J. Clin. Oncol. **38**(10), 1019–1029 (2020). https://doi.org/10.1200/JCO.19.02767
11. Mansouri, A., et al.: Stereotactic radiosurgery for patients with brain metastases: current principles, expanding indications and opportunities for multidisciplinary care. Nat. Rev. Clin. Oncol. **22**(5), 327–347 (2025). https://doi.org/10.1038/s41571-025-01013-1
12. Rozenshtein, A., Findeiss, L.K., Wood, M.J., Shih, G., Parikh, J.R.: The U.S. radiologist workforce: *AJR* expert panel narrative review. AJR Am. J. Roentgenol. **224**(5), e2432085 (2025). https://doi.org/10.2214/AJR.24.32085. Epub 2024 Dec 18. PMID: 39692304
13. Consortium, T.M.: Project MONAI (Version 0.4.0) [Computer software]. Zenodo (2020). https://doi.org/10.5281/ZENODO.4323059

14. Myronenko, A., Yang, D., He, Y., Xu, D.: Automated 3D Segmentation of Kidneys and Tumors in MICCAI KiTS 2023 Challenge (Version 1). arXiv (2023). https://doi.org/10.48550/ARXIV.2310.04110
15. Zhou, Z., et al.: MetNet: computer-aided segmentation of brain metastases in post-contrast T1-weighted magnetic resonance imaging. Radiother. Oncol. **153**, 189–196 (2020). https://doi.org/10.1016/j.radonc.2020.09.016
16. Moawad, A.W., et al.: The brain tumor segmentation-metastases (brats-mets) challenge 2023: Brain metastasis segmentation on pre-treatment mri. ArXiv, pp.arXiv-2306 (2024)
17. Wang, T.-W., et al.: Brain metastasis tumor segmentation and detection using deep learning algorithms: a systematic review and meta-analysis. Radiother. Oncol. **190**, 110007 (2024)
18. He, Y., Yang, D., Roth, H., Zhao, C., Xu, D.: DiNTS: differentiable neural network topology search for 3D medical image segmentation. In: 2021 IEEE/CVF Conference on Computer Vision and Pattern Recognition (CVPR) (2021)
19. Hsu, C., Chang, C., Chen, T., Tsai, H.S., Wang, W.: Brain Tumor Segmentation (BraTS) challenge short paper: improving three-dimensional brain tumor segmentation using SegResnet and hybrid boundary-dice loss (2021)https://doi.org/10.1007/978-3-031-09002-8_30
20. Myronenko, A., Siddiquee, M., Yang, D., He, Y., Xu, D.: Automated head and neck tumor segmentation from 3D PET/CT (2022). https://doi.org/10.48550/arXiv.2209.10809
21. Angona, T., Mondal, M.: An attention based residual U-Net with swin transformer for brain MRI segmentation. Array **25** (2025). https://doi.org/10.1016/j.array.2025.100376

Taking Advantage of MONAI and DiNTS Frameworks to Develop a State-of-the-Art Algorithm for Automatic Segmentation of Brain Metastases

Fabian Umeh[1], Nikolay Y. Yordanov[2](✉), Nazanin Maleki[3], Raisa Amiruddin[3], Ahmed Moawad[4], Monika Pytlarz[3], Crystal Chukwurah[5], and Mariam Aboian[3]

[1] Teesside University, Middlesbrough, UK
[2] Department of Neurointensive Care, Multiprofile Hospital for Active Treatment in Neurology and Psychiatry "St. Naum", Sofia, Bulgaria
102500@students.mu-sofia.bg
[3] Department of Radiology, Children's Hospital of Philadelphia, Philadelphia, PA, USA
[4] Department of Radiology, Division of Neuroradiology, Perelman School of Medicine at the University of Pennsylvania, Philadelphia, PA, USA
[5] Yale School of Medicine, New Haven, CT, USA

Abstract. Brain metastases are the most common intracranial tumors. Volumetric assessment of the lesions is crucial for stereotactic radiosurgery planning. However, manual annotation of the lesions is time-consuming and prone to error. Automated, reliable solutions have the potential to overcome those barriers. A DiNTS-based 3D segmentation model of brain metastases MRI cases, trained on the Brain Tumor Segmentation (BraTS) – Metastases 2025 Lighthouse Challenge dataset was developed and presented in this study. MONAI and DiNTS frameworks with combined Dice and Focal loss were utilized to develop the model that achieved mean Dice coefficients of 0.692 (WT), 0.718 (TC), and 0.687 (ET) on a validation set of 130 cases. These scores indicate the model's performance across tumor subregions.

Keywords: brain metastases · image segmentation · magnetic resonance imaging · artificial intelligence

1 Introduction

The most frequently diagnosed brain tumors is a metastases originating from a primary cancer [1]. Additionally, it is estimated that brain metastatic disease occurs as a complication in at least 10 percent of patients with solid tumors, with varying incidence depending on the type of the primary malignant process [2]. Schnurman et al. found that despite the advancements in diagnosis and treatment of brain metastatic disease, approximately 10 percent of the patients with brain metastases die secondary to the central nervous system spread of the primary malignance [3]. These data indicate the clinical burden of brain metastatic disease and underscore the need for further improving diagnosis, treatment and follow-up of patients with brain metastases.

S. Bakas et al. (Eds.): MICCAI 2025, LNCS 16376, pp. 182–189, 2026.
https://doi.org/10.1007/978-3-032-16365-3_17

Accurate lesion detection, volume assessment, and longitudinal tracking are necessary for stereotactic radiosurgery planning, decision-making and management of patients with brain metastases [4]. Manual completion of these tasks is time-consuming and laborious, rater-dependent, and prone to errors [5, 6]. Artificial intelligence tools have emerged as a promising solution for automating the volumetric analysis of brain tumors, including brain metastases [7].

U-Net is an example of a commonly used artificial neural network architecture for the segmentation of biomedical images and can be trained on a variety of datasets, adapted for 3D imaging, and applied to various tasks [8, 9]. Isensee et al. developed a framework based on U-Net that self-configures itself to be applicable to any new biomedical image segmentation tasks [10]. Another volumetric convolutional neural network, proposed by Mulletari et al., is V-Net, which was further developed by Hua et al. and applied to a brain tumor segmentation task [11, 12]. Both U-Net and V-Net methods follow an encoder-decoder structure and allow for fine-tuning and architectural modifications aimed at enhancing the accuracy and precision of the model for the specific medical image segmentation task [13].

We took advantage of the DiNTS architecture with combined Dice and Focal loss to develop a model for 3D segmentation of MRI brain metastases cases. We present the strategy employed for creating the model, as well as the results obtained via testing the model on 130 validation cases.

2 Methods

The dataset utilized for the model training was curated from the Medical Image Computing and Computer Assisted Intervention Society (MICCAI) Brain Tumor Segmentation (BraTS) – Metastases 2025 Lighthouse Challenge training dataset, comprising multimodal pre-operative MRI scans of brain metastases (BM): T1-weighted with contrast enhancement (T1C), native T1-weighted (T1N), T2-weighted (T2W), and T2-FLAIR. The sequences for each case were co-registered in either native space or SRI24 multichannel atlas of the brain [14]. The dataset underwent a 5-step annotation pipeline, for which a 4-label system for image annotation was used [15]. The necrotic core of the tumor is labelled with Label 1 (Non-enhancing tumor core, NETC), the peritumoral edema with Label 2 (Surrounding non-enhancing FLAIR hyperintensity, SNFH), the enhancing portion of the tumor with Label 3 (Enhancing tumor, ET), and the resection cavity (in case of a post-treatment study) with Label 4 (Resection cavity, RC). The tumor core (TC) comprises Label 2 (ET) plus Label 1 (NETC). The whole tumor (WT) comprises TC plus Label 3 (SNFH). All scans and labels were resampled to 1mm isotropic resolution, and although missing cases were designed to be excluded, there were no missing cases during metadata generation. Dataset splits for training and testing were assigned using a simple fold assignment via case indexing, resulting in an approximately balanced distribution of cases across five folds. Metadata and fold assignments were programmatically encoded for reproducibility.

Preprocessing and data augmentation were performed using the MONAI framework [16, 17]. The pipeline included loading images as float32 and masks as unit8, reorienting to RAS, and intensity normalizing channel-wise over nonzero voxels. Volumes and labels were resampled to [1.0, 1.0, 1.0]mm resolution and padded/cropped to a fixed voxel ROI. The tumor masks represent the extent of the tumor, and each pixel in the mask has one of the labels mentioned in the previous paragraph assigned to it. The masks were converted to multi-channel one-shot representations for whole tumor (WT), tumor core (TC), and enhancing tumor (ET) prediction. Training patches were sampled with 'RandCropByLabelClassesd' to enforce class balance. Augmentations included random affine transformations (rotation, zoom), intensity perturbations (scaling, shifting, Gaussian noise, smoothing), and spatial flips, with automatic parameter selection from a search space preconfigured by MONAI.

The Differentiable Neural Architecture Search (DiNTS) model was employed for 3D segmentation. DiNTS optimizes network topology by searching a space of 12 blocks across 4 depth levels with downsampling [18]. The search space consisted of eight primitive operations, including separable convolutions (3x3x3, 5x5x5, 7x7x7), dilated convolution, max and average pooling, identity connections, and zero operation. The search used MONAI's TopologySearch with Adam for architecture weights and stochastic gradient descent (SGD) for model weights. The selected topology was instantiated and fine-tuned using SGD, with DiceFocal loss to address class imbalance and focus learning on challenging voxels in tumor regions by combining volumetric overlap with hard example emphasis, improving overall prediction compared to using them individually [19]. The model accepts four-channel MRI inputs and outputs three segmentation classes via sigmoid activation. An overview of the pipeline is demonstrated in Fig. 1.

Training involved random patch sampling (2–14 patches per image) to balance GPU memory of a 15GB Nvidia Tesla T4 GPU. For the final training, a polynomial learning rate scheduler with a power of 0.5 decayed the initial learning rate of 0.2, and the SGD optimizer used a momentum of 0.9 and weight decay of 4.0e-05 over 66 epochs. Automatic mixed precision was used. Validation occurred every 1–2 epochs, with early stopping based on Dice score stagnation (patience up to 30 epochs). All operations were automated via MONAI's Auto3DSeg AutoRunner.

Performance was evaluated using mean volumetric Dice coefficients and region-wise overlap statistics across the selected cross-validation folds, adhering to BraTS leaderboard requirements. The best performing checkpoint was saved for inference. All pipelines are encoded in version-controlled YAML configs and scripts, publicly available in the code repository.

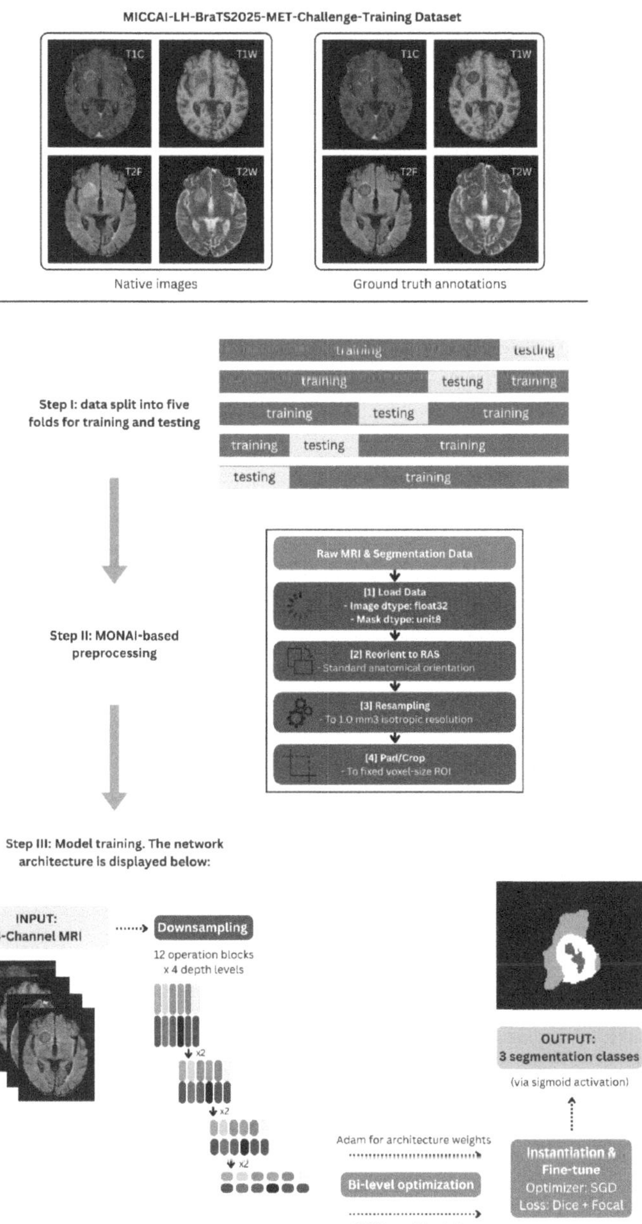

Fig. 1. Graphical representation of the methodology for creating the medical image segmentation model

3 Results

We evaluated our DiNTS-based segmentation model on a validation set of 130 cases from the BraTS-METS 2025 dataset. The segmentation quality was assessed using the Dice Similarity Coefficient (Dice score) for each primary tumor subregion: whole tumor (WT), tumor core (TC), and enhancing tumor (ET). The mean scores for each label are provided in Table 1.

Table 1. Mean Dice coefficients for every tumor region

Tumor Region	Mean Dice Coefficient ± SD (validation set)	Mean Dice Coefficient ± SD (official testing set)
Whole Tumor (WT)	0.692 ± 0.256	0.692 ± 0.256
Tumor Core (TC)	0.718 ± 0.235	0.718 ± 0.235
Enhancing Tumor (ET)	0.687 ± 0.238	0.687 ± 0.238

The model achieved Dice scores above 0.68 across all tumor subregions, indicating consistent segmentation performance. The Dice + Focal Loss contributed to delineation of smaller and more irregular regions, as reflected by the relative scores on the enhancing tumor class despite its smaller volume and weaker contrast. Figure 2 provides a visual representation of the model's performance.

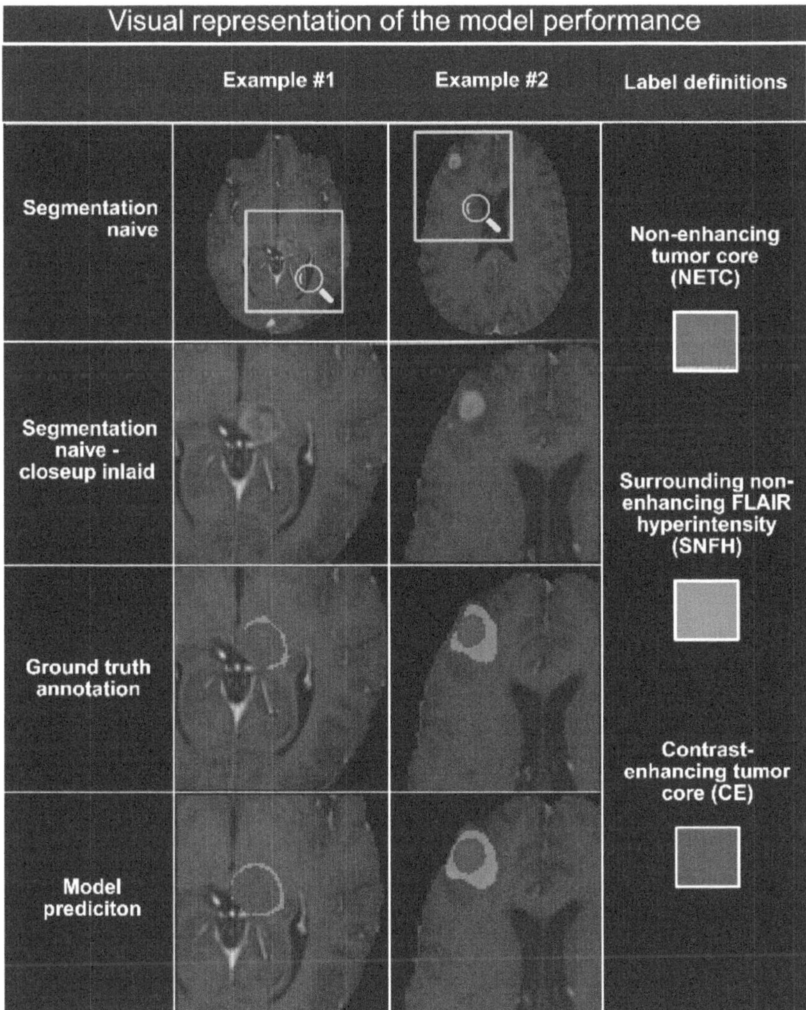

Fig. 2. Examples of validation cases with corresponding ground truth and model predictions.

4 Clinical Implications

Volumetric assessment of brain metastatic lesions using automated segmentation tools is a crucial step in the development of algorithms that support the physicians in stereotactic surgery planning, treatment-response assessment, and management decision making.

Disclosure of Interests. We have no conflicts of interest to disclose.

References

1. Ostrom, Q.T., Wright, C.H., Barnholtz-Sloan, J.S.: Brain metastases: epidemiology. Handb. Clin. Neurol. **149**, 27–42 (2018). https://doi.org/10.1016/b978-0-12-811161-1.00002-5
2. Lamba, N., Wen, P.Y., Aizer, A.A.: Epidemiology of brain metastases and leptomeningeal disease. Neuro-Oncol. **23**, 1447–1456 (2021). https://doi.org/10.1093/neuonc/noab101
3. Schnurman, Z., et al.: Causes of death in patients with brain metastases. Neurosurgery **93**, 986–993 (2023). https://doi.org/10.1227/neu.0000000000002542
4. Wang, J.-Y., et al.: Stratified assessment of an FDA-cleared deep learning algorithm for automated detection and contouring of metastatic brain tumors in stereotactic radiosurgery. Radiat. Oncol. **18**, 61 (2023). https://doi.org/10.1186/s13014-023-02246-z
5. Andrearczyk, V., et al.: Automatic detection and multi-component segmentation of brain metastases in longitudinal MRI. Sci. Rep. **14** (2024). https://doi.org/10.1038/s41598-024-78865-7
6. Machura, B., et al.: Deep learning ensembles for detecting brain metastases in longitudinal multi-modal MRI studies. Comput. Med. Imaging Graph. **116**, 102401 (2024). https://doi.org/10.1016/j.compmedimag.2024.102401
7. Grøvik, E., Yi, D., Iv, M., Tong, E., Rubin, D., Zaharchuk, G.: Deep learning enables automatic detection and segmentation of brain metastases on multisequence MRI. J. Magn. Reson. Imaging **51**, 175–182 (2020). https://doi.org/10.1002/jmri.26766
8. Bousabarah, K., et al.: Deep convolutional neural networks for automated segmentation of brain metastases trained on clinical data. Radiat. Oncol. **15** (2020). https://doi.org/10.1186/s13014-020-01514-6
9. Duong, M.T., et al.: Convolutional neural network for automated FLAIR lesion segmentation on clinical brain MR imaging. Am. J. Neuroradiol. **40**, 1282–1290 (2019). https://doi.org/10.3174/ajnr.a6138
10. Abstract: nnU-Net: Self-adapting Framework for U-Net-Based Medical Image Segmentation. In: Informatik aktuell, p. 22. Springer Fachmedien Wiesbaden, Wiesbaden (2019). https://doi.org/10.1007/978-3-658-25326-4_7
11. Milletari, F., Navab, N., Ahmadi, S.-A.: V-Net: fully convolutional neural networks for volumetric medical image segmentation. In: 2016 Fourth International Conference on 3D Vision (3DV), pp. 565–571. IEEE, Stanford (2016). https://doi.org/10.1109/3dv.2016.79
12. Hua, R., et al.: Segmenting brain tumor using cascaded v-nets in multimodal MR images. Front. Comput. Neurosci. **14** (2020). https://doi.org/10.3389/fncom.2020.00009
13. Tran, M., Vo-Ho, V.-K., Le, N.T.H.: 3DConvCaps: 3DUnet with convolutional capsule encoder for medical image segmentation. In: 2022 26th International Conference on Pattern Recognition (ICPR), pp. 4392–4398. IEEE, Montreal (2022). https://doi.org/10.1109/icpr56361.2022.9956588
14. Rohlfing, T., Zahr, N.M., Sullivan, E.V., Pfefferbaum, A.: The SRI24 multichannel atlas of normal adult human brain structure. Hum. Brain Mapp. **31**, 798–819 (2010). https://doi.org/10.1002/hbm.20906
15. Maleki, N., et al.: Analysis of the MICCAI brain tumor segmentation -- metastases (BraTS-METS). In: 2025 Lighthouse Challenge: Brain Metastasis Segmentation on Pre- and Post-treatment MRI (2025). https://arxiv.org/abs/2504.12527. https://doi.org/10.48550/ARXIV.2504.12527
16. Cardoso, M.J., et al.: MONAI: An open-source framework for deep learning in healthcare (2022). https://arxiv.org/abs/2211.02701. https://doi.org/10.48550/ARXIV.2211.02701
17. Consortium, T.M.: Project MONAI (2020). https://zenodo.org/record/4323059. https://doi.org/10.5281/ZENODO.4323059

18. He, Y., Yang, D., Roth, H., Zhao, C., Xu, D.: DiNTS: differentiable neural network topology search for 3D medical image segmentation (2021). https://arxiv.org/abs/2103.15954. https://doi.org/10.48550/ARXIV.2103.15954
19. Agravat, R., Raval, M.S.: 3D semantic segmentation of brain tumor for overall survival prediction (2020). https://doi.org/10.48550/ARXIV.2008.11576

Challenge 5 – BraTS-Africa

Ensembling CNN, Transformer, and Mamba with Stacking for Brain Tumor Segmentation

Trung D. Q. Dang, Huy Hoang Nguyen(✉), and Aleksei Tiulpin

University of Oulu, Oulu, Finland
{trung.ng,huy.nguyen,aleksei.tiulpin}@oulu.fi

Abstract. In this study, we explore the effectiveness of a stacking ensemble approach for brain tumor segmentation by combining three distinct deep neural network architectures: nnU-Net (based on convolutional neural network, SwinUNETR (based on transformer), and LoG-VMamba (based on VMamba). Each model offers unique representational strengths that, when integrated through ensemble learning, enhance overall segmentation performance. To enable robust fusion, our model utilizes two core components: (1) label noise modeling through signed soft labels and (2) stacking-based model fusion. All models, including ensembles, are evaluated on two tasks of the BraTS 2025 challenge: Task 1 (pre- and post-treatment glioma in adults) and Task 5 (glioma segmentation within a Sub-Saharan African patient population). Our results show that SwinUNETR consistently performs below nnU-Net and LoG-VMamba on both tasks. The ensemble method surpasses all individual models according to both regional and boundary-aware metrics, demonstrating improved accuracy and robustness. Our findings underscore the value of architectural diversity and ensemble learning in advancing medical image segmentation.

Keywords: Semantic segmentation · Soft label · Ensemble

1 Introduction

Glioma, the most common type of brain tumor in adults, is a major contributor to cancer-related mortality, particularly in men under 40 years of age and women under 20 years of age [25]. Accurate segmentation of gliomas plays a critical role in diagnosis, treatment planning, and longitudinal monitoring. Due to its high soft tissue contrast and non-invasive nature, magnetic resonance imaging (MRI) is the main imaging modality used for the evaluation of brain tumors [28]. However, manual segmentation of gliomas in MRI is time consuming, labor intensive, and subject to interobserver variability. As such, there has been an increasing interest in developing Deep Learning (DL)-based automated segmentation methods to support clinical workflows. These methods aim to delineate tumor

S. Bakas et al. (Eds.): MICCAI 2025, LNCS 16376, pp. 193–204, 2026.
https://doi.org/10.1007/978-3-032-16365-3_18

subregions—such as the enhancing tumor core, edema, and necrotic tissue—directly from multi-modal MRI data [12,13,27,32]. Delineation is an instance of Semantic segmentation (SSEG) problem.

SSEG is a core task in computer vision, where the objective is to assign a class label to each voxel (or pixel) in an image, enabling fine-grained delineation of structures. It has broad applications, from autonomous driving to medical imaging. In the medical domain, in particular, SSEG is essential for analyzing complex anatomical and pathological structures in 3D volumes. During the past decade, deep learning (DL) has become the dominant approach to this problem.

Early DL-based SSEG methods relied primarily on convolutional neural networks (CNNs), which effectively model local spatial hierarchies through convolutional filters. However, CNNs struggle to capture long-range dependencies due to their inherently limited receptive field. To address this limitation, transformer-based models adapted from natural language processing have been applied to vision tasks, leveraging self-attention mechanisms to model the global context. Notable examples include Swin UNETR [13] and TransBTS [30], which integrate transformer layers into U-Net-like architectures. More recently, state-space models (SSMs) such as Mamba have been proposed as a new modeling paradigm, combining the global modeling capacity of transformers with improved efficiency. Architectures like LoG-VMamba [9] exemplify this direction, achieving strong performance while keeping linear complexity in the number of tokens.

Recent developments in brain tumor segmentation have focused on three key research directions. The first explores architectural innovations, including hybrid CNN-transformer models [12,13,24,30,34], and more recently SSM-based architectures [9]. The second line of work emphasizes the design of loss functions, in order to better align the training objective with segmentation evaluation metrics such as Dice and IoU [4,5,23,31,32]. The third explores alternative ground truth (GT) representations, moving beyond hard binary labels to soft labels or regression-based formulations that better reflect the uncertainty of the annotation and the ambiguity of the boundaries [8,18,27].

In this work, we utlize the benefits of CNN, Transformer, and VMamba to develop an ensemble model. Following Dang *et al.* [8], we formulate semantic segmentation as a voxel-wise regression task to mitigate the issue of label noise. Specifically, binary ground truth masks are first transformed into signed "soft labels" using the signed normalized geodesic distance transform. The ensemble is then trained on the outputs of individual models to produce the final tumor segmentation masks. We evaluate our method on multiple tasks from the BraTS-Lighthouse 2025 Challenge.

2 Methods

2.1 Overview

We employ an ensemble-based framework for brain tumor segmentation that benefits from architectural diversity with robust training strategies (see Fig. 1). Specifically, our approach integrates predictions from M different DL models, each trained using K-fold cross-validation. This results in a total of $M \times K$ predicted segmentation masks per subject, which are subsequently fused to produce the final output. This ensemble strategy, presented in Sect. 2.4, is designed to reduce the variance of the final prediction and improve the robustness of segmentation in different subregions of the tumor.

Rather than formulating segmentation as a voxel-wise classification task, we follow the recent paradigm introduced by Dang *et al.* [8], and recast it as a *voxel-level regression problem* (see Sect. 2.2). This formulation enables the models to generate continuous-valued output, offering improved spatial precision and better uncertainty modeling at tissue boundaries compared to conventional classification-based approaches. To exploit the complementary strengths of different neural network architectures, we incorporate models from three major design families (see Sect. 2.3):

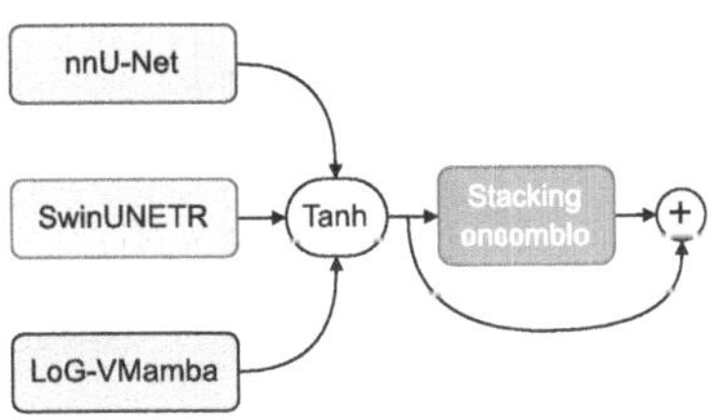

Fig. 1. Overview of the ensemble architecture

- **nnU-Net** [14]: a CNN framework that adapts dynamically to dataset-specific properties and has demonstrated strong performance across medical imaging benchmarks;
- **SwinUNETR** [12]: a transformer-based architecture that leverages self-attention mechanisms to model long-range dependencies and global context;
- **LoG-VMamba** [9]: a recent architecture based on the VMamba design, which combines state-space modeling with gated MLP mechanisms to efficiently capture both local and global features.

2.2 Signed Normalized Geodesic Regression

Signed Normalized Geodesic Transform. Instead of assigning discrete class labels to each voxel, Dang *et al.* [8] propose the Signed Normalized Geodesic Transform (SiNG), which encodes each binary voxel as a signed real-valued distance to the nearest region boundary, normalized across the volume (see Fig. 2). Specifically, foreground regions (e.g., tumor volumes) are represented by non-negative values in $[0, 1]$, with boundary voxels taking a value of zero. In contrast, background voxels are assigned to values in $[-1, 0)$. For those voxels significantly distant from the boundary are set to -1.

Formally, given an input image I with spatial dimensions $H \times W \times L$ and a region $R \subset \Omega = [H] \times [W] \times [L]$, the *unsigned geodesic distance transform* (GeoDT) from a point $i \in \Omega$ to R is defined as [26,29]:

$$G^{\lambda}(i; R, I) = \min_{j \in R} D^{\lambda}(i, j, I), \tag{1}$$

$$D^{\lambda}(i, j; I) = \min_{p \in P_{i,j}} \int_0^1 (1-\lambda)\|p'(s)\|_1 + \lambda \|\nabla I(p(s)) \cdot u(s)\|_1, \tag{2}$$

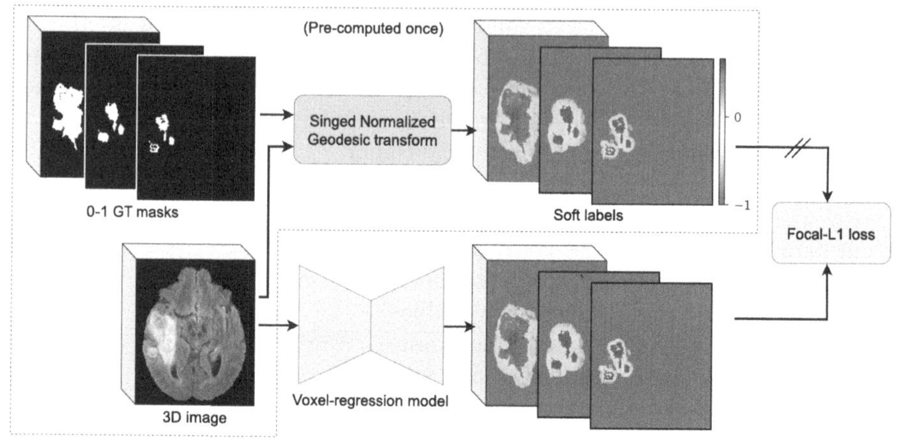

Fig. 2. Framework for signed normalized geodesic regression [8].

where $\lambda \in [0, 1]$ balances spatial and image gradient costs, $P_{i,j}$ is the set of all paths from i to j, $u(s) = \frac{p'(s)}{\|p'(s)\|_1}$, and $\nabla I(p(s))$ is the image gradient. GeoDT assigns zero distance for all $i \in R$. Though accurate, this transform is computationally expensive—scaling with the size of R and I.

The *signed GeoDT* is typically computed by applying GeoDT to foreground and background regions separately [10], which is costly. To reduce computation, we instead apply unsigned GeoDT to a boundary set R_B, extracted from a segmentation mask M via the Canny edge detector [6]. For simplicity, we write $G_i^\lambda := G^\lambda(i; R_B, I)$. The signed distance is then:

$$s_i G_i^\lambda, \quad \text{where } s_i = \text{sign}(2M_i - 1).$$

To focus on annotation uncertainty near object boundaries, we ignore distant regions by setting $\lambda = 0$ and defining:

$$\mathcal{B} = \left\{ i \in \Omega \mid G_i^0 \leq \beta \right\}, \tag{3}$$

$$\beta = \max_{i \in \Omega : M_i = 1} G_i^0. \tag{4}$$

Finally, we define the *SiNG transform*:

$$\mathcal{S}_i = \begin{cases} \frac{1}{\tau}(1-\delta) s_i G_i^\lambda + \delta s_i & \text{if } i \in \mathcal{B}, \\ -1 & \text{otherwise}, \end{cases} \tag{5}$$

where $\tau = \max_{j \in \mathcal{B}} G_j^\lambda$ normalizes the distance and $\delta \in [0, 1)$ controls the margin between foreground and background.

Focal-L1 Loss. Dang *et al.* [8] formulate the tumor segmentation task as an image-level regression problem rather than a voxel classification task, the latter of which typically employs cross-entropy (CE) or focal loss for optimization [16]. Accordingly, the regression loss is designed to prioritize hard regions over easy ones. Drawing inspiration from the CE-based focal loss [16], the authors introduce a novel L1-based focal loss, termed Focal-L1, tailored for the regression task.

For an arbitrary pair of inputs (I, M), the authors apply the SiNG transformation to generate a corresponding map $\mathcal{S}$ with a specified parameter λ. Furthermore, given a parametric function f_θ with parameters θ, where $f_\theta(I)$ represents a mask predicted from the input image I, the authors use the tanh function to transform the values of $f_\theta(I)$ into the range $[-1, 1]$, denoted $\mathcal{Z} = \tanh(f_\theta(I))$. To this end, the Focal-L1 loss is defined as follows [8]:

$$\mathcal{L}_{\text{FocalL1}}(\mathcal{S}, \mathcal{Z}; \theta) = \frac{1}{|\Omega|} \sum_{i \in \Omega} |\mathcal{S}_i - \mathcal{Z}_i| \underbrace{\frac{|\mathcal{S}_i - \mathcal{Z}_i|^{\gamma \mathbb{I}(\mathcal{S}_i \mathcal{Z}_i \geq 0)}}{\max(|\mathcal{S}_i|, |\mathcal{Z}_i|) + \varepsilon}}_{\text{Sample weighting}}, \tag{6}$$

where ε is a positive constant to prevent numerical instability, γ is a positive hyperparameter, and $\mathbb{I}(\cdot)$ is the indicator function.

2.3 Models

nnU-Net [14] represents a robust and fully automated solution for biomedical image segmentation, distinguished not by architectural novelty but by its comprehensive self-configuration capabilities. This framework systematically adapts its architecture, preprocessing, training, and inference procedures to the characteristics of each target dataset, thereby eliminating the need for manual tuning and domain-specific heuristics.

At its core, nnU-Net employs the standard U-Net architecture [22]. The network consists of a symmetric encoder-decoder design, where the encoder extracts increasingly abstract feature representations through a series of convolutional blocks and strided downsampling operations, while the decoder restores spatial resolution via upsampling and skip connections that concatenate corresponding encoder features. For 3D data, each convolutional block typically comprises two convolutional layers with kernel size $3 \times 3 \times 3$, followed by instance normalization and leaky rectified linear unit (Leaky ReLU) activation functions. The number of filters per layer, network depth, and other architectural parameters are not fixed but are instead derived automatically based on the input data properties and available computational resources.

SwinUNETR [12] is a transformer-based segmentation model with hierarchical encoding. It is a U-shaped segmentation architecture that integrates a Swin Transformer encoder [17] with a convolutional decoder, designed specifically for volumetric medical image segmentation. Unlike conventional CNN-based encoders, the Swin Transformer captures long-range dependencies via window-based self-attention, applied hierarchically across multiple scales. The input volume is divided into non-overlapping 3D patches, linearly embedded, and passed through a series of Swin Transformer blocks, which employ both windowed and shifted window self-attention to balance efficiency and context modeling. Patch merging operations between stages reduce spatial resolution and expand the feature dimension, forming a natural multiscale representation.

The decoder mirrors the hierarchical encoder, using convolutional blocks with upsampling layers to reconstruct high-resolution segmentation maps. Feature maps from corresponding encoder stages are fused via skip connections, enabling the model to combine global contextual information with local spatial detail. Residual connections and standard 3D convolutions (with instance normalization and Leaky ReLU) further stabilize training.

LoG-VMamba [9] is a vision DL architecture that extends the Mamba framework [11,19] – a selective state space model—by effectively integrating local and global spatial context for high-resolution medical image segmentation. The inherently sequential nature of Mamba poses challenges in preserving fine-grained local dependencies among neighboring voxels in 3D data, as well as capturing long-range relationships across distant regions. LoG-VMamba [9] overcomes these limitations through a dual-branch design that concurrently extracts local and global tokens. Its segmentation model is based on U-Mamba [19], embedding LoG-VMamba blocks within the U-shaped architecture of U-Net [22] to enable multi-scale feature fusion.

2.4 Stacking Ensemble

Data Construction. We adopt the stacking strategy to construct a model ensemble [33] and aggregate predictions from multiple models. The dataset is partitioned into K disjoint chunks, denoted $\mathcal{D}_1, \ldots, \mathcal{D}_K$. Let $\{f_{m,k}\}_{m \in [M], k \in [K]}$ denote a collection of trained models, where $[M] = \{1, \ldots, M\}$ indexes different model architectures, and $[K] = \{1, \ldots, K\}$ corresponds to data folds. For instance, $f_{m,1}$ denotes model architecture m trained on the data chunks $\mathcal{D}_2, \ldots, \mathcal{D}_K$ and validated on $\mathcal{D}_1$. For each fold k, we define the set of validation predictions as $\mathcal{F}_k = \{[f_{m,k}(\mathbf{x})]_{m=1}^M \mid \mathbf{x} \in \mathcal{D}_k, \}$, from which we construct the training and validation sets as follows:

$$\hat{\mathcal{D}}_k^{\text{train}} = \bigcup_{i \in [K] \setminus \{k\}} \mathcal{F}_i = \left\{[f_{m,i}(\mathbf{x})]_{m=1}^M \mid \mathbf{x} \in \mathcal{D}_i, i \in [K] \setminus \{k\}\right\} \tag{7}$$

$$\hat{\mathcal{D}}_k^{\text{val}} = \mathcal{F}_k = \left\{[f_{m,k}(\mathbf{x})]_{m=1}^M \mid \mathbf{x} \in \mathcal{D}_k\right\}. \tag{8}$$

We then concatenate the predictions from different models, $[f_{m,k}(\mathbf{x})]_{m=1}^M$, along the channel axis. As a result, each element in the resulting set has dimensions $C \times M \times H \times W \times D$, where C denotes the number of classes in the segmentation task.

Ensembling Model. Given M segmentation models, each trained with K-fold cross-validation, our goal is to fuse the M predicted masks produced for each fold $k \in [K]$. We propose a lightweight ResNet-inspired architecture to combine the M predictions per class $c \in [C]$. Let $\mathbf{x}_c \in \mathbb{R}^{M \times H \times W \times D}$ denote the stacked logits for class c from all M models. A class-specific sub-network θ_c processes these logits as follows:

$$\mathbf{z} = \tanh(\mathbf{x}_c) \tag{9}$$

$$\mathbf{h}_1 = \tanh(\phi_1(\mathbf{z})) \tag{10}$$

$$\mathbf{h}_2 = \tanh(\phi_2(\mathbf{h}_1)) \tag{11}$$

$$\tilde{\mathbf{y}}_c = \mathbf{h}_2 + \mathbf{z} \tag{12}$$

where ϕ_1 is a 3D convolutional layer mapping from M input channels to 64, and ϕ_2 maps from 64 to M. The resulting tensor $\tilde{\mathbf{y}}_c$ is then averaged along the model dimension to produce the final output $\mathbf{y}_c \in \mathbb{R}^{1 \times H \times W \times D}$, representing the fused prediction for class c. Subsequently, we concatenate the fused outputs across all classes to obtain the normalized prediction for fold $k \in [K]$:

$$\mathbf{y}^{(k)} = \text{Concat}(\mathbf{y}_1, \ldots, \mathbf{y}_C) \in [-1, 1]^{C \times H \times W \times D}. \tag{13}$$

At deployment time, we average the normalized predictions across all K folds to obtain the final output:

$$\mathbf{y} = \frac{1}{K} \sum_{k=1}^{K} \mathbf{y}^{(k)}. \tag{14}$$

3 Experiments

3.1 Datasets

We conducted our experiments on the following segmentation tasks of the BraTS-Lighthouse 2025 challenge:

- (Task 1) Glioma segmentation on pre- and post-treatment MRI [2,3,20][1];
- (Task 5) Segmentation of brain glioma in Sub-Saharan Africa patient population [1].

The data description of the three tasks is presented in Table 1. For simplicity, from this point forward, we will reference the datasets using the task index.

Table 1. Description of datasets

Index	Name	Classes	Samples	Crop size	Std spacing (mm)
Task 1	PRE	3	1251	128 × 128 × 128	1 × 1 × 1
Task 5	SSA	3	60	128 × 128 × 128	1 × 1 × 1

[1] We only work on the pre-treatment data.

3.2 Experimental Setups

Implementation Details. All experiments were conducted on AMD MI250x GPUs. The codebase was developed using PyTorch [21] and MONAI [7]. MRI scans and corresponding masks were resampled to an isotropic resolution of $1 \times 1 \times 1$ mm. During training, we applied data augmentations including foreground cropping, random flipping, intensity scaling, and shifting. Each random $128 \times 128 \times 128$ crop was normalized for intensity. Ground-truth masks were converted into three standard classes: enhancing tumor (ET), tumor core (TC), and whole tumor (WT). For optimization, we utilized the Adam algorithm [15].

Training and Evaluation Protocols. We performed 5-fold cross-validation on each dataset. For every fold, nnU-Net, SwinUNETR, and LoG-VMamba were trained independently. Their predictions were then used to train the stacking ensemble described in Sect. 2.4. Model performance was evaluated using the Dice score, 95% Hausdorff Distance (HD95), and Normalized Surface Dice (NSD) with a threshold of 1.

3.3 Results

Task 1. We present the fold-level results of Task 1 in Table 2. The nnU-Net model consistently yields strong Dice scores, especially on Folds 0 and 2, while LoG-VMamba shows competitive performance with a slight advantage in NSD on Fold 3. SwinUNETR trails behind in both metrics, suggesting that transformer-based approaches may require further optimization for this specific task. Overall, the ensemble method achieves the highest performance across nearly all folds, outperforming individual models and their averaged performances in both Dice and NSD metrics.

The class-wise results are presented in Table 3. Among the individual methods, nnU-Net and LoG-VMamba achieve comparable performance in terms of Dice and NSD, with LoG-VMamba exhibiting a slight advantage in HD95, indicating more accurate boundary delineation. In contrast, SwinUNETR shows lower performance across all metrics, particularly in the tumor core (TC) region, suggesting potential limitations in its representational capacity for this task. The ensemble method, which integrates the strengths of all three architectures, consistently outperforms the individual models across all evaluated metrics—Dice, HD95, and NSD. The performances of the ensemble model on the test set are presented in Table 6.

Task 5. The fold-level results for Task 5, presented in Table 4, demonstrate that the ensemble method consistently achieves the highest Dice and NSD scores across most folds. Among the standalone models, LoG-VMamba and nnU-Net show similar performance trends, with LoG-VMamba slightly outperforming nnU-Net in NSD across several folds. SwinUNETR performs comparably in Dice for Fold 0 but shows a marked decline in both Dice and NSD for Fold 4, suggesting reduced consistency and generalizability across validation subsets.

Table 2. Per-fold comparison of segmentation methods across Dice, and NSD on Task 1.

Method	Dice (%)					NSD (%)				
Fold	0	1	2	3	4	0	1	2	3	4
nnU-Net	**89.6**	88.9	**89.1**	89.9	89.4	85.2	83.8	84.2	84.9	85.1
SwinUNETR	87.8	87.1	87.6	88.2	88.6	82.3	81.2	82.1	81.7	83.7
LoG-VMamba	89.1	88.7	88.4	90.0	89.1	85.1	83.8	83.8	85.5	84.8
Average	88.8	88.2	88.4	89.4	89.0	84.2	83.0	83.4	84.0	84.5
Ensemble	**89.6**	**89.0**	89.0	**90.3**	**89.6**	**85.5**	**84.1**	**84.7**	**85.6**	**85.4**

Table 3. Comparison of segmentation methods across Dice, HD95, and NSD on Task 1.

Method	Dice (%)				HD95 (mm)				NSD (%)			
	ET	TC	WT	Avg	ET	TC	WT	Avg	ET	TC	WT	Avg
nnU-Net	85.8	89.8	92.6	89.4	**4.0**	4.7	6.2	5.0	86.2	83.5	84.2	84.6
SwinUNETR	84.5	87.4	91.6	87.9	5.2	6.2	7.5	6.3	84.4	79.9	82.4	82.2
LoG-VMamba	85.1	89.5	92.5	89.1	4.2	4.6	5.8	4.8	86.3	83.2	84.2	84.6
Average	85.2	88.9	92.2	88.8	4.5	5.1	6.5	5.4	85.6	82.2	83.6	83.8
Ensemble	**85.9**	**90.0**	**92.7**	**89.5**	**4.0**	**4.4**	**5.5**	**4.7**	**86.7**	**83.8**	**84.7**	**85.1**

The class-wise performance in Table 5 further highlights the strength of the ensemble approach, which achieves the highest average Dice (82.1%), lowest HD95 (8.6 mm), and best NSD (70.2%) across all tumor subregions (ET, TC, WT). LoG-VMamba attains the best Dice for TC (78.3%) among individual models and also demonstrates superior boundary accuracy with lower HD95 and higher NSD for TC and WT compared to nnU-Net and SwinUNETR. While nnU-Net matches LoG-VMamba in overall Dice, its higher HD95 suggests less precise boundary localization. SwinUNETR lags behind across all classes and metrics, particularly in TC segmentation, aligning with its weaker fold-level performance. The results of the ensemble model on the private test set are shown in Table 6.

4 Discussion

We propose a stacking ensemble model designed to take advantage of the complementary strengths of diverse deep learning architectures: nnU-Net, SwinUNETR, and LoG-VMamba, representing convolutional, transformer-based, and VMamba-based paradigms, respectively. By integrating the outputs of these heterogeneous models, the ensemble consistently outperforms all individual models, as well as their unweighted averages. These results suggest that architectural diversity enhances feature representation and contributes to improved generalization in multi-class tumor segmentation.

Table 4. Per-fold comparison of segmentation methods across Dice, and NSD on Task 5.

Method	Dice (%)					NSD (%)				
Fold	0	1	2	3	4	0	1	2	3	4
nnU-Net	75.1	88.5	81.5	78.1	**84.5**	64.5	75.3	70.0	68.0	71.8
SwinUNETR	79.8	85.3	81.7	76.3	72.1	**67.8**	70.1	69.9	64.5	57.4
LoG-VMamba	76.9	88.4	80.5	78.4	83.2	65.3	75.8	70.4	68.3	68.8
Average	77.3	87.4	81.3	77.6	79.9	65.9	73.7	70.1	66.9	66.0
Ensemble	**79.3**	**88.7**	**82.1**	**79.2**	81.3	**67.8**	**76.2**	**71.8**	**69.8**	**65.5**

Table 5. Comparison of segmentation methods across Dice, HD95, and NSD on the validation sets of Task 5.

Method	**Dice (%)**				**HD95 (mm)**				**NSD (%)**			
	ET	TC	WT	Avg	ET	TC	WT	Avg	ET	TC	WT	Avg
nnU-Net	77.5	77.9	89.2	81.5	8.9	13.7	10.0	10.9	72.0	62.7	75.0	69.9
SwinUNETR	75.0	73.8	88.5	79.1	8.9	12.6	10.0	10.5	68.2	55.4	74.2	65.9
LoG-VMamba	76.8	**78.3**	89.3	81.5	8.4	10.5	9.0	9.3	70.3	**62.9**	76.0	69.7
Average	76.4	76.7	89.0	80.7	8.7	12.3	9.7	10.2	70.2	60.3	75.1	68.5
Ensemble	**78.3**	78.2	**89.8**	**82.1**	**8.2**	**9.8**	**7.8**	**8.6**	**72.2**	62.0	**76.5**	**70.2**

Table 6. Evaluation results of the ensemble model on the private test sets.

Task	**Dice (%)**				**NSD (%)**			
	ET	RC	TC	WT	ET	RC	TC	WT
1	$74.4_{\pm 30.1}$	$59.5_{\pm 49.1}$	$74.1_{\pm 32.3}$	$83.2_{\pm 21.3}$	$78.3_{\pm 29.1}$	$59.5_{\pm 49.1}$	$73.5_{\pm 30.6}$	$78.3_{\pm 21.9}$
5	$75.8_{\pm 27.1}$	–	$76.7_{\pm 29.8}$	$85.4_{\pm 20.9}$	$68.9_{\pm 25.6}$	–	$62.4_{\pm 27.3}$	$73.4_{\pm 22.6}$

References

1. Adewole, M., et al.: The brain tumor segmentation (BRaTS) challenge 2023: Glioma segmentation in Sub-Saharan Africa patient population (BRaTS-Africa). arXiv pp. arXiv–2305 (2023)
2. Baid, U., et al.: The RSNA-ASNR-MICCAI BRaTS 2021 benchmark on brain tumor segmentation and radiogenomic classification. arXiv preprint arXiv:2107.02314 (2021)
3. Bakas, S., et al.: Advancing the cancer genome atlas glioma MRI collections with expert segmentation labels and radiomic features. Sci. Data **4**(1), 1–13 (2017)
4. Berman, M., Triki, A.R., Blaschko, M.B.: The lovász-softmax loss: a tractable surrogate for the optimization of the intersection-over-union measure in neural networks. In: Proceedings of the IEEE Conference on Computer Vision and Pattern Recognition, pp. 4413–4421 (2018)
5. Bertels, J., et al.: Optimizing the dice score and Jaccard index for medical image segmentation: theory and practice. In: Shen, D., et al. (eds.) MICCAI 2019. LNCS, vol. 11765, pp. 92–100. Springer, Cham (2019). https://doi.org/10.1007/978-3-030-32245-8_11
6. Canny, J.: A computational approach to edge detection. IEEE Trans. Pattern Anal. Mach. Intell. **6**, 679–698 (1986)
7. Cardoso, M.J., et al.: MONAI: an open-source framework for deep learning in healthcare. arXiv preprint arXiv:2211.02701 (2022)
8. Dang, T., Nguyen, H.H., Tiulpin, A.: SiNGR: brain tumor segmentation via signed normalized geodesic transform regression. In: Linguraru, M.G., et al. (eds.) MICCAI 2024. LNCS, vol. 15009, pp. 593–603. Springer, Cham (2024). https://doi.org/10.1007/978-3-031-72114-4_57
9. Dang, T.D.Q., Nguyen, H.H., Tiulpin, A.: LoG-VMAmba: local-global vision mamba for medical image segmentation. In: Proceedings of the Asian Conference on Computer Vision, pp. 548–565 (2024)
10. Fu, K., Gu, I.Y., Ödblom, A., Liu, F.: Geodesic distance transform-based salient region segmentation for automatic traffic sign recognition. In: 2016 IEEE Intelligent Vehicles Symposium (IV), pp. 948–953. IEEE (2016)
11. Gu, A., Dao, T.: Mamba: linear-time sequence modeling with selective state spaces. arXiv preprint arXiv:2312.00752 (2023)
12. Hatamizadeh, A., Nath, V., Tang, Y., Yang, D., Roth, H.R., Xu, D.: Swin UNETR: swin transformers for semantic segmentation of brain tumors in mri images. In: Crimi, A., Bakas, S. (eds.) BrainLes 2021. LNCS, vol. 12962, pp. 272–284. Springer, Cham (2021). https://doi.org/10.1007/978-3-031-08999-2_22
13. Hatamizadeh, A., et al.: UNETR: transformers for 3D medical image segmentation. In: Proceedings of the IEEE/CVF Winter Conference on Applications of Computer Vision, pp. 574–584 (2022)
14. Isensee, F., Jaeger, P.F., Kohl, S.A., Petersen, J., Maier-Hein, K.H.: nnU-net: a self-configuring method for deep learning-based biomedical image segmentation. Nat. Methods **18**(2), 203–211 (2021)
15. Kingma, D.P., Ba, J.: Adam: a method for stochastic optimization. arXiv preprint arXiv:1412.6980 (2014)
16. Lin, T.Y., Goyal, P., Girshick, R., He, K., Dollár, P.: Focal loss for dense object detection. In: Proceedings of the IEEE International Conference on Computer Vision, pp. 2980–2988 (2017)

17. Liu, Z., Lin, Y., Cao, Y., Hu, H., Wei, Y., Zhang, Z., Lin, S., Guo, B.: Swin transformer: hierarchical vision transformer using shifted windows. In: Proceedings of the IEEE/CVF International Conference on Computer Vision, pp. 10012–10022 (2021)
18. Ma, J., Wang, C., Liu, Y., Lin, L., Li, G.: Enhanced soft label for semi-supervised semantic segmentation. In: Proceedings of the IEEE/CVF International Conference on Computer Vision, pp. 1185–1195 (2023)
19. Ma, J., Li, F., Wang, B.: U-mamba: enhancing long-range dependency for biomedical image segmentation. arXiv preprint arXiv:2401.04722 (2024)
20. Menze, B.H., et al.: The multimodal brain tumor image segmentation benchmark (BRaTS). IEEE Trans. Med. Imaging **34**(10), 1993–2024 (2014)
21. Paszke, A., et al.: PyTorch: an imperative style, high-performance deep learning library. In: Advances in Neural Information Processing Systems, vol. 32 (2019)
22. Ronneberger, O., Fischer, P., Brox, T.: U-net: convolutional networks for biomedical image segmentation. In: Navab, N., Hornegger, J., Wells, W.M., Frangi, A.F. (eds.) MICCAI 2015. LNCS, vol. 9351, pp. 234–241. Springer, Cham (2015). https://doi.org/10.1007/978-3-319-24574-4_28
23. Salehi, S.S.M., Erdogmus, D., Gholipour, A.: Tversky loss function for image segmentation using 3D fully convolutional deep networks. In: Wang, Q., Shi, Y., Suk, H.-I., Suzuki, K. (eds.) MLMI 2017. LNCS, vol. 10541, pp. 379–387. Springer, Cham (2017). https://doi.org/10.1007/978-3-319-67389-9_44
24. She, D., Zhang, Y., Zhang, Z., Li, H., Yan, Z., Sun, X.: EoFormer: edge-oriented transformer for brain tumor segmentation. In: Greenspan, H., et al. (eds.) MICCAI 2023. LNCS, vol. 14223, pp. 333–343. Springer, Cham (2023). https://doi.org/10.1007/978-3-031-43901-8_32
25. Siegel, R.L., Miller, K.D., Fuchs, H.E., Jemal, A.: Cancer statistics, 2022. CA: Can. J. Clinic. **72**(1), 7–33 (2022)
26. Toivanen, P.J.: New geodosic distance transforms for gray-scale images. Pattern Recogn. Lett. **17**(5), 437–450 (1996)
27. Vasudeva, S.A., Dolz, J., Lombaert, H.: Geols: geodesic label smoothing for image segmentation. In: Medical Imaging with Deep Learning, pp. 468–478. PMLR (2024)
28. Verduin, M., et al.: Noninvasive glioblastoma testing: multimodal approach to monitoring and predicting treatment response. Dis. Mark. **2018** (2018)
29. Wang, G., et al.: DeepIGeoS: a deep interactive geodesic framework for medical image segmentation. IEEE Trans. Pattern Anal. Mach. Intell. **41**(7), 1559–1572 (2018)
30. Wang, W., Chen, C., Ding, M., Yu, H., Zha, S., Li, J.: TransBTS: multimodal brain tumor segmentation using transformer. In: de Bruijne, M., et al. (eds.) MICCAI 2021. LNCS, vol. 12901, pp. 109–119. Springer, Cham (2021). https://doi.org/10.1007/978-3-030-87193-2_11
31. Wang, Z., Blaschko, M.B.: Jaccard metric losses: optimizing the Jaccard index with soft labels. arXiv preprint arXiv:2302.05666 (2023)
32. Wang, Z., Popordanoska, T., Bertels, J., Lemmens, R., Blaschko, M.B.: Dice semimetric losses: optimizing the dice score with soft labels. arXiv preprint arXiv:2303.16296 (2023)
33. Wolpert, D.H.: Stacked generalization. Neural Netw. **5**(2), 241–259 (1992)
34. Xing, Z., Yu, L., Wan, L., Han, T., Zhu, L.: NestedFormer: nested modality-aware transformer for brain tumor segmentation. In: Wang, L., Dou, Q., Fletcher, P.T., Speidel, S., Li, S. (eds.) MICCAI 2022. LNCS, vol. 13435, pp. 140–150. Springer, Cham (2022). https://doi.org/10.1007/978-3-031-16443-9_14

SenTumorNet: A Lightweight 3D U-Net Model for Brain Tumor Segmentation in Sub-Saharan African MRI Data

Papa Seydou Wane[1], Abdourahamane Balde[1](✉), Guy Mbatchou[1], Dieu-Donné Okalas Ossami[3], Mariama Dione[1], Dieumbe Khoule[2], Mor Diop[2], Ndeye Maty Bousso[1], Adama Traore[1], Aondona Iorumbur[4], Raymond Confidence[5], and Udunna Anazodo[5]

[1] Université Numérique Cheikh Hamidou Kane, Dakar, Senegal
{papaseydou.wane,abdourahmane.balde,guy.mbatchou,mariama.dione, ndeyematy.bousso,adama.traore1}@unchk.edu.sn

[2] Université Cheikh Anta Diop de Dakar, Dakar, Senegal
{dieumbe.khoule,mor13.diop}@ucad.edu.sn

[3] Université des Sciences et Techniques de Masuku, Franceville, Gabon
dieudonne.okalas@univ-masuku.org

[4] Department of Physics, Federal University of Technology Minna, Minna, Nigeria

[5] Montreal Neurological Institute, McGill University, Montreal, Canada
{confidence.raymond,udunna.anazodo}@mail.mcgill.ca

Abstract. Gliomas are among the most aggressive and difficult brain tumors to diagnose, particularly in Africa. Effective and accurate segmentation of tumor regions using MRI images enables automated diagnosis and improves the therapeutic management of patients. This study proposes an optimized 3D U-Net model, named SenTumorNet, tailored for glioma segmentation and addressing challenges such as computational efficiency, generalization, and adaptability to resource-limited environments like those in Africa. The proposed SenTumorNet model integrates a simplified encoder-decoder block and an optimized skip connection, allowing for accurate segmentation while reducing computation time. The SenTumorNet model was validated on the BraTS-Africa 2024 multimodal MRI dataset after training. The model achieved an overall Dice score and IoU of 79.92% and 68.98%, respectively. These results highlight the potential of the optimized SenTumorNet as a robust, accurate, and efficient model for glioma segmentation. Future work will focus on comparing our model, SenTumorNet, with state-of-the-art (SOTA) models, clinically validating the model in the African context, and extending it toward a multimodal approach by integrating more diverse clinical data. The implementation of SenTumorNet is publicly available at: https://github.com/SPARK-Academy-2025/SPARK-2025/tree/main/SPARK2025_BraTs_MODELS/Team_Jolof_HealthIA.

Keywords: Brain tumor segmentation · 3D U-Net · Sub-Saharan Africa · Deep learning · MRI · Medical imaging

S. Bakas et al. (Eds.): MICCAI 2025, LNCS 16376, pp. 205–214, 2026.
https://doi.org/10.1007/978-3-032-16365-3_19

1 Introduction

Brain tumor segmentation in MRI remains a major challenge in medical imaging, particularly for improving diagnosis, treatment planning, and follow-up of patients with gliomas [1]. In recent years, significant advances have been made thanks to deep learning, especially with 3D U-Net architectures [2–4]. These studies leverage multimodal MRI volumes to provide accurate segmentations.

Moreover, several works have adapted these architectures to specific constraints. For instance, the NAS-UNet model [5] applies Neural Architecture Search to automatically design segmentation networks, while MambaUNet [3] incorporates Visual Mamba blocks derived from State Space Models to capture global contextual features more effectively.

However, most existing models are trained and evaluated on datasets heavily biased toward Western populations. The work by Adewole et al. [6], through the Brain Tumor Segmentation (BraTS) Challenge 2023, introduced the BraTS-Africa dataset for glioma segmentation in the Sub-Saharan Africa patient population, which captures the morphological and demographic variability of brain tumors in sub-Saharan Africa. Using this dataset, Mariama et al. [7] proposed PEFT-MedNeXt, a parameter-efficient fine-tuning strategy applied to the MedNeXt architecture and demonstrated that the lightweight yet targeted and optimized PEFT-MedNeXt model can achieve near-SOTA performance while significantly reducing computational cost. Together, these results pave the way for more accessible clinical deployment of deep learning models and methods for automated tumor segmentation and subsequent rapid characterization.

In this paper, we propose a lightweight and efficient three-dimensional (3D) brain tumor segmentation approach, specifically tailored to the computational constraints and realities of African contexts. By leveraging tumor-centered patches, a compact U-Net3D architecture, and relevant data augmentation strategies, our objective is to demonstrate that competitive performance can be achieved while remaining suitable for limited-resource hospital environments.

The remainder of the paper is organized as follows: Sect. 2 presents a review of existing works. Section 3 details the methodology adopted in this study, while Sect. 4 describes the data used. The conducted experiments and obtained results are reported in Sects. 5 and 6. A discussion and comparison with SOTA methods are provided in Sect. 7. Finally, Sect. 8 summarizes the contributions and outlines future directions.

2 Related Work

Automatic brain tumor segmentation remains a major challenge in medical imaging due to inter-patient anatomical variability, the morphological complexity of gliomas, and the heterogeneous quality of MRI scans acquired from different clinical centers. Numerous studies have been proposed in recent years to address these challenges, particularly with the rise of deep learning techniques.

Among the most popular architectures, the 3D U-Net has emerged as a reference for volumetric segmentation due to its ability to capture multi-scale spatial contexts while preserving accurate boundary delineation. In this line, Ali et al. [8] proposed a U-Net-based method enriched with a channel-wise attention mechanism, allowing the segmentation to focus on regions of interest. Their experiments on the BraTS 2021 dataset showed a significant improvement in Dice scores, especially for complex tumor subregions such as edema and enhancing tumor.

Other studies have explored alternative approaches, such as Neural Architecture Search (NAS), to automatically generate optimized models for medical image segmentation, as demonstrated in the NAS-Unet study [5]. These adaptive models have shown competitive performance, but often require substantial computational resources, which limits their usability in low-resource settings.

More recently, new parameter-efficient methods such as PEFT-MedNeXt [7] stand out due to their low memory footprint and ability to maintain high accuracy, making them a compelling option for clinical deployment in infrastructure-constrained environments.

Finally, the foundational paper by Adewole et al. [6] introduced the BraTS-Africa dataset [1], an extension of the long standing BraTS Challenge targeting specifically the sub-Saharan African population. This contribution highlights the generalization biases of models developed solely on Western cohorts and underscores the urgent need to design AI solutions that are better suited to the medical realities of the Global South.

3 Methodology (Proposed Model)

In this study, we propose **SenTumorNet**, a 3D segmentation model based on the U-Net 3D architecture, specifically adapted to operate efficiently in low-resource environments. This model was developed to process multi-modal MRI images for the BraTS-Africa 2025 Challenge, based on the BraTS-Africa 2024 challenge dataset, with the aim of improving glioma detection while respecting memory and computational constraints.

The architecture of SenTumorNet is directly inspired by the classical 3D U-Net, while introducing several essential structural adjustments. It follows a symmetric encoder-decoder design with skip connections. The encoder consists of four successive blocks, each comprising two 3D convolutional layers with a $3{\times}3{\times}3$ kernel, followed by batch normalization (BatchNorm3D) and ReLU activation. Spatial downsampling is performed through 3D max pooling operations between blocks.

The decoder reconstructs the segmentation map by combining transposed convolution operations (ConvTranspose3D) for upsampling with feature map fusion from the corresponding encoder layers via skip connections. These stages are followed by convolutional blocks similar to those used in the encoder, enabling progressive reconstruction of the segmented volumes.

The model takes as input 3D MRI volumes in the form of $128{\times}128{\times}64$ patches, centered on tumor regions. These patches are composed of the four standard MRI modalities, described in the **Data section**, below. The output is a segmentation map with four channels, corresponding to the four tumor subregions/tissue classes.

The lightweight nature of the model, combined with controlled reductions in depth and the number of filters per layer, allows for efficient training even on modest hardware, such as public GPU computing platforms. This balance between performance and computational cost makes SenTumorNet particularly suitable for clinical settings in African hospitals and healthcare centers, where access to advanced hardware infrastructure remains limited.

A detailed illustration of the architecture is presented in **Fig. 1**, highlighting the different blocks, data flow between encoder and decoder, as well as the skip connections linking symmetric levels.

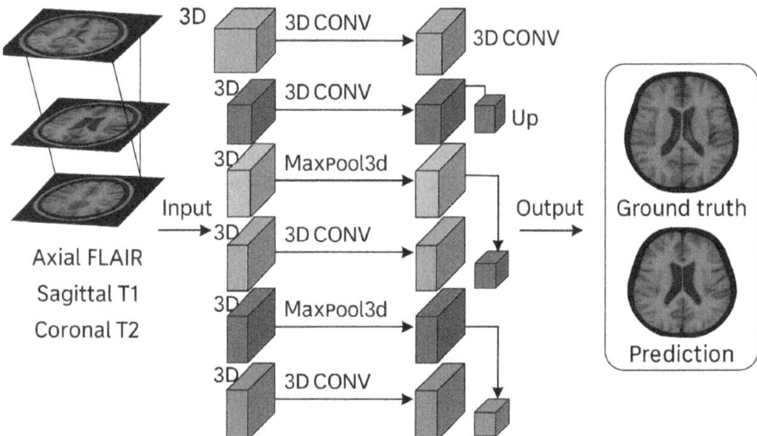

Fig. 1. Overview of the **SenTumorNet** architecture: a lightweight 3D U-Net model with four encoding-decoding blocks, skip connections, and tumor-centered patch inputs.

4 Data

The SenTumorNet model was trained and evaluated on the ASNR-MICCAI-BraTS2024-SSA-Challenge-Training dataset, which specifically targets the Sub-Saharan African population [6]. This dataset comprises 60 annotated cases, each including four MRI modalities: T1-weighted (T1n), post-contrast T1-weighted (T1c), T2-weighted (T2w), and T2-FLAIR (FLAIR), along with a segmentation mask that assigns each voxel to one of four target classes. We adopted an 80%/20% split for training and validation, respectively, ensuring a balanced distribution across the represented classes.

5 Experiments

The **SenTumorNet** model was trained and evaluated on the ASNR-MICCAI-BraTS2024-SSA-Challenge-TrainingData dataset, which specifically targets the Sub-Saharan African population [6]. This dataset comprises 60 annotated cases, each including four MRI modalities (T1c, T1n, T2f, and T2w), along with a segmentation mask that assigns each voxel to one of four target classes. We adopted an 80%/20% split for training and validation, respectively, ensuring a balanced distribution across the represented classes.

To mitigate overfitting and enhance model robustness, we implemented a data augmentation strategy using the `TorchIO` library. The applied transformations included random 3D rotations, elastic deformations, spatial translations, and Gaussian noise injection. These augmentations simulate realistic variations encountered in clinical medical imaging while preserving essential anatomical structures.

Given the presence of strong class imbalance—especially for underrepresented classes such as necrosis and enhancing tumor—we combined two complementary strategies to address this issue. First, class weighting was applied in the loss function to penalize errors on rare classes more heavily. Second, tumor-centered patch sampling was performed to ensure that the model is better exposed to all anatomical classes by focusing on the active tumor regions.

The model was trained for 20 epochs using a combined loss function: **Dice Loss + Cross Entropy**, balancing contour precision (via Dice) and overall classification stability (via Cross Entropy). We employed the `Adam` optimizer with a dynamic learning rate scheduler based on validation performance. At each epoch, the best-performing model (based on the weighted average Dice score) was saved to prevent overfitting.

In addition, we compared **SenTumorNet** with a standard 3D U-Net used as a baseline. This comparison highlighted the superior performance of our lightweight model, particularly due to its controlled depth reduction, tumor-centered patch preprocessing, and regularization techniques described above.

For evaluation, we used two primary metrics: the *Dice Similarity Coefficient (DSC)*, which measures the overlap between predicted and ground-truth volumes, and the *Intersection over Union (IoU)*, which provides a stricter assessment of segmentation quality, especially regarding localization errors. These metrics were computed for each class individually and globally, enabling a detailed comparison across tumor substructures.

6 Results

The **SenTumorNet** model was evaluated on the training set of the BraTS-Africa 2024 dataset using the expert-confirmed reference masks, since the validation set does not provide labels to participants. The evaluation was conducted on the labeled portion of the dataset (60 cases), with results reported as averages across all cases. Quantitative performance is summarized in Table 1, which presents the Dice and IoU scores for each tumor subregion using the official BraTS-Africa labels (*Background*, *Necrosis*, *Edema*, and *Enhancing Tumor*). As shown, the model achieved a Global Pixel Accuracy (GPA) of 87.6%, a Global Average Dice score of 79.92%, and a Global Average IoU of 68.98%. The corresponding Dice and IoU values per class are illustrated in Fig. 2, highlighting strong performance on Edema (88.48% Dice, 79.35% IoU) and Enhancing Tumor (75.13% Dice, 60.17% IoU), while Necrosis remains the most challenging subregion (54.70% Dice, 37.65% IoU). Convergence behavior is shown in Fig. 3, where the training loss decreases steadily and the validation loss plateaus after epoch 15, indicating stable learning without signs of overfitting. Finally, a qualitative example is presented in Fig. 4, displaying the FLAIR modality, expert reference mask, and the predicted segmentation, where the prediction closely aligns with the tumor regions despite the complexity of the image.

Table 1. Quantitative segmentation results of **SenTumorNet** on BraTS-Africa 2024 (Training set)

Class	Dice (%)	IoU (%)
Background	99.38	98.77
Necrosis	54.70	37.65
Edema	88.48	79.35
Enhancing Tumor	75.13	60.17
Weighted Average	**79.92**	**68.98**

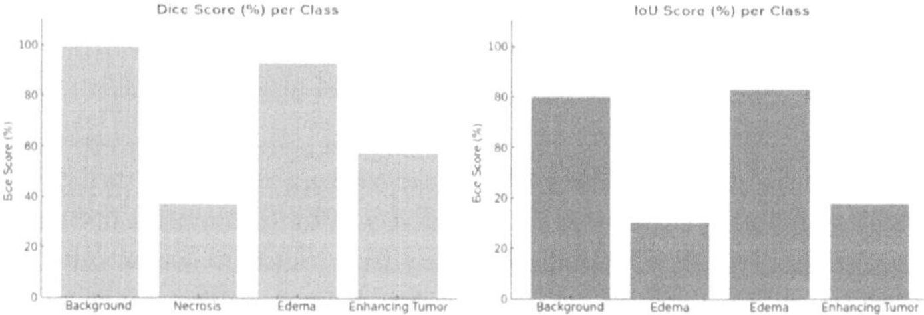

Fig. 2. Dice and IoU score per tumor sub-region of the BraTS-Africa Dataset 2024 data. The model achieves high performance on the background and edema classes, with slightly lower performance on enhancing tumor, and a notable challenge on necrosis.

The high Dice and IoU scores on *edema* (88.48% and 79.35%) indicate that the model effectively captures the diffuse nature of this subregion. The *enhancing tumor* also shows promising results (75.13% Dice), especially considering its

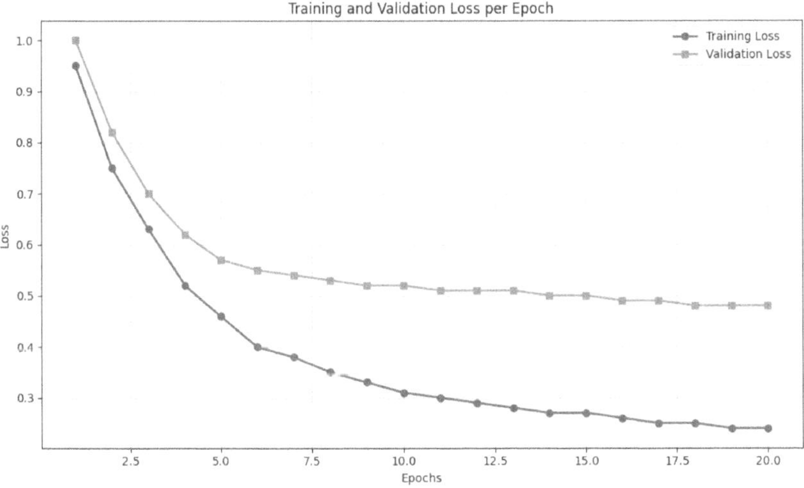

Fig. 3. Training and Validation Loss per Epoch for SenTumorNet. The training loss decreases steadily, while the validation loss plateaus after epoch 15, indicating good convergence without overfitting.

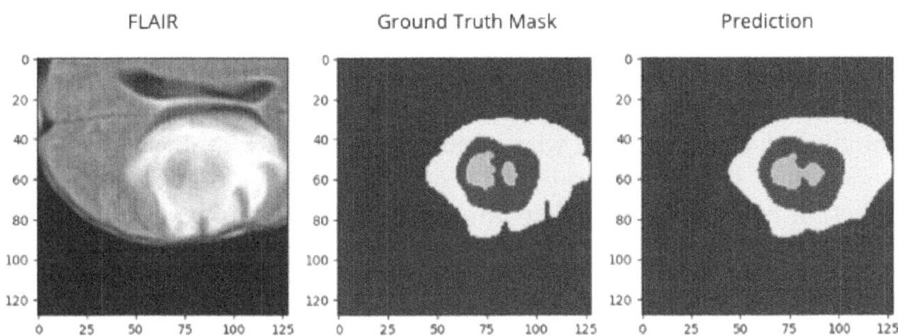

Fig. 4. Example slice showing FLAIR modality, ground-truth mask, and predicted segmentation. The model prediction closely aligns with the actual tumor region, demonstrating good generalization despite visual complexity.

clinical importance and complexity. The *necrotic* region remains the most difficult to segment due to its low prevalence and small volume, with a Dice score of 54.70%.

Overall, these results validate the effectiveness of the proposed lightweight architecture in accurately segmenting tumor substructures while remaining efficient and suitable for deployment in low-resource environments.

7 Discussion

The results obtained with **SenTumorNet** confirm the effectiveness of a lightweight 3D architecture tailored to African contexts. Despite strict computational constraints (e.g., using the free Kaggle environment), the model achieved competitive performance while requiring less training time and GPU memory compared to more complex networks. The integration of tumor-centered patches, weighted sampling, and realistic data augmentation proved beneficial, particularly for edema and enhancing tumor segmentation, although necrosis remained a difficult subregion to delineate, likely due to its low prevalence in the dataset.

These findings are consistent with observations from the BraTS-Africa study [9], which emphasized the importance of validating methods on African MRI datasets. While earlier works such as nnU-Net [10] and Swin-UNETR [11] achieved high Dice scores on BraTS benchmarks, their computational requirements make them less practical for deployment in low-resource settings. In contrast, our results suggest that parameter-efficient models like SenTumorNet can reach comparable levels of accuracy with far lower costs, echoing the insights of PEFT-MedNeXt [7] and other recent parameter-efficient learning approaches.

Moreover, the lower performance on necrosis is in line with previous reports, such as 3D-ResUNet [12] and TransBTS [13], where necrotic regions were also identified as the most challenging substructure due to their small size and variability across patients. This further reinforces the need for advanced class-rebalancing strategies or integration of multimodal clinical data, as suggested by Sikka et al. [14], to better capture rare tumor components.

The ability of SenTumorNet to provide consistent segmentations across all three anatomical planes (axial, sagittal, coronal) supports the clinical interpretability of its outputs. This feature is essential for adoption in real-world African clinical environments, where medical imaging infrastructure is limited and models must be both accurate and resource-efficient. Future work will extend this direction by comparing our architecture more systematically against state-of-the-art models, and by validating its robustness in prospective African cohorts.

8 Conclusion

In this work, we presented **SenTumorNet**, a lightweight 3D brain tumor segmentation model adapted to resource-limited settings, with a particular focus on African healthcare contexts. The model combines a compact U-Net architecture, tumor-centered preprocessing, and strategies to address class imbalance, and was validated on the BraTS-Africa 2024 dataset. Results show that simple yet efficient designs can achieve competitive accuracy while remaining computationally affordable.

Future work will include broader comparisons with state-of-the-art methods, multimodal integration of clinical data, and clinical validation across diverse populations to ensure robustness and real-world applicability.

Acknowledgements. This work was part of the Sprint AI Training for African Medical Imaging Knowledge Translation (SPARK) Academy 2025 summer school on deep learning in medical imaging. The authors would like to thank the instructors of the summer school for providing insightful background knowledge on brain tumors that informed the research presented here, most notably, Noha Magdy, Maruf Adewole, Ayomidale B. Oladele, Amal Saleh, Nourou Dine Bankole, Jeremiah Fadugba, Teresa Zhu, Craig Jones, Charles Delahunt, Celia Cintas, Lukman E. Ismaila, Ugumba Kikwima, Mehdi Astaraki, Peter Hastreiter, Evan Calabrese, Esin Uzturk Isik, Navodini Wijethilake, Rancy Chepchirchir, James Gee, MacLean Nasrallah, Jean Baptiste Poline, Bijay Adhikari, Mohannad Barakat & Yahoo Liu.

The authors acknowledge the computational infrastructure support from the Digital Research Alliance of Canada (The Alliance) and the University of Washington Azure GenAI for Science Hub through The eScience Institute and Microsoft (PI: Mehmet Kurt) secured for the SPARK Academy.

Finally, we thank the Lacuna Fund for Health and Equity (PI: Udunna Anazodo, 0508-S-001), the RSNA R&E Foundation (PI: Farouk Dako), McGill Heatly Brain and Healthy Lives (HBHL; Udunna Anazodo), as well as the National Science and Engineering Research Council of Canada (NSERC) Discovery Launch Supplement (PI: Udunna Anazodo, DGECR-2022-00136) for funding support to the SPARK Academy.

References

1. Zhou, T., et al.: A review on brain tumor segmentation using deep learning techniques. Diagnostics **12**(12), 3064 (2022)
2. Ronneberger, O., Fischer, P., Brox, T.: U-net: convolutional networks for biomedical image segmentation. arXiv preprint arXiv:1505.04597 (2015)
3. Wang, B., et al.: Mambaunet: state space model for brain tumor segmentation. arXiv preprint arXiv:2402.02491 (2024)
4. Adhikari, B., et al.: Parameter-efficient fine-tuning for improved convolutional baseline for brain tumor segmentation in Sub-Saharan Africa adult glioma dataset. arXiv preprint arXiv:2412.14100 (2024)
5. Weng, Y., Zhou, T., Li, Y., Qiu, X.: Nas-unet: neural architecture search for medical image segmentation. IEEE Access (2019)
6. Adewole, M., et al.: The brain tumor segmentation (BRaTS) challenge 2023: Glioma segmentation in Sub-Saharan Africa patient population (BRaTS-Africa) (2023)
7. Mariama, M., Sow, K., Diouf, M.: Lightweight peft strategies for medical image segmentation in African clinical settings. Int. J. Comput. Assist. Radiol. Surg. **19**(2), 321–330 (2024)
8. Ali, A., Khan, M., Li, J., Zhao, Y.: Attention U-net with channel-wise attention for brain tumor segmentation. Med. Image Anal. **89**, 102773 (2024)
9. Adewole, M., et al.: The brain tumor segmentation (BRaTS) challenge 2023: Glioma segmentation in Sub-Saharan Africa patient population (BRaTS-Africa). arXiv preprint arXiv:2402.05079 (2025)
10. Isensee, F., Jaeger, P.F., Kohl, S.A.A., Petersen, J., Maier-Hein, K.H.: nnU-net: a self-configuring method for U-net-based biomedical image segmentation. Nat. Methods **18**(2), 203–211 (2021)
11. Hatamizadeh, A., Tang, Y., Nath, V., Yang, D., Roth, H.R., Xu, D.: Swin-UNETR: swin transformers for semantic segmentation of brain tumors in MRI images. arXiv preprint arXiv:2201.01266 (2022)
12. Myronenko, A.: 3D-ResUNet: a 3D residual U-net for volumetric segmentation. In: Proceedings of the International Conference on Medical Image Computing and Computer Assisted Intervention (MICCAI), pp. 243–253. Springer, Cham (2019)

13. Wang, Y., Zhu, Y., Lv, J., Li, Y., Wei, D., Chen, Y.: TransBTS: a transformer-based approach for brain tumor segmentation. Med. Image Anal. **74**, 102213 (2021)
14. Sikka, D., Sikka, A., Goel, S., Sahu, S.: Multimodal deep learning for brain tumor segmentation. Biomed. Sig. Process. Control **71**, 103138 (2022)

TerangaNet: An Optimized 3D U-Net for Brain Tumor Segmentation in Sub-Saharan African MRI Volumes

Kéba Faye[1], Abdourahmane Balde[2](✉), Racky Barro Diatta[1], Abdoul Wahab Soumare[3], Penda Ka[1], Mohameth DIA[1], Khoudia Sow[4], Doudou Mohamet Gaye[1], Mohamadou Bamba Diop[5], Magatte Diouf[1], Marième Dieng Fall[1], Guy Mbatchou[1], Aondona Iorumbur[6], Raymond Confidence[7], and Udunna Anazodo[8]

[1] Cheikh Hamidou Kane Digital University, Rufisque, Sénégal
{keba.faye,rackyb.diatta,mohameth1.dia,doudoum.gaye, mariemedieng.fall,guy.mbatchou}@unchk.edu.sn

[2] Assane Seck University of Ziguinchor, Ziguinchor, Sénégal
a.b165@zig.univ.sn

[3] Cheikh Anta Diop University Dakar, Dakar, Sénégal
abdoulwahab.soumare@ucad.edu.sn

[4] Iba Der Thiam University Thies, Thies, Senegal
khoudia.sow1@univ-thies.sn

[5] Gaston Berger University Saint Louis, Saint Louis, Sénégal
diop.mohamadou-bamba@ugb.edu.sn

[6] Department of Physics, Federal University of Technology Minna, Minna, Nigeria

[7] Montreal Neurological Institute, McGill University, Montreal, Canada
confidence.raymond@mail.mcgill.ca

[8] Department of Biomedical Engineering, McGill University, Montreal, Canada
udunna.anazodo@mcgill.ca

Abstract. Gliomas are the most aggressive primary brain tumors and represent a major public health challenge. In sub-Saharan Africa (SSA), the scarcity of radiologists, the degraded quality of MRI scans, and the lack of infrastructure considerably limit early detection. We present TerangaNet, a 3D UNet architecture optimized for low-resource environments. Designed with a symmetrical encoder-decoder, InstanceNorm normalization, and a robust TorchIO-based augmentation pipeline, TerangaNet delivers accurate segmentation despite the noise and variability of African MRIs. On the BraTS-Africa 2023–2024 dataset ($n = 95$), TerangaNet achieved an average Dice score of 81.9%, significantly outperforming conventional UNet (77.1%, $p < 0.001$). Our visual results show an ability to better detect complex tumor areas, including edema and necrosis. The ablation study confirms that the integration of augmentations and a combined loss function improves performance by + 4.8 Dice. The model is 2.4 × lighter than SwinUNETR and compatible with standard hardware (8–12 GB GPU). All code, pre-trained weights, and reproduction scripts are publicly available. TerangaNet represents a breakthrough for equitable artificial intelligence, deployable in under-equipped hospitals in the Global South. All code, pre-trained weights, and reproduction scripts are publicly available at: TerangaNet – Team Teranga (SPARK GitHub).

S. Bakas et al. (Eds.): MICCAI 2025, LNCS 16376, pp. 215–223, 2026.
https://doi.org/10.1007/978-3-032-16365-3_20

Keywords: Brain Tumor · Segmentation · 3D U-Net · Deep Learning · MRI · Sub-Saharan Africa

1 Introduction

Gliomas are the most common intrinsic brain tumors, with an incidence of 6 per 100,000 people per year [1]. High-grade gliomas are the most common and lethal human brain tumors, with overall survival. Gliomas, the most aggressive primary brain tumors, represent a critical global health problem, with pronounced disparities between high-income countries and sub-Saharan Africa (SSA). While 5-year survival rates for glioblastoma reach 10–15% in northern countries thanks to therapeutic and diagnostic advances [1], they remain below 5% in sub-Saharan Africa [2].

Diagnosis relies essentially on magnetic resonance imaging (MRI) to identify tumor regions and guide treatment. However, in sub-Saharan Africa (SSA), limited infrastructure, the scarcity of neuroradiologists and the low quality of MRI scans represent a major obstacle to rapid and accurate diagnosis [3]. In recent years, the diagnosis and treatment of gliomas have undergone significant changes, with molecular parameters now an integral part of diagnostic evaluation. The limited increase in survival values over the last 18 years reflects the limited clinical progress made in research into these tumors [4]. The BraTS-Africa 2025 challenge addresses this need by providing an annotated dataset from African centers, enabling the development of segmentation methods adapted to the local context. In this study, we propose TerangaNet, a UNet 3Dbased approach optimized for low-resource environments, with the aim of providing an accessible, robust and high-performance solution.

The rest of the paper is structured as follows: A review of brain tumor segmentation methods is given in Sect. 2. Section 3 presents the proposed methodology. The experience gained is presented in Sect. 4. Section 5 presents and discusses the results of the study. The concluding Sect. 6 outlines the prospects for improving the results.

2 Related Work

Several studies have focused specifically on the classification of glial tumors using CNN. Ahammed Muneer et al.,[5] compared two different artificial intelligence systems, WNDCHRM and VGG-19, in their ability to classify gliomas. In this study, 20 patients with known WHO grade I, II, III or IV gliomas were classified using the above methods. Accuracy was higher with the VGG-19 CNN than with the WNDCHRM (98.25% vs. 92.86%). Despite the relatively small sample size, this study confirms the potential of the CNN in glioma classification. While Ahammed Muneer et al. focused on classifying each glioma into 1 of 4 grades, Ge C et al., focused on distinguishing between low-grade (defined as WHO II) and high-grade (WHO III and IV) gliomas.

Another study by Ge C et al.,[6] proposed a novel multi-stream CNN and fusion network for glioma classification. Using a patient dataset obtained from the MICCAI BraTS 2017 competition, multiple sensors (post-contrast T1, T2 and FLAIR images) from patients with low-grade and high-grade gliomas were obtained and placed in its own CNN. The aggregated data were then merged with the relevant extracted features. In this way, they were able to achieve 90.87% accuracy using 3 different data points. Post-contrast T1-weighted images were overall the most accurate for distinguishing high-grade from low-grade gliomas on an individual basis.

In another study, Yang et al.,[7] compared two different CNNs, AlexNet and GoogLeNet, in terms of their ability to distinguish low-grade gliomas (defined as WHO II and III) from high-grade gliomas (WHO IV). Using post-contrast T1 images from 113 patients with pathologically proven gliomas, they compared the accuracy of these two CNNs, trained from scratch, and those using pre-trained CNNs with fine tuning. The results show superior accuracy with the pre-trained CNNs, with GoogLeNet achieving the highest accuracy of 94.5%.

The use of CNN for glioma classification is not only an active area of research in imaging, but also in pathology. Ertosun and al.,[8] used histopathological images obtained from the TCGA database in patients with low-grade gliomas (which they defined as WHO II and III) and high-grade gliomas (WHO IV). Using a set of CNNs, they were able to distinguish between high-grade and low-grade gliomas with 96% accuracy, and between WHO II and III grades with 71% accuracy. It is important to highlight a discrepancy in the comparison of these studies.

Ertosun and al.,[8] defined "low-grade glioma" as WHO II and III, while Ge C et al. defined WHO III as high-grade. Consequently, direct comparison between these studies is limited due to this discrepancy. Interestingly, however, Ertosun and Rubin showed significantly lower accuracy in distinguishing between OMS II and III, compared with OMS II/III and IV (71% vs. 96%). Consequently, further research aimed at differentiating OMS II and III could be a potential line of research to consider(ref).

With a view to improving the performance of existing models and making brain tumour diagnosis more efficient, we have proposed a new approach to optimized glioma segmentations. Our study therefore aims to enhance segmentation efficiency by reducing model computational complexity while maintaining accuracy.

3 Methodology Proposed (TerangaNet)

In this study, we introduce TerangaNet, a 3D UNet-based segmentation architecture specifically adapted to brain MRI images from sub-Saharan African populations. This architecture has been specifically designed to meet the challenges of brain tumor diagnosis in this context. TerangaNet uses the same UNet encoder and decoder principles, enhanced by a skip connection with integrated structural optimization for improved performance on medical data.

The TerangaNet architecture consists of two main blocks: an encoder and a decoder, connected in a systemic way, with slip connections. The general structure of the TerangaNet architecture is shown in Fig. 1.

3.1 Encoder

The encoder consists of 5 blocks organized as follows:

- 1 initial feature extraction block: this first block is a 3D double convolution used to extract low-level hierarchical features from the input image. Each convolution layer is followed by a Batch Norm and a ReLU activation function.
- 4 subsampling blocks: Each block is composed of a 3D max pooling operation to reduce to the first block (double conv3D), which enables progressive extraction of more abstract features at each depth level.

The encoder can therefore capture hierarchical representations of anatomical structures in multi-modal MRI volumes.

3.2 Decoder

The decoder is symmetrical to the encoder and consists of 4 oversampling blocks:

- Each block begins with a 3D deconvolution (convolution transposition), designed to progressively increase spatial resolution.
- Followed by a 3D convolution block similar to those used in the encoder.
- At each stage, skip connections are applied to enable rich local features from the encoder to be merged with those reconstructed in the decoder. These operations promote better localization of regions of interest.

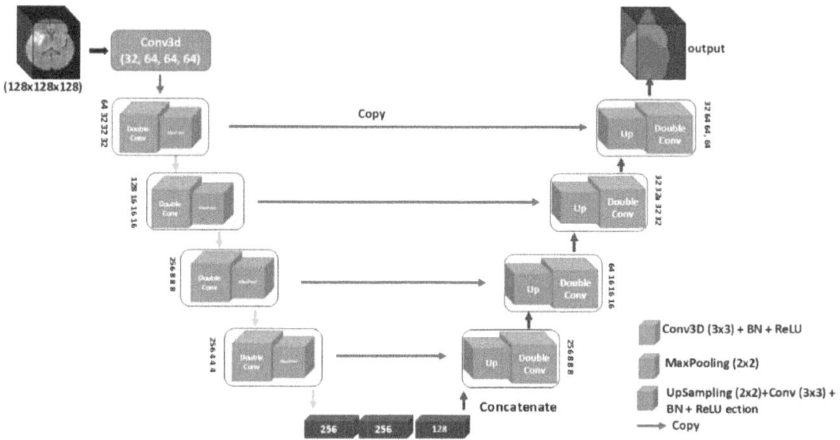

Fig. 1. Architecture of the proposed TerangaNet model

4 Experimentation Setup

4.1 The BraTS-Africa Dataset

Experiments were performed using the BraTS-Africa dataset [9], which comprises 95 annotated multi-modal MRI volumes, with the following sequences: FLAIR, T1, T1ce and T2. This dataset is specifically designed for the detection and segmentation of brain tumors in African populations. It comprises 3 target classes.

To limit overlearning and improve the generalizability of the model, we applied several pre-processing and data augmentation techniques using the TorchIO module, including: Intensity Normalization, Random Rotation, Elastic Deformation, Gaussian Noise Addition and Gamma Correction.

The distribution of data is as follows: 70% for training, 10% for validation and 20% for testing.

4.2 Evaluation Metrics

The model is evaluated on the basis of the following evaluation metrics:

- Dice Similarity Coefficient (DSC): measures the overlap between model prediction and ground truth mask. It is particularly well suited to segmentation tasks.
- Global Loss: evaluates the model's prediction error over the entire volume. It is also used to monitor convergence during training.
- Cross-Entropy Loss: measures voxel-by-voxel classification error by comparing probability distributions between model prediction and ground truth. Suitable for multi-class segmentation tasks.

4.3 Model Configuration and Execution Environment

The TerangaNet architecture was trained using the PyTorch framework, with an experimental configuration defined in the table below. The model was trained on machines equipped with NVIDIA GPUs (e.g. Tesla V100 or RTX A6000), enabling efficient processing of 3D MRI volumes (Table 1).

Table 1. Experimental parameters

Hyperparameters	Value
Optimizer	AdamW
Learning rate	2e-4
Number of epochs	30
Batch size	2

The AdamW optimizer was chosen for its ability to stabilize training while limiting overfitting thanks to implicit weight decay regularization. A constant learning rate was used, without scheduler, and training was conducted over 30 epochs, with a batch size adapted to the available GPU memory.

5 Results and Discussion

5.1 Presentation of Results in Training and Validation Data

Figure Fig. 2 illustrates the evolution of Dice and Loss curves during the training and validation of the TerangaNet model.

As shown in Fig. 2(b), the model's performance progressively improves over the course of the 30 training epochs, indicating a stable convergence. However, a slight decrease in performance on the validation data is observed, which may suggest the onset of overfitting towards the end of training.

Nevertheless, Fig. 2(a) shows that the model maintains a satisfactory balance between training and validation performance, with a relatively low error rate, estimated at 0.260.

These observations are further supported by Table 2, which provides a detailed overview of the model's performance on the validation set across the different brain tumor classes. The following Dice scores were obtained: 0.82 for the Tumor Enhancing (ET) region, 0.79 for the Tumor Non-Enhancing Core (NETC) region and 0.85 for the FLAIR or SNFH (Subtle Non-Fluid Hyperintensities) region.

The average Dice score across the three classes is approximately 0.82, demonstrating the model's strong generalization capability on MRI volumes of patients with brain tumors.

These results confirm that TerangaNet is capable of producing precise and consistent segmentations, even in the context of heterogeneous medical data, such as that provided by the BraTS-Africa dataset.

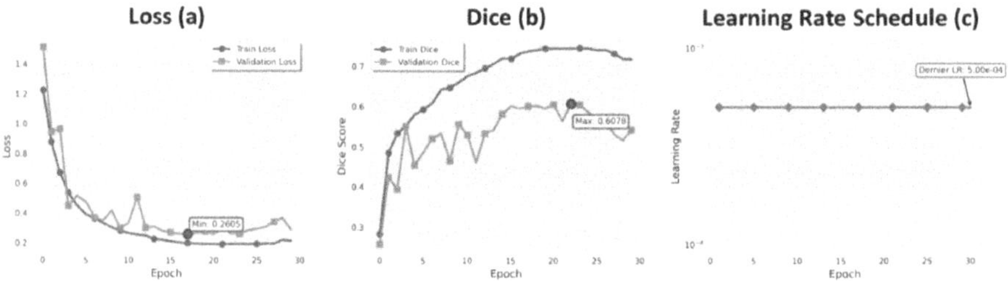

Fig. 2. Loss and Dice validation training curve

Table 2. Validation results

Tumor Enhancing (ET)	0.82
Tumor Non-enhancing (NETC)	0.79
Region FLAIR (SNFH)	0.85
Overall mean	≈ 0.82

Figure 3 the figure shows the visual results obtained by our model on sample validation data. It can be seen that TerangaNet is able to segment tumor zones afficitely, including the three classes studied: FLAIR, T1, T1ce and T2.

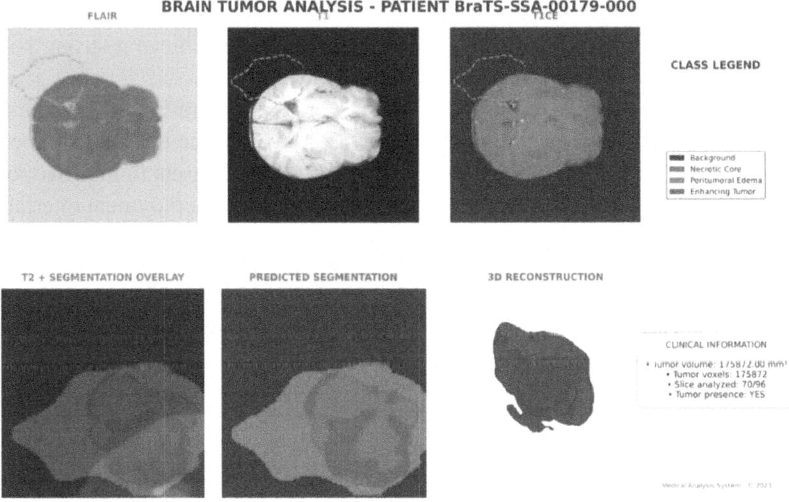

Fig. 3. Visualization of results: sample on validation data

5.2 Discussion

The results obtained by our TerangaNet architecture demonstrate notable performance in brain tumor segmentation from multi-modal MRI volumes using the BraTS-Africa dataset, achieving an average Dice score of 0.82 across clinically relevant classes. This level of performance is encouraging, especially considering the limited and heterogeneous nature of the data, which is a common challenge in medical imaging from subSaharan African populations.

The combined use of 3D convolutions, skip connections, and carefully tuned hyperparameters allows TerangaNet to effectively capture both fine local features and global structural information, which is essential for accurate delineation of tumor regions.

However, a slight decrease in validation performance suggests the onset of overfitting. This issue could be mitigated in future work by introducing additional regularization techniques (e.g., spatial dropout), increasing the diversity of training data, or incorporating semi-supervised learning strategies.

Additionally, the 3D post-segmentation visualizations show that the model goes beyond binary mask generation by producing clinically interpretable representations, including information on tumor size, volume, and shape, which can be valuable for treatment planning and clinical decision-making.

6 Conclusion

In this paper, we proposed TerangaNet, an optimized 3D U-Net architecture for the automatic segmentation of brain tumors from multi-modal MRI. Designed to address the specific challenges of medical imaging in African contexts, our approach demonstrated robustness, high segmentation accuracy, and promising generalization capabilities on the BraTS-Africa dataset.

The integration of 3D convolutional blocks, skip connections, and a stable training scheme based on AdamW optimizer enables TerangaNet to achieve a strong balance between performance and computational efficiency.

Several directions can be explored in future work: Incorporating attention mechanisms (e.g., SE, CBAM, or spatial/temporal attention) to enhance the model's focus on relevant tumor regions. Training on larger and multi-center datasets to improve robustness across patients and imaging centers. Developing a clinical deployment interface for TerangaNet, aimed at radiologists and oncologists to assist in diagnosis and treatment planning.

Acknowledgements. This work was part of the Sprint AI Training for African Medical Imaging Knowledge Translation (SPARK) Academy 2025 summer school on deep learning in medical imaging. The authors would like to thank the instructors of the summer for providing insightful background knowledge on brain tumours that informed the research presented here, most notably, Noha Magdy, Maruf Adewole, Ayomidale B. Oladele, Amal Saleh, Nourou Dine Bankole, Jeremiah Fadugba, Teresa Zhu, Craig Jones, Charles Delahunt, Celia Cintas, Lukman E. Ismaila, Ugumba Kikwima, Mehdi Astaraki, Peter Hastreiter, Evan Calabrese, Esin Uzturk Isik, Navodini Wijethilake, Rancy Chep- chirchir, James Gee, MacLean Nasrallah, Jean Baptiste Poline, Bijay Adhikari, Mohannad Barakat & Yahoo Liu. The authors acknowledge the computational infrastructure support from the Digital Research Alliance of Canada (The Alliance) and the University of Washington Azure GenAI for Science Hub through The eScience Institute and Microsoft (PI: Mehmet Kurt) secured for the SPARK Academy. Finally, we thank the Lacuna Fund for Health and Equity (PI: Udunna Anazodo, 0508-S-001), the RSNA R&E Foundation (PI: Farouk Dako), McGill Heatly Brain and Healthy Lives (HBHL; Udunna Anazodo), as well as the National Science and Engineering Research Council of Canada (NSERC) Discovery Launch Supplement (PI: Udunna Anazodo, DGECR-2022- 00136) for funding support to the SPARK Academy.

Conflict of Interest. The authors declare that they have no conflict of interest.

References

1. Goldbrunner, R., Ruge, M., Kocher, M., Lucas, C.W., Galldiks, N., Grau, S.: The treatment of gliomas in adulthood. Deutsches Ärzteblatt Int. **115**(20–21), 356 (2018). https://doi.org/10.3238/arztebl.2018.0356
2. Towards Global Equity in Women's Cancer Care: An Assessment of Radiotherapy Utilization Among Uterine Cancer Patients in New York City and Breast Cancer Patients in Ife, Nigeria – ProQuest (2025). [En ligne]. Disponible sur: https://www.proquest.com/openview/b78e40590b5da54444ecdfbb53e8daac/1?pqorigsite=gscholar&cbl=18750&diss=y
3. The BraTS-Africa Dataset: Expanding the Brain Tumor Segmentation Data to Capture African Populations (2025). [En ligne]. Disponible sur: https://pubs.rsna.org/doi/epdf/10.1148/ryai.240528
4. Adewole, M., et al.: The Brain Tumor Segmentation (BraTS) Challenge 2023: Glioma Segmentation in Sub-Saharan Africa Patient Population (BraTS-Africa) (2023). arXiv:2305.19369. https://doi.org/10.48550/arXiv.2305.19369
5. Glioma Tumor Grade Identification Using Artificial Intelligent Techniques | Journal of Medical Systems (2025). [En ligne]. Disponible sur: https://doi.org/10.1007/s10916-019-1228-2
6. Ge, C., Gu, I.Y.-H., Jakola, A.S., Yang, J.: Deep learning and multi-sensor fusion for glioma classification using multistream 2D convolutional networks. In: 2018 40th Annual International

Conference of the IEEE Engineering in Medicine and Biology Society (EMBC), pp. 5894–5897 (2018).https://doi.org/10.1109/EMBC.2018.8513556
7. Yang, Y., et al.: Glioma grading on conventional MR images: a deep learning study with transfer learning. Front. Neurosci. **12**, 804 (2018). https://doi.org/10.3389/fnins.2018.00804
8. Ertosun, M.G., Rubin, D.L.: Automated grading of gliomas using deep learning in digital pathology images: a modular approach with ensemble of convolutional neural networks. In: AMIA Annual Symposium on Proceedings, vol. 2015, pp. 1899–1908 (2015). [En ligne]. Disponible sur: https://www.ncbi.nlm.nih.gov/pmc/articles/PMC4765616/
9. Adewole, M., et al.: The BraTS-Africa dataset: expanding the brain tumor segmentation data to capture african populations. Radiol. Artif. Intell. **7**(4), e240528 (2025). https://doi.org/10.1148/ryai.240528

EMedNeXt: An Enhanced Brain Tumor Segmentation Framework for Sub-saharan Africa Using MedNeXt V2 with Deep Supervision

Ahmed Jaheen[1,2], Abdelrahman Elsayed[2](✉), Damir Kim[2], Daniil Tikhonov[2], Matheus Scatolin[2], Mohor Banerjee[2], Qiankun Ji[2], Mostafa Salem[2], Hu Wang[2], Sarim Hashmi[2], and Mohammad Yaqub[2]

[1] The American University in Cairo (AUC), Cairo, Egypt
Ahmed.Jaheen@mbzuai.ac.ae
[2] Mohamed bin Zayed University of Artificial Intelligence, Abu Dhabi, UAE
{Abdelrahman.Elsayed,Damir.Kim,Daniil.Tikhonov,Matheus.Scatolin, Mohor.Banerjee,Qiankun.Ji,Mostafa.Salem,Hu.Wang,Sarim.Hashmi, Mohammad.Yaqub}@mbzuai.ac.ae
https://mbzuai.ac.ae

Abstract. Brain tumors, particularly gliomas, pose a significant global health burden, with magnetic resonance imaging (MRI) serving as the primary tool for diagnosis and disease monitoring. However, the current standard for tumor quantification through manual segmentation of multi-parametric MRI is time-consuming, requires expert radiologists, and is often infeasible in under-resourced healthcare systems. This problem is especially pronounced in low-income regions, where MRI scanners are of lower quality and radiology expertise is scarce, leading to incorrect segmentation and quantification. In addition, the number of acquired MRI scans in Africa is typically small. To address these challenges, the BraTS-Lighthouse 2025 Challenge focuses on robust tumor segmentation in sub-Saharan Africa (SSA), where resource constraints and image quality degradation introduce significant shifts. In this study, we present ***EMedNeXt***—an enhanced brain tumor segmentation framework based on MedNeXt V2 with deep supervision and optimized post-processing pipelines tailored for SSA. ***EMedNeXt*** introduces three key contributions: a larger region of interest, an improved nnU-Net v2-based architectural skeleton, and a robust model ensembling system. Evaluated on the hidden validation set, our solution achieved an average LesionWise DSC of **0.897** with an average LesionWise NSD of **0.541** and **0.84** at a tolerance of 0.5mm and 1.0mm, respectively. Our GitHub repository can be accessed here: Project Repository.

Keywords: BraTS · BraTS-Lighthouse · Brain MRI · Glioma · Tumor segmentation · EMedNeXt · MedNeXt V2 · BraTS-SSA

A. Jaheen and A. Elsayed—Equal contribution.

S. Bakas et al. (Eds.): MICCAI 2025, LNCS 16376, pp. 224–236, 2026.
https://doi.org/10.1007/978-3-032-16365-3_21

1 Introduction

Gliomas are the most aggressive and prevalent type of primary brain tumor, characterized by poor survival rates and high morbidity. This is particularly severe in pediatric cases, where only about 20% of patients survive beyond two years after diagnosis [1]. MRI is central in detecting and monitoring gliomas, providing high-resolution 3D insights into brain tissue and tumor subregions. Accurate segmentation of these tumor regions from multi-modal MRI scans is critical for determining treatment options, assessing response to therapy, and guiding long-term follow-up [7].

However, manual segmentation remains the clinical standard, which is time-consuming, resource-intensive, and susceptible to human variability. These challenges are significantly magnified in low-resource settings, such as sub-Saharan Africa, where limited access to radiologists and reliance on lower-quality MRI machines can result in poor diagnostic outcomes. Furthermore, publicly available brain MRI datasets from African populations are scarce, which limits the generalizability of current state-of-the-art machine learning models [10].

To address these limitations, the BraTS-Lighthouse 2025 Challenge introduced a new task focused on brain tumor segmentation in sub-Saharan African (SSA) patients hosted by the Medical Image Computing and Computer Assisted Interventions (MICCAI) conference, which annually hosts various medical imaging competitions that draw research teams internationally, including the BraTS challenge [4]. This task addresses a critical gap in current research—developing robust models that can generalize across domain shifts introduced by demographic, anatomical, and acquisition variability. Compared to previous years that focused on Global North adult glioma segmentation [8,9], this challenge prioritizes equity in AI development by evaluating segmentation methods on data from underserved populations (e.g., in sub-Saharan Africa), where automated solutions could provide the most clinical benefit.

Deep learning remains the standard for brain tumor segmentation, with most top-performing solutions based on U-Net-style architectures since the BraTS 2014 challenge [2,3]. Recent work has focused on enhancing these architectures through better feature encoding, skip connections, attention mechanisms, and normalization strategies. One such advancement is the MedNeXt architecture, which adapts ConvNeXt blocks into a 3D U-Net-like framework [11,12].

In this paper, we present our state-of-the-art segmentation pipeline ***EMedNeXt*** based on MedNeXt V2, designed specifically for the SSA task in BraTS-Lighthouse 2025. ***EMedNeXt*** introduces three key improvements over its predecessor: (1) a larger region of interest (ROI) for better contextual learning, (2) an updated architectural skeleton inspired by nnU-Net v2, and (3) a framework for ensembling the model to enhance prediction robustness. We also explore deep supervision, training optimizations, and post-processing strategies tailored to this domain. The data used for performance assessment was obtained from standard clinical care for brain tumors and was annotated by radiologists and reviewed by neurologists to ensure accuracy [5,13]. Our results on the hidden validation set that exceeded the best model of last year demonstrate the effectiveness of our pipeline in addressing real-world distribution shifts and resource constraints. The remainder of this paper is organized as follows. The methods, including the datasets used, the architecture, and the framework training flow, are discussed in Sect. 2. The results and discussion, including the performance evaluation, are presented in Sect. 3. Finally, the conclusion and future work are summarized in Sect. 4.

2 Methods

In this section, we outline the datasets used, the architectural backbone of our model, and the comprehensive training paradigm employed to build our segmentation system.

2.1 Data

In this study, we utilize two different datasets to train and evaluate our tumor segmentation pipeline, both provided as part of the BraTS-Lighthouse 2025 Challenge. Due to the limited number of samples (60 patients) in the Sub-Saharan African (SSA) dataset (Task #5), we also incorporate data from the Pre- and Post-Treatment Adult Glioma (PPTAG) dataset (Task #1), with a uniform size of $240 \times 240 \times 155$.

2.1.1 BraTS Sub-saharan African Dataset

The SSA dataset consists of multi-parametric MRI scans acquired from clinical sites in sub-Saharan Africa, specifically Nigeria. Each case includes four MRI modalities—T1-weighted (T1), T1 with contrast enhancement (T1c), T2-weighted (T2), and Fluid-Attenuated Inversion Recovery (FLAIR)—along with expert-annotated tumor segmentation masks. This dataset captures the real-world variability and noise introduced by low-resource imaging settings, such as low-field MRI scanners and diverse patient demographics. It includes 60 patients' training and 35 validation brain MRI scans. An example case is shown in Fig. 1.

2.1.2 Pre and Post-treatment Adult Glioma Dataset

The PPTAG dataset contains high-quality MRI scans of adult glioma patients captured before and after treatment. Like the SSA dataset, it includes all four standard modalities and expert annotations. However, due to differences in imaging quality, the dataset underwent a preprocessing pipeline involving denoising, intensity normalization, and spatial resampling to better align with the SSA distribution. Given the limited number of SSA cases, we augment our training set by merging the PPTAG samples with SSA data. It includes 1195 training and 219 validation brain MRI scans. An example from the PPTAG dataset is shown in Fig. 2.

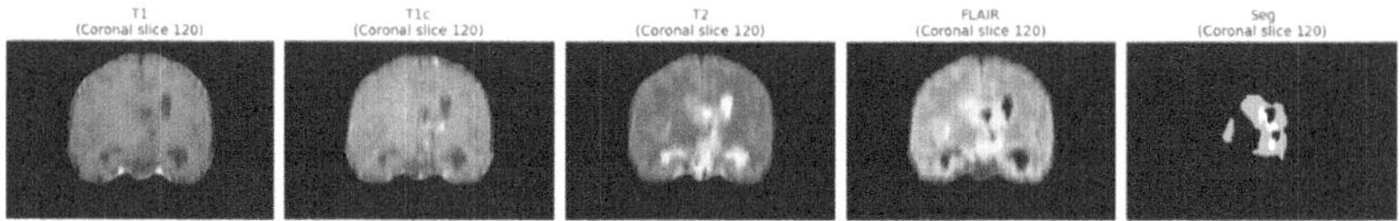

Fig. 1. Cross sections of the four modalities obtained from a sample data-point from the SSA dataset along with the corresponding segmentation masks.

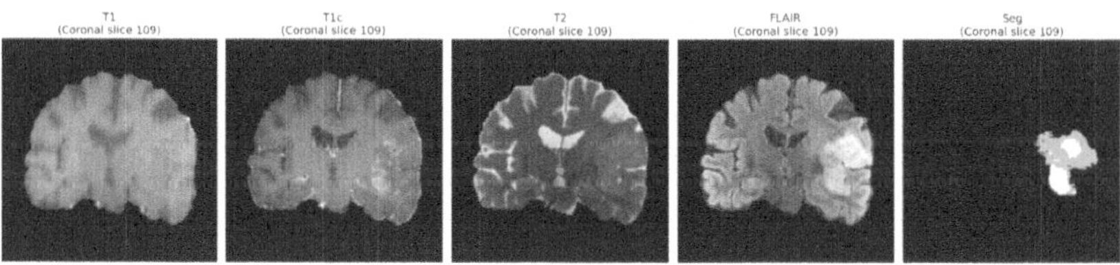

Fig. 2. Cross sections of the four modalities obtained from a sample data-point from the PPTAG dataset along with the corresponding segmentation masks.

2.2 MedNeXt V2

Having established the datasets, we now describe the core segmentation architecture used in ***EMedNeXt***: MedNeXt V2, which enhances the original MedNeXt V1 for improved accuracy and robustness through several key upgrades:

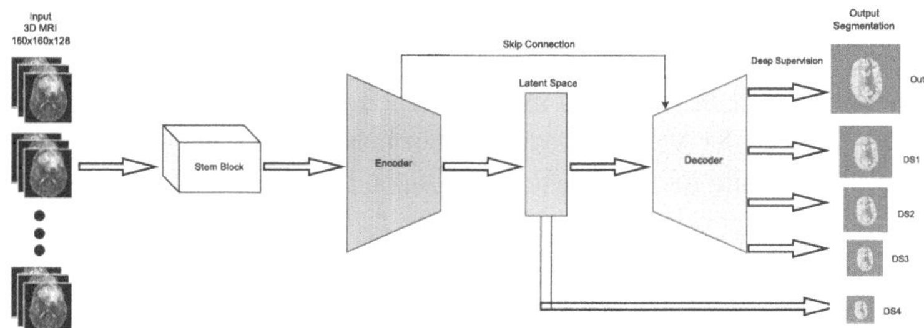

Fig. 3. MedNeXt V2: High-level architecture. A 4-channel 3D MRI input ($160 \times 160 \times 128$) is processed through a stem block, followed by an encoder that extracts hierarchical features, a bottleneck, and a decoder that reconstructs segmentation maps.

(i) **Adopting nnU-Net V2:** A dynamic, data-driven framework for segmentation without manual tuning.

(ii) **Kernel Size Unification:** All depthwise convolutions now use a fixed $3 \times 3 \times 3$ kernel instead of variable kernel sizes with channel expansion ($C \times R$) and compression (C) are explicitly performed using $1 \times 1 \times 1$ convolutions after depth-wise convolutions.

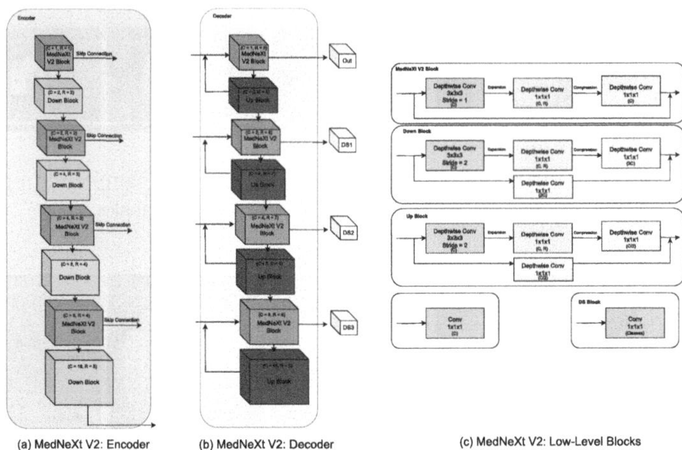

Fig. 4. Detailed MedNeXt V2 architecture: (a) encoder path, (b) decoder path, and (c) low-level block components.

(iii) **Larger Field of View:** The input patch size is increased to $160 \times 160 \times 128$ to provide the network with more contextual information.
(iv) **Deep Supervision:** Enhanced Auxiliary outputs are introduced at multiple decoder levels to improve gradient flow and training stability.
(v) **Improved Skip Connections:** Enhanced skip connections are used to better preserve spatial alignment between encoder and decoder features.

Figure 3 provides the high-level layout; architectural details of the encoder, decoder, and block design appear in Fig. 4c. The encoder (Fig. 4a) is composed of alternating MedNeXt V2 blocks and Down blocks, each progressively reducing spatial resolution while increasing feature depth. The decoder (Fig. 4b) symmetrically mirrors the encoder using Up blocks followed by MedNeXt V2 blocks. It integrates skip connections from the encoder and produces four outputs: one final segmentation map and three intermediate outputs for deep supervision.

2.3 EMedNeXt Training Flow

Having outlined the architecture, we now present our complete training workflow for ***EMedNeXt***. The pipeline is designed to effectively handle heterogeneous and limited-resource MRI datasets. Figure 5 illustrates the two-phase training paradigm: initial pre-training using diverse datasets followed by specialized fine-tuning on the SSA dataset. The robustness of this pipeline is further enhanced through additional steps including model ensembling, inference, postprocessing, and evaluation.

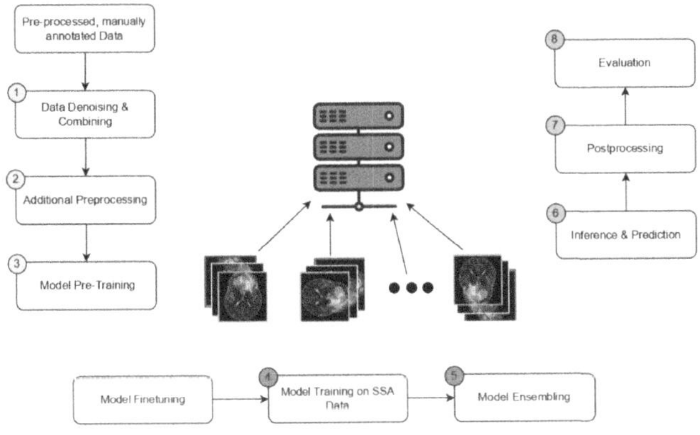

Fig. 5. EMedNeXt: Training Flow.

2.3.1 Data Denoising and Combining

To prepare the training dataset, we merged the SSA dataset and the PPTAG dataset, as detailed in Subsect. 2.1. This integration addresses the limited size of the SSA dataset by incorporating additional annotated examples while aiming to preserve domain relevance. The raw NIfTI volumes from all patients were first denoised and intensity-standardized. Each modality (FLAIR, T1, T1c, T2) was loaded and cast to `int16`, with negative outliers clipped and extreme values reset to zero to suppress scanner artifacts. To harmonize the intensity distributions, we applied channel-wise normalization limited to nonzero voxels, ensuring that each modality contributes comparably to the downstream model and that background regions do not skew the normalization statistics. Finally, all image volumes were resampled to a fixed voxel spacing of $(1.0, 1.0, 1.0)$ and a target shape of $160 \times 160 \times 128$ using cubic interpolation. The resulting unified dataset contained 1,255 preprocessed training cases with corresponding multi-class tumor segmentation masks.

2.3.2 Additional Preprocessing

Following denoising and normalization, we applied structural preprocessing to localize and standardize the region of interest. Using MONAI's spatial bounding box utilities, we identified the tightest enclosing box around all nonzero voxels in each scan and cropped both the image and its corresponding segmentation label accordingly. To ensure uniform input size for training, the cropped images were padded (or further cropped if needed) to $160 \times 160 \times 128$ using symmetric padding centered on the brain. Next, all four MRI modalities were stacked into a single 4-channel volume. We also added a fifth channel representing the aggregated foreground mask across modalities, which helps the model distinguish brain tissue from background. Segmentation masks underwent identical transformations to maintain spatial alignment. All outputs, preprocessed images, masks, and metadata (such as bounding boxes and original shapes), were stored as NumPy arrays in a designated directory. To accelerate the pipeline, we parallelized the process using Python's `multiprocessing` library across CPU cores.

2.3.3 Model Pre-training

As we described earlier, we first merge and preprocess the SSA and PPTAG datasets to increase training diversity. Building on this, we perform a preliminary pre-training stage on the combined dataset to provide the model with a broader distribution of tumor cases and imaging conditions. This stage serves to initialize the model with robust feature representations, which led to an effective fine-tuning when the model is later trained on the SSA dataset.

2.3.4 Data Augmentation

To enhance the robustness and generalization of the model, we applied both spatial and intensity-based augmentations during training. Spatial augmentations included random cropping of regions of interest (ROIs) with dimensions (r_x, r_y, r_z) and random flips along the sagittal, coronal, and axial axes with a probability of $p = 0.5$, thereby increasing anatomical variability. Intensity augmentations consisted of random scaling (factor ± 0.1) and shifting (offset ± 0.1) of image intensities, each applied with probability $p = 1.0$, to simulate inter-patient and inter-scanner variations. Collectively, these augmentations improve model generalization while preserving clinically relevant features.

2.3.5 Model Finetuning and Training on SSA Dataset

Given the limited size and domain shift of the SSA dataset, we adopt a lightweight adaptation strategy that focuses training primarily on the *decoder*. This allows us to preserve *encoder* features learned during pre-training while tailoring the decoder to SSA-specific imaging artifacts and tumor patterns. Hence, we implemented a *structured freezing strategy*:

(i) Freeze *all* encoder parameters to retain generic representations.
(ii) Unfreeze the last k decoder blocks, all upsamplers, and the 3 segmentation heads (main and two deep supervision outputs).
(iii) Optionally, unfreeze the deepest 2 encoder stages to enable minor low-level domain adaptation.

This setup ensures that a small subset of the model remains trainable, typically no more than $X\%$ ($X \in \{34.8\%, 38.7\%\}$) of the total parameters, helping avoid overfitting. We, then, optimize the model using AdamW Schedule-Free [6], with distinct learning rates for different parameter groups:

- Main body: $\eta = 1.0 \times 10^{-4}$
- Decoder blocks: $\eta_{\text{dec}} = \eta$

- Segmentation heads: $\eta_{\text{head}} = 2\eta$
- Unfrozen encoder stages (optional): $\eta_{\text{enc}} = 0.1\eta$

This configuration removes the need for explicit learning-rate schedules, as the optimizer adapts the step size automatically. Training proceeds in two phases: (i) **pre-training** on the merged SSA+PPTAG dataset for 150 epochs, and (ii) **fine-tuning** on the SSA dataset for 50 epochs under the structured freezing strategy. Both stages use 160×160×128 voxel patches, batch size 3, and mixed precision.

To enhance boundary quality, which is crucial for *Normalised Surface Dice* (NSD), we utilized a hybrid boundary-aware loss: the standard Dice–Focal loss with a 3D boundary term. Let $\mathbf{p} \in [0,1]^{C\times H\times W\times D}$ be the predicted probabilities and $\mathbf{g} \in \{0,1\}^{C\times H\times W\times D}$ be the one-hot ground truth. The total loss becomes:

$$\mathcal{L}_{\text{total}} = \mathcal{L}_{\text{Dice–Focal}} + \alpha\,\mathcal{L}_{\text{boundary}}, \qquad \alpha = 0.5 \tag{1}$$

The boundary loss term is defined as:

$$\mathcal{L}_{\text{boundary}} = \|\nabla_{\text{Sobel}}\mathbf{p} - \nabla_{\text{Sobel}}\mathbf{g}\|_2^2 \tag{2}$$

where ∇_{Sobel} denotes a 3D Sobel operator applied channel-wise. The total loss is computed across all decoder outputs with deep supervision weights $w_i = 2^{-i}$ (finest resolution $i{=}0$), emphasizing the finer-resolution outputs.

2.3.6 Model Ensembling and Inference

Following the fine-tuning stage, we further boost segmentation robustness by aggregating predictions from multiple MedNeXt variants. As observed in preliminary experiments, individual checkpoints tend to inconsistently over- or under-segment certain tumor sub-regions, which ensembling helps mitigate. To achieve this, we apply late fusion at the probability level, where each model m produces a soft probability map $P_m \in [0,1]^{C\times D\times H\times W}$ over the $C = 3$ BraTS tumor classes: whole tumor (WT), tumor core (TC), and enhancing tumor (ET). Each model is assigned a non-negative weight vector $\mathbf{w}_m = (w_{m,1}, w_{m,2}, w_{m,3})$, and the ensemble probability for voxel (x,y,z) and class c is calculated via a weighted average:

$$\hat{P}_c(x,y,z) = \frac{\sum_{m=1}^{M} w_{m,c}\, P_{m,c}(x,y,z)}{\sum_{m=1}^{M} w_{m,c}}, \qquad c \in \{\text{WT},\text{TC},\text{ET}\}. \tag{3}$$

In our implementation, we use uniform weights $\mathbf{w}_m = (1,1,1)$ across all models, yielding an arithmetic mean.[1] To reduce memory requirements and support arbitrary ensemble sizes, we adopt a two-pass inference strategy:

[1] The framework allows class- or model-specific weighting, useful for discounting noisy channels or low-performing models, by adjusting $w_{m,c}$ in Eq. (3).

(i) **Per-model inference.** Each checkpoint is processed independently using sliding-window inference (patch size 160×160×128, with 50% overlap), combined with 7-way test-time augmentation (TTA) via flipping.
(ii) **Normalization pass.** Once all M models have been evaluated, we normalize the accumulated predictions using a multiprocessing pool, dividing by the sum of weights as per Eq. (3), yielding the final ensemble output $\hat{P} \in \mathbb{R}^{3 \times D \times H \times W}$.

This strategy requires only the memory of a single model at runtime and avoids synchronization overhead. Also, the modular design enables seamless integration of additional checkpoints in future ensemble configurations.

2.3.7 Postprocessing

To further refine the segmentation predictions obtained from the ensemble stage, we apply a tailored postprocessing pipeline that restores anatomical consistency and suppresses residual false positives. The ensemble inference outputs a three-channel probability tensor

$$\mathbf{P} = \{P_{\mathrm{TC}}, P_{\mathrm{WT}}, P_{\mathrm{ET}}\} \in [0,1]^{3 \times D \times H \times W},$$

for each subject, representing soft predictions for the TC, WT, and ET classes. Although the finetuned MedNeXt V2 backbone incorporates deep supervision, raw outputs still contain numerous sub-millimetric false positives. The postprocessing pipeline described below mitigates these issues:

(i) **Independent hard thresholding:** Each probability map is binarized using class-specific thresholds:

$$\tau_{\mathrm{TC}} \in \{0.5, 0.7\}, \quad \tau_{\mathrm{WT}} \in 0.5, \quad \tau_{\mathrm{ET}} \in \{0.5, 0.7\}.$$

The elevated threshold for ET reduces low-confidence activations that would otherwise degrade the NSD score.
(ii) **Connected-component (CC) pruning:** For each class $c \in \{\mathrm{TC}, \mathrm{WT}, \mathrm{ET}\}$, we extract 26-connected components $\mathcal{C} = \{C_1, \ldots, C_K\}$ and retain components satisfying:

$$|C_k| \geq \gamma_c \quad \text{and} \quad \bar{P}_c(C_k) = \frac{1}{|C_k|} \sum_{x \in C_k} P_c(x) \geq \eta_c, \tag{4}$$

where $(\gamma_c, \eta_c) = (150, 0.1)$ for TC, $(500, 0.1)$ for WT, and $(100, 0.1)$ for ET. If more than 10 components pass the filter (4), we retain only the largest 10 per class.
(iii) **Hierarchical enforcement:** To ensure topological correctness, we enforce the anatomical hierarchy ET $\subseteq$ TC $\subseteq$ WT by propagating accepted ET masks into TC, and TC into WT. We then reapply the connected-component filter (4) to restore structural coherence and improve boundary-sensitive metrics.

(iv) **Label fusion with priority rules:** Finally, the three refined binary masks are merged into a single label map $S \in \{0, 1, 2, 3\}^{D \times H \times W}$ using a fixed priority: ET $\triangleright$ TC $\triangleright$ WT:

$$S(x) = \begin{cases} 3 & \text{if } \mathrm{ET}(x) = 1, \\ 2 & \text{else if } \mathrm{TC}(x) = 1, \\ 1 & \text{else if } \mathrm{WT}(x) = 1, \\ 0 & \text{otherwise.} \end{cases}$$

2.3.8 Evaluation and Experimental Setup

To ensure fair evaluation, we followed the official BraTS 2025 SSA protocol. During model development, we performed K-fold cross-validation (K=5) on the SSA training set (60 cases), using 80% of cases for training and 20% for internal validation in each fold. This procedure helped stabilize training and guide hyperparameter selection. For final reporting, models pre-trained on the combined SSA+PPTAG training data were retrained on the full SSA training set and evaluated on the hidden BraTS-SSA validation set (35 cases). We assess the segmentation quality using the DSC and NSD metrics, both at global and lesion-wise levels, as defined in the challenge guidelines. All training and inference experiments were conducted on a cluster with 4 NVIDIA A6000 GPUs using mixed precision. We trained our model using the AdamW optimizer with a learning rate of $2.8e^{-3}$ and ScheduleFree scheduling for a total of 150 epochs of pre-training followed by 50 epochs of fine-tuning, enabling deep supervision. Other key configurations include a batch size of 3, weight decay of $1e^{-6}$, and using MedNeXt-B variant with a kernel size of 3.

3 Results and Discussion

With the training setup and evaluation methodology established, we now present the results of our experiments. We analyze the effectiveness of each component in our pipeline, from architectural upgrades to post-processing refinements. Table 1 summarizes the lesion-wise Dice Similarity Coefficient (DSC) and Normalized Surface Dice (NSD) achieved by successive versions of our framework. Starting from the original *MedNeXt V1* baseline, each component we introduced gives a boost in our segmentation quality:

(i) **Backbone upgrade (V1 → V2).** Replacing the V1 encoder–decoder with the larger-receptive-field *MedNeXt V2* architecture ("Base= 5") lifts the mean DSC from **0.839** to **0.873** and the mean $\mathrm{NSD}_{0.5}$ from **0.395** to **0.472**. The gains are maximized for enhancing-tumour (ET) class.

(ii) **Domain-adaptive fine-tuning.** Freezing the encoder and re-training only the decoder on the SSA dataset with the boundary loss improves boundary alignment with the ground-truth. Mean DSC is slightly pushed to **0.884**,

Table 1. Lesion-wise segmentation performance on the BraTS-SSA hidden validation set and our best performing model on the test set (higher is better). Best values are **bolded**.

Model	Dice ↑			$NSD_{0.5}$ ↑			$NSD_{1.0}$ ↑		
	ET	TC	WT	ET	TC	WT	ET	TC	WT
Baseline (MedNeXt V1)	0.822	0.815	0.881	0.424	0.378	0.383	0.764	0.698	0.728
MedNeXt V2 (B=5)	0.845	0.860	0.914	0.501	0.470	0.444	0.822	0.776	0.796
FT MedNeXt V2 (B=5)	0.870	0.863	0.919	0.570	0.513	0.499	0.863	0.798	0.821
MedNeXt V2 (B=3)	0.860	0.832	0.904	0.569	0.479	0.487	0.852	0.763	0.809
FT MedNeXt V2 (B=3)	0.873	0.835	0.927	0.569	0.472	0.498	0.869	0.769	0.830
Ensemble (B=3)	0.883	0.873	0.933	0.579	0.519	0.520	0.873	0.806	0.839
Ensemble + PP*	**0.883**	**0.873**	**0.933**	**0.580**	**0.522**	**0.521**	**0.873**	**0.806**	**0.839**
Test-phase Results									
Ensemble + PP (Mean)	0.8597	0.8821	0.9298	–	–	–	0.8534	0.8182	0.8544
Ensemble + PP (Std)	0.1612	0.1749	0.1147	–	–	–	0.1558	0.1908	0.1316

* Post-processing: thresholds $\tau_{ET} = \tau_{TC} = 0.625$ and connected-component filter $|CC_{ET}| \geq 30$ voxels.

and mean $NSD_{0.5}$ to **0.518**. Therefore, fine-tuning allows the model to learn SSA-specific intensity profiles while avoiding over-fitting to the small training set.

(iii) **Base architecture variant with kernel size of 3.** Narrowing the channel width gave us a boost in performance. After fine-tuning, the "Base=3" model attains a DSC of **0.878** and an $NSD_{0.5}$ of **0.513**.

(iv) **Ensembling.** Averaging the logits of 5 our best base with fine-tuned checkpoints of the kernel size 3 model pushed the mean DSC to **0.896** and the $NSD_{0.5}$ to **0.537**. Ensemble voting mitigates individual checkpoint biases.

(v) **Post-processing optimization.** Adjusting the hard-threshold for ET/TC to 0.625 and relaxing the ET component-size filter (from 100 to 30 voxels) recovers additional small lesions, raising the final $NSD_{0.5}$ to **0.541** and $NSD_{1.0}$ to **0.84**, while leaving the already high DSC unchanged. Similarly, we used these settings along with our ensembling approach for our final submission in the test-phase.

In general, the proposed ***EMedNeXt*** pipeline delivers an average Lesion-Wise DSC of **0.897** with solid boundary alignment performance. These gains translate to visibly cleaner segmentation and fewer noisy fragments, as illustrated in Fig. 6. The qualitative sample highlights the advantages of the ensemble of models (right) over the single fine-tuned *B5* model (left). The *B5* model fails to capture several small, isolated enhancing tumor regions (orange contours) along the inferior margin of the lesion and within the necrotic core. These regions are consistently recovered by the ensemble, reflecting the improvement in ET-wise NSD reported in Table 1. Furthermore, the set provides a more precise whole tumor envelope (green), with noticeably tighter adherence to the actual tumor boundaries.

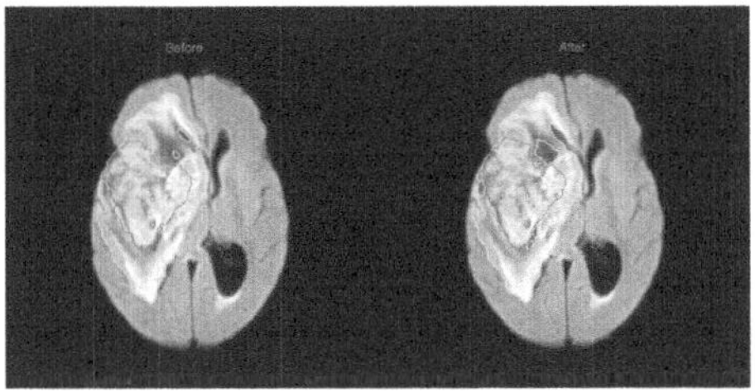

Fig. 6. Comparison between Finetuned MedNext with B=5 and our final ensemble of models qualitative predictions.

4 Conclusion

In this work, we presented ***EMedNeXt***, a MedNeXt V2-based framework for brain tumor segmentation tailored to the BraTS-Lighthouse 2025 SSA task. Our pipeline integrates a larger field of view, structured decoder fine-tuning via encoder freezing, and a class-specific post-processing strategy. To address domain shifts and data scarcity, we employed pretraining on PPTAG data followed by fine-tuning on SSA scans. Ensembling and optimized post-processing further improved lesion boundary quality. Our final model achieved an average Lesion-Wise Dice of **0.897**, with NSD scores of **0.541** (0.5mm) and **0.84** (1.0mm), demonstrating strong performance in low-resource settings. Future work will extend this framework to pediatric data and explore new architectures for the segmentation framework.

References

1. Mesfin, F.B., aet al.: Gliomas. StatPearls [Internet], StatPearls Publishing, Treasure Island (2024). Accessed 20 May 2023. https://www.ncbi.nlm.nih.gov/books/NBK441874/
2. Ferreira, A., Solak, N., Li, J., Dammann, P., Kleesiek, J., Alves, V., Egger, J.: How we won BraTS 2023 Adult Glioma challenge? Just faking it! Enhanced Synthetic Data Augmentation and Model Ensemble for brain tumour segmentation (2024). https://arxiv.org/abs/2402.17317
3. Ronneberger, O., Fischer, P., Brox, T.: U-net: convolutional networks for biomedical image segmentation. In: Navab, N., Hornegger, J., Wells, W.M., Frangi, A.F. (eds.) MICCAI 2015. LNCS, vol. 9351, pp. 234–241. Springer, Cham (2015). https://doi.org/10.1007/978-3-319-24574-4_28
4. Menze, B.H., et al.: The multimodal brain tumor image segmentation benchmark (BRATS). IEEE Trans. Med. Imaging **34**(10), 1993–2024 (2014)

5. Adewole, M., et al.: The Brain Tumor Segmentation (BraTS) Challenge 2023: Glioma Segmentation in Sub-Saharan Africa Patient Population (BraTS-Africa) (2023). https://arxiv.org/abs/2305.19369
6. Defazio, A., Mehta, H., Mishchenko, K., Khaled, A., Cutkosky, A., et al.: The Road Less Scheduled. arXiv preprint arXiv:2405.15682 (2024)
7. Owrangi, A.M., Greer, P.B., Glide-Hurst, C.K.: MRI-only treatment planning: benefits and challenges. Phys. Med. Biol. **63**(5), 05TR01 (2018)
8. Bakas, S., et al.: Advancing the cancer genome atlas glioma MRI collections with expert segmentation labels and radiomic features. Sci. Data **4**(1), 1–13 (2017)
9. Bakas, S., et al.: Segmentation labels and radiomic features for the pre-operative scans of the TCGA-LGG collection. Cancer Imag. Arch. **286** (2017)
10. Adewole, M., et al.: The brain tumor segmentation (BraTS) challenge 2023: Glioma segmentation in Sub-Saharan Africa patient population (BraTS-Africa). ArXiv (2023)
11. Roy, S., et al.: MedNeXt: Transformer-driven Scaling of ConvNets for Medical Image Segmentation. arXiv preprint arXiv:2303.09975 (2023)
12. Liu, Z., Mao, H., Wu, C.-Y., Feichtenhofer, C., Darrell, T., Xie, S.: A ConvNet for the 2020s. In: CVPR, pp. 11976–11986 (2022)
13. Adewole, M., Rudie, J. D., Gbadamosi, A., et al.: The BraTS-Africa dataset: expanding the brain tumor segmentation (BraTS) data to capture African populations. Radiol. Artif. Intell. (2025). https://doi.org/10.1148/ryai.240528

Improving Pre-trained Adult Glioma Segmentation Models Using only Post-processing Techniques

Abhijeet Parida[1,2], Daniel Capellán-Martín[1,2], Zhifan Jiang[1], Nishad Kulkarni[1], Krithika Iyer[1], Austin Tapp[1], Syed Muhammad Anwar[1,3], María J. Ledesma-Carbayo[2], and Marius George Linguraru[1,3](✉)

[1] Sheikh Zayed Institute for Pediatric Surgical Innovation, Children's National Hospital, Washington, DC, USA

[2] Universidad Politécnica de Madrid and CIBER-BBN, ISCIII, Madrid, Spain

[3] School of Medicine and Health Sciences, George Washington University, Washington, DC, USA

mlingura@childrensnational.org

Abstract. Gliomas are the most common malignant brain tumors in adults and are among the most lethal. Despite aggressive treatment, the median survival rate is less than 15 months. Accurate multiparametric MRI (mpMRI) tumor segmentation is critical for surgical planning, radiotherapy, and disease monitoring. While deep learning models have improved the accuracy of automated segmentation, large-scale pre-trained models generalize poorly and often underperform, producing systematic errors such as false positives, label swaps, and slice discontinuities in slices. These limitations are further compounded by unequal access to GPU resources and the growing environmental cost of large-scale model training. In this work, we propose adaptive post-processing techniques to refine the quality of glioma segmentations produced by large-scale pretrained models developed for various types of tumors. We demonstrated the techniques in multiple BraTS 2025 segmentation challenge tasks, with the ranking metric improving by 14.9 % for the sub-Saharan Africa challenge and 0.9% for the adult glioma challenge. This approach promotes a shift in brain tumor segmentation research from increasingly complex model architectures to efficient, clinically aligned post-processing strategies that are precise, computationally fair, and sustainable.

Keywords: Brain MRI · BraTS Challenge · Glioma segmentation · Medical image analysis · Resource-aware AI

1 Introduction

Gliomas are the most common malignant brain tumors in adults and remain among the deadliest among cancer types. Despite aggressive treatment strategies (maximal surgical resection, chemotherapy, radiotherapy), median overall

A. Parida, D. Capellán-Martín and Z. Jiang—These authors contributed equally.

S. Bakas et al. (Eds.): MICCAI 2025, LNCS 16376, pp. 237–247, 2026.
https://doi.org/10.1007/978-3-032-16365-3_22

survival duration is around 15 months. Malignant gliomas collectively account for approximately 2.5% of all cancer-related deaths [26]. Considering these alarming facts, there is a pressing need for tools that enable earlier detection, accurate characterization, and effective treatment planning to improve patient outcomes. Central to the clinical management of gliomas is multi-parametric magnetic resonance imaging (mpMRI), which provides non-invasive, high-resolution visualization of tumor anatomy and physiology. mpMRIbased tumor segmentation of tumors is routinely used to: (i) guide surgical resection margins [27], (ii) paint radiotherapy dose [8], and (iii) monitor volumetric disease progression [10]. Despite its critical importance, tumor segmentation is still performed manually: an iterative and labor intensive process that can consume substantial expert time per case [4]. In addition, the manual segmentation process is highly subjective, reducing the reproducibility between observers. Several deep learning models have recently been proposed to segment various pathologies [1,30]. Automating the tumor segmentation step with deep learning models promises significant time savings and greater standardization across centers.

Since 2012, Brain Tumor Segmentation (BraTS) challenges, held in conjunction with the International Conference on Medical Image Computing and Computer Assisted Intervention (MICCAI), have become a leading contributor towards the development and benchmarking of automated tumor segmentation models by providing large, expertly annotated, and standardized datasets. The 2025 edition introduced the largest expert-annotated glioma data set and standardized lesion-wise normalized surface distance (NSD) metrics [5,22]. During this period, the best performing methods have primarily relied on the nnU-Net framework [14], which extends the original U-Net architecture [24] with modality- and dataset-specific adaptations to deliver state-of-the-art performance for 3D biomedical image tasks. In contrast, large-scale pre-trained models underperform in glioma segmentation and may perform inconsistently and generalize poorly even after light fine-tuning [12]. Their residual errors (tiny false positive islands), segmentation label swaps, or slicewise discontinuities are systematic and easily correctable. Previous BraTS winners have shown that post-processing steps such as ensemble voting [21], size-sensitive connected component filtering [9], ET-to-NCR relabeling heuristics [9], and adaptive refinement [16,23] can significantly improve segmentation accuracy.

Beyond the choice of model and post-processing algorithms, socioeconomic conditions also strongly affect the challenge outcomes. Access to GPUs remains highly unequal, with recent surveys showing that GPU resources are highly concentrated in high-income settings, leaving researchers, especially in low and middle-income countries, without adequate resources [19]. Moreover, training complex deep learning models on GPUs consumes considerable energy; therefore, the environmental impact of using GPUs is becoming impossible to ignore. However, post hoc refinement using simple image-processing techniques typically requires only a few CPU hours. Thus, adaptive post-processing offers a compute-democratic path, allowing all steps to run on commodity CPUs.

This can broaden meaningful participation in BraTS while simultaneously shrinking the carbon footprint of medical-AI research.

Taken together, the saturation of performance gains in large-scale pre-trained segmentation model architectures, the unequal access to computational resources, and the environmental costs of large-scale training underscore the need for more efficient alternatives. Therefore, this article proposes samplewise adaptive post-processing techniques on foundation models for the segmentation of adult gliomas (**GLI**) and adult gliomas in sub-Saharan African patients (**SSA**). We show performance gains over the base foundation model without additional GPU training. We advocate a shift in brain MRI segmentation research from ever deeper backbones toward smarter, greener, and clinically aligned post-processing – promoting accuracy, computational equity, and sustainability.

2 Previous Work

2.1 Glioma Segmentation Models

The *BraTS orchestrator* [18] provides dockerized access to the best performing solutions from previous BraTS challenges, enabling fair, side-by-side evaluation of winning models. Since these models generalize well and have been trained on large datasets using the best practices to get the best performance, they are considered our large-scale pre-trained segmentation models. For pretreatment adult glioma (**GLI-pre**), the BraTS 2023 winner combined SwinUNETR [13] and nnU-Net [14] in an ensemble trained on real and GAN-augmented data [11]. A closely related ensemble from the same group secured the first place in the post-treatment GLI (**GLI-post**) task at BraTS 2024.

For adult glioma in sub-Saharan African patients (**SSA**), the leading model of BraTS 2024 first pre-trained on the large GLI-pre cohort and then fine-tuned on the modest SSA dataset, using a MedNeXT [25]nnU-Net ensemble [23]. Although these architectures differ in backbone details, their training recipes converge on heavy GPU usage, large-scale augmentation, and multifold ensembling to squeeze out the last increments in Dice.

2.2 Adaptive Post-processing

To mitigate systematic residual errors that survive end-to-end training, several groups have proposed *adaptive post-processing*, i.e., selecting sample-specific refinements rather than applying a fixed post-processing pipeline to every case. Jiang *et al.* [15] formalized the concept and demonstrated that radiomic features of the predicted mask can guide which operations (connected-component filtering, ET→NCR relabeling, etc.) maximize Dice gain for a given sample. Follow-up work clustered cases in radiomic space to learn cluster-wise thresholds for component removal [16], and Parida *et al.* [23] also applied similar heuristic rules to win the BraTS 2024 SSA challenge. These refinements run entirely on CPUs and boost generalization.

3 Challenge and Data Description

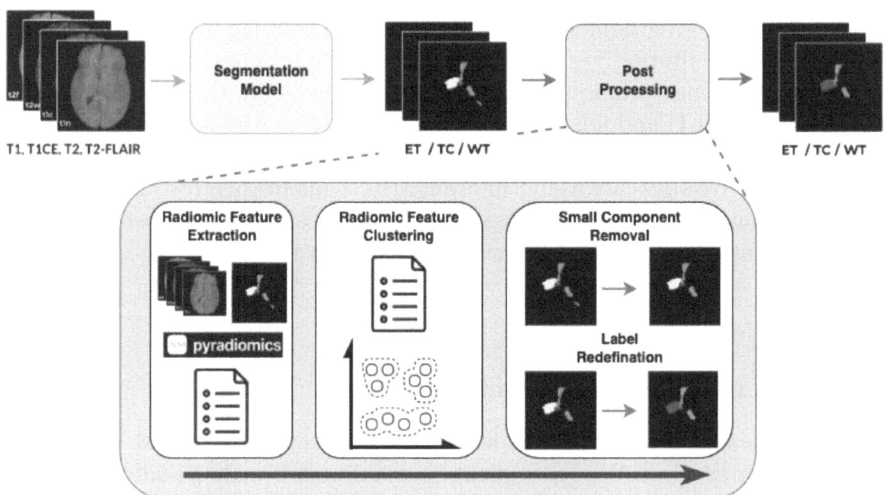

Fig. 1. The process pipeline shows the high-level overview of our proposed post-processing pipeline. It shows the major steps of PyRadiomics-based feature extraction, clustering of samples based on the radiomic signature, removal of small components, and small label redefinition to get the final segmentation.

BraTS 2024 GLI [6,7,29] aims at automatic segmentation of diffuse gliomas on multi-institutional, clinically acquired pre and post-treatment mpMRI scans. Each case provides four sequences collected routinely: precontrast T1-weighted (T1), contrast-enhanced T1-weighted (T1CE), T2-weighted (T2), and T2-weighted fluid-attenuated inversion recovery (T2-FLAIR). The current version contains 1,251 GLI-pre and 1,350 GLI-post training cases. For the validation set, there are 219 GLI-pre and 188 GLI-post cases. Ground truth annotations cover six clinically relevant regions: non-enhancing tumor core (NETC, label 1), surrounding non-enhancing FLAIR hyperintensity (SNFH, label 2), enhancing tumor tissue (ET, label 3), resection cavity (RC, label 4), the tumor core (TC = ET + NETC), and the whole tumor (WT = ET + SNFH + NETC). The challenge ranking is based on the Dice and the normalized surface distance (NSD) computed per lesion.

BraTS 2024 SSA [2,3] is the largest public collection of annotated pretreatment glioma scans from adult African patients, including low-grade gliomas and glioblastomas. It uses four MRI sequences (T1, T1CE, T2, T2-FLAIR) and the same label taxonomy (NETC, SNFH, ET, TC, WT) as the GLI task. The data set comprises 60 training and 35 validation cases; test labels are withheld. Evaluation employs identical Dice/NSD metrics.

4 Methods

We built on large-scale pre-trained segmentation networks and included a task specific, three stage post-processing pipeline (Fig. 1). The stages were (i) *radiomic feature extraction and case clustering*, (ii) *thresholding to delete small, isolated components*, and (iii) *thresholding to fix label mix-ups*.

We optimized the thresholds and chose the best model with the ranking approach proposed by the BraTS team LaBella *et al.* [20]. LaBella *et al.* stated - "The evaluation is done in a hidden test set, computing lesion-wise metrics in all regions and comparing ranks of all the submissions rather than the metrics". We folowed the idea and replicated this procedure, we built an internal ranking metric that produced a single score. The ranking metric was optimized for a lower score where a smaller value means better performance on Dice and NSD at the 0.5 and 1 mm thresholds for each of the regions. The code is available on GitHub [2].

The ranking metric approach was chosen because it was robust to outlier predictions. Further, the ranking metric allowed us to optimize for a single value while aligning with the contest evaluation pipeline.

Radiomic Feature Extraction and Clustering: For the prediction of the WT ensemble, we calculated 386 radiomic features using *PyRadiomics* [28], following the protocol of Jiang *et al.* [17]. Therefore, each case had- 14 shape descriptors that capture tumor geometry, and 93 intensity & texture descriptors- for each of the four MRI sequences (T1, T1Gd, T2, FLAIR). Using principal component analysis (PCA), we retained the principal components that explain 90 % of the variance and then partitioned the cases with k means clustering [15,16]. The optimal number of clusters was determined by maximizing the silhouette coefficient in the training folds. Each new case was assigned to the nearest cluster at test time, allowing for the post-processing to be applied on the basis of its radiomic signature.

Threshold Identification for Removing Small Components (p_{cc}): Within each cluster and for each label (NETC, SNFH, ET, and RC), we performed a grid search over minimum size thresholds to retain the lesion [23]. Each threshold was evaluated on a cross-validated ranking metric; the threshold that minimized the ranking metrics was selected. The application of a sample-specific cluster p_{cc} removed tiny disconnected islands, noise that would otherwise inflate the false positive count.

Threshold Identification for Label Redefinition ($lblredef$): A second adaptive search fine-tuned the consistency between labels. Jiang *et al.* [15] suggested a similar approach after the removal of the noisy component. For example, if the enhancing tumor fraction fell below its cluster-specific cut-off point, ET voxels were relabeled as non-enhancing core or surrounding edema; an analogous

[2] https://github.com/Pediatric-Accelerated-Intelligence-Lab/BraTS-Unofficial-Ranker

rule was applied to ED when its share of WT was too small. We propose correcting systematic label confusions in a data-driven way. After removing small components, we built a confusion matrix over all cross-validated predictions to identify pairs of frequently swapped labels. For every such pair (lbl_x, lbl_y), we searched, within each cluster, for the cut-off point on the ratio lbl_x/WT that minimizes the ranking metric. If a new case fell below this cutoff point, all lbl_x voxels are converted to lbl_y. This ratio-based *lblredef* step enforced anatomically plausible label volumes and improved the performance on the BraTS metrics at the lesion level.

5 Implementation Details

For each task, we used the best segmentation models from the previous BraTS edition (see Sect. 2.1). These models were trained on BraTS 2024 datasets, which is identical to the current edition BraTS 2025 data. GLI-pre and GLI-post were treated as separate tasks for post-processing (GLI-post included RC). The labels being the same, the SSA task used the same pipeline for hyperparameter search as GLI-pre. The post-processing used the binary labels produced by the segmentation models as input.

6 Results

Table 1 provides an overview of the performance evaluation of our post-processed models for the validation set of the GLI and SSA tasks. Additionally, results on the testing set are included in Table 2. The reported numbers are obtained from the automatic pipeline setup in the BraTS 2025 digital platform with no access to the ground truth of the validation set and no access to any testing data including

Table 1. Quantitative results on the validation subset of GLI and SSA. Lesion-wise (LW) Dice coefficients and Normalized Surface Distance (NSD) with thresholds of 1.0 mm were computed for enhancing tumor (ET), tumor core (TC), whole tumor (WT), non-enhancing tumor core (NETC), surrounding non-enhancing FLAIR hyperintensity (SNFH), and resection cavity (RC), respectively. (↑) represents a metric where a higher value is better and (↓) represents a metric where a lower value is better. The best performing ranking metric for each task is highlighted in **bold**. SM: segmentation model.

Task	Model	GPU Time(hrs)	Ranking Metric(↓)	LW Dice(↑)						LW NSD(↑)					
				ET	TC	WT	NETC	SNFH	RC	ET	TC	WT	NETC	SNFH	RC
GLI (n = 407)	SM	401[§]	1.137	0.794	0.798	0.881	0.756	0.823	0.858	0.838	0.782	0.832	0.770	0.819	0.860
	SM + p_{cc}	0	1.129	0.794	0.798	0.881	0.756	0.824	0.859	0.838	0.782	0.832	0.770	0.819	0.862
	SM + p_{cc} + *lblredef*	0	**1.127**	0.794	0.798	0.881	0.757	0.824	0.859	0.838	0.782	0.832	0.771	0.819	0.862
SSA (n = 35)	SM	168	1.729	0.870	0.865	0.926				0.871	0.812	0.849			
	SM + p_{cc}	0	1.629	0.870	0.865	0.927				0.872	0.812	0.849			
	SM + p_{cc} + *lblredef*	0	**1.471**	0.870	0.865	0.927				0.872	0.812	0.849			

[§] estimated based on the segmentation models used; does not include synthetic data generation training images and labels. Submission-related CSVs were downloaded from the platform and used to obtain the ranking metric. Figure 2 illustrated qualitative results on validation cases for SSA and GLI.

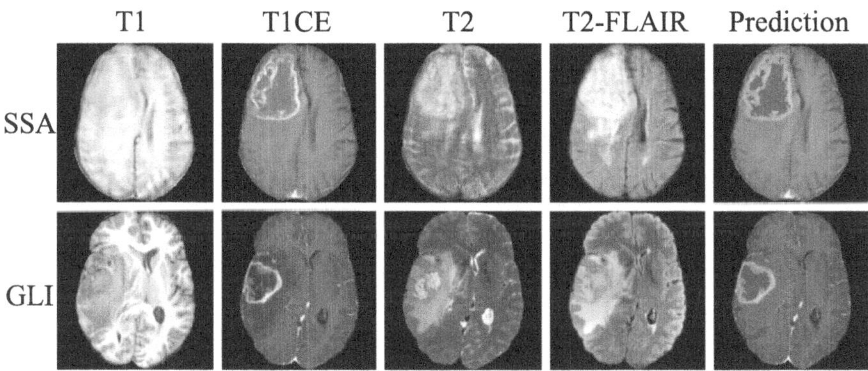

Fig. 2. Qualitative results showing median lesion-wise Dice of the whole tumor. SSA: 0.959, orange = ED, blue = NCR, green = ET; GLI: 0.947, orange = SNFH, blue = NETC, green = ET. (Color figure online)

Table 2. Quantitative results on the test subset of GLI and SSA. These results were calculated on a hidden test set and provided by the organizers post-challenge. Lesion-wise (LW) Dice coefficients and Normalized Surface Distance (NSD) with thresholds of 1.0 mm were computed for enhancing tumor (ET), tumor core (TC), whole tumor (WT), non-enhancing tumor core (NETC), surrounding non-enhancing FLAIR hyper-intensity (SNFH), and resection cavity (RC), respectively. (↑) represents a metric where a higher value is better and (↓) represents a metric where a lower value is better. SM: segmentation model.

Task	Model	LW Dice(↑)				LW NSD(↑)			
		ET	TC	WT	RC	ET	TC	WT	RC
GLI	SM + p_{cc} + *lblredef*	0.813	0.813	0.882	0.894	0.855	0.821	0.851	0.892
SSA	SM + p_{cc} + *lblredef*	0.900	0.912	0.934		0.904	0.865	0.872	

For the GLI task in Table 1, the lesion-wise Dice scores increase from 0.756 to 0.757 for NETC, 0.823 to 0.824 for SNFH and 0.858 to 0.859 for RC due to post-processing. Lesion-wise NSD also improves, from 0.770 to 0.771 for NETC and 0.860 to 0.862 for RC. Together, these refinements reduce the overall ranking metric from 1.137 to 1.127, showing that the post-processed results perform better than the original segmentation model.

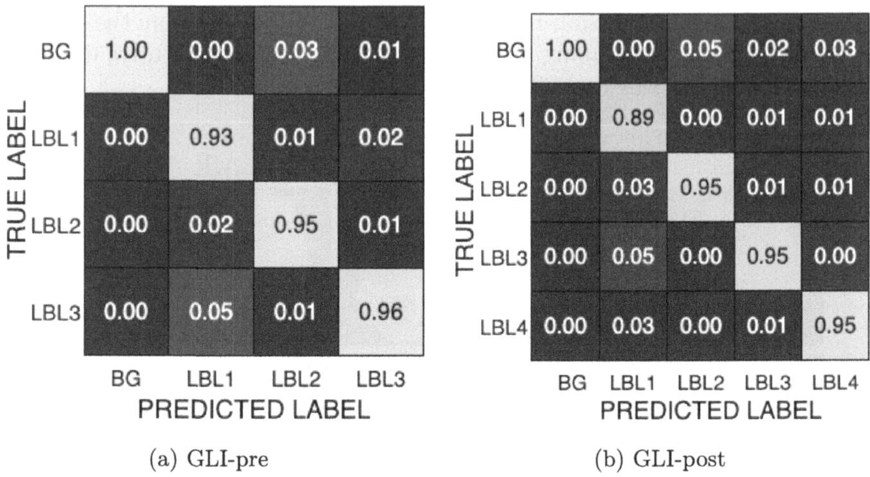

(a) GLI-pre

(b) GLI-post

Fig. 3. Confusion matrices illustrating systematic label confusions across cross-validated predictions of GLI-pre and GLI-post after pp_{cc}. These confusion matrices are used to identify the labels that are redefined as part of $lblredef$. For example in GLI-pre lbl_1 is redefined to lbl_3 based on the lbl_1/WT ratio.

Also, in Table 1 for the SSA task, post-processing improves the lesion-wise Dice of the WT from 0.926 to 0.927 and the lesion-wise NSD for the ET from 0.871 to 0.872. The ranking metric improved from 1.729 to 1.471.

In Fig. 3a, we see the confusion matrix for the GLI-pre cross-validated set after the pp_{cc} step. We see that the biggest error is lbl_3 falsely predicted as lbl_1. Similarly, in Fig. 3b for GLI-post the biggest errors are lbl_3 falsely predicted as lbl_1. These error regions are the focus of $lblredef$, where lbl_1/WT are identified as $lbl_1 \rightarrow lbl_3$ for each of the clusters.

7 Discussion

For the GLI validation set, adaptive post-processing nudged metrics only slightly (NETC Dice +0.001, SNFH Dice +0.001, RC NSD +0.002), improving the BraTS ranking score by just 0.9 % (1.137 → 1.127). The ensemble is therefore already near the task ceiling; further gains will likely need (i) stronger anatomical priors for smoother boundaries or (ii) fine-tuning on the few failure cases.

In the resource-limited SSA cohort, the Dice scores were unchanged ($\leq$ 0.001), but the ranking score improved by 14.9 % (1.729 → 1.471). Because this metric penalizes severely poor segmented subjects, radiomics-guided threshold tuning helped improve the segmentation scores for outliers. This could be largely attributed to the poor quality of SSA data acquisition, leading to more false positives in the segmentations from the pre-trained model. This leads to better result improvement after applying the post-processing strategies.

Training the full ensemble models costs 401 GPU hours (GLI) and 168 GPU hours (SSA). In contrast, the entire post-processing pipeline–PyRadiomics feature extraction, k means clustering, and a grid search over p_{cc} and $lblredef$ thresholds–ran on CPUs and did not use any GPU time.

It is important to note that the optimization for the tasks was tailored to improve the BraTS ranking score, which does not necessarily translate into clinically better segmentations. For medical relevance, optimizing directly for Dice or NSD, or a combination of both, may be more meaningful than maximizing challenge ranking, as these metrics better capture overlap and boundary accuracy in a clinical setting.

The rules of connected component and volume ratio appear saturated in GLI; integrating shape descriptors, vascular atlases, or uncertainty maps could further smooth out the boundaries. Because radiomics are derived from predicted masks, an iterative loop that alternates segmentation and feature extraction is another avenue for improvement. Further improvement in radiomics extraction can be improved by calculating the radiomics on the WT of a lesion instead of the WT of the entire case.

Finally, to facilitate reproducibility and extend the utility of our adaptive post-processing approach, we have made the complete pipeline publicly available as easy-to-use Docker containers and a webapp. This enables researchers and clinicians to easily deploy, test, and build on our methods without the need for complex setups. The Docker images are hosted at: https://hub.docker.com/r/aparida12/brats2025 and the webapp is accessible at: https://segmenter.hope4kids.io/.

8 Conclusion

We demonstrated that an adaptive, radiomic-based postprocessing pipeline improved the accuracy of brain segmentation models on multiple BraTS 2025 glioma segmentation tasks with zero additional GPU hours. These findings promote shifting the focus from building increasingly larger models or further resource intensive training schemes, towards data-driven efficient post-processing strategies. By fine-tuning large-scale segmentation models using adaptive post-processing, we can make automated brain tumor segmentation both accurate and equitable.

Acknowledgments. This work was supported by the National Cancer Institute (UG3 CA236536), the Spanish Ministerio de Ciencia e Innovación, the Agencia Estatal de Investigación, NextGenerationEU grants PDC2022-133865-I00 and PID2022-141493OB-I00, and the EUCAIM project co-funded by the European Union (Grant Agreement #101100633). The authors acknowledge the Universidad Politécnica de Madrid for providing computing resources on the Magerit Supercomputer.

References

1. Abidin, Z.U., Naqvi, R.A., Haider, A., Kim, H.S., Jeong, D., Lee, S.W.: Recent deep learning-based brain tumor segmentation models using multi-modality magnetic resonance imaging: a prospective survey. Front. Bioeng. Biotechnol. **12**, 1392807 (2024)
2. Adewole, M., et al.: The BraTS-Africa dataset: expanding the brain tumor segmentation data to capture African populations. Radiol. Artif. Intell. **7**(4), e240528 (2025)
3. Adewole, M., et al.: The brain tumor segmentation (BraTS) challenge 2023: Glioma segmentation in sub-saharan Africa patient population (BraTS-Africa). ArXiv pp. arXiv–2305 (2023)
4. Anantharajan, S., Gunasekaran, S., Subramanian, T., R, V.: MRI brain tumor detection using deep learning and machine learning approaches. Meas. Sensors **31**, 101026 (2024). https://doi.org/10.1016/j.measen.2024.101026. https://www.sciencedirect.com/science/article/pii/S2665917424000023
5. Baid, U., et al.: The RSNA-ASNR-MICCAI BraTS 2021 benchmark on brain tumor segmentation and radiogenomic classification. CoRR arxiv:2107.02314 (2021)
6. Baid, U., et al.: The rsna-asnr-miccai brats 2021 benchmark on brain tumor segmentation and radiogenomic classification (2021). https://arxiv.org/abs/2107.02314
7. Bakas, S., et al.: Advancing the cancer genome atlas glioma mri collections with expert segmentation labels and radiomic features. Sci. Data **4**(1), 1–13 (2017)
8. Brighi, C., et al.: Repeatability of radiotherapy dose-painting prescriptions derived from a multiparametric magnetic resonance imaging model of glioblastoma infiltration. Phys. Imaging Radiat. Oncol. **23**, 8–15 (2022)
9. Capellán-Martín, D., et al.: Model ensemble for brain tumor segmentation in magnetic resonance imaging. In: International Challenge on Cross-Modality Domain Adaptation for Medical Image Segmentation, pp. 221–232. Springer, Heidelberg (2023). https://doi.org/10.1007/978-3-031-76163-8_20
10. Climent Pardo, J.C., et al.: Deep learning volumetrics reveal distinct clinical trajectories for pediatric low-grade gliomas under surveillance: a multicenter study. Neuro-Oncol. Adva. vdaf145 (2025)
11. Ferreira, A., Solak, N., Li, J., Dammann, P., Kleesiek, J., Alves, V., Egger, J.: How we won BraTS 2023 adult glioma challenge? Just faking it! enhanced synthetic data augmentation and model ensemble for brain tumour segmentation. arXiv preprint arXiv:2402.17317 (2024)
12. Fu, G., et al.: Comparing foundation models and nnU-Net for segmentation of primary brain lymphoma on clinical routine post-contrast T1-weighted MRI. In: Gimi, B.S., Krol, A. (eds.) Medical Imaging 2025: Clinical and Biomedical Imaging, vol. 13410, p. 1341019. International Society for Optics and Photonics, SPIE (2025). https://doi.org/10.1117/12.3044679
13. Hatamizadeh, A., Nath, V., Tang, Y., Yang, D., Roth, H.R., Xu, D.: Swin unetr: swin transformers for semantic segmentation of brain tumors in MRI images. In: International MICCAI Brainlesion Workshop, pp. 272–284. Springer, Heidelberg (2021). https://doi.org/10.1007/978-3-031-76163-8_20
14. Isensee, F., Jaeger, P.F., Kohl, S.A., et al.: nnU-Net: a self-configuring method for deep learning-based biomedical image segmentation. Nat. Methods **18**(2), 203–211 (2021)

15. Jiang, Z., et al.: Enhancing generalizability in brain tumor segmentation: model ensemble with adaptive post-processing. In: 2024 IEEE International Symposium on Biomedical Imaging (ISBI), pp. 1–4. IEEE (2024)
16. Jiang, Z., Capellán-Martín, D., Parida, A., Tapp, A., Liu, X., Ledesma-Carbayo, M.J., Anwar, S.M., Linguraru, M.G.: Magnetic resonance imaging feature-based subtyping and model ensemble for enhanced brain tumor segmentation. arXiv preprint arXiv:2412.04094 (2024)
17. Jiang, Z., et al.: Automatic visual acuity loss prediction in children with optic pathway gliomas using magnetic resonance imaging. In: 2023 45th Annual International Conference of the IEEE Engineering in Medicine & Biology Society (EMBC), pp. 1–5. IEEE (2023)
18. Kofler, F., et al.: BraTS orchestrator: democratizing and disseminating state-of-the-art brain tumor image analysis. arXiv preprint arXiv:2506.13807 (2025)
19. Kudiabor, H.: AI's computing gap: academics lack access to powerful chips needed for research. Nature **636**(8041), 16–17 (2024)
20. LaBella, D., et al.: Analysis of the BraTS 2023 intracranial meningioma segmentation challenge. J. Mach. Learn. Biomed. Imaging **3**(March 2025), 38–58 (2025)
21. Maani, F., Hashmi, A.U.R., Aljuboory, M., Saeed, N., Sobirov, I., Yaqub, M.: Advanced tumor segmentation in medical imaging: an ensemble approach for BraTS 2023 adult glioma and pediatric tumor tasks. In: International Challenge on Cross-Modality Domain Adaptation for Medical Image Segmentation, pp. 264–277. Springer, Heidelberg (2023). https://doi.org/10.1007/978-3-031-76163-8_24
22. Menze, B.H., et al.: The multimodal brain tumor image segmentation benchmark (BraTS). IEEE Trans. Med. Imaging **34**(10), 1993–2024 (2015). https://doi.org/10.1109/TMI.2014.2377694
23. Parida, A., et al.: Adult Glioma Segmentation in Sub-Saharan Africa using Transfer Learning on Stratified Finetuning Data. arXiv preprint arXiv:2412.04111 (2024)
24. Ronneberger, O., Fischer, P., Brox, T.: U-net: convolutional networks for biomedical image segmentation. In: Navab, N., Hornegger, J., Wells, W.M., Frangi, A.F. (eds.) MICCAI 2015. LNCS, vol. 9351, pp. 234–241. Springer, Cham (2015). https://doi.org/10.1007/978-3-319-24574-4_28
25. Roy, S., et al.: Mednext: transformer-driven scaling of convnets for medical image segmentation. In: International Conference on Medical Image Computing and Computer-Assisted Intervention, pp. 405–415. Springer, Heidelberg (2023). https://doi.org/10.1007/978-3-031-43901-8_39
26. Sabouri, M., Dogonchi, A.F., Shafiei, M., Tehrani, D.S.: Survival rate of patient with glioblastoma: a population-based study. Egypt. J. Neurosurg. **39**(1), 42 (2024)
27. Shaver, M.M., et al.: Optimizing neuro-oncology imaging: a review of deep learning approaches for glioma imaging. Cancers **11**(6), 829 (2019)
28. Van Griethuysen, J.J., et al.: Computational radiomics system to decode the radiographic phenotype. Can. Res. **77**(21), e104–e107 (2017)
29. de Verdier, M.C., et al.: The 2024 brain tumor segmentation (BraTS) challenge: glioma segmentation on post-treatment MRI. arXiv preprint arXiv:2405.18368 (2024)
30. Verma, A., Yadav, A.K.: Brain tumor segmentation with deep learning: current approaches and future perspectives. J. Neurosci. Methods 110424 (2025)

Domain Adaptation for Adult Glioma Segmentation in Sub-Saharan Africa: An Ensemble of nnU-Net v2 and MedNeXt

Willem P. E. Boonzaier[1,2(✉)], Farhana Moosa[2], Kagiso Lebang[2,3], Hanifa Jabaar[2], Aondona Iorumbur[2,4], Dong Zhang[2,6,7], and Confidence Raymond[2,5,7,8]

[1] Department of Medical Physics, University of the Free State, Bloemfontein, South Africa

[2] SPRINT AI Training for African Medical Imaging Knowledge Translation (SPARK) Program, Montreal, Canada

boonzaierwpe@ufs.ac.za, donzhang@ece.ubc.ca

[3] Department of Medical Physics, University of the Witwatersrand, Johannesburg, South Africa

[4] Department of Physics, Federal University of Technology, Minna, Nigeria

[5] Montreal Neurological Institute, McGill University, Montreal, Canada

confidence.raymond@mail.mcgill.ca

[6] Department of Electrical and Computer Engineering, University of British Columbia, Vancouver, Canada

[7] Medical Artificial Intelligence Laboratory, Lagos, Nigeria

[8] Department of Biomedical Engineering, McGill University, Montreal, Canada

Abstract. Deep learning models for brain tumour segmentation have shown remarkable performance in curated datasets from high-resource settings. However, these models often underperform when applied to magnetic resonance imaging (MRI) scans acquired in low- and middle-income regions due to domain shifts caused by differences in scanner hardware, acquisition protocols, and population-specific characteristics. In this paper, we investigate domain adaptation strategies–specifically transfer learning and the augmentation of training data using MRI characteristics from African data–to improve generalization to scans from Sub-Saharan Africa. Using the BraTS-Africa 2025 dataset as a benchmark, and the nnU-Net v2 and MedNeXt architectures, we develop and compare domain-specific augmentation strategies guided by global image statistics and local artifact patterns. We show that applying transfer learning and augmentation techniques to high-resource training data enables models to better generalize to African MRI datasets. Our results indicate that augmentation can reduce 95% Hausdorff distance (HD95) by up to 11 mm, while transfer learning improves both Dice scores (by up to 5%) and HD95 (by up to 13 mm). These improvements are particularly notable for tumour core and enhancing tumour subregions, which are the most sensitive to domain shift. These findings represent a step toward more equitable AI by addressing performance gaps in glioma segmentation for underrepresented populations. While our approach improves

S. Bakas et al. (Eds.): MICCAI 2025, LNCS 16376, pp. 248–261, 2026.
https://doi.org/10.1007/978-3-032-16365-3_23

model performance in resource-constrained imaging settings, further validation across diverse African cohorts and clinical contexts is necessary to assess its broader generalizability and clinical utility.

Keywords: Glioma · Brain tumour segmentation · Sub-Saharan Africa · Deep learning · nnU-Net · MedNeXt · Low-resource settings

1 Introduction

Gliomas account for approximately 80% of all malignant primary brain tumours and are responsible for the majority of deaths from primary brain cancer [17]. Among these, glioblastoma is the most aggressive subtype, with an overall median survival of just 12 to 15 months despite current treatment efforts [14]. Although outcomes for glioma patients have improved by up to 30% in high-income countries over recent decades, mortality rates in Sub-Saharan Africa (SSA) have increased by approximately 25% [7]. This disparity may be attributed to delayed presentation, limited access to imaging resources, and a shortage of specialized medical expertise, further compounded by a high prevalence of comorbidities [1].

Accurate glioma segmentation from multiparametric magnetic resonance imaging (mpMRI) is essential for determining prognosis, guiding treatment planning, and monitoring response to therapy. However, manual delineation by experts is time-consuming, resource-intensive, and susceptible to inter- and intra-observer variability [5,16]. These limitations have driven the development of automated segmentation methods, particularly those based on deep learning, which aim to achieve expert-level accuracy while substantially reducing clinical workload. Convolutional neural networks (CNNs) and in particular U-Netbased architectures have emerged as leading approaches in this domain, demonstrating strong performance across various segmentation tasks. Such tools are particularly valuable in low-resource settings, such as SSA, where limited access to trained radiologists makes reliable and efficient tumour delineation an urgent need.

The Brain Tumour Segmentation (BraTS) Challenge has played an instrumental role in advancing automated glioma segmentation [6]. Since its inception in 2012, BraTS has provided a large, publicly available dataset of glioma cases with expert annotations, enabling the development and benchmarking of segmentation algorithms designed to delineate tumour sub-regions [11]. However, these datasets primarily reflect high-quality imaging and patient populations from high-income countries, introducing a bias that raises concerns about their applicability in SSA, where MRI is often performed using lower-quality imaging equipment with reduced contrast and resolution. Additionally, delayed presentation and potentially differing tumour characteristics in SSA populations

W. P. E. Boonzaier and F. Moosa—These authors contributed equally to this work.

present further challenges. To address this gap, the BraTS-Africa Challenge was launched in 2023, providing the first publicly available, annotated glioma MRI dataset from adult patients in SSA [1].

Recent top-performing submissions to the BraTS-Africa 2024 Challenge have demonstrated the effectiveness of transfer learning and modern architectures such as nnU-Net [9] and MedNeXt [15] for glioma segmentation in SSA. The top-ranked team, Parida et al. [13], employed stratified fine-tuning by pretraining nnU-Net and MedNeXt on glioma MRI data from the Global North and fine-tuning on the SSA dataset, incorporating radiomics-informed fold design, model ensembling, and adaptive postprocessing. Similarly, Zhao et al. [18] showed that transfer learning from high-quality data significantly outperformed SSA-only training. Their solution extended the nnU-Net framework by expanding the network architecture and replacing batch normalization with group normalization. Hashmi et al. [8] adopted MedNeXt with a schedule-free optimizer and systematically evaluated fine-tuning and ensembling strategies. In addition, Adhikari et al. [2] introduced parameter-efficient fine-tuning for MedNeXt, achieving comparable performance to full fine-tuning while reducing computational overhead. Collectively, these studies highlight transfer learning, combined with state-of-the-art architectures, as a promising approach for addressing domain shift and data scarcity in SSA.

Inspired by the winning solution from the BraTS-Africa 2024 Challenge, which combined transfer learning with an ensemble of nnU-Net and MedNeXt, we extend this approach in our participation in the BraTS-Africa 2025 Lighthouse Challenge by focusing on targeted, high-intensity data augmentations designed to better reflect the noise profiles, resolution limitations, and artifact patterns commonly observed in MRI scans from SSA. These adaptations aim to improve domain alignment and enhance segmentation reliability in low-resource imaging settings.

2 Methods

2.1 Data Description

This study utilizes two publicly available datasets: the RSNA-ASNR-MICCAI BraTS 2021 dataset[1] and the MICCAI-CAMERA-Lacuna Fund BraTS-Africa 2025 Challenge dataset[2]. Both datasets consist of mpMRI scans of pre-operative glioma cases with four modalities: T1-weighted (T1), post-contrast T1-weighted (T1Gd), T2-weighted (T2), and T2 Fluid Attenuated Inversion Recovery (T2-FLAIR). All images were preprocessed by the respective challenge organizers and include co-registration to the SRI24 anatomical template, skull stripping, and resampling to 1mm^3 isotropic resolution. Tumour subregions, including the enhancing tumour (ET), non-enhancing tumour core (NETC), and surrounding FLAIR hyperintensity (SNFH) were annotated by radiologists with varying levels of experience and subsequently validated by certified neuroradiologists with

[1] https://www.cancerimagingarchive.net/analysis-result/rsna-asnr-miccai-brats2021.
[2] https://www.cancerimagingarchive.net/collection/bratsafrica.

more than 5 years of experience. A detailed description of the datasets can be found in [1,3,4,12].

The BraTS 2021 dataset comprises 1251 cases collected from multiple institutions in the Global North. From this dataset, a representative subset of 250 cases (hereafter referred to as the GLI dataset) was used for pretraining. The BraTS-Africa 2025 dataset (referred to as the SSA dataset) contains 146 cases from multiple imaging centers in SSA, including 60 cases with training labels and an additional 35 cases without ground truth designated for validation. The remaining 51 cases are part of the full dataset but were not included in the training or validation sets provided to participants. A visual comparison between the two datasets is given in Fig. 1.

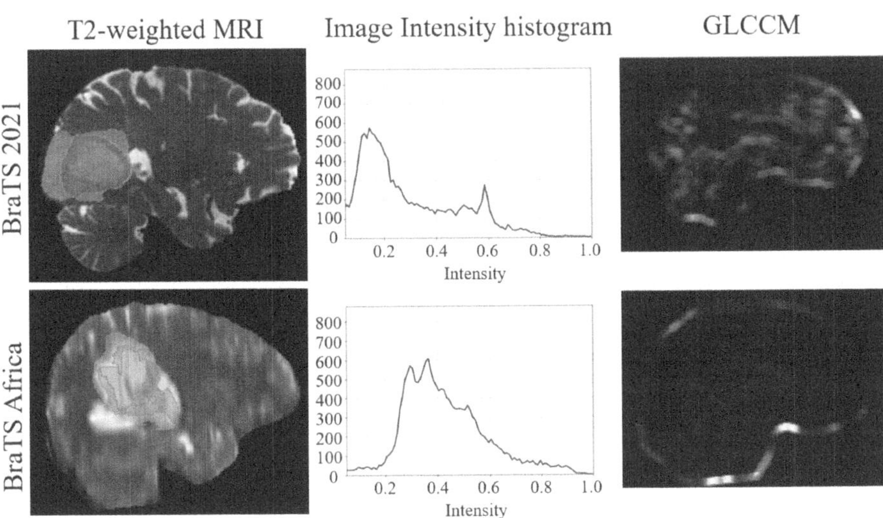

Fig. 1. Visual comparison of T2-weigthed MRI in the sagittal plane in a representative BraTS 2021 (GLI) case and a representative BraTS-Africa (SSA) case. The tumour segmentations overlayed in green for surrounding FLAIR hyperintensity (SNFH), blue for enhancing tumor (ET) and red for non-enhancing tumour core (NETC) and the image intensity histogram and a gray level co- occurrence contrast matrix (GLCCM) estimated from the cases are highlighted. High GLCCM values indicate high contrast. (Color figure online)

2.2 Deep Learning Frameworks

nnU-Net is a state-of-the-art deep learning framework for biomedical image segmentation [9]. It automatically configures its architecture, preprocessing, training, and postprocessing pipelines based on the properties of a given dataset. All configurations originate from a fixed U-Net template, with adaptations to patch size, batch size, and network topology guided by GPU memory constraints and dataset-specific image spacing. The architecture employs instance normalization, leaky ReLU activations, and deep supervision to ensure stable training and effective gradient flow. Training typically uses a combined Dice and cross-entropy loss with on-the-fly data augmentation, while inference employs a sliding window and Gaussian-weighted softmax aggregation. The nnU-Net v2 framework was adopted in this study for all nnU-Net experiments [10], with the main architectural modification being the introduction of a residual encoder.

MedNeXt is a convolution-based segmentation architecture designed to replicate the large receptive fields of transformer models while preserving the efficiency and inductive biases of convolutional networks [15]. Developed with data-sparse medical imaging tasks in mind, MedNeXt adopts an architecture based on the U-Net design, featuring distinct encoder, bottleneck, and decoder components composed entirely of MedNeXt blocks. Each encoder block integrates a depth-wise convolution with kernel size $k \in \{3, 5, 7, 9\}$, followed by a channel expansion and subsequent compression via $1 \times 1 \times 1$ convolutions. Decoder blocks mirror this structure but employ transposed convolutions for upsampling. Deep supervision is applied at intermediate decoder stages to improve gradient flow and training stability.

2.3 Model Development

To develop a robust and generalizable glioma segmentation pipeline for low-resource imaging environments, we implemented a four-phase framework comprising: (1) identification of domain differences, (2) design of dataset-specific augmentations, (3) model training and transfer learning, and (4) final model ensembling.

Domain-Difference Identification. To characterize the domain gap between the GLI and SSA datasets, we performed a detailed image-quality analysis prior to model training. Quantitative metrics included mean image intensity and the average gray-level co-occurrence contrast matrix (GLCCM) to capture intensity-histogram shifts and differences in contrast. Additionally, the medical physics team visually inspected each MRI scan in the SSA dataset to document the presence, extent, and prevalence of artifacts such as motion, bias fields, and slice-thickness inconsistencies. Insights from this analysis directly informed the design of dataset-specific augmentations.

Dataset-Specific Augmentation. The nnU-Net v2 framework applies a standard set of spatial and intensity augmentations during training, including elastic deformations, random rotations and anisotropic scaling, mirroring across axes, Gaussian noise and blur, brightness and contrast adjustments, gamma augmentation, and simulated low-resolution sampling. MedNeXt implements a comparable augmentation pipeline through its default configuration, provided in the `get_moreDA_augmentation` function within the MedNeXt codebase[3]. In addition

[3] https://github.com/MIC-DKFZ/MedNeXt.

to this default configuration, MedNeXt also includes an Insane Data Augmentation (IDA) strategy, implemented in the `get_insaneDA_augmentation` class. To better accommodate the domain shift observed between the GLI and SSA datasets, we applied both the IDA strategy and an African-Specific Augmentation (ASA) strategy that we designed based on empirical observations from the SSA brain MRI dataset. ASA increases the probability of low-resolution simulation for T1, T2, and T2-FLAIR modalities and introduces sinusoidal field bias to T1 and T1Gd images, while leaving other modalities unchanged. Table 1 summarizes the augmentation functions, probabilities, and modality-specific settings for ASA and IDA.

Table 1. Comparison of augmentation strategies used in experiments, showing probabilities and affected modalities.

Augmentation	IDA	ASA	
	Probability	Probability	Modalities
Gaussian noise	0.15	–	–
Gaussian blur	0.20	–	–
Intensity shift	0.15	0.25	T2, T2-FLAIR
Contrast adjustment	0.15	–	–
Low resolution/Slice averaging	0.25	0.60	T1, T2, T2-FLAIR
Sinusoidal field bias	–	0.15	T1, T1Gd

Note. Probabilities are applied per sample.

Experimental Framework. Baseline performance was first established by training nnU-Net v2 and MedNeXt independently on the SSA dataset using their respective default augmentation pipelines. To simulate scenarios where no SSA data is available, both architectures were also trained exclusively on the GLI dataset, using either IDA or ASA in separate training runs. Transfer learning experiments were then performed by first pretraining on the GLI dataset with either IDA or ASA, followed by fine-tuning on SSA. Finally, we ensembled the softmax probabilities of the top nnU-Net v2 and MedNeXt models. We compared non-weighted, model-weighted, and class-weighted averaging and, based on validation performance, selected the class-weighted scheme. The weights were selected by grid search on the validation set, assigning larger weights to better-performing modelclass pairs. A diagram of the final training and inference pipeline[4] is shown in Fig. 2.

Training Setup. All models trained solely on a single dataset (SSA or GLI) were run for 200 epochs. For transfer learning, each model was first pretrained

[4] https://github.com/SPARK-Academy-2025/SPARK-2025/tree/main/SPARK2025_BraTs_MODELS/Team_Sparkans.

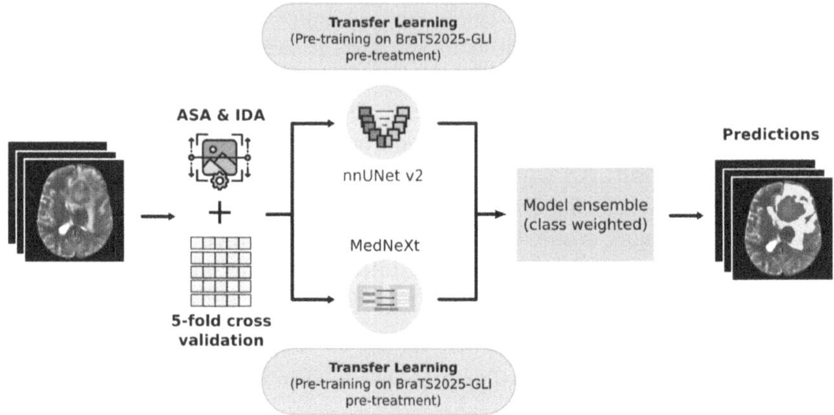

Fig. 2. Diagram showing experimental setup for final ensembled model creation.

on the GLI dataset for 100 epochs and then fine-tuned on the SSA dataset for an additional 100 epochs. The nnU-Net v2 experiments employed the medium residual encoder configuration, while MedNeXt was implemented using the small variant with a kernel size of $k = 3$ unless otherwise stated. Both nnU-Net v2 and MedNeXt were trained in their 3D full-resolution configuration using the default optimizer and learning-rate schedule provided by the respective implementations. MedNeXt models were trained using Kaggle's cloud-based environment with dual NVIDIA T4 GPUs (16 GB VRAM each), while nnU-Net v2 models were trained on the University of the Free State's High Performance Computing (HPC) cluster using dual NVIDIA Tesla V100 GPUs (16 GB VRAM each).

Evaluation Protocol. Performance was evaluated on the SSA validation set via the BraTS-Africa 2025 Lighthouse Challenge validation (Synapse) platform using blinded testing[5]. The performance metrics were based on the two BraTS-Africa benchmarking metrics - lesion-wise Dice and the 95th percentile Hausdorff Distance (HD95) [11]. Results for ET, NETC and SNFH classes are presented in Table 2. Statistical significance between results was determined using Welch's t-test with a p-value threshold of p smaller than or equal to 0.05.

3 Results

3.1 Model Development

Manual evaluation of the SSA dataset by our medical physics team revealed that motion or ghosting artifacts were present in T1-weighted images, affecting 11.67%(7) of cases. Bias artifacts were confined to T1 images, observed in 25%(15) of T1 scans and 13.33%(8) of T1Gd scans. Visibly noisy images were

[5] https://www.synapse.org/Synapse:syn64153130/wiki/631251.

uncommon, occurring in only 1.63.33%(1–2) of slices across all modalities. Slice thickness artifacts were identified in all T1, T2-FLAIR, and T2 images, while 96.67%(58) of contrast-enhanced T1 images exhibited such artifacts. Furthermore, in qualitative analysis, the SSA dataset exhibited a 72.04% higher variability in the standard deviation of image intensities compared to the GLI dataset, particularly in the T2 and T2-FLAIR sequences. In addition, a quantitative analysis of the GLCCM revealed that the mean contrast in the SSA dataset is only approximately 59.35% of that observed in the GLI dataset. Figure 3 illustrates qualitative differences between the SSA and GLI datasets and demonstrates how specific augmentations can alter the GLI dataset to more closely resemble the characteristics of the SSA dataset.

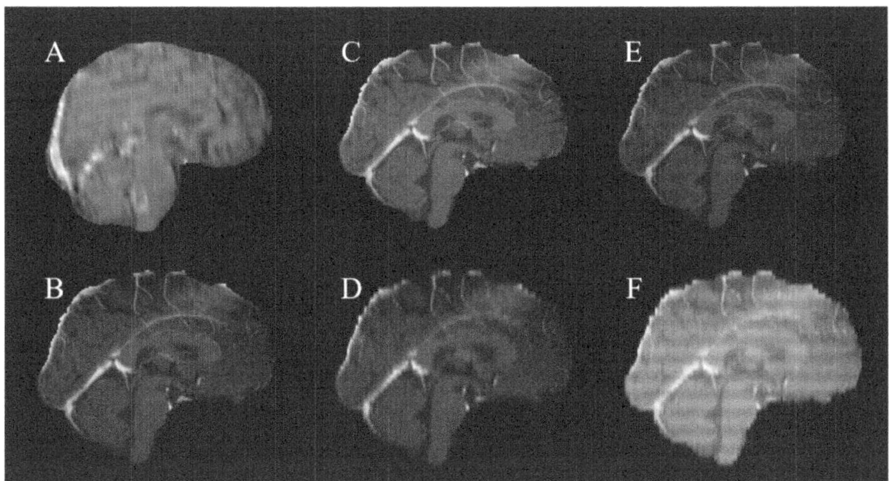

Fig. 3. Augmentation influence on BraTS 2021 GLI dataset. A) Sagittal T1 MRI of a patient in the SSA dataset. B) Sagittal T1 MRI of a patient in the GLI dataset. C) Random intensity shift applied to B. D) Slice thickness averaging (3mm) applied to B (1mm). E) Sinusoidal field bias applied to B. F) Random intensity shift, slice thickness averaging, and field bias applied to B.

In the experimental case where no SSA dataset is available and training happens solely on the GLI dataset with augmentation to bridge the domain gap, the IDA augmentations provided better HD95 scores overall at the cost of ET Dice score, while the ASA augmentations improved even further on ET and NETC HD95 at a cost of SNFH HD95 score and ET Dice.

When introducing transfer learning with the assumption that an SSA and GLI dataset exists, both nnU-Net v2 and MedNeXt showed improved Dice scores in all classes. For nnU-Net v2, this was at a cost of HD95 of the SNFH, where MedNext had experienced no tradeoff as visualised in Table 2.

Caution should be exercised when evaluating model performance solely on mean quantitative scores, as is evident from Fig. 4 and Fig. 5, where the potential

Table 2. Segmentation performance (lesion-wise Dice and HD95) for experiments leading up to model ensembling. None of the observed differences compared to the baseline were statistically significant (Welch's t-test, $p > 0.05$).

Model	Description	Dataset(s)	Dice ↑			HD95 (mm) ↓		
			ET	NETC	SNFH	ET	NETC	SNFH
nnU-Net v2	Baseline	SSA	0.83	0.81	0.89	37.02	43.82	14.85
	Insane DA	GLI	0.79	0.81	0.89	31.46	35.77	11.43
	ASA	GLI	0.79	0.82	0.88	26.42	32.63	16.91
	Transfer	Both	0.86	0.85	0.89	23.89	30.62	24.63
	Transfer & ASA	Both	0.84	0.84	0.89	31.27	34.56	24.49
MedNeXt	Baseline	SSA	0.82	0.81	0.88	37.19	44.03	25.06
	Insane DA	GLI	0.81	0.80	0.87	42.44	49.34	29.94
	Base Transfer	Both	0.83	0.83	0.93	34.60	37.92	9.01
	Medium Transfer	Both	0.84	0.84	0.92	30.36	33.65	14.14

population benefit in HD95 and Dice scores is shown for our domain adaptation strategies.

Additionally, Table 3 shows the lesion-wise scores obtained through ensembling. Class-weighted ensembling showed the best average performance across all classes when weight was distributed 60%: 40% between nnU-Net v2 and MedNeXt for the ET and NETC classes and 48%: 52% for the SNFH class. Final model performance against ground truth for one patient case in the training population is also presented in Fig. 6 for visual inspection.

Table 3. Lesion-wise Dice and HD95 (mm) for ensemble strategies. None of the observed differences compared to the baseline were statistically significant (Welch's t-test, $p > 0.05$).

Method	Dice ↑			HD95 (mm) ↓		
	ET	NETC	SNFH	ET	NETC	SNFH
Non-weighted	0.85	0.84	0.90	24.92	28.28	14.38
Model-weighted	0.85	0.84	0.88	24.92	28.27	19.70
Class-weighted	0.86	0.86	0.89	23.11	26.43	19.66

The final model mean and standard deviation lesion-wise Dice scores on the unseen BraTS Africa 2025 test dataset are shown in Table 4. These results are consistent with validation scores.

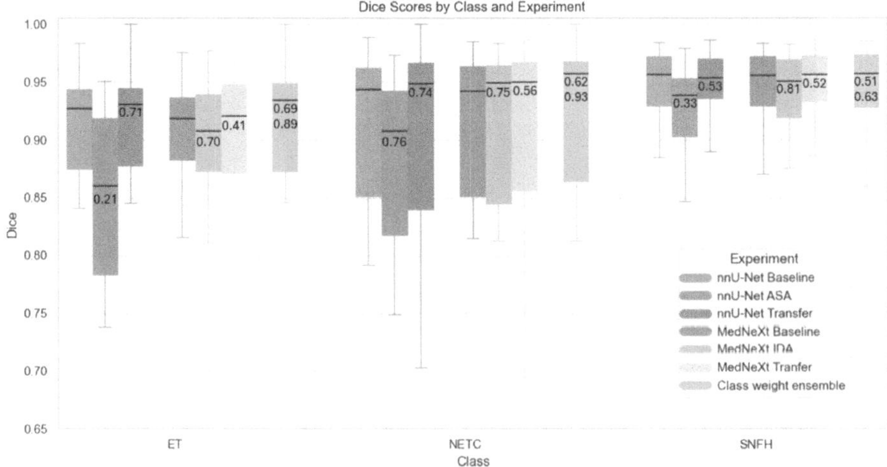

Fig. 4. Box and whisker plot of dice scores excluding outliers of experiments in domain adaptation. Data labels show p-values compared to the baseline with Welch's t-test.

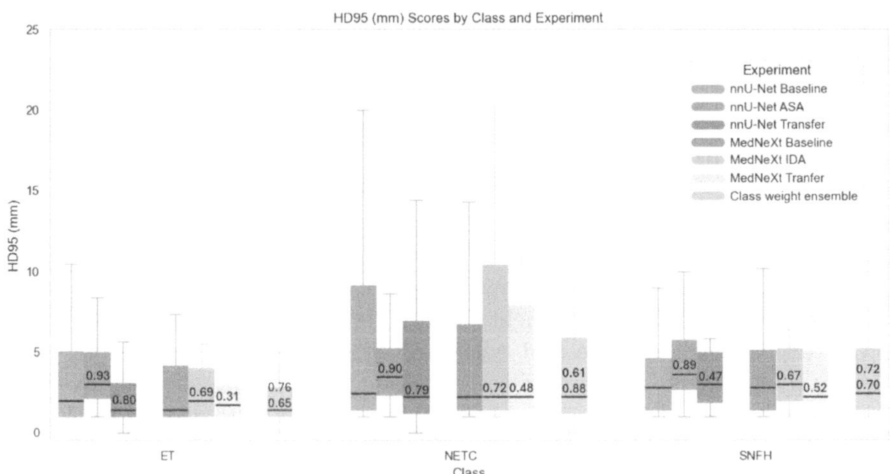

Fig. 5. Box and whisker plot of HD95 excluding outliers of experiments in domain adaptation. Data labels show p-values compared to the baseline with Welch's t-test.

Table 4. Lesion-wise Dice scores on the unseen test population set.

Metric	ET	NETC	SNFH
Mean	0.89	0.90	0.89
Std	0.12	0.13	0.18

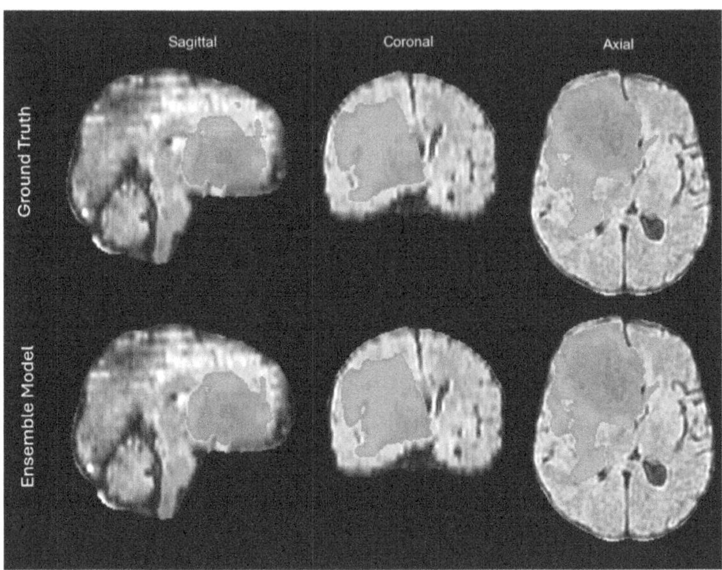

Fig. 6. Visual comparison of ground truth and final ensembled tumour segmentations overlayed in green for surrounding FLAIR hyperintensity (SNFH), blue for enhancing tumor (ET) and red for non-enhancing tumour core (NETC) T2-weighted MRI in all three cardinal planes for a single patient in the SSA dataset. (Color figure online)

4 Discussion

Our analysis of data quality underscored significant differences between the SSA and GLI datasets. The SSA dataset exhibited higher variability in image intensity and contrast, suggesting lower texture information, potentially due to prevalent artifacts, including motion, field bias, and slice thickness averaging.

Our experiments indicate that when an SSA dataset is not available, data augmentation can be used to bridge the domain gap quite successfully with a loss of 4% to ET Dice scores. Additionally, training with higher resolution data, such as the GLI dataset, enhances the HD95 when compared to training on lower quality datasets such as the SSA. Figure 5 additionally indicates that when applying augmentation, the variability in HD95 could be lowered, with the ASA augmentations showing the smallest variability in NETC HD95 scores. This seems to come at a non-statistically significant cost of a lower dice score on all classes as can be seen in Fig. 4.

Additionally, our experiments revealed that transfer learning provided a performance gain, with Dice improvements of approximately 3% to 5% across all regions and potential reductions in HD95 of up to 16 mm. Although adding ASA whilst performing transfer learning doesn't seem to prove beneficial from the mean Dice and HD95 scores, deeper analysis suggests that it could improve HD95 variability in all classes, as seen in Fig. 5.

When comparing predictions from both nnU-Net and MedNeXt models, nnU-Net seems to be more accurate in predicting smaller volume classes like ET and NETC, while MedNeXt outperforms nnU-Net for SNFH. When ensembling these two models, the best ensemble model was produced by doing class-weight-based ensembling. None of the observed differences in any experiment compared to the baseline were statistically significant (Welch's t-test, $p > 0.05$).

Collectively, our results suggest that successful domain adaptation for glioma segmentation requires strategies beyond architectural tuning, including domain-aware transfer learning and careful consideration of data artifacts and intensity distributions, depending on the availability of data in the target population, but that high quality models can be obtained by various techniques of varying contributions of african and non-african data.

Lastly, on the unseen test set, all classes performed comparably to or better than validation, indicating no loss of performance on held-out data.

5 Conclusion

In this work, we evaluated the effect of augmentation and transfer learning techniques on domain adaptation using nnU-Net v2 and MedNeXt architectures for glioma segmentation on the SSA and GLI datasets. Our findings suggest that data augmentation may be beneficial to domain adaptation when no African dataset is available. This has a significant potential benefit for low-resource settings. When GLI and SSA datasets are available, combining information from both datasets via transfer learning provides the best results overall for nnU-Net v2 and MedNeXt. A deeper analysis of our results confirmed that the use of domain-specific augmentation leads to the best performance for the NETC class compared to standard augmentations. Additionally, there might be a population that might benefit from robustness when augmenting during transfer learning. These insights emphasise the critical role of transfer learning and dataset-specific augmentation in addressing domain shifts in neuro-oncological imaging. We therefore propose three equivalent techniques for automated glioma segmentation in the SSA environment for varying levels of data and resource availability. Future work should explore more sophisticated domain adaptation techniques and evaluate their generalization across diverse global imaging datasets.

Acknowledgements. This work was part of the Sprint AI Training for African Medical Imaging Knowledge Translation (SPARK) Academy 2025 summer school on deep learning in medical imaging. The authors would like to thank the instructors of the summer for providing insightful background knowledge on brain tumours that informed the research presented here, most notably: Maruf Adewole, Mohannad Barakat, Craig Jones, Noha Magdy, Tinashe Mutsvangwa, MacLean Nasrallah, Nicephorus Boniface Rutabasibwa, Charles Delahunt, Celia Cintas, Evan Calabrese, and Amal Saleh. The authors acknowledge the funding support provided to SPARK through the Lacuna Fund for Health and Equity (PI: Udunna Anazodo), the RSNA R&E Foundation (PI: Farouk Dako), the University of Washington Population Health Initiative Tier 2 Grant

(PI: Mehmet Kurt), McGill University Healthy Brain and Healthy Lives (HBHL, Anazodo), and the National Science and Engineering Research Council of Canada (NSERC) Discovery Launch Supplement (PI: Udunna Anazodo, DGECR-2022- 00136).

References

1. Adewole, M., Rudie, J.D., Gbadamosi, A., et al.: The brain tumor segmentation (brats) challenge 2023: Glioma segmentation in Sub-Saharan Africa patient population (brats-africa). ArXiv:2305.19369 [eess.IV] (2023)
2. Adhikari, B., et al.: Parameter-efficient fine-tuning for improved convolutional baseline for brain tumor segmentation in Sub-Saharan Africa adult glioma dataset. arXiv preprint arXiv:2412.14100 (2024)
3. Baid, U., et al.: The rsna-asnr-miccai brats 2021 benchmark on brain tumor segmentation and radiogenomic classification. arXiv preprint arXiv:2107.02314 (2021)
4. Bakas, S., et al.: Advancing the cancer genome atlas glioma mri collections with expert segmentation labels and radiomic features. Sci. Data **4**, 170117 (2017). https://doi.org/10.1038/sdata.2017.117
5. Baskar, R., Lee, K.A., Yeo, R., Yeoh, K.W.: Cancer and radiation therapy: current advances and future directions. Int. J. Med. Sci. **9**(3), 193 (2012)
6. Bonato, B., Nanni, L., Bertoldo, A.: Advancing precision: a comprehensive review of mri segmentation datasets from brats challenges (2012–2025). Sensors (Basel, Switzerland) **25**(6), 1838 (2025)
7. Patel, A.P., et al.: GBD 2016 brain and other CNS cancer collaborators: global, regional, and national burden of brain and other cns cancer, 1990–2016: a systematic analysis for the global burden of disease study 2016. Lancet Neurol. **18**, 376–393 (2019)
8. Hashmi, S., et al.: Optimizing brain tumor segmentation with mednext: brats 2024 SSA and pediatrics. arXiv preprint arXiv:2411.15872 (2024)
9. Isensee, F., Jaeger, P.F., Kohl, S.A., Petersen, J., Maier-Hein, K.H.: nnu-net: a self-configuring method for deep learning-based biomedical image segmentation. Nat. Methods **18**(2), 203–211 (2021)
10. Isensee, F., et al.: nnu-net revisited: A call for rigorous validation in 3d medical image segmentation. In: International Conference on Medical Image Computing and Computer-Assisted Intervention, pp. 488–498. Springer, Heidelberg (2024). https://doi.org/10.1007/978-3-031-72114-4_47
11. Menze, B.H., et al.: The multimodal brain tumor image segmentation benchmark (brats). IEEE Trans. Med. Imaging **34**(10), 1993–2024 (2014). https://doi.org/10.1109/TMI.2014.2377694
12. Menze, B.H., et al.: The multimodal brain tumor image segmentation benchmark (brats). IEEE Trans. Med. Imaging **34**(10), 1993–2024 (2015). https://doi.org/10.1109/TMI.2014.2377694
13. Parida, A., et al.: Adult glioma segmentation in Sub-Saharan Africa using transfer learning on stratified finetuning data. arXiv preprint arXiv:2412.04111 (2024)
14. Poursaeed, R., Mohammadzadeh, M., Safaei, A.A.: Survival prediction of glioblastoma patients using machine learning and deep learning: a systematic review. BMC Cancer **24**(1), 1581 (2024)
15. Roy, S., et al.: Mednext: transformer-driven scaling of convnets for medical image segmentation. In: International Conference on Medical Image Computing and Computer-Assisted Intervention, pp. 405–415. Springer, Heidelberg (2023). https://doi.org/10.1007/978-3-031-43901-8_39

16. Vorwerk, H., et al.: Protection of quality and innovation in radiation oncology: the prospective multicenter trial the german society of radiation oncology (degro-quiro study). Evaluation of time, attendance of medical staff, and resources during radiotherapy with imrt. Strahlentherapie und Onkologie **190** (2014)
17. Weller, M., et al.: Glioma. Nat. Rev. Dis. Primers **10**(1), 33 (2024)
18. Zhao, Y., Bai, L., Zhang, Z., Wu, Y., Islam, M., Ren, H.: Transferring knowledge from high-quality to low-quality mri for adult glioma diagnosis. arXiv preprint arXiv:2410.18698 (2024)

GLIMS-MedNeXt: An Ensemble Framework for Brain MRI Segmentation in Sub-Saharan Africa

Ali Azmoudeh[1(✉)], İlkay Öksüz[1], and Hazım Kemal Ekenel[1,2]

[1] Department of Computer Engineering, Istanbul Technical University, Istanbul, Turkey
{azmoudeh22,oksuzilkay,ekenel}@itu.edu.tr
[2] Division of Engineering, NYU Abu Dhabi, Abu Dhabi, UAE
he2244@nyu.edu

Abstract. Segmentation of brain magnetic resonance imaging is essential for precise diagnosis, effective treatment planning, and monitoring of neurological disorders. However, low and middle income countries often face significant limitations due to resource constraints and the low quality of imaging. To address these challenges, we propose a hybrid ensemble model combining two advanced segmentation architectures, GLIMS and MedNeXt. By utilizing transfer learning from high-quality datasets, comprehensive fine-tuning, and ensemble fusion techniques, our approach achieves superior performance in segmenting tumors under low-quality imaging conditions. Experimental validation using the BraTS-SSA dataset highlights improvements in accuracy and robustness, positioning this approach as a clinically viable solution for enhancing diagnostic accuracy in resource-limited settings. https://github.com/AliAZ98/GLIMS-MedNeXt.

Keywords: Hybrid Deep Learning Models · Sub-Saharan Africa · Low Quality Brain MR Image

1 Introduction

Brain MRI segmentation is a critical task in medical imaging, essential for accurate diagnosis, effective treatment planning, and monitoring of neurological conditions such as tumors, stroke, and neurodegenerative diseases. Precise segmentation delineates pathological regions of healthy tissues, providing clinicians with detailed anatomical insights crucial for surgical intervention, radiation therapy, and patient prognosis. Accurate segmentation has a significant impact on clinical outcomes, reducing intra- and inter-observer variability and enhancing diagnostic consistency [2].

However, sub-Saharan African countries face substantial challenges in medical imaging, primarily due to limited access to high-quality imaging equipment, trained experts, and robust healthcare infrastructure. Low-field MRI scanners,

S. Bakas et al. (Eds.): MICCAI 2025, LNCS 16376, pp. 262–273, 2026.
https://doi.org/10.1007/978-3-032-16365-3_24

outdated technology, and inconsistent imaging protocols often result in compromised image quality, which restricts accurate tumor segmentation [3]. These limitations significantly impact diagnostic accuracy and the efficacy of subsequent treatments, underscoring the need for specialized methodologies that are robust in low-quality imaging conditions.

Recent advancements in deep learning have significantly impacted brain MRI segmentation, introducing powerful algorithms that can extract complex features and adapt to varying imaging conditions. Convolutional Neural Networks (CNNs) and Vision Transformers (ViTs) [6] have demonstrated exceptional capabilities in capturing detailed spatial contexts, generalizing across diverse datasets, and improving segmentation accuracy even under challenging imaging scenarios [13]. Techniques such as transfer learning, attention mechanisms [16], and ensemble modeling further enhance model robustness, making them key in resource-constrained healthcare settings [11].

In this study, we introduce a hybrid ensemble model that employs the strengths of two state-of-the-art segmentation architectures, GLIMS [18] and MedNeXt [15], to address the specific challenges posed by low-quality MRI scans prevalent in sub-Saharan Africa. Our approach integrates transfer learning strategies from high-quality datasets, fine-tuning, and ensemble fusion techniques, significantly improving segmentation accuracy and generalizability across different quality standards. This combination aims to establish a reliable and clinically practical solution for enhancing diagnostic precision in resource-limited settings.

2 Related Works

Recent studies have focused on overcoming the specific challenges posed by low-quality imaging conditions through innovative transfer learning and model ensembling techniques.

Zhao et al. [19] developed a transfer learning strategy specifically designed to improve glioma diagnosis from low-quality MRI scans in the Brats SSA [1] dataset. Their approach involved initially training a segmentation model on the high-quality BraTS-GLI 2021 [4] dataset and subsequently fine-tuning it on SSA-specific data. They also experimented with super-resolution enhancements to improve the visual quality of images, emphasizing the advantage of integrating prior knowledge from high-quality datasets into resource-constrained subjects.

Hashmi et al. [7] and Maani et al. [12] utilized the MedNeXt [15] architecture for brain tumor segmentation tasks, particularly highlighting its capability to process volumetric medical imaging data efficiently. MedNeXt combines the strengths of convolutional networks and transformer-inspired designs, incorporating residual connections, iterative kernel scaling, and post-processing methods. Their methodologies included sophisticated preprocessing and extensive model ensembling, enhancing model reliability and robustness across diverse patient demographics and varying image quality standards.

Parida et al. [14] introduced a novel stratified fine-tuning and ensemble approach explicitly designed to address the limitations inherent in low-quality and limited SSA MRI datasets. This approach utilizes radiomic analysis to generate representative training folds and employs advanced segmentation architectures, including nnU-Net [9] and MedNeXt. Their adaptive post-processing and ensembling further improved generalizability and segmentation accuracy, demonstrating substantial robustness in practical healthcare scenarios.

Yazici et al. [18] developed GLIMS, a lightweight hybrid architecture that combines CNNs and transformers, designed explicitly for volumetric semantic segmentation. GLIMS incorporates Dilated Feature Aggregator Convolutional Blocks and a Swin Transformer-based [8] bottleneck, enhanced with Channel and Spatial-Wise Attention Blocks for accurate localization of tumor boundaries. This design efficiently balances model complexity and accuracy, achieving significant improvements in inter-class segmentation clarity and feature representation, thus demonstrating substantial applicability in medical image analysis tasks.

These methods demonstrate the importance of using ensemble models and hybrid architectures to capture global and local features in 3D brain MRI scans. Specifically, the limited data in Medical imaging requires specific architecture designs for adapting to medical tasks and generalizability across various data with diverse quality.

3 Methods

In this section, we describe the two main architectures employed in our study: GLIMS [18] and MedNeXt [15]. Both are advanced models designed for volumetric medical and 3D brain MR images segmentation, taking advantage of different architectural paradigms. In the following, we will describe these two methods.

3.1 GLIMS

The GLIMS [18] architecture is a hybrid segmentation network designed to exploit the strengths of both CNNs and ViTs. The architecture explicitly addresses the challenge of efficiently capturing local and global features simultaneously for volumetric semantic segmentation. GLIMS comprises four major modules: Dilated Feature Aggregator Convolutional Blocks (DACB), Swin Transformer-based bottleneck, Channel and Spatial-Wise Attention Blocks (CSAB), and depth-wise multi-scale upsampling (DMSU).

Figure 1 demonstrates the overall architecture of the GLIMS. DACB modules are crucial for accurately capturing both local and global feature correlations. These blocks incorporate parallel dilated convolutions, enabling GLIMS to extract fine grained local features while preserving global context through depth-wise operations. The use of dilated kernels increases receptive fields without significant computational cost, thereby maintaining the segmentation accuracy and clarity of the boundaries. The Swin Transformer-based bottleneck bridges the local-global feature gap efficiently by utilizing shifted window multi-head self-attention (SW-MSA) to capture long-range dependencies effectively.

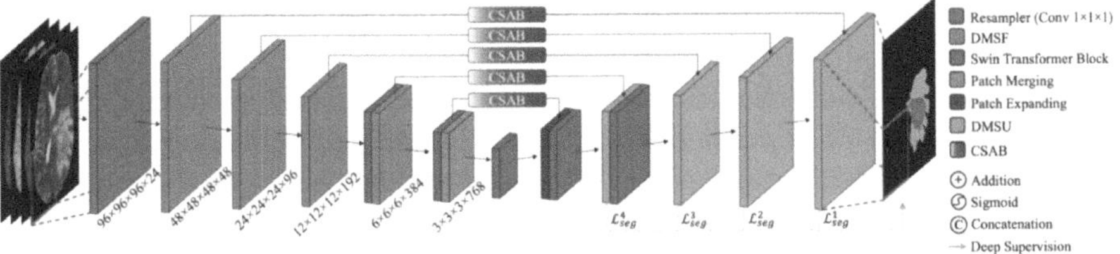

Fig. 1. GLIMS architecture overview. The network combines Dilated Feature Aggregator Convolutional Blocks and a Swin Transformer bottleneck to capture both local details and global context. Channel and Spatial-Wise Attention Blocks in the skip connections focus on the most relevant features, while depth-wise multi-scale upsampling in the decoder, with deep supervision at several scales, produces precise volumetric segmentation masks. [18]

Additionally, GLIMS utilizes CSAB in its skip connections, which significantly enhances segmentation performance. The CSAB module independently processes spatial and channel-wise attention to emphasize important regions and suppress irrelevant features. This mechanism enhances localization, which is crucial for accurately segmenting tumor boundaries and distinguishing between classes. The decoder branch utilizes DMSU blocks for efficient upsampling, combining the attention-enhanced high-resolution features from the encoder branch to generate precise and refined segmentation masks. The overall structure integrates deep supervision at multiple intermediate layers to ensure robust training and accurate segmentation results.

3.2 MedNeXt

MedNeXt [15] is a convolutional network architecture inspired by transformer-based designs optimized explicitly for medical image segmentation tasks. Its unique design features a fully convolutional 3D encoder-decoder structure, utilizing ConvNeXt [10] blocks derived from the Transformer architecture to balance the model's inductive biases and scalability effectively. The key components of MedNeXt include Residual Inverted Bottleneck blocks, iterative kernel scaling, and compound scaling across network depth, width, and receptive fields.

The ConvNeXt blocks in MedNeXt adopt a transformer-like inverted bottleneck structure, comprising a depthwise convolution layer followed by an expansion and compression layer. The depthwise convolution layer utilizes large kernels to mimic transformer attention windows, capturing extensive spatial context. These blocks maintain computational efficiency through channel-wise normalization, which limits computational overhead and facilitates training on data-limited medical datasets. Residual Inverted Bottleneck blocks specifically support semantic richness during resampling, preserving feature details through both downsampling and upsampling layers, thereby enhancing segmentation performance.

A distinctive feature of MedNeXt is the iterative kernel scaling method. This method incrementally increases kernel sizes (UpKern), initializing larger kernel networks with the weights from previously trained smaller kernel models. UpKern effectively prevents performance saturation common in medical imaging tasks with limited dataset sizes. Furthermore, MedNeXt utilizes compound scaling, simultaneously optimizing the network's depth, channels, and receptive fields. This approach achieves balanced scalability and robust performance, which is crucial to handling diverse and challenging segmentation tasks in medical imaging.

In summary, while GLIMS and MedNeXt share goals of enhancing segmentation accuracy through robust feature extraction and attention mechanisms, their primary differences lie in the architectural choices. GLIMS adopts a hybrid CNN-transformer approach, emphasizing attention-driven fine-grained feature localization. In contrast, MedNeXt utilizes scalable convolutional blocks with transformer-inspired mechanisms, focusing on inductive bias and computational efficiency for medical datasets.

3.3 Model Ensembling

To further enhance segmentation performance, two ensemble strategies were explored: a fusion-based model and an averaging-based model. Both GLIMS and MedNeXt generate multi-scale outputs with 3-channel prediction maps corresponding to the tumor subregions. In the fusion-based ensemble approach, the 3-channel outputs from both models at corresponding resolution levels are concatenated along the channel dimension, resulting in 6-channel feature maps. These concatenated outputs are then fed into a lightweight convolutional fusion block composed of three sequential convolutional layers. This fusion head was trained from scratch during ensemble training, enabling the model to learn effective combinations of complementary features from both architectures.

In contrast, the averaging ensemble strategy directly computes the mean of the probability maps from GLIMS and MedNeXt without introducing additional trainable parameters. This approach is computationally efficient and yields stable predictions, making it particularly useful during early fine-tuning phases to improve convergence. The fusion ensemble was primarily used in the later training stages, as it can actively learn explicit integration mappings to exploit architectural diversity better.

Selective freezing experiments were conducted to assess the balance between generalization and computational efficiency. In these configurations, certain pre-trained layers were frozen to explore whether high segmentation accuracy could be maintained under reduced training resource constraints. Figure 2 illustrates the ensemble strategies employed in this study.

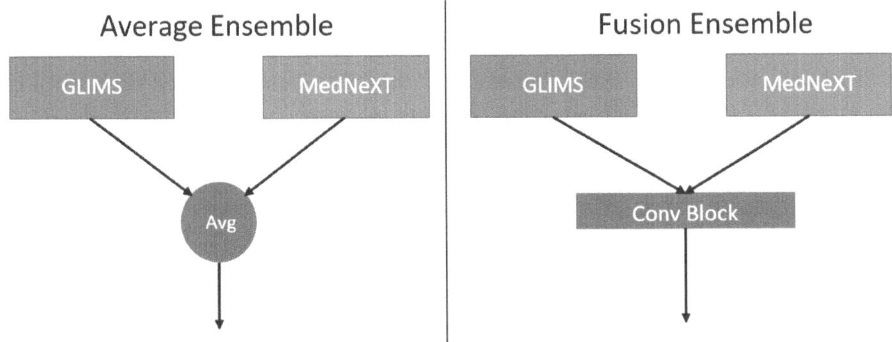

Fig. 2. Ensemble strategies for GLIMS and MedNeXt. The averaging ensemble (left), the fusion ensemble (right)

4 Datasets

4.1 BraTS-SSA 2023

The BraTS-SSA 2023 [1] dataset enables brain tumor segmentation research in low-resource settings with low-quality MRI scans. It includes 60 training cases (240 volumes across T1, T1ce, T2, FLAIR) and 35 unlabeled validation cases. Scans, acquired from Sub-Saharan institutions using low-field MRI, are provided in 3D NIfTI format with a resolution of $1 \times 1 \times 1$ mm^3 and a volume size of $240 \times 240 \times 155$. Training masks label enhancing tumor (ET), tumor core (TC), and whole tumor (WT) for robust model evaluation (Fig. 3).

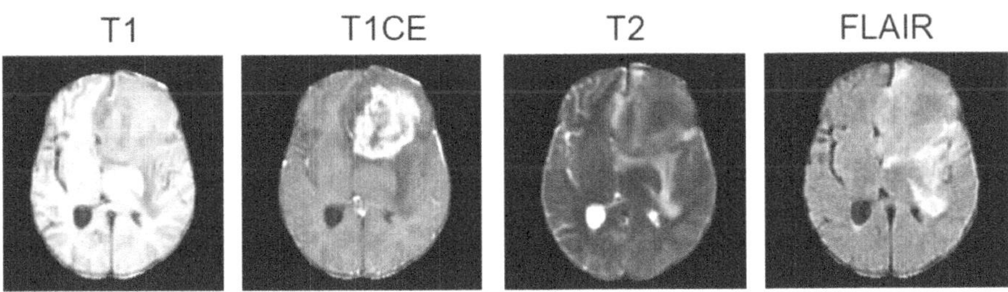

Fig. 3. Example axial slices from BraTS-SSA 2023 in T1, T1ce, T2, and FLAIR modalities used for tumor segmentation.

4.2 BraTS-GLI

The BraTS-GLI [17] dataset features 1,251 high-quality brain MRI cases from advanced medical centers, following standardized protocols. Each case includes

T1, T1ce, T2, and FLAIR modalities, preprocessed with skull-stripping, co-registration, isotropic resampling ($1 \times 1 \times 1$ mm^3), and intensity normalization. It provides segmentation masks for ET, TC, and WT regions. Used for pretraining, BraTS-GLI enables strong spatial feature learning, improving generalization when fine-tuning on the lower-quality BraTS-SSA data.

5 Experimental Setup

GLIMS training involved fine-tuning publicly available pre-trained weights on the BraTS-SSA dataset at a learning rate of 1×10^{-7}. MedNeXt training comprised two phases: initial pretraining on BraTS-GLI at 1×10^{-3}, followed by fine-tuning on BraTS-SSA at 1×10^{-8}. Both models were trained using the AdamW optimizer and a warmup cosine learning rate scheduler. Training was performed on an NVIDIA RTX 3090 GPU with a batch size of 2.

The ensemble model was fine-tuned on the BraTS-SSA dataset using pre-trained GLIMS and MedNeXt backbones, with a learning rate of 1×10^{-7} for the main architecture and 1×10^{-4} for the fusion head. All models were trained for 1000 epochs using a combined loss function: the average of Dice loss and Cross-Entropy loss. Ensemble training followed the same optimizer and scheduler setup and was conducted on an NVIDIA A100 GPU with a batch size of 2.

To improve generalization on limited and low-quality data, extensive data augmentation was applied using the MONAI [5] library. The transformations included random spatial cropping, foreground cropping, random flipping across all spatial axes, histogram intensity shifting, intensity normalization, random intensity scaling and shifting, contrast adjustments, Gaussian noise, and Gaussian smoothing. All models were trained using a window size of $96 \times 96 \times 96$, uniformly applied to crop 3D input volumes from the preprocessed MRI scans, which included all four modalities: T1-weighted (T1), contrast-enhanced T1 (T1ce), T2-weighted (T2), and FLAIR.

We evaluated the models using three metrics: Dice Score (DCS), Lesion-wise Dice Score, and 95th percentile Hausdorff Distance (HD95). The Dice Score was computed on a per-structure basis across the entire 3D volume and reflects the overall overlap between predicted and ground truth segmentations. In contrast, the lesion-wise dice score individually evaluates each connected lesion component, providing more sensitivity to smaller or fragmented lesions, which is particularly useful in low-quality MRI contexts. HD95 measures boundary-level segmentation accuracy by calculating the 95th percentile of surface distances between prediction and ground truth contours. Lesion-wise DCS and HD95 evaluations were conducted only on the official validation set of the BraTS-SSA dataset, for which the ground truth annotations were provided only on the submission platform by the challenge organizers.

To ensure consistent comparison across all models, a single validation fold was selected from a 6-fold split of the BraTS-SSA training set and used throughout all experiments. This was a fixed validation strategy, not a cross-validation process, enabling fair benchmarking under uniform evaluation conditions.

6 Results

6.1 Quantitative Results

To ensure consistent and fair evaluation of all models, we divided the BraTS-SSA training set into six folds and selected one fold as a fixed validation set for all experiments. Importantly, this was not a cross-validation procedure; instead, we consistently used the same fold for validation throughout all training runs, while the remaining five folds were used for training. This setup allowed for reliable comparison of model performance under identical data conditions and training protocols.

Table 1 summarizes the segmentation results achieved on this fixed internal validation fold. The "Pre-trained" column indicates the dataset on which each model (or model component) was initially trained before fine-tuning. Specifically, "GLI" refers to pretraining on the high-quality BraTS-GLI dataset, while "SSA" indicates that the model was trained on BraTS-SSA data (the pre-trained model on the BraTS-SSA dataset was previously pre-trained on the BraTS-GLI dataset). The best-performing model was the Ensemble-Fuse model pre-trained on BraTS-GLI, with all layers fine-tuned on BraTS-SSA. This model achieved a Mean Dice Score (MeanDCS) of 88.73, outperforming all other configurations. It showed consistently high segmentation performance across all tumor subregions–WT (93.52), TC (85.51), and ET (85.61)–highlighting the effectiveness of comprehensive fine-tuning and the benefit of initializing from a high-quality pretraining dataset.

In comparison, standalone GLIMS and MedNeXt models performed well, with MeanDCS values of 87.34 and 85.67, respectively. An ensemble using simple averaging achieved a moderate improvement (MeanDCS of 86.33). Fusion-based ensembles that included partial freezing of encoder or decoder layers achieved slightly lower scores, underscoring the importance of full fine-tuning in maximizing performance. These findings confirm that the combination of architectural diversity, full end-to-end fine-tuning, and strong pretraining from high-quality datasets significantly contributes to segmentation robustness. As a result, the Ensemble-Fuse model pre-trained on BraTS-GLI and fully fine-tuned on SSA was selected for final testing and submission to the BraTS 2025 Lighthouse Challenge.

Following submission, the organizers' blinded evaluation reported lesion-wise Dice of 0.830 ± 0.204 (ET), 0.848 ± 0.221 (TC), and 0.844 ± 0.201 (WT), together with Normalized Surface Dice (NSD) at 1 mm of 0.800 ± 0.206 (ET), 0.746 ± 0.229 (TC), and 0.745 ± 0.201 (WT). These results are consistent with our internal ranking, showing reliable performance on ET and WT, with a slightly lower boundary agreement for TC. Overall, the lesion-wise Dice and NSD demonstrate that the submitted model achieves both solid volumetric segmentation and reliable boundary alignment at a clinically meaningful tolerance.

Table 2 presents a detailed comparison between the GLIMS model and the best-performing Ensemble-Fuse model, evaluated on a consistently selected internal validation fold derived from the BraTS-SSA training set. The Ensemble-Fuse

Table 1. Achieved results utilizing GLIMS and MedNeXt models on selected fold validation data from the BraTS-SSA train set. This table compares individual model performance and various ensemble strategies. Among them, the Ensemble-Fuse model pre-trained on BraTS-GLI achieved the best results across all tumor subregions (WT, TC, ET) and overall segmentation performance (MeanDCS).

Model	Pre-trained	Frozen Encoder	Frozen Decoder	WT	TC	ET	MeanDCS
GLIMS	GLI			91.33	83.73	84.9	87.34
MedNeXT	GLI			89.74	83.82	81.11	85.67
Ensemble-avg	GLI			90.57	81.79	84.4	86.33
Ensemble-Fuse	SSA	✓	✓	92.64	83.59	83.28	87.06
Ensemble-Fuse	SSA	✓		91.67	82.91	82.3	86.45
Ensemble-Fuse	SSA			92.06	83.59	83.91	87.21
Ensemble-Fuse	GLI			**93.52**	**85.51**	**85.61**	**88.73**

model, which combines multi-scale outputs from both GLIMS and MedNeXt through a convolutional fusion head, demonstrates superior performance across all lesion-wise and global metrics. In particular, it shows marked improvements in Dice scores for the Whole Tumor (WT), Tumor Core (TC), and Enhancing Tumor (ET) regions, as well as significant reductions in Hausdorff Distance (HD95) values. These consistent gains underline the effectiveness of the ensemble strategy in addressing low-quality imaging conditions and highlight its robustness in tumor subregion segmentation.

Table 2. Detailed comparison of segmentation performance between the GLIMS model and the Ensemble-Fuse architecture on the BraTS-SSA validation set. Metrics include lesion-wise Dice Score (DCS), standard Dice Score, and Hausdorff 95 distance (HD95) for three tumor subregions: Whole Tumor (WT), Tumor Core (TC), and Enhancing Tumor (ET). The Ensemble-Fuse approach significantly improves lesion-level accuracy and boundary precision, achieving superior performance across all evaluated metrics.

Model	Lesionwise DCS WT	Lesionwise DCS TC	Lesionwise DCS ET	DCS WT	DCS TC	DCS ET	HD95 WT	HD95 TC	HD95 ET	Mean Lesionwise DCS	Mean DCS	Mean HD95
GLIMS	83.5	72	77.3	91.98	87.2	85.77	9.08	19.6	14.15	77.6	88.32	14.28
Ensemble-Fuse	**87.86**	**83.5**	**84.05**	**93.78**	**91.06**	**90.1**	**5.31**	**5.36**	**3.15**	**85.14**	**91.65**	**4.61**

6.2 Qualitative Results

The qualitative results in Fig. 4 illustrate the segmentation differences among the proposed models in two representative cases. Ground truth labels show the complete and precise segmentation of the tumor subregions. The individual models, GLIMS and MedNeXt, provide accurate and reliable segmentations but with occasional misses or over-segmentation at tumor boundaries. The fusion ensemble approach exhibits improved consistency, minimizing outliers in segmentation but sometimes blending boundaries. In contrast, the fusion-based ensemble delivers the most refined results, closely matching the ground truth in both tumor boundary clarity and overall completeness, validating its superior segmentation capability.

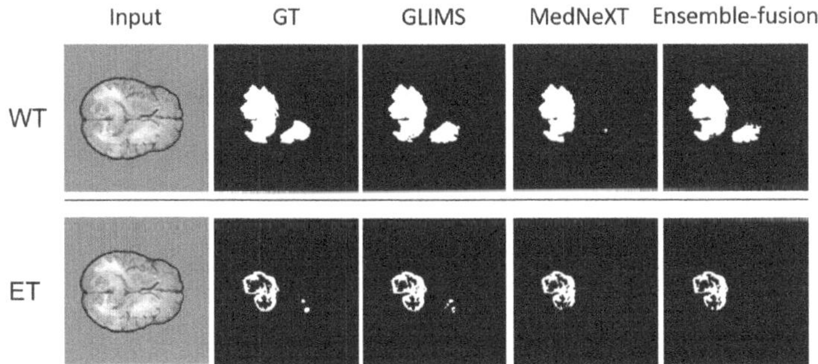

Fig. 4. Qualitative comparison of segmentation results for two example cases from the BraTS-SSA dataset. The fusion-based ensemble shows better performance in segmenting tumor subregions (WT and ET) compared to individual and averaging-based models.

7 Discussion

This study demonstrates improvements in brain tumor segmentation accuracy using a hybrid ensemble approach designed for low-quality MRI data. Despite promising results, several limitations exist. One notable challenge is the limited availability of publicly accessible pre-trained models specifically designed for volumetric 3D brain MRI segmentation, which restricts extensive experimentation and may impact optimal model initialization. Additionally, variations in image acquisition protocols across sub-Saharan institutions introduce data heterogeneity that may affect model generalizability. For future work, expanding the availability of diverse pre-trained models extensively trained on high-quality datasets, such as BraTS-GLI, is critical. This would facilitate comprehensive evaluations and further enhance the effectiveness of fine-tuning resource-limited datasets, such as BraTS-SSA, ultimately improving segmentation accuracy and clinical applicability.

8 Conclusion

This study presents a hybrid ensemble method specifically designed to address the challenges of brain tumor segmentation in low-resource sub-Saharan African healthcare settings. By combining the strengths of GLIMS and MedNeXt architectures through strategic transfer learning, fine-tuning, and fusion ensemble methods, our model achieved superior segmentation accuracy and robustness. These results validate the potential of designed deep learning strategies to significantly enhance medical imaging quality and diagnostic performance, providing a practical solution for resource-constrained environments.

Acknowledgment. This work was partially funded by the ITU-Turkcell research scholarship and benefited from ITU BAP research funds (Project ID: 47363). The computing resources used in this work were provided by the National Center for High Performance Computing of Türkiye (UHeM) under grant number 4022542025.

References

1. Adewole, M., et al.: The brain tumor segmentation (brats) challenge 2023: Glioma segmentation in Sub-Saharan Africa patient population (brats-africa). ArXiv pp. arXiv–2305 (2023)
2. Akter, A., et al.: Robust clinical applicable cnn and u-net based algorithm for mri classification and segmentation for brain tumor. Expert Syst. Appl. **238**, 122347 (2024)
3. Anazodo, U.C., et al.: A framework for advancing sustainable magnetic resonance imaging access in Africa. NMR Biomed. **36**(3), e4846 (2023)
4. Baid, U., et al.: The rsna-asnr-miccai brats 2021 benchmark on brain tumor segmentation and radiogenomic classification. arXiv preprint arXiv:2107.02314 (2021)
5. Cardoso, M.J., et al.: Monai: an open-source framework for deep learning in healthcare. arXiv preprint arXiv:2211.02701 (2022)
6. Dosovitskiy, A., et al.: An image is worth 16x16 words: transformers for image recognition at scale. arXiv preprint arXiv:2010.11929 (2020)
7. Hashmi, S., et al.: Optimizing brain tumor segmentation with mednext: brats 2024 ssa and pediatrics. arXiv preprint arXiv:2411.15872 (2024)
8. He, Y., Nath, V., Yang, D., Tang, Y., Myronenko, A., Xu, D.: Swinunetr-v2: stronger swin transformers with stagewise convolutions for 3d medical image segmentation. In: International Conference on Medical Image Computing and Computer-Assisted Intervention, pp. 416–426. Springer, Heidelberg (2023). https://doi.org/10.1007/978-3-031-43901-8_40
9. Isensee, F., et al.: nnu-net: self-adapting framework for u-net-based medical image segmentation. arXiv preprint arXiv:1809.10486 (2018)
10. Liu, Z., Mao, H., Wu, C.Y., Feichtenhofer, C., Darrell, T., Xie, S.: A convnet for the 2020s. In: Proceedings of the IEEE/CVF Conference on Computer Vision and Pattern Recognition, pp. 11976–11986 (2022)
11. Ma, C., Wang, Z.: Semi-mamba-unet: pixel-level contrastive and cross-supervised visual mamba-based unet for semi-supervised medical image segmentation. Knowl.-Based Syst. **300**, 112203 (2024)
12. Maani, F.A., Hashmi, A.U.R., Saeed, N., Yaqub, M.: On enhancing brain tumor segmentation across diverse populations with convolutional neural networks. In: 2024 IEEE International Symposium on Biomedical Imaging (ISBI), pp. 1–4. IEEE (2024)
13. Nizamani, A.H., Chen, Z., Nizamani, A.A., Bhatti, U.A.: Advance brain tumor segmentation using feature fusion methods with deep u-net model with cnn for mri data. J. King Saud Univ.-Comput. Inf. Sci. **35**(9), 101793 (2023)

14. Parida, A., et al.: Adult glioma segmentation in Sub-Saharan Africa using transfer learning on stratified finetuning data. arXiv preprint arXiv:2412.04111 (2024)
15. Roy, S., et al.: Mednext: transformer-driven scaling of convnets for medical image segmentation. In: International Conference on Medical Image Computing and Computer-Assisted Intervention, pp. 405–415. Springer, Heidelberg (2023). https://doi.org/10.1007/978-3-031-43901-8_39
16. Vaswani, A., et al.: Attention is all you need. Adv. Neural Inf. Process. Syst. **30** (2017)
17. de Verdier, M.C., et al.: The 2024 brain tumor segmentation (brats) challenge: glioma segmentation on post-treatment mri. arXiv preprint arXiv:2405.18368 (2024)
18. Yazıcı, Z.A., Öksüz, İ, Ekenel, H.K.: Glims: attention-guided lightweight multi-scale hybrid network for volumetric semantic segmentation. Image Vis. Comput. **146**, 105055 (2024)
19. Zhao, Y., Bai, L., Zhang, Z., Wu, Y., Islam, M., Ren, H.: Transferring knowledge from high-quality to low-quality mri for adult glioma diagnosis. arXiv preprint arXiv:2410.18698 (2024)

MAPS-Glioma: Modality-Specific Augmentation and Tissue-Adaptive Postprocessing for Robust Glioma Segmentation in Resource-Limited Settings

Ayomide B. Oladele[1], Helena Machibya[2,3], Mariam Kaoneka[4], Frederick Lyimo[5], Debora Hoza[2], Immaculata Kafumu[2], Idris Olalekan[6], Jeremiah Fadugba[7], Dong Zhang[8], Aondona Iorumbur[9], Raymond Confidence[10,11], Nicephorus Rutabasibwa[12], and Ugumba M. Kwikima[12](✉)

[1] Medical Artificial Intelligence Laboratory (MAI Lab), Lagos, Nigeria
[2] Temeke Regional Referral Hospital, Dar Es Salaam, Tanzania
[3] Muhimbili University of Health and Allied Sciences (MUHAS), Dar Es Salaam, Tanzania
[4] Mwananyamala Regional Referral Hospital, Dar Es Salaam, Tanzania
[5] Muhimbili National Hospital, Dar Es Salaam, Tanzania
[6] PublicaAI, Lagos, Nigeria
[7] University of Ibadan, Ibadan, Nigeria
[8] Department of Electrical and Computer Engineering, University of British Columbia, Vancouver, Canada
[9] Department of Physics, Federal University of Technology, Minna, Nigeria
[10] Montreal Neurological Institute, McGill University, Montreal, Canada
[11] Department of Biomedical Engineering, McGill University, Montreal, Canada
[12] Muhimbili Orthopedic and Neurosurgery Institute, Dar Es Salaam, Tanzania
drkwik80@gmail.com

Abstract. Gliomas are by far the most frequent primary tumors affecting the central nervous system (CNS). In Sub-Saharan Africa (SSA), gliomas pose a significant health burden due to high mortality rates that are caused by the late presentation of the disease and limited access to advanced diagnostic imaging. The prevailing state-of-the-art brain tumor segmentation algorithms designed for rapid automated lesion characterization are largely trained on datasets from high-income countries, limiting their general application in Sub-Saharan African (SSA) populations. These models frequently encounter challenges in SSA settings due to the region's lower-quality MRI scans, which present with poor image contrast and resolution, as well as distinct disease characteristics like the late-stage presentation of tumors.

In this study, we proposed a deep learning framework that shifts the focus from a model-centric approach to a data processing focused approach, for accurate segmentation of the brain glioma sub-regions. The study made use of the BraTS-Africa 2025 Challenge dataset from SSA populations. Our approach combines modality-specific data augmentation and a tissue-adaptive postprocessing technique, built upon an optimized 3D U-Net architecture. Preliminary results demonstrate promising Dice scores of 0.74 for the enhancing tumor (ET), 0.75 for the tumor core (TC), and 0.85 for the whole tumor (WT), as well as HD95 values

S. Bakas et al. (Eds.): MICCAI 2025, LNCS 16376, pp. 274–283, 2026.
https://doi.org/10.1007/978-3-032-16365-3_25

of 13.2, 14.5, and 14.8 for the ET, TC, and WT respectively, suggesting improved robustness and spatial accuracy on SSA-specific data. This work represents a step toward reducing global health disparities and advancing precision medicine for glioma patients in SSA.

Keywords: BraTS · 3D UNet · convolutional neural network · deep learning · glioma · magnetic resonance imaging · segmentation · Low-resource

1 Introduction

Representing the most frequent type of primary tumor affecting the central nervous system (CNS), gliomas are understood to arise from neural stem or progenitor cells that have undergone tumor-initiating genetic alterations. These tumors can manifest as either well-defined, circumscribed masses or as diffusely infiltrative lesions that can affect any area of the brain [1]. The World Health Organization (WHO) provides a formal classification system that grades gliomas from 1 to 4, establishing a spectrum that ranges from low-grade to the highest level of malignancy based on microscopic and molecular characteristics [2–4]. Gliomas are a significant health challenge in Sub-Saharan Africa (SSA). The region's officially low brain cancer incidence (0.8 per 100,000 persons) is likely underestimated, masking the true burden. Such figures may result from inadequate data collection and surveillance methods. Limited access to advanced diagnostics like MRI and specialized care in SSA contributes to significant underdiagnosis. This diagnostic gap forces patients to present at later stages, leading to higher morbidity and mortality rates compared to high-income countries [5].

Addressing the diagnostic challenges and resource limitations in SSA, this study proposes a deep learning framework for rapid and automated lesion segmentation. The framework focused on modality-specific data augmentation and tissue-adaptive post-processing techniques, built upon an optimized 3D U-Net architecture. This approach is designed to enhance the robustness and accuracy of glioma sub-region segmentation in brain MRI scans, particularly under conditions of variable image quality, heterogeneous tumor presentation and low-computational resource.

2 Research Landscape

Deep learning, a key pillar of artificial intelligence, has revolutionized medical image analysis, especially in brain glioma segmentation. While convolutional neural networks (CNNs) have historically played a central role, the U-Net architecture has emerged as a particularly powerful and widely adopted approach for medical image segmentation tasks [6].

The application of convolutional neural networks (CNNs) in medical image segmentation has seen substantial advancements. Initially, two-dimensional CNNs (2D-CNNs) were employed, framing segmentation as a classification problem. These models would look at small sections of 2D images from different MRI modalities, classifying the central voxel of each patch into specific tumor sub-regions, such as edema, enhancing tumors, or necrosis [7, 8]. However, a key drawback of 2D methods was their failure to fully exploit the volumetric information inherent in MRI data. Processing the brain slice-by-slice meant losing valuable spatial context between slices. To overcome this limitation, research rapidly shifted to three-dimensional CNNs (3D-CNNs). First utilized for gliomas by Urban et al. [9], these models directly process volumetric 3D image patches. This approach allows them to learn from the complete spatial and contextual information of the tumor, proving more effective for the task of brain glioma segmentation [10].

Among the different types of CNN architectures, U-Net and its variations have become essential for segmenting medical images, including brain gliomas. The standard 3D U-Net, which combines an encoder–decoder structure with skip connections, effectively preserves fine-grained spatial details while capturing global contextual information [11]. However, the complex and heterogeneous nature of gliomas demands further enhancements to this baseline.

Recent research has focused on enhancing 3D U-Net architectures to improve their ability to delineate challenging tumor sub-regions. For instance, Futrega et al. [12] proposed deeper encoder designs and optimized convolutional filter configurations, while Wang et al. [13] incorporated Atrous Spatial Pyramid Pooling (ASPP) modules and Multi-scale Fusion Attention Blocks (MFAB) to better capture multi-scale features and emphasize critical tumor regions. Additionally, advanced loss functions—such as combinations of Dice loss and Focal loss—have been introduced to mitigate severe class imbalance in tumor segmentation [14]. Together, these innovations have improved the delineation of critical tumor compartments, including the whole tumor (WT), tumor core (TC), and enhancing tumor (ET) [9].

Despite these advances, a critical research gap remains: most state-of-the-art U-Net models are trained and validated on datasets from high-income countries, where MRI machines are high-quality, patients are diagnosed earlier, and disease presentation differs. This raises serious concerns about whether these models can generalize to Sub-Saharan Africa (SSA), where imaging quality is lower, tumor morphology may differ, and patients often present at more advanced stages [5]. This "data gap" raises concerns about their clinical applicability in SSA. Recent studies have begun addressing this issue. For example, Amod et al. [15]examined U-Net generalization to SSA data, while Barakat et al. [16] explored using Segment Anything Models (SAM) for tumor segmentation in this context. Although promising, these efforts demonstrate the importance of models specifically tailored and validated on African data.

3 Methods

3.1 Dataset

The dataset used for model training was acquired from the MICCAI-CAMERA-Lacuna Fund BraTS-Africa 2025 Challenge [17]. The data consists of an annotated retrospective cohort of routine multi-parametric MRI (mpMRI) clinical scans acquired as part of standard clinical care of pre-operative glioma in adult Africans. The cohort comprises cases of both low-grade glioma (LGG) and glioblastoma or high-grade glioma

(GBM/HGG), gathered from various institutions following standard brain tumor imaging protocols. Each mpMRI study includes T1 weighted (T1), contrast enhanced T1 weighted (T1Gd), T2 weighted (T2), and T2 FLAIR sequences (Fig. 1). All scans were reviewed by board certified radiologists, then manually annotated and preprocessed to form the final training, validation, and test datasets [18].

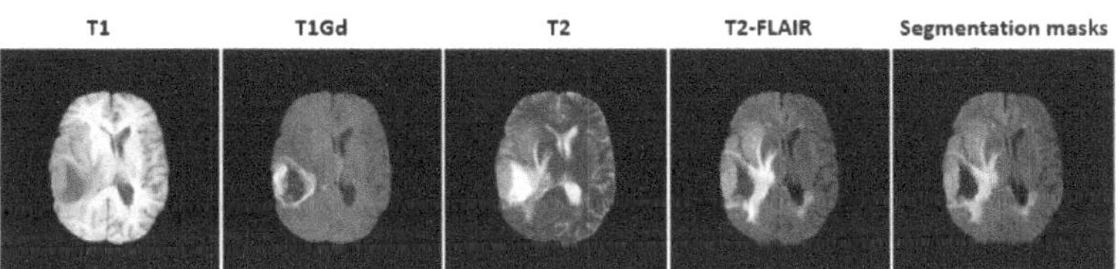

Fig. 1. MRI sequences (T1, T1Gd, T2, T2-FLAIR) and the corresponding segmentation mask; whole tumor (WT) consists of the necrotic part (NCR, dark-red color), the enhancing tumor part (ET, light-yellow color), and the peritumoral edematous tissue (ED, green color). The tumor core (TC) consists of the NCR, and the ET. Adapted and modified from Li. et al. [19].

3.2 Dataset Preparation and Processing

We implemented an advanced preprocessing pipeline to standardize MRI data and avoid biases. Background voxels were converted to NaNs before Z-score normalization, so the normalization can be computed on meaningful tissue regions. Intensities were dynamically rescaled and clipped to the 1st–99th percentile to reduce outliers while preserving relevant signals. Reversible center-cropping ensured spatial consistency and allowed restoration during inference. A tailored, modality-specific augmentation strategy was designed to improve generalization. This included elastic deformations, Rician noise (especially for T1), aggressive contrast and brightness changes (T1c), and bias field simulation (T2-FLAIR). Cutout and motion artifacts were added to increase robustness to missing data and patient movement.

To refine segmentation outputs, we applied a hierarchical, tissue-aware postprocessing strategy. False-positive suppression was performed using 3D connected-component analysis with region-specific thresholds (ET: 30 voxels, TC: 50 voxels, WT: 75 voxels), balancing sensitivity and specificity across tumor sub-regions. Topology-preserving hole-filling was used to maintain anatomical plausibility, employing adaptive connectivity rules (6- to 26-neighborhoods depending on the subregion). Finally, a multi-stage relabeling process corrected misclassified voxels introduced during false-positive removal, ensuring continuity and morphological consistency within tumor structures. The full data processing strategy used is shown in Fig. 2.

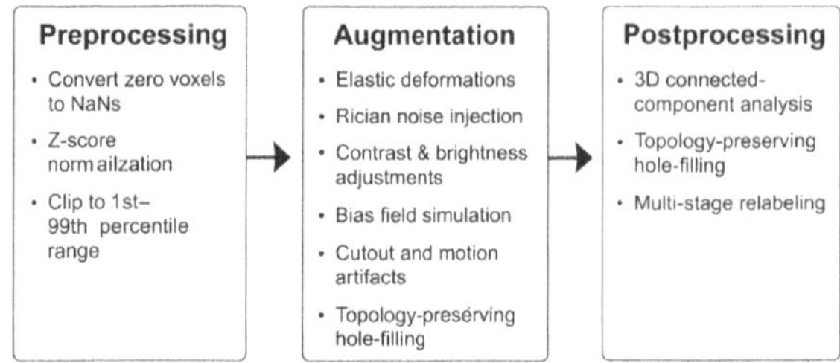

Fig. 2. A schematic diagram of the Data Processing techniques utilized in this study

3.3 Model Architecture

An optimized 3D U-Net-style encoder-decoder architecture developed by Futrega et al. [12] was implemented in this study (see Fig. 3). The encoder progressively down samples the input volume, reducing spatial resolution by a factor of 2 at each level, while simultaneously expanding the channels from 16 to 256. Each encoding block consists of 3D convolutions, instance normalization, and ReLU activations.

The decoder mirrors the encoder structure, using transposed convolutions for up sampling and integrating high-resolution features via skip connections from corresponding encoder layers. To improve stability in deeper layers, Leaky ReLU ($\alpha = 0.01$) is used in the bottleneck and decoder blocks, reducing the risk of dead neurons and improving gradient flow.

The deepest layer (bottleneck module) captures global contextual information at a resolution of 1/64 of the input size. A final sigmoid activation is applied at the output layer to produce voxel-wise probabilities, enabling binary classification in segmentation tasks. We also experimented with varying the number of filters (8 to 32), depending on available computing resources.

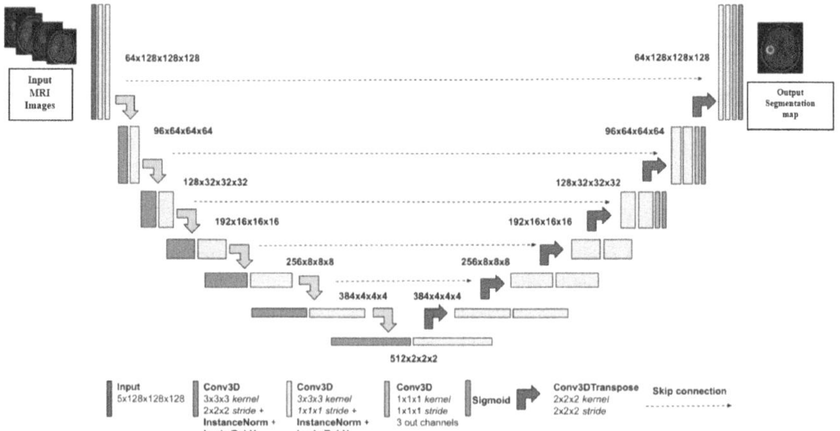

Fig. 3. Architecture of the optimized 3D U-Net model for brain tumor segmentation from MRI scans. Adapted and Modified from Futrega et al. [12]

3.4 Model Training

Our model was trained with a hybrid loss function that combine Dice-Cross-Entropy loss (weighted at 70%) for accurate overlap and pixel-level precision, and Focal Loss (30%, $\gamma = 2.0$) to emphasize hard-to-classify tumor voxels. Class weights [1.0, 2.0, 3.0] are used to address imbalance among non-enhancing core (NCR/NE), edema (ED), and enhancing tumor (ET). The pipeline was optimized with AdamW (with initial learning rate 3×10^{-4}, weight decay $1e^{-5}$, AMSGrad), ReduceLROnPlateau scheduler to make the training adapt learning rates dynamically. An exponential decay rate of 0.995 per epoch was added for stable convergence. The model was trained on the entire training data with no validation strategy implemented due to time constraints, and yet we got a promising result.

Our source code can be found here.

4 Results

4.1 Segmentation Performance of MAPS-Glioma U-Net Model

After training the model on 60 glioma cases for 150 epochs with a batch size of 1 on 8GB NVIDIA GeForce RTX 2080, the proposed MAPS-Glioma framework was evaluated on a validation cohort comprising 35 glioma cases from the BraTS-Africa 2025 dataset. The segmentation performance was quantitatively assessed using the mean Dice similarity coefficient (DSC) and the 95th percentile Hausdorff distance (Hausdorff95) for each tumor subregion: enhancing tumor (ET), tumor core (TC), and whole tumor (WT). The detailed results are summarized in Table 1.

Table 1. Segmentation performance metrics (mean ± standard deviation) for enhancing tumor (ET), tumor core (TC), and whole tumor (WT) on 35 validation data.

Metric	ET	TC	WT
Dice Score	0.74 ± 0.21	0.75 ± 0.23	0.85 ± 0.19
Hausdorff95	11.62 ± 13.68 mm	13.97 ± 13.12 mm	14.87 ± 8.04 mm

The results indicate that the model achieved the highest segmentation accuracy on the whole tumor (WT) segmentation, with a mean Dice score of 0.872 ± 0.17 and a mean Hausdorff95 of 8.86 ± 8.04 mm, showing the robust delineation of the tumor's full extent despite image variability. For the enhancing tumor (ET) and tumor core (TC), the model achieved moderate segmentation performance, with Dice scores of 0.75 ± 0.22 and 0.73 ± 0.25, respectively. Corresponding Hausdorff95 distances for these subregions (11.62 ± 13.68 mm for ET and 13.97 ± 13.12 mm for TC) reflect slightly less precise boundary agreement, suggesting residual challenges in segmenting these more heterogeneous and less well-defined areas (Fig. 4).

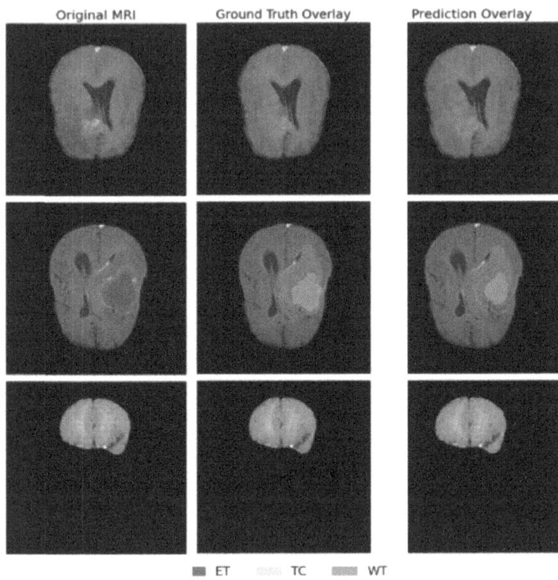

Fig. 4. A visual comparing our model's segmentation versus the ground truth

4.2 Comparative Analysis with Other Architecture

The performance of our framework was benchmarked against other segmentation models that trained on similar cohorts from BraTS 2024 Africa dataset. The comparative analysis includes a baseline 3D U-Net model (Degu et al. [20]) and the state-of-the-art (SOTA) MedNeXt architecture [21], which was a top-performing entry in the BraTS 2024 SSA challenge. The results are summarized in Table 2.

Table 2. Comparison of a baseline 3D U-Net model, SOTA model and our model.

Model / Study	Metric	ET	TC	WT
Our Study	Dice Score	0.75 ± 0.22	0.73 ± 0.25	0.872 ± 0.17
	Hausdorff95	11.62 ± 13.68 mm	13.97 ± 13.12 mm	8.86 ± 8.04 mm
Degu et al. [20],	Dice Score	0.84	0.81	0.84
	Hausdorff95	–	–	–
MedNeXt (BraTS 2024 SSA) [21]	Dice Score	0.82	0.82	0.88
	Hausdorff95	14.248 mm	21.028 mm	8.770 mm

Although the MedNeXt model achieved marginally higher Dice scores, particularly for WT, this performance came at the expense of substantially higher Hausdorff95 distances, most notably for ET and TC, indicating less precise spatial boundary alignment. In contrast, our model maintains competitive Dice performance, especially on whole tumor segmentation, while demonstrating superior spatial accuracy through consistently lower Hausdorff95 scores across all tumor subregions.

5 Discussion

Result from our study shows that applying modality-specific augmentation and tissue-postprocessing to a 3D U-Net, provides substantial improvements in glioma subregion segmentation, showing a competitive segmentation performance while maintaining a superior spatial accuracy compared to existing state-of-the-art methods. On the validation cohort of 35 glioma cases from the BraTS-Africa 2025 dataset, our model achieved a mean Dice score of 0.75 ± 0.22 for ET and 0.73 ± 0.25 for TC, a moderate performance that presents room for improvement. A key strength of our approach lies in the consistently lower Hausdorff95 distances for ET (11.62 ± 13.68 mm) and TC (13.97 ± 13.12 mm) compared to the MedNeXt baseline architecture.

In addition to these gains in ET and TC segmentation, the model maintained excellent performance on the whole tumor (WT), achieving a Dice score of 0.8723 ± 0.17 and a Hausdorff95 of 8.86 ± 8.04 mm. This consistently high WT performance underscores the model's overall robustness and its ability to accurately capture the global tumor extent across heterogeneous MRI scans. While the improvements in ET and TC segmentation are encouraging, there remains room for further enhancement, particularly in reducing variability across individual cases as reflected in the standard deviations.

The computational design of MAPS-Glioma prioritizes efficiency and scalability. Trained on an 8GB GPU and optimized for environments with limited resources, our model shows the feasibility of deploying high-quality AI solutions in under-resourced healthcare systems without a trade-off on performance. The results of our study reinforce the value of context-aware model development that considers local data, pathology presentation and infrastructure realities.

6 Conclusion

In this study, we developed MAPS-Glioma, a computationally efficient and region-adapted deep learning pipeline for glioma segmentation in SSA MRI datasets. By integrating modality-specific data augmentation and tissue-adaptive postprocessing into an optimized 3D U-Net architecture, our framework achieved robust and consistent performance across all tumor subregions, including the typically challenging enhancing tumor (ET) and tumor core (TC).

The results demonstrate that MAPS-Glioma not only excels in accurately segmenting the whole tumor region but also significantly improves segmentation precision in difficult subregions, offering an important advantage over many existing state-of-the-art (SOTA) methods. In addition to the segmentation performance, the pipeline's computational efficiency makes it highly suitable for deployment in resource-constrained clinical environments, where access to advanced computational infrastructure is limited.

The result from our study holds a promising future for the enhancement of diagnostic accuracy and the enablement of more precise, personalized treatment planning for glioma patients in SSA. Most importantly for us, the development and application of MAPS-Glioma represent an important step toward reducing global health disparities and supporting equitable access to high-quality neuro-oncological care worldwide.

Acknowledgments. This work was part of the Sprint AI Training for African Medical Imaging Knowledge Translation (SPARK) Academy 2025 summer school on deep learning in medical imaging. The authors would like to thank the instructors of the summer school for providing insightful background knowledge on brain tumours that informed the research presented here, most notably: Maruf Adewole, Mohannad Barakat, Craig Jones, Noha Magdy, Tinashe Mutsvangwa, MacLean Nasrallah, Evan Calabrese, Celia Cintas, Charles Delahunt, Nicephorus Boniface Rutabasibwa and Amal Saleh. The authors acknowledge computational infrastructure support from the Digital Research Alliance of Canada (The Alliance) and Muhimbili Orthopedic and Neurosurgery Institute, which has been the site for the Hackathon for Team Tanzania.

Finally, we thank the Lacuna Fund for Health and Equity, the RSNA R&E Foundation (PI: Farouk Dako), McGill University Healthy Brains and Healthy Lives (HBHL), and NSERC Discovery Launch Supplement for their grant support. Lacuna Fund for Health and Equity (PI: Udunna Anazodo, 0508-S-001) as well as the National Science and Engineering Research Council of Canada (NSERC) Discovery Launch Supplement (PI: Udunna Anazodo, DGECR-2022- 00136).

Disclosure of Interests. The authors have no competing interests to declare that are relevant to the content of this article.

References

1. Tonn, J.-C., Westphal, M., Rutka, J.T., Grossman, S.A.: Neuro-Oncology of CNS Tumors. Springer, Heidelberg (2006)
2. Weller, M., et al.: Glioma. Nat. Rev. Dis. Primers **10**, 33 (2024). https://doi.org/10.1038/s41572-024-00516-y
3. Rasmussen, B.K., et al.: Epidemiology of glioma: clinical characteristics, symptoms, and predictors of glioma patients grade I-IV in the the Danish Neuro-Oncology Registry. J. Neurooncol **135**, 571–579 (2017). https://doi.org/10.1007/s11060-017-2607-5
4. Mesfin, F.B., Karsonovich, T., Al-Dhahir, M.A.: Gliomas. In: StatPearls. StatPearls Publishing, Treasure Island (2025)
5. Adewole, M., et al.: The Brain Tumor Segmentation (BraTS) Challenge 2023: Glioma Segmentation in Sub-Saharan Africa Patient Population (BraTS-Africa). ArXiv. arXiv:2305.19369v1 (2023)
6. Azad, R., et al.: Medical image segmentation review: the success of U-Net. IEEE Trans. Pattern Anal. Mach. Intell. **46**, 10076–10095 (2024). https://doi.org/10.1109/TPAMI.2024.3435571
7. Prastawa, M., Bullitt, E., Ho, S., Gerig, G.: A brain tumor segmentation framework based on outlier detection. Med. Image Anal. **8**, 275–283 (2004). https://doi.org/10.1016/j.media.2004.06.007
8. Ronneberger, O., Fischer, P., Brox, T.: U-Net: Convolutional Networks for Biomedical Image Segmentation, http://arxiv.org/abs/1505.04597, (2015). https://doi.org/10.48550/arXiv.1505.04597
9. Urban, G., Bendszus, M., Hamprecht, F.A., Kleesiek, J.: Multi-modal brain tumor segmentation using deep convolutional neural networks. In: MICCAI BraTS (Brain Tumor Segmentation) Challenge. Proceedings, Winning Contribution, pp. 31–35 (2014)

10. Çiçek, Ö., Abdulkadir, A., Lienkamp, S.S., Brox, T., Ronneberger, O.: 3D U-net: learning dense volumetric segmentation from sparse annotation. In: Ourselin, S., Joskowicz, L., Sabuncu, M.R., Unal, G., Wells, W. (eds.) Medical Image Computing and Computer-Assisted Intervention – MICCAI 2016, pp. 424–432. Springer, Cham (2016). https://doi.org/10.1007/978-3-319-46723-8_49
11. Attention 3D U-Net with Multiple Skip Connections for Segmentation of Brain Tumor Images. https://www.mdpi.com/1424-8220/22/17/6501. Accessed 12 July 2025
12. Futrega, M., Milesi, A., Marcinkiewicz, M., Ribalta, P.: Optimized U-Net for Brain Tumor Segmentation. http://arxiv.org/abs/2110.03352 (2021). https://doi.org/10.48550/arXiv.2110.03352
13. Wang, T., et al.: 3D-MRI brain glioma intelligent segmentation based on improved 3D U-net network. PLoS ONE **20**, e0325534 (2025). https://doi.org/10.1371/journal.pone.0325534
14. Eelbode, T., et al.: Optimization for medical image segmentation: theory and practice when evaluating with dice score or jaccard index. IEEE Trans. Med. Imaging **39**, 3679–3690 (2020). https://doi.org/10.1109/TMI.2020.3002417
15. Bridging the Gap: Generalising State-of-the-Art U-Net Models to Sub-Saharan African Populations. https://www.researchgate.net/publication/387444048_Bridging_the_Gap_Generalising_State-of-the-Art_U-Net_Models_to_Sub-Saharan_African_Populations. Accessed 12 July 2025
16. Mohannad, B., et al.: Towards SAMBA: Segment Anything Model for Brain Tumor Segmentation in Sub-Sharan African Populations. https://arxiv.org/abs/2312.11775. Accessed 12 July 2025
17. Aboian, M., et al.: MICCAI 2025 lighthouse challenge: brain tumor segmentation cluster of challenges (BraTS) (2024)
18. Adewole, M., et al.: The BraTS-Africa dataset: expanding the brain tumor segmentation data to capture African populations. Radiol. Artif. Intell. **7**, e240528 (2025). https://doi.org/10.1148/ryai.240528
19. Li, Y., et al.: Radiomics-Based Method for Predicting the Glioma Subtype as Defined by Tumor Grade, IDH Mutation, and 1p/19q Codeletion (2022). https://www.researchgate.net/publication/359655249_Radiomics-Based_Method_for_Predicting_the_Glioma_Subtype_as_Defined_by_Tumor_Grade_IDH_Mutation_and_1p19q_Codeletion?_tp=eyJjb250ZXh0Ijp7ImZpcnN0UGFnZSI6InB1YmxpY2F0aW9uIiwicGFnZSI6Il9kaXJlY3QifX0. Accessed 30 July 2025
20. Degu, M.Z., Raymond, C., Zhang, D., Saleh, A., Anazodo, U.C., Simegn, G.L.: Optimized brain tumor segmentation for resource constrained settings: VGG-infused U-net approach. In: Medical Information Computing - First MICCAI Meets Africa Workshop, MImA 2024, and First MICCAI Student Board Workshop on Empowering Medical Information Computing and Research through Early-Career Expertise, EMERGE 2024, Held in Conjunction with MICCAI 2024, Revised Selected Papers, pp. 14–23. Springer, Heidelberg (2025). https://doi.org/10.1007/978-3-031-79103-1_2
21. Hashmi, S., Lugo, J., et al.: Optimizing brain tumor segmentation with MedNeXt: BraTS 2024 SSA and Pediatrics (2024). https://www.researchgate.net/publication/386378863_Optimizing_Brain_Tumor_Segmentation_with_MedNeXt_BraTS_2024_SSA_and_Pediatrics. Accessed 30 July 2025

BRAIN-CATS: Brain Tumour Reliability-Aware Imaging with Neural Networks Using Calibration-Aware Training and Segmentation

Abba Mohammed[1], Zulyadaini Muhammad Aminu[1], Ummulkhairi Ibrahim[1,2,3], Amina Suleiman Damo[1,4], Theodore Barfoot[5], Alexander Hammers[5], Raymond Confidence[1,6,7], Aondona Iorumbar[1,6,8], Abdulrazaq Zubair[1,3,4], and Mubaraq Yakubu[1,4,5,6(✉)]

[1] SPARK Academy, Lagos, Nigeria
{muhammadabba9741,zulyadainimuhammad2,ummkhairi16, aminasuleimandamo11}@gmail.com, aondona.lorumbar@macgill.ca, abdulrazaq.zubair@nkdc.ng
[2] Federal University of Health Sciences Teaching Hospital Azare, Azare, Bauchi State, Nigeria
[3] Federal University of Health Sciences Azare, Azare, Bauchi State, Nigeria
[4] Aminu Kano Teaching Hospital, Kano, Kano State, Nigeria
[5] King's College London, London, UK
{theodore.d.barfoot,alexander.hammers,mubaraq.yakubu}@kcl.ac.uk
[6] Medical Artificial Intelligence Laboratory, Lagos, Lagos State, Nigeria
[7] McGill University, Montreal, Canada
confidence.raymond@mcgill.ca
[8] Federal University of Technology Minna, Minna, Nigeria

Abstract. Accurate and reliable brain tumour segmentation from MRI remains a clinical challenge, particularly in low-resource settings such as Sub-Saharan Africa (SSA). We present BRAIN-CATS, a segmentation framework that combines the Attention U-Net architecture with calibration-aware training to improve both accuracy and model reliability. Our approach is specifically optimized for low-resolution, multi-modal MRI data typical in under-resourced environments.

We trained the model using 5-fold cross-validation on n = 60 patients from the BraTS-Africa 2023 dataset, employing advanced preprocessing techniques, data augmentation, and a composite loss function that includes Dice, Binary Cross-Entropy, Focal Loss, and the marginal L1 Average Calibration Error (mL1-ACE). The calibration-aware component penalizes miscalibrated predictions, improving confidence estimates across tumour boundaries.

The model achieved an average Dice score of 90.38% for edema (ED), 81.94% for enhancing tumour (ET) and 78.88% for the tumour core (TC) across the folds. On external validation using 35 held-out cases, mean Dice scores were 65.30% (ET), 66.50% (TC) and 50.80% for whole tumour (WT), confirming the model's ability to generalize to unseen data

S. Bakas et al. (Eds.): MICCAI 2025, LNCS 16376, pp. 284–295, 2026.
https://doi.org/10.1007/978-3-032-16365-3_26

despite limited training resources. Early stopping between epochs 36–39 prevented overfitting, and stochastic weight averaging further improved generalization.

Ensemble inference using all fold checkpoints yielded smooth, consistent predictions on validation data. Visual and quantitative evaluations confirm BRAIN-CATS as a practical and resource-efficient solution for glioma segmentation in challenging imaging contexts.

Keywords: Brain tumour Segmentation · Attention-UNet · Calibration-Aware Training · mL1-ACE Loss · Low-Resource Settings

1 Introduction

Gliomas are the most common and aggressive form of primary brain tumours, contributing significantly to cancer-related morbidity and mortality worldwide, especially in Sub-Saharan Africa [22]. Magnetic Resonance Imaging (MRI) remains the gold standard for visualizing glioma boundaries and surrounding brain tissue [11]. Accurate segmentation of these tumours is essential for treatment planning, disease monitoring, and prognostication [14,18].

However, achieving high-precision segmentation in low-resource environments presents challenges. These include limited access to MRI scanners, lower-resolution imaging, and restricted computational capacity [10,16]. Existing models trained on high-quality datasets often underperform on local datasets due to these domain-specific limitations [9].

To address this, we propose a segmentation framework based on Attention-UNet [13], optimized for low-resolution, multi-modal MRI data typical in Sub-Saharan Africa. Attention mechanisms improve feature extraction and focus on relevant tumour regions, enhancing performance in complex scenes [19].

We further introduce calibration-aware training using the marginal L1 Average Calibration Error (mL1-ACE) loss function [7], targeting the reliability of model outputs – a critical requirement for clinical translation. Unlike most segmentation studies, we emphasize both pixel-wise accuracy and confidence calibration to ensure the model not only segments tumours well but also provides trustworthy uncertainty estimates.

These efforts culminate in our proposed framework, Brain Tumour Reliability-Aware Imaging with Neural networks using Calibration-Aware Training and Segmentation (BRAIN-CATS). Its contributions are as follows: (1) we fine-tune Attention-UNet on African glioma MRI datasets; (2) we apply calibration-aware training to improve model reliability; and (3) we use preprocessing and optimization techniques suited for resource-limited environments.

2 Methodology

2.1 Dataset

The dataset used in this study is the ASNR-MICCAI-BraTS2023-SSA-Challenge-Training Data (SSA), released as part of the MICCAI-CAMERA-

Lacuna Fund BraTS-Africa 2025 Challenge [2]. It consists of multi-institutional, multi-modal MRI scans of glioma patients, totaling 60 subject folders containing axial 2D slices. Each case includes four standard MRI modalities:

- T1: Pre-contrast T1-weighted image
- T1CE: Contrast-enhanced T1-weighted image
- T2: T2-weighted image
- FLAIR: Fluid-attenuated inversion recovery image

The dataset includes 60 annotated glioma cases, each comprising the full set of expert-labeled segmentation masks. An additional held-out validation set consisting of 35 unseen cases from BraTS-Africa 2024 Training and Validation Dataset. [1] was used for external evaluation. The ground truth segmentation includes:

- Label 0: Background
- Label 1: tumour core (TC)
- Label 2: Peritumoural edema (ED)
- Label 3: Gadolinium-enhancing tumour (ET)

For training, we employed an 80/20 train-validation split using 5-fold cross-validation (e.g., Fold 1) to enhance robustness and generalization.

Preprocessing and Adaptation to Low-Resolution Data. Given the challenges posed by low-resolution MRI data and limited computational resources, several preprocessing and data adaptation strategies were employed to enhance segmentation accuracy and training efficiency:

1. **Standardization with Percentile Clipping**: Intensity values were clipped to the 1st and 99th percentiles of non-zero voxels to remove outliers. Z-score normalization was then applied (mean 0, standard deviation 1) to ensure consistent intensity scaling across scans.
2. **Gaussian Denoising**: To reduce random image noise without significant computational overhead, Gaussian denoising was enabled.
3. **3D Intelligent Cropping and Resizing**: Volumes were center-cropped around the tumour region using bounding box heuristics, leveraging ground truth segmentation and resized to fixed dimensions (256×256).

Data Augmentation. To improve model robustness and prevent overfitting on the relatively small dataset, we applied the following data augmentation strategies:

1. **Expanded Affine Transformations**: Random translations, scaling, and shear operations were applied to simulate anatomical variability and patient misalignment in real-world clinical scenarios.

2. **Per-Channel Photometric Adjustments**: To simulate scanner-specific intensity variability, we applied random brightness, contrast, and gamma adjustments independently to each modality (T1, T1CE, T2, FLAIR). Gamma correction introduced nonlinear brightness transformations, enabling robustness to variations in image contrast across scanners and acquisition settings.

2.2 Model Architecture

We adopt the Attention U-Net architecture [13] for multi-class glioma segmentation. This architecture builds upon the original U-Net by integrating attention mechanisms that enhance focus on tumour regions while suppressing irrelevant background features. Its design is particularly suited to low-resolution and noisy MRI data, common in resource-limited settings.

The architecture consists of the following components:

- **Encoder:** A series of convolutional blocks followed by down-sampling operations to extract hierarchical semantic features from the input MRI slices.
- **Attention Gates:** Incorporated into each skip connection between the encoder and decoder. These gates adaptively weight spatial features, allowing the network to concentrate on tumour-relevant regions and ignore irrelevant or noisy areas.
- **Decoder:** Mirrors the encoder structure, with up-sampling layers that reconstruct the spatial resolution. Skip connections from the encoder are gated and concatenated to refine spatial detail in the output.
- **Final Layer:** A 1×1 convolution followed by a softmax activation function outputs voxel-wise class probabilities across the defined tumour subregions.

This architecture enables the model to selectively propagate features relevant to tumour regions. The configuration supports segmentation of multiple glioma components.

2.3 Calibration-Aware Loss Function

To improve both segmentation accuracy and model confidence calibration, we combine traditional segmentation objectives with a calibration-aware loss formulation [7].

The loss function is defined as:

$$\mathcal{L}_{\text{seg}} = \lambda_1 \cdot \text{Dice Loss} + \lambda_2 \cdot \text{Binary Cross Entropy} + \lambda_3 \cdot \text{Focal Loss}$$

where:

- **Dice Loss:** Encourages high overlap between predicted and ground truth masks, particularly useful for medical image segmentation.
- **Binary Cross Entropy (BCE):** Provides pixel-wise supervision and helps optimize probabilistic outputs.

- **Focal Loss:** Addresses class imbalance and reduces overconfidence by focusing more on hard-to-classify pixels.
- $\lambda_1, \lambda_2, \lambda_3$ are weighting coefficients set to 0.6, 0.3, and 0.1 based on prior work and preliminary validation [15].

Marginal L1 Average Calibration Error (mL1-ACE). As an extension, we incorporated the marginal L1 Average Calibration Error (mL1-ACE) [7] as an auxiliary calibration-aware loss term during training. This loss function directly optimizes pixel-wise calibration without requiring surrogate soft binning techniques.

The mL1-ACE loss measures the discrepancy between predicted confidence and observed accuracy over hard bins, while remaining differentiable and computationally tractable. Given a predicted confidence map and corresponding accuracy map across all pixels, the mL1-ACE is defined as:

$$\text{mL1-ACE} = \frac{1}{B} \sum_{b=1}^{B} |\text{conf}_b - \text{acc}_b|$$

where B is the number of bins, conf_b is the average predicted confidence within bin b, and acc_b is the empirical accuracy for that bin. Despite using hard binning, the loss remains differentiable due to a reformulated aggregation mechanism [8].

In our setting, this term can be combined with the main segmentation loss as follows:

$$\mathcal{L}_{\text{total}} = \mathcal{L}_{\text{seg}} + \lambda_4 \cdot \text{mL1-ACE}$$

where λ_4 controls the influence of the calibration loss.

2.4 Training Strategy

To ensure robust model training and generalization across diverse glioma cases, we employed a comprehensive training strategy incorporating cross-validation, optimizer scheduling, and regularization techniques.

- **K-Fold Cross-Validation (K = 5):** The dataset was divided into five folds, with each fold used once for validation while the remaining four served for training. This strategy improves robustness and reduces performance variance from any single train-validation split [17].
- **Optimizer and Scheduler:** We used the Adam optimizer with an initial learning rate of 1×10^{-4}. Learning rate was dynamically adjusted using either the ReduceLROnPlateau or Cosine Annealing scheduler based on validation loss trends [12].
- **Epochs and Early Stopping:** The model was trained for up to 50 epochs using a patience threshold of 7 epochs, based on validation Dice performance. Early stopping was enabled to halt training when validation performance plateaued, preventing overfitting [5].

- **Batch Size:** A batch size of 8 was used for 2D slice-based training, balancing memory constraints with stable optimization.
- **Stochastic Weight Averaging (SWA):** SWA was enabled starting from the midpoint of training (i.e., epoch 15), averaging model weights across subsequent epochs. This encourages convergence to flatter minima, often improving generalization on unseen data [21].
- **Model Checkpointing:** During training, the model's weights were saved at each epoch. The checkpoint corresponding to the highest validation Dice score was selected as the final model. This approach ensures that the model used at inference time reflects the best generalization performance observed during training, rather than relying on the final epoch, which may be affected by overfitting or instability.

As illustrated in Fig. 1, the BRAIN-CATS pipeline integrates attention-based segmentation and calibration-aware loss design for improved accuracy and reliability in tumour delineation (Table 1).

3 Results

The model was trained using 5-fold cross-validation on 60 annotated glioma cases from the BraTS-Africa 2023 dataset. Each fold consisted of approximately 48 training and 12 validation cases.

Table 2 shows the training performnce for tumour sub-region. Training progress across folds showed early convergence, with training Dice scores exceed-

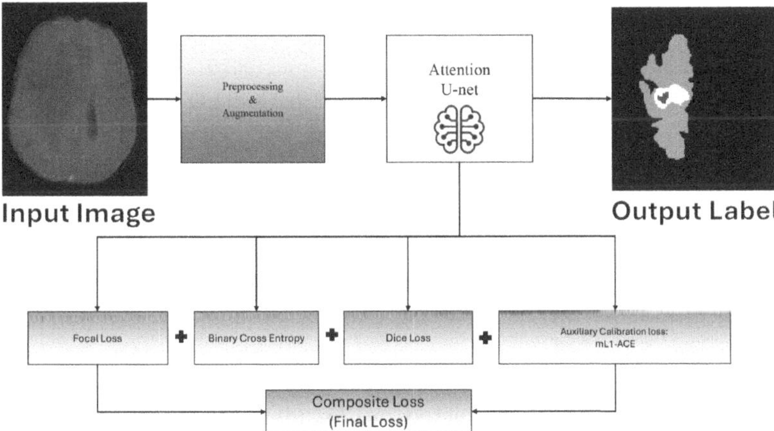

Fig. 1. Overview of the BRAIN-CATS segmentation pipeline. The input MRI slice undergoes preprocessing before being passed into the Attention U-Net model. The model is trained using a composite segmentation loss (Dice, BCE, Focal) and a calibration-aware loss (mL1-ACE), resulting in well-calibrated tumour segmentation output.

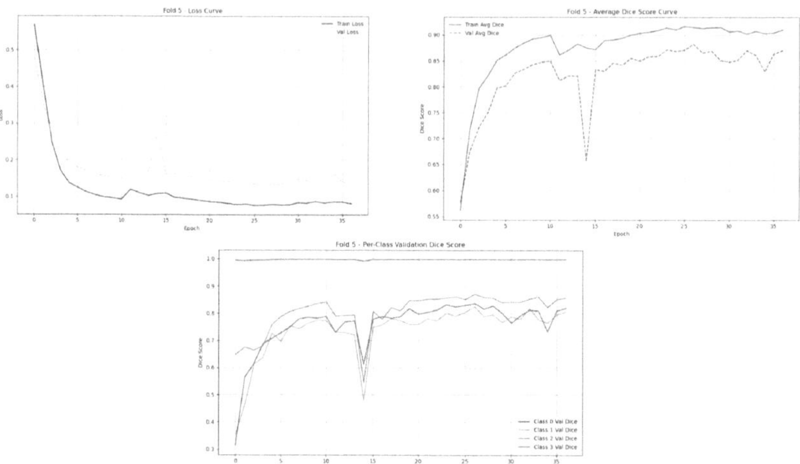

Fig. 2. Training dynamics for Fold 5. The composite figure illustrates (1) training and validation loss curves, (2) average Dice scores, and (3) per-class validation Dice across epochs. Convergence is observed around epoch 20, with early stopping triggered between epochs 3639 to prevent overfitting.

Table 1. 5-Fold cross-validation Dice performance (% ± SD) per tumour sub-region.

Fold	TC	ED	ET
Fold 1	78.7	90.4	81.9
Fold 2	77.3	89.8	82.5
Fold 3	79.1	90.1	80.2
Fold 4	80.4	91.0	82.1
Fold 5	78.9	90.6	83.0
Mean ± SD	**78.88 ± 1.07**	**90.38 ± 0.45**	**81.94 ± 1.04**

ED - Edema, ET Enhancing Tumour, TC Tumour Core

ing 90%. Early stopping was triggered between epochs 36 and 39 due to plateauing or increasing validation loss.

Figure 2 summarizes the training behavior for Fold 5, which recorded the highest overall performance. The model reached loss convergence by epoch 20. Mild oscillations in validation loss were observed beyond epoch 30. Per-class validation Dice scores (TC, ED, ET) remained stable throughout training.

External validation was conducted on 35 unseen test cases using region-wise and lesion-wise evaluation metrics. Results for Enhancing tumour (ET), tumour Core (TC), and Whole tumour (WT) are summarized in Table 2. Mean Dice scores were 65.30% (ET), 66.50% (TC), and 50.80% (WT). Corresponding median Dice scores, Normalized Surface Dice (NSD), interquartile ranges, and Hausdorff Distance (HD95) are also reported. Noticeably, the external validation, which was conducted by the challenge organizers, excludes reporting on surrounding ED and includes WT,

Table 2. External validation performance metrics per tumour sub-region.

Metric	Mean Dice ± SD	Median Dice (Q1Q3)	Dice IQR	Mean NSD	**HD95**
ET	0.653 ± 0.250	0.756 (0.4360.866)	0.430	0.299 ± 0.167	81.4 ± 105.4
TC	0.665 ± 0.271	0.718 (0.4590.922)	0.463	0.264 ± 0.171	84.3 ± 107.5
WT	0.508 ± 0.302	0.465 (0.2300.816)	0.586	0.161 ± 0.095	160.4 ± 128.3

ET Enhancing Tumour, NSD - Normalized Surface Dice, TC Tumour Core, WT Whole Tumour

4 Discussion

This study presents BRAIN-CATS, a brain tumour segmentation framework tailored for resource-constrained settings, leveraging the strengths of Attention-UNet and calibration-aware training. Designed in response to challenges posed by low-quality imaging, limited data availability, and constrained computational resources, this approach targets real-world clinical bottlenecks in underserved environments. Through extensive 5-fold cross-validation on the BraTS-Africa 2023 dataset, our model achieved training segmentation performance across all tumour subregions – with average Dice scores of 90.38% for ED, 81.94% for ET and 78.88% for TC. These results reflect the model's ability to handle heterogeneity in glioma presentations, even under data and hardware constraints.

A key innovation in this work is the integration of the marginal L1 Average Calibration Error (mL1-ACE) as an auxiliary loss for BraTS-Africa 2023 dataset segmentation. This addition theoretically improves the reliability of the model's confidence estimates [8]– a critical factor in clinical applications where overconfident incorrect predictions can lead to harmful consequences. Calibration-aware training not only enhances the trustworthiness of model outputs but also encourages robust learning in data-constrained settings [7].

Despite being trained on only 60 annotated cases without external pretraining, our model achieved encouraging segmentation performance. This contrasts with findings in prior work such as [6], which reported near-chance-level performance (50% Dice) when training on the same dataset. Our results – with Dice scores exceeding 65% for Enhancing tumour (ET) and tumour Core (TC) – highlight the effectiveness of our tailored strategy combining calibration-aware losses and lightweight architectural choices.

Similarly, [4] reported training Dice scores in the range of 0.800.87 using a generative augmentation approach. While their performance was impressive, it was achieved through data augmentation pipelines and potentially greater computational resources. In contrast, our work prioritized low-compute efficiency, ensuring feasibility for deployment in resource-limited African clinical environments.

The SAMBA framework [3] achieved higher Dice performance (84.6%) on the BraTS-Africa dataset. However, their framework incorporated advanced data augmentation, larger-scale optimization, and more expressive model architectures, benefiting from greater access to compute infrastructure. Our relatively modest setup, constrained by hardware limitations and limited training size, still produced stable and generalizable performance – demonstrating that with careful design, reliability and segmentation quality can be achieved without expensive computational budgets.

Our model leveraged preprocessing techniques such as percentile clipping, Gaussian denoising, and photometric augmentation to address the challenges of low-resolution and noisy MRI inputs – a common limitation in data sourced from low-resource environments. These strategies contributed to stable learning across folds and facilitated meaningful feature extraction, particularly for ED segmentation, which exhibited the most consistent performance. In contrast, ET segmentation remained the most variable, likely influenced by contrast inconsistencies in T1CE modalities. Compared to the model presented by [20] which achieved a higher Dice score (84%) for whole tumour segmentation using a 2D U-Net trained and tested on the BraTS-Africa dataset, our performance was lower. However, it is important to note that their evaluation was conducted on only 12 validation cases, whereas our model was tested on a larger cohort of 35 patients, providing a more comprehensive performance assessment.

In our approach, the ensemble prediction strategy consolidated the strengths of individual folds, reducing prediction variance and enhancing robustness. Altogether, BRAIN-CATS represents a practical step toward democratizing access to reliable brain tumour segmentation tools in underserved regions. It directly addresses challenges stemming from a low number and low quality of annotated training data, as well as limited computational resources – conditions that often hinder performance in low-resource settings. By doing so, our approach helps bridge the gap left by models developed exclusively on high-resource datasets.

4.1 Limitations

One key limitation of this study is the absence of ablation experiments to evaluate the individual contribution of each loss function used during training. This was primarily due to restricted access to computational resources. Additionally, we were unable to perform pre-training using external glioma datasets, which might have further enhanced model performance. Compounding these issues, unstable internet connectivity occasionally interrupted access to remote compute resources, further delaying experimentation and limiting the ability to iterate on model improvements. These challenges collectively constrained the scope of our experimentation.

5 Conclusion

This study presents BRAIN-CATS, a lightweight and reliability-aware segmentation framework developed as part of the BraTS-Africa 2025 Challenge to address the unique constraints of low-resource healthcare settings in Sub-Saharan Africa. Our approach is specifically tailored to operate under three major limitations: a small number of annotated cases, low-quality and noisy MRI inputs, and restricted access to computational infrastructure. By combining an attention-enhanced U-Net architecture with calibration-aware training and resource-efficient preprocessing, BRAIN-CATS demonstrates reasonable generalization and reliable performance, underscoring the potential for deploying trustworthy deep learning models in real-world, under-resourced environments.

Acknowledgements. This work was part of the Sprint AI Training for African Medical Imaging Knowledge Translation (SPARK) Academy 2025 summer school on deep learning in medical imaging. The authors would like to thank the instructors of the summer school for providing insightful background knowledge on brain tumours that informed the research presented here, most notably: Maruf Adewole, Mohannad Barakat, Craig Jones, Noha Magdy, Tinashe Mutsvangwa, MacLean Nasrallah, Nicephorus Boniface Rutabasibwa, Charles Delahunt, Celia Cintas, Evan Calabrese, and Amal Saleh.

The authors acknowledge the funding support provided to SPARK through the Lacuna Fund for Health and Equity (PI: Udunna Anazodo), the RSNA R&E Foundation (PI: Farouk Dako), the University of Washington Population Health Initiative Tier 2 Grant (PI: Mehmet Kurt), McGill University Healthy Brain and Healthy Lives (HBHL, Anazodo), and the Natural Sciences and Engineering Research Council of Canada (NSERC) Discovery Launch Supplement (PI: Udunna Anazodo, DGECR-2022-00136).

We also extend our sincere gratitude to the NSIA Kano Diagnostic Center (NKDC) for institutional support, and to Prof. Muhammad Abba Suwaid and Dr. Abbas Rabiu for their guidance and encouragement. Special thanks to Dr. Navodini Wijethilake for her crucial support in resolving technical challenges during model development and training.

Author contributions. AM[1] & ZM[2]: co-first authorship; conceptualization, methodology, software implementation, training strategy design, validation, results interpretation, writing–original draft preparation.

UI[3] & ASD[4]: data curation, result formatting, manuscript editing, and internal review.

TB[5]: support for containerizing model predictions and Docker-based evaluation submission.

AH[6]: manuscript structure guidance, iterative revision, and critical review.

RC[7] & AI[8]: data curation, conceptualization (SPARK Practicum - BraTS challenge).

AZ[9] & MY[10]: senior authorship; project supervision, conceptualization, methodology, technical validation, training and loss design guidance, manuscript writing, review and correspondence handling.[1](Abba Mohammed) [2](Zulyadaini Muhammad Aminu) [3](Ummulkhairi Ibrahim) [4](Amina Suleiman Damo) [5](Theodore Barfoot)

[6](Alexander Hammers) [7](Raymond Confidence) [8](Aondona Iorumbur) [9](Abdulrazaq Zubair) [10](Mubaraq Yakubu)

Disclosure of Interests. The authors have no competing interests to declare that are relevant to the content of this article. The training code is publicly available at: https://github.com/SPARK-Academy-2025/Attention-Unet-Model-Team-Nigerian-North-East-Savannah-AI-

References

1. Adewole, M., et al.: The brats-Africa dataset: expanding the brain tumor segmentation data to capture African populations. Radiol. Artif. Intell. **7**(4), e240528 (2025)
2. Adewole, M., et al.: The brain tumor segmentation (brats) challenge 2023: Glioma segmentation in Sub-Saharan Africa patient population (brats-africa). ArXiv pp. arXiv–2305 (2023)
3. Afolabi, B., et al.: Samba: style-aware multi-task brain analysis for glioma subregion segmentation. arXiv preprint arXiv:2307.10947 (2023)
4. Ali, Z., Stojanov, A., et al.: Generative style for robustness: domain generalization for medical image segmentation on limited data. Med. Image Anal. **80**, 102538 (2023). https://doi.org/10.1016/j.media.2022.102538
5. Anam, M.K., Defit, S., Haviluddin, H., Efrizoni, L., Firdaus, M.B.: Early stopping on cnn-lstm development to improve classification performance. J. Appl. Data Sci. **5**(3), 1175–1188 (2024)
6. Antwi, Y., Zhang, D., Confidence, R., Rethnakaran, P., Anazodo, U., et al.: Bridging the gap between deep learning and sparse data for brain tumor segmentation. arXiv preprint arXiv:2311.16101 (2023)
7. Barfoot, T., Garcia-Peraza-Herrera, L.C., Akcay, S., Glocker, B., Vercauteren, T.: Average calibration losses for reliable uncertainty in medical image segmentation. arXiv preprint arXiv:2506.03942 (2025)
8. Barfoot, T., Garcia Peraza Herrera, L.C., Glocker, B., Vercauteren, T.: Average calibration error: a differentiable loss for improved reliability in image segmentation. In: International Conference on Medical Image Computing and Computer-Assisted Intervention, pp. 139–149. Springer, Heidelberg (2024). https://doi.org/10.1007/978-3-031-72114-4_14
9. Chen, X., Singh, M.M., Geyer, P.: Utilizing domain knowledge: robust machine learning for building energy performance prediction with small, inconsistent datasets. Knowl.-Based Syst. **294**, 111774 (2024)
10. JS, N.: Brain tumor segmentation using multi-scale attention u-net with efficientnetb4 encoder for enhanced mri analysis. Sci. Rep. **15**(1), 9914 (2025)
11. Kalpathy-Cramer, J., Gerstner, E.R., Emblem, K.E., Andronesi, O.C., Rosen, B.: Advanced magnetic resonance imaging of the physical processes in human glioblastoma. Can. Res. **74**(17), 4622–4637 (2014)
12. Lee, M.H.: Learning rate schedules and optimizers, a game changer for deep neural networks. In: Advances in Intelligent Computing Techniques and Applications, p. 327 (2023)
13. Li, X., Lu, Q., Li, Y., Li, M., Qi, Y.: Optimized unet with attention mechanism for multi-scale semantic segmentation. arXiv preprint arXiv:2502.03813 (2025)
14. Miller, K.D., et al.: Brain and other central nervous system tumor statistics, 2021. CA: Canc. J. Clin. **71**(5), 381–406 (2021)

15. Müller, R., Kornblith, S., Hinton, G.E.: Calibration of modern neural networks is improved by use of label smoothing and mixup. Nat. Commun. **12**(1), 1–10 (2021). https://doi.org/10.1038/s41467-021-20979-5
16. Murali, S., et al.: Bringing mri to low-and middle-income countries: directions, challenges and potential solutions. NMR Biomed. **37**(7), e4992 (2024)
17. Nti, I.K., Nyarko-Boateng, O., Aning, J., et al.: Performance of machine learning algorithms with different k values in k-fold cross-validation. Int. J. Inf. Technol. Comput. Sci. **13**(6), 61–71 (2021)
18. Rasool, N., Bhat, J.I.: A critical review on segmentation of glioma brain tumor and prediction of overall survival. Arch. Comput. Methods Eng. 1–45 (2024)
19. Sun, Y., Bi, F., Gao, Y., Chen, L., Feng, S.: A multi-attention unet for semantic segmentation in remote sensing images. Symmetry **14**(5), 906 (2022)
20. Toufiq, M., et al.: A hybrid approach for tumor segmentation in brain mri: bridging performance and interpretability. arXiv preprint arXiv:2310.11638 (2023)
21. Wang, P., Shen, L., Tao, Z., He, S., Tao, D.: Generalization analysis of stochastic weight averaging with general sampling. In: Forty-First International Conference on Machine Learning (2024)
22. Yevudza Jr, W.E., Buckman, V., Darko, K., Banson, M., Totimeh, T.: Neuro-oncology access in Sub-Saharan Arica: a literature review of challenges and opportunities. Neuro-Oncol. Adv. **6**(1), vdae057 (2024)

How We Won BraTS-SSA 2025: Brain Tumor Segmentation in the Sub-Saharan African Population Using Segmentation-Aware Data Augmentation and Model Ensembling.

Claudia Takyi Ankomah[1(✉)], Livingstone Eli Ayivor[1], Ireneaus Nyame[2], Leslie Wambo[1], Patrick Yeboah Bonsu[3], Aondona Moses Iorumbur[5], Raymond Confidence[4], and Toufiq Musah[1]

[1] Kwame Nkrumah University of Science and Technology, Kumasi, Ghana
ctankomah@st.knust.edu.gh
[2] University of Cape Coast, Cape Coast, Ghana
[3] University of Toronto, Toronto, Canada
[4] Department of Biomedical Engineering, McGill University, Montreal, Canada
[5] Department of Physics, Federal University of Technology, Minna, Nigeria

Abstract. Brain tumors, particularly gliomas, pose significant challenges due to their complex growth patterns, infiltrative nature, and the variability in brain structure across individuals, which makes accurate diagnosis and monitoring difficult. Deep learning models have been developed to accurately delineate these tumors. However, most of these models were trained on relatively homogenous high-resource datasets, limiting their robustness when deployed in underserved regions. In this study, we performed segmentation-aware offline data augmentation on the BraTS-Africa dataset to increase the data sample size and diversity to enhance generalization. We further constructed an ensemble of three distinct architectures, MedNeXt, SegMamba, and Residual-Encoder U-Net, to leverage their complementary strengths. Our best-performing model, MedNeXt, was trained on 1000 epochs and achieved the highest average lesion-wise dice and normalized surface distance scores of 0.86 and 0.81 respectively. However, the ensemble model trained for 500 epochs produced the most balanced segmentation performance across the tumor subregions. This work demonstrates that a combination of advanced augmentation and model ensembling can improve segmentation accuracy and robustness on diverse and underrepresented datasets. Code available at: https://github.com/SPARK-Academy-2025/SPARK-2025/tree/main/SPARK2025_BraTs_MODELS/SPARK_NeuroAshanti.

Keywords: Brain Tumor Segmentation · Deep Learning · Ensembling · Data augmentation

S. Bakas et al. (Eds.): MICCAI 2025, LNCS 16376, pp. 296–306, 2026.
https://doi.org/10.1007/978-3-032-16365-3_27

1 Introduction

Brain tumors, particularly gliomas, represent a significant challenge in neuro-oncology due to their infiltrative nature, histological heterogeneity, and variable prognosis [1]. Gliomas originate from glial cells such as astrocytes and oligodendrocytes and are categorized by the World Health Organization (WHO) into grades I to IV based on histological and molecular features [2]. While low-grade gliomas (LGGs) tend to grow slowly and are sometimes curable via surgery, high-grade gliomas (HGGs), including glioblastoma multiforme (GBM), are aggressive and associated with poor outcomes. Despite standard-of-care therapies, median survival for GBM patients remains approximately 16 months [3].

These tumors pose additional challenges due to their complex growth patterns and the variability in brain structure across individuals, which makes accurate diagnosis and monitoring difficult. Timely and precise tumor segmentations from magnetic resonance imaging (MRI) scans are important for improving patient outcomes through better treatment planning and response assessment [4].

Manual segmentation of gliomas from multimodal MRI is considered the clinical gold standard. It is however time-consuming, labor-intensive, and prone to inter- and intra-observer variability [5]. To overcome these limitations, deep learning-based approaches have been employed, demonstrating superior performance and efficiency compared to traditional image processing methods [6,7]. The Brain Tumor Segmentation (BraTS) Challenge has played a pivotal role in benchmarking and advancing automated glioma segmentation since 2012, offering a standardized dataset that includes preprocessed T1-weighted, T1Gd, T2-weighted, and T2-FLAIR sequences, with expert annotations for enhancing tumor (ET), necrotic and non-enhancing tumor core (NCR/NET), and peritumoral edema (ED) [8].

Despite progress, a persistent bottleneck in deploying deep learning models for clinical segmentation remains the limited size and diversity of training datasets. This problem becomes especially pronounced when models are applied to out-of-distribution populations [9]. The recently introduced BraTS-Africa dataset begins to address this gap by providing multimodal MRI scans of glioma patients from healthcare institutions in sub-Saharan Africa. It includes 146 annotated cases, 95 adult diffuse gliomas, and 51 other central nervous system neoplasms. [10,11]. The BraTS-Africa dataset is relatively small, and the variability in scanner quality, clinical settings, and imaging protocols presents further challenges. As a result, training highly accurate and robust segmentation models in these settings remains an open problem, especially under data-limited conditions and diverse real-world constraints.

1.1 Related Works

Over the past decade, convolutional neural networks (CNNs) have emerged as the predominant approach for brain tumor segmentation, particularly in benchmark challenges such as BraTS [8,12]. Among these, U-Net and its many derivatives have become foundational, since the launch of the BraTS challenge in 2014, due to their encoder-decoder architecture with skip connections, which help preserve spatial information critical for accurate medical image segmentation [13]. To improve performance, these models have been progressively enhanced with architectural innovations such as attention gates, residual connections, and cascaded refinement stages [14,15]. Over time, top-performing solutions began to integrate ensemble learning techniques by combining predictions from multiple U-Net variants to reduce model variance and enhance generalization [16,17].

A major advancement was made with the introduction of nnU-Net. It has been the base model of winning solutions in BraTS 2020 [18], 2021 [19], and 2022 [20]. By 2023, this trend evolved further, with the winning team employing an ensemble of a SwinUNETR and nnU-Net to improve tumor subregion segmentation. Complementary strategies like aggressive augmentation, GAN-generated data, and ensemble-based label refinement have also been used to address class imbalance and reduce overfitting [1]. Modern segmentation models such as MedNeXt [21] have moved beyond the traditional U-net architecture. The model was validated across multiple benchmarks, including BraTS, showing that MedNeXt matches or surpasses nnU-Net in accuracy while maintaining scalability and robustness across diverse tumor types and imaging conditions [21]. Newer approaches such as the State Space based [22] SegMamba have been proposed address the high computational demands of the Transformer-based models like SwinUNETR.

Our approach builds on recent advances by exploring both model diversity and advanced data augmentation strategies. We ensemble three distinct architectures; MedNeXt, SegMamba, and Residual-Encoder U-Net (ResEnc U-Net), to leverage the complementary strengths of convolutional neural networks and state-space models. To address limited data sample size and variability, we implement a segmentation-aware offline data augmentation pipeline that combines standard geometric and intensity-based transformations together with a custom label-masked elastic deformation to generate diverse and anatomically plausible samples. The label-masked transform applies aggressive elastic deformations specifically to the tumor regions. This targeted augmentation increases variability within the lesion context, thereby enhancing model generalization in data-limited settings such as those represented in the BraTS-Africa dataset.

2 Methods

2.1 Data Description

This study utilized the BraTS-Africa dataset from the MICCAI-CAMERA-Lacuna Fund BraTS-Africa 2025 Challenge, which comprises 95 preoperative glioma cases (60 for training and 35 for validation) [10,11]. Each case consists of four MRI sequences: T1-weighted (T1), T1-Contrast Enhanced (T1-CE), T2-weighted (T2), and T2-Fluid Attenuated Inversion Recovery (T2-FLAIR). These modalities provide complementary structural and pathological details that are important for accurate tumor assessment and segmentation. The corresponding ground truth labels were manually annotated by expert radiologists and define three tumor subregions, namely the Enhancing tumor (ET), Non-enhancing tumor Core (TC), and Whole tumor (WT). ET represents regions with contrast uptake on post-contrast T1 images, TC includes necrotic or cystic components that lack enhancement, and WT corresponds to peritumoral edema, which is visible on FLAIR sequences.

2.2 Data Expansion

Given the limited sample size of the dataset, segmentation-aware offline data augmentation pipeline was implemented. This approach was adopted to increase the number of data samples, thereby enhancing model generalizability and robustness across varied anatomical presentations of brain tumors, which are important for brain tumor segmentation.

Segmentation-Aware Offline Data Augmentation. This augmentation pipe-line combines affine, flip, bias-field, and elastic deformation transforms from the TorchIO [23] library, and a custom label-mask transform. All the transforms were chained, and predefined probabilities were assigned to all except the label-mask transform, which was applied deterministically. This introduced controlled variation and generation of new samples with realistic brain anatomical characteristics as seen in Fig. 1(b).

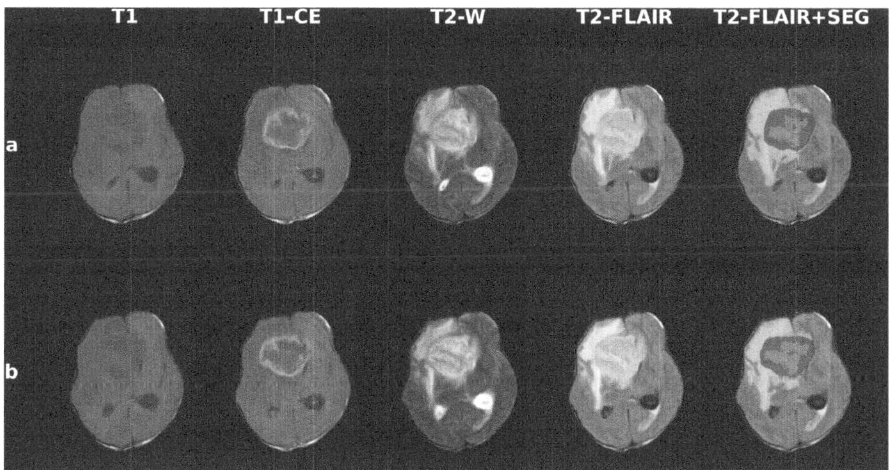

Fig. 1. Axial slices of multi-parametric MRI sequences from the BraTS-Africa dataset. (a) Original sample (BraTS-SSA-00007-000).(b) Augmented version of (a) using segmentation-aware offline data augmentation. Columns show T1, T1CE, T2-W, T2-FLAIR, and T2-FLAIR with segmentation overlay, where the ET, TC and WT are represented in blue, red, and green respectively. (Color figure online)

Complementing the whole-brain transformations, the label-mask transform applied elastic deformation exclusively within the tumor regions. This preserved the structural integrity of surrounding brain tissue while introducing controlled morphological variability to the tumor shape and boundary. In contrast to conventional elastic transforms that distort the entire brain volume and often produce unrealistic anatomical changes, our approach confines variability to regions where it is clinically meaningful for segmentation.

2.3 Models

Multiple segmentation models were selected to explore how variations in their strengths contribute to brain tumor segmentation. All models were trained using the nnU-Net framework to utilize its streamlined pipeline for data preprocessing, training, and inference. Additionally, an ensemble of the selected models was implemented to harness the distinct advantages of each architecture.

SegMamba: SegMamba is a novel 3D medical image segmentation model that incorporates a U-shaped architecture with Mamba, a state space model designed for long-range dependency modelling [24]. Unlike transformer-based approaches, SegMamba can efficiently capture both global and multiscale features from an entire input volumetric space with less computational overhead. The architecture consists of a 3D encoder with multiple Tri-orientated Spatial Mamba (TSMamba) blocks for multiscale global feature modelling, a convolution-based decoder, and skip connections with Feature-level Uncertainty Estimation (FUE) modules to refine features from the encoder that are fed to the upsampling path.

MedNeXt: MedNeXt is a fully convolutional segmentation model that employs ConvNeXt blocks in its encoder and decoder, combining the inherent inductive bias of convolutional networks with the scalable design principles of Transformer architectures [21]. The model replaces conventional upsampling and downsampling layers with residual inverted bottlenecks to preserve semantic feature details, leverages an upsampling-based kernel to smoothly transfer pretrained weights from smaller to larger kernels, and supports compound scaling in depth, width, and kernel size for flexible adaptability across diverse segmentation tasks. In this study, the MedNeXt medium variant with a kernel size of 3 was utilized.

Residual-Encoder U-NET: Residual-Encoder U-Net is a derivative of the original nnU-Net framework that introduces residual connections into the encoder pathway [25]. This architectural network replaces the plain convolutional blocks in the encoder with residual blocks, which reinforce feature representations and gradient flow in deep networks. The decoder structure and overall topology remain consistent with the standard implementation, ensuring compatibility with the self-adapting configuration pipeline of nnU-Net. This modification helps improve learning efficiency and model performance, particularly in deep networks, and it is well-suited for challenging segmentation tasks such as brain tumor segmentation, where detecting subtle variations in tumor appearance is important.

2.4 Experiments

A series of experiments were conducted to evaluate the performance of our selected models on the BraTS-Africa dataset along with the augmented datasets. Each model was initially trained from scratch for 50 epochs using the original BraTS-Africa dataset. Training continued for 500, and then a 1000 epochs using the best saved model weights checkpoint to assess the impact of extended training durations on segmentation performance. All models were trained in a 5-fold cross validation manner, using a composite loss function of Dice and Cross-Entropy loss to balance region-level and voxel-wise accuracy. Stochastic Gradient Descent (SGD) was employed as the optimizer, with a cosine annealing learning rate schedule initialized at 1e-4.

In creating the offline augmented dataset, transformations were applied 5 times per sample to the training set, forming a total of 300 cases.

Segmentation performance was evaluated using standard metrics, including Lesion-Wise Dice (LSD) and Normalized Surface Distance (NSD) at 1.00 mm for the Enhancing Tumor (ET), Non-enhancing Tumor Core (TC), and Whole Tumor (WT) subregions. Model predictions on the 35 validation cases were submitted to the synapse platform for evaluation.

3 Results

3.1 Segmentation Performance

Tables 1 and 2 summarize the segmentation performance of SegMamba, MedNeXt, Residual-Encoder U-Net, and the ensemble across different training configurations on the validation set.

Test Set Performance: The final ensemble was evaluated on the BraTS-Africa 2025 test set. The evaluation reported the mean and standard deviation of the Lesion-wise Dice (LSD) and Normalized Surface Distance (NSD) at 1.00 mm across the tumor subregions. For LSD, the model achieved ET $= 0.893 \pm 0.10$, TC $= 0.904 \pm 0.12$, and WT $= 0.918 \pm 0.15$. Corresponding NSD scores were ET $= 0.890 \pm 0.10$, TC $= 0.847 \pm 0.14$, and WT $= 0.867 \pm 0.13$ (Fig. 2).

Table 1. Results of the experiments comparing individual model performance (LSD - Lesion-Wise Dice and NSD_1.0 mm - Normalized Surface Distance at 1.00 mm) across the tumor subregions Enhancing Tumor (ET), Tumor Core (TC), and Whole Tumor (WT), as well as their overall average (AVG), under different training durations and settings. Each method is denoted by its initial: S for SegMamba, M for MedNeXt, and R for Residual-Encoder U-Net, followed by the corresponding training configuration. Best results per column are in **Bold**.

Method	LSD				NSD_1.0 mm			
	ET	TC	WT	AVG	ET	TC	WT	AVG
S_{50e}	0.796	0.790	0.877	0.821	0.786	0.714	0.777	0.759
M_{50e}	0.799	0.794	0.879	0.824	0.793	0.729	0.790	0.771
R_{50e}	0.791	0.787	0.881	0.820	0.777	0.704	0.783	0.755
${S^{aug}}_{50e}$	0.799	0.785	0.871	0.818	0.761	0.770	0.699	0.743
${M^{aug}}_{50e}$	0.804	0.790	0.887	0.827	0.782	0.715	0.776	0.758
${R^{aug}}_{50e}$	0.791	0.783	0.857	0.810	0.835	0.770	**0.823**	0.809
S_{500e}	0.806	0.790	0.892	0.829	0.795	0.717	0.797	0.770
M_{500e}	0.836	0.831	**0.912**	0.860	0.789	0.725	0.778	0.764
R_{500e}	0.801	0.798	0.866	0.822	0.789	0.725	0.778	0.764
S_{1000e}	0.801	0.781	0.893	0.825	0.792	0.715	0.801	0.769
M_{1000e}	**0.855**	**0.844**	0.896	**0.865**	**0.846**	**0.775**	0.808	**0.810**
R_{1000e}	0.800	0.796	0.864	0.820	0.790	0.726	0.778	0.765
${M^{aug}}_{1000e}$	0.836	0.838	0.876	0.850	0.831	0.775	0.775	0.794

Table 2. Results of the ensemble experiments (LSD - Lesion-Wise Dice and NSD_1.0 mm - Normalized Surface Distance at 1.00 mm) across the tumor subregions Enhancing Tumor (ET), Tumor Core (TC), and Whole Tumor (WT), as well as their overall average (AVG). Ensembles are denoted by listing their constituent models: S (SegMamba), M (MedNeXt), and R (Residual-Encoder U-Net). Best results are in **Bold**.

Ensemble Method	LSD				NSD_1.0 mm			
	ET	TC	WT	AVG	ET	TC	WT	AVG
$S + M + R_{50e}$	0.795	0.787	0.881	0.821	0.787	0.717	0.791	0.765
$S + M + R_{500e}$	0.846	0.843	0.896	0.861	0.839	0.775	0.812	0.809
$S + M + R_{1000e}$	0.857	0.842	0.883	0.861	0.847	0.772	0.798	0.806
$S + M_{1000e}$	0.824	0.810	0.895	0.843	0.814	0.740	0.806	0.787
$M + R_{1000e}$	**0.860**	**0.846**	0.897	**0.867**	**0.852**	**0.780**	0.812	**0.815**
$M + R + {M^{aug}}_{1000e}$	0.848	0.843	**0.898**	0.863	0.843	**0.780**	**0.816**	0.813

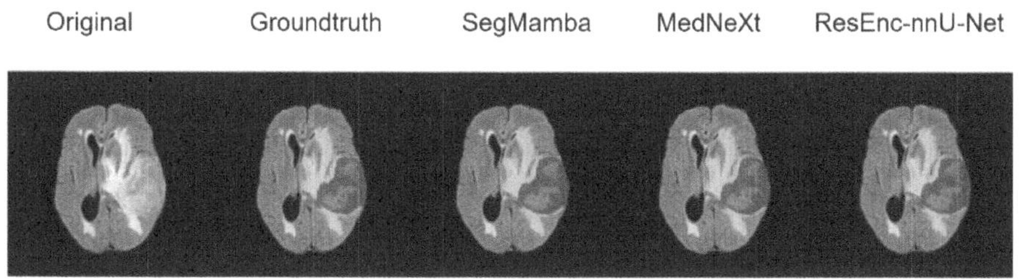

Fig. 2. Predictions of the three tumor subregions (TC in red, ET in blue, WT in green) by each of the models. Order of images: Original, Ground truth, SegMamba, MedNeXt, Residual-Encoder U-Net, from sample BraTS-SSA-00141-000. (Color figure online)

4 Discussion and Conclusion

This study investigated the segmentation performance of three distinct deep learning models, MedNeXt, SegMamba, and ResEnc U-Net and their ensemble, on the BraTS-Africa dataset under varying training setups. The findings reveal that the model architecture, augmentation approach, training configuration and integration strategy play a significant role in determining segmentation accuracy, particularly within data-limited and anatomically diverse cases.

Training duration had a notable impact on model performance. Across all architectures, extending training epochs generally led to improved segmentation results. This trend was apparent in the MedNeXt model, which recorded the highest average LSD of **0.865** and NSD of **0.810** at 1000 epochs (M_{1000e}). Interestingly, the best WT segmentation performance in terms of LSD, with a score of **0.912**, was achieved by the MedNeXt-model trained for 500 epochs (M_{500e}). This suggests that optimal performance on individual tumor subregions may not always correlate linearly with increased training duration. In contrast, SegMamba showed diminishing results beyond 500 epochs, suggesting that optimal training duration may vary depending on architectural characteristics and convergence behavior.

We performed statistical significance testing on the in-training validation set of fold-0, using per-patient results from the 1000-epoch runs. Across the three architectures, MedNeXt achieved the highest mean Dice scores for ET and WT, whereas Residual Encoder U-Net slightly surpassed it for TC. However, paired t-tests indicated that these differences were not statistically significant ($p > 0.05$), except for the TC subregion where Residual-Encoder U-Net significantly outperformed SegMamba ($p = 0.042$). SegMamba demonstrated competitive performance, particularly in WT segmentation, but its differences with MedNeXt ($p = 0.849$) and Residual Encoder U-Net ($p = 0.985$) were not significant. Overall, the models performed comparably across tumor subregions, suggesting that observed variations in mean performance should be interpreted with caution.

The segmentation-aware augmented dataset yielded NSD improvements for some models compared to their baselines. The $R^{aug}{}_{50e}$ recorded NSD scores of **0.835**, **0.770**, and **0.823** for ET, TC, and WT respectively, with its WT score being the highest among all models and its average NSD increasing from **0.755** to **0.809**. $S^{\text{aug}}{}_{50\text{e}}$ showed a notable increase in TC NSD, although its overall average NSD declined slightly. Meanwhile, $M^{\text{aug}}{}_{50\text{e}}$ exhibited a small decrease in average NSD, suggesting that augmentation may not consistently benefit all architectures. While its effects varied across models, the observed improvements highlight the benefit of targeted augmentation in improving boundary-level segmentation performance.

The ensemble models consistently outperformed their individual counterparts in both LSD and NSD metrics, confirming the benefit of combining diverse architectural representations. The $M+R_{1000\text{e}}$ configuration achieved the highest average NSD of **0.815** and tied for the highest LSD of **0.867**. The Residual-Encoder U-Net was initially excluded from the ensemble (results indicated by $S+M_{1000\text{e}}$) based on the assumption that its standalone performance was inferior to the other models. However, its inclusion was later shown to enhance overall ensemble performance, suggesting that it contributed meaningfully to the final predictions. Another noteworthy observation was that, although SegMamba achieved competitive standalone performance, its removal from the ensemble unexpectedly led to a slight improvement in overall results. This outcome suggests that not all high-performing models contribute positively when combined, and that ensemble behavior may depend on how different architectures how they interpret MRI modalities differently, as shown by Ren et al. [26]. Future work should examine how these differences affect ensemble performance. Collectively, these findings suggest that integrating multiple architectures produces a more balanced and generalizable model and highlights its potential for use in clinical contexts where these attributes are essential.

Although increasing training duration generally improved model performance, the variation in fold usage and training epochs from 50 to 1000 may have led to unstable learning in certain configurations. A more uniform strategy, such as training all models on the same folds and applying a cosine annealing schedule with warm restarts, could have yielded smoother convergence and better generalization. Future work can explore such dynamic scheduling approaches to stabilize training across folds and enhance performance without significantly increasing runtime.

Overall, the findings demonstrate that brain tumor segmentation performance is influenced by the type of model architecture, training configuration, augmentation strategy, and ensemble learning. Leveraging these factors collectively in this study supports the development of robust brain tumor segmentation models with improved generalizability, suitable for deployment in Sub-Saharan Africa and other resource-limited medical imaging settings.

Acknowledgments. The authors would like to thank the following instructors of the Sprint AI Training for African Medical Imaging Knowledge Translation (SPARK) Academy 2025 summer school on deep learning in medical imaging for providing insightful background knowledge on brain tumors that informed the research presented here; Noha Magdy, Maruf Adewole, Ayomidale B. Oladele, Amal Saleh, Nourou Dine Bankole, Jeremiah Fadugba, Iorumbur Moses Aondona, Toufiq Musah, Teresa Zhu,

Craig Jones, Confidence Raymond, Lukman E. Ismaila, Ugumba Kikwima, Mehdi Astaraki, Peter Hastreiter, Evan Calabrese, Esin Uzturk Isik, Navodini Wijethilake, Rancy Chepchirchir, James Gee, MacLean Nasrallah, Jean Baptiste Poline, Bijay Adhikari, Kenneth Agu, Mohannad Barakat & Yahoo Liu. The authors would also like to thank Linshan Liu for administrative assistance in supporting the SPARK Academy training and capacity-building activities, which the authors immensely benefited from. The authors acknowledge the computational infrastructure support from the Digital Research Alliance of Canada (The Alliance) and the University of Washington Azure GenAI for Science Hub through The eScience Institute and Microsoft (PI: Mehmet Kurt) secured for the SPARK Academy. Finally, we would like to thank the Lacuna Fund for Health and Equity, the Radiological Society of North America (RSNA), the Research & Education (R&E) Foundation Derek Harwood-Nash International Education Scholar Grant, the McGill University Healthy Brain and Healthy Lives (HBHL) and the National Science and Engineering Research Council of Canada (NSERC) Discovery Launch Supplement for making the SPARK Academy possible via research grant supports.

Disclosure of Interests. The authors have no competing interests to declare that are relevant to the content of this article

References

1. Ferreira, A., et al.: How we won brats 2023 adult glioma challenge? just faking it! enhanced synthetic data augmentation and model ensemble for brain tumour segmentation. arXiv preprint arXiv:2402.17317 (2024)
2. Bhimavarapu, U., Chintalapudi, N., Battineni, G.: Brain tumor detection and categorization with segmentation of improved unsupervised clustering approach and machine learning classifier. Bioengineering **11**(3), 266 (2024)
3. Louis, D.N., et al.: The 2016 world health organization classification of tumors of the central nervous system: a summary. Acta Neuropathol. **131**(6), 803–820 (2016)
4. Neetha, K.S., Narayan, D.L.: Segmentation and classification of brain tumour using LRIFCM and LSTM. Multimedia Tools Appli. **83**(31), 76705–76730 (2024)
5. Foster, B., et al.: A review on segmentation of positron emission tomography images. Comput. Biol. Med. **50**, 76–96 (2014)
6. Huang, S.-Y., et al.: Fully convolutional network for the semantic segmentation of medical images: a survey. Diagnostics **12**(11), 2765 (2022)
7. Kamnitsas, K., et al.: Efficient multi-scale 3D CNN with fully connected CRF for accurate brain lesion segmentation. Med. Image Anal. **36**, 61–78 (2017)
8. Menze, B.H., et al.: The multimodal brain tumor image segmentation benchmark (BRATS). IEEE Trans. Med. Imaging **34**(10), 1993–2024 (2014)
9. Kelly, C.J., et al.: Key challenges for delivering clinical impact with artificial intelligence. BMC Med. **17**(1), 195 (2019)
10. Adewole, M., et al.: The brain tumor segmentation (brats) challenge 2023: Glioma segmentation in sub-saharan africa patient population (bratsafrica). arXiv–2305 (2023)
11. Adewole, M., et al.: The BraTS-africa dataset: expanding the brain tumor segmentation data to capture african populations. Radiol. Artifi. Intell. **7**(4), e240528 (2025)

12. Bakas, S., et al.: Identifying the best machine learning algorithms for brain tumor segmentation, progression assessment, and overall survival prediction in the BRATS challenge. arXiv preprint arXiv:1811.02629 (2018)
13. Ronneberger, O., Fischer, P., Brox, T.: U-Net: convolutional networks for biomedical image segmentation. In: Navab, N., Hornegger, J., Wells, W.M., Frangi, A.F. (eds.) MICCAI 2015. LNCS, vol. 9351, pp. 234–241. Springer, Cham (2015). https://doi.org/10.1007/978-3-319-24574-4_28
14. Oktay, O., et al.: Attention u-net: Learning where to look for the pancreas. arXiv preprint arXiv:1804.03999 (2018)
15. Li, Z., et al.: Residual-attention UNet++: a nested residual-attention Unet for medical image segmentation. Appl. Sci. **12**(14), 7149 (2022)
16. Isensee, F., et al.: nnU-Net: a self-configuring method for deep learning based biomedical image segmentation. Nat. Methods **18**(2), 203–211 (2021)
17. Myronenko, A.: 3D MRI brain tumor segmentation using autoencoder regularization. In: Crimi, A., Bakas, S., Kuijf, H., Keyvan, F., Reyes, M., van Walsum, T. (eds.) BrainLes 2018. LNCS, vol. 11384, pp. 311–320. Springer, Cham (2019). https://doi.org/10.1007/978-3-030-11726-9_28
18. Isensee, F., Jäger, P.F., Full, P.M., Vollmuth, P., Maier-Hein, K.H.: nnU-net for brain tumor segmentation. In: Crimi, A., Bakas, S. (eds.) BrainLes 2020. LNCS, vol. 12659, pp. 118–132. Springer, Cham (2021). https://doi.org/10.1007/978-3-030-72087-2_11
19. Luu, H.M., Park, SH.: Extending nn-UNet for brain tumor segmentation. In: International MICCAI Brainlesion Workshop, pp. 173–186. Springer (2021). https://doi.org/10.1007/978-3-031-09002-8_16
20. Zeineldin, R.A., Karar, M.E., Burgert, O., Mathis-Ullrich, F.: Multimodal CNN networks for brain tumor segmentation in MRI: A BraTS 2022 Challenge Solution. In: Bakas, S., et al. (eds.) BrainLes 2022. LNCS, vol 13769. Springer, Cham (2023). https://doi.org/10.1007/978-3-031-33842-7_11
21. Roy, S. et al.: MedNeXt: transformer-driven scaling of ConvNets for medical image segmentation. In: Greenspan, H., et al. (eds.) MICCAI 2023. LNCS, vol. 14223. Springer, Cham (2023). https://doi.org/10.1007/978-3-031-43901-8_39
22. Gu, A., Dao, T.: Mamba: Linear-time sequence modeling with selective state spaces. arXiv preprint arXiv:2312.00752 (2023)
23. Pérez-García, F., Sparks, R., Ourselin, S.: TorchIO: a Python library for efficient loading, preprocessing, augmentation and patch-based sampling of medical images in deep learning. Comput. Methods Programs Biomed. **208**, 106236 (2021)
24. Xing, Z., Ye, T., Yang, Y., Liu, G., Zhu, L.: SegMamba: long-range sequential modeling mamba for 3D medical image segmentation. In: Linguraru, M.G., et al. (eds.) MICCAI 2024. LNCS, vol. 15008. Springer, Cham (2024). https://doi.org/10.1007/978-3-031-72111-3_54
25. Ji, K., Wu, Z., Han, J., Jia, J., Zhai, G., Liu, J.: Application of 3D nnU-Net with residual encoder in the 2024 MICCAI head and neck tumor segmentation challenge. In: Wahid, K.A., Dede, C., Naser, M.A., Fuller, C.D. (eds.) HNTSMRG 2024. LNCS, vol. 15273. Springer, Cham (2025). https://doi.org/10.1007/978-3-031-83274-1_20
26. Ren, T., et al.: Here Comes the Explanation: A Shapley Perspective on Multi-contrastMedical Image Segmentation. arXiv preprint arXiv:2504.04645 (2025)

Training Beyond Convergence: Grokking nnU-Net for Glioma Segmentation in Sub-Saharan MRI

Mohtady Barakat[1](✉), Omar Salah[1], Ahmed Yasser[1], Mostafa Ahmed[1], Zahirul Arief[1], Waleed Khan[1], Dong Zhang[2,3], Aondona Iorumbur[4], Confidence Raymond[3,5,6], Mohannad Barakat[7], and Noha Magdy[7]

[1] Faculty of Engineering, Multimedia University, Cyberjaya, Selangor, Malaysia
barakat.mohtady@gmail.com
[2] Department of Electrical and Computer Engineering, University of British Columbia, Vancouver, Canada
[3] Montreal Neurological Institute, McGill University, Montreal, QC, Canada
[4] Department of Physics, Federal University of Technology Minna, Minna, Nigeria
[5] Department of Biomedical Engineering, McGill University, Montreal, Canada
[6] Medical Artificial Intelligence Laboratory, Lagos, Nigeria
[7] Department of Computer Science, Friedrich-Alexander-Universität, Erlangen, Germany

Abstract. Gliomas are placing an increasingly clinical burden on Sub-Saharan Africa (SSA). In the region, the median survival for patients remains under two years, and access to diagnostic imaging is extremely limited. These constraints highlight an urgent need for automated tools that can extract the maximum possible information from each available scan, tools that are specifically trained on local data, rather than adapted from high-income settings where conditions are vastly different. We utilize the Brain Tumor Segmentation (BraTS) Africa 2025 Challenge dataset, an expert annotated collection of glioma MRIs. Our objectives are: (i) establish a strong baseline with nnUNet on this dataset, and (ii) explore whether the celebrated "grokking" phenomenon an abrupt, late training jump from memorization to superior generalization can be triggered to push performance without extra labels. We evaluate two training regimes. The first is a fast, budget-conscious approach that limits optimization to just a few epochs, reflecting the constrained GPU resources typically available in African institutions. Despite this limitation, nnUNet achieves strong Dice scores: 92.3% for whole tumor (WH), 86.6% for tumor core (TC), and 86.3% for enhancing tumor (ET). The second regime extends training well beyond the point of convergence, aiming to trigger a grokking-driven performance leap. With this approach, we were able to achieve grokking and enhanced our results to higher Dice scores: 92.2% for whole tumor (WH), 90.1% for tumor core (TC), and 90.2% for enhancing tumor (ET).

Keywords: nnUNet · BraTS · model grokking · Glioma · MRI · Africa

M. Barakat and O. Salah\x97Equal contribution.

S. Bakas et al. (Eds.): MICCAI 2025, LNCS 16376, pp. 307–317, 2026.
https://doi.org/10.1007/978-3-032-16365-3_28

1 Introduction

Brain tumors constitute a significant global health burden, with more than 300,000 new cases and 250,000 deaths recorded worldwide in 2020 alone [1]. Within this group, gliomas represent the second most common primary brain neoplasm, accounting for roughly one-quarter of all cases, and are responsible for the vast majority of malignant presentations [2].

Magnetic Resonance Imaging (MRI) plays a central role in neuro-oncology, offering rich, multiparametric views of brain tumors through sequences like T1-weighted (T1), T1 post- contrast, T2-weighted (T2), and Fluid-Attenuated Inversion Recovery (FLAIR). These scans capture different aspects of tumor structure and behavior, making MRI an essential tool for diagnosis, treatment planning, and monitoring. However, transforming these detailed images into precise, usable measurements still depends heavily on manual effort. Experts often spend over an hour per case carefully outlining tumor regions, and even then, results can vary significantly between individuals [3]. Automated segmentation promises to relieve this burden.

The Brain Tumor Segmentation (BraTS) Challenge has played a pivotal role in advancing machine learning (ML) applications for glioma diagnosis, by providing open-access MRI data, expert annotations, and standardized evaluation metrics. However, it remains uncertain whether ML models trained on BraTS data primarily from high-income settings can generalize to clinical environments in Sub-Saharan Africa [4, 5]. Challenges such as fewer annotated cases, lower-resolution imaging, and differing clinical workflows raise important concerns about model transferability [6], In this study, we address these gaps by leveraging the newly released BraTS-Africa dataset [6], designed specifically to reflect the realities of Sub-Saharan clinical imaging.

1.1 Related Works

Maruf Adewole [6] implemented an nnU-Net approach for glioma brain tumour segmentation on the BraTS 2021 dataset. Furthermore, Zhao et al. [7] tested whether a BraTS 2021 Challenge (BraTS-GLI 2021) champion-grade nnU-Net method can be adapted to the lower resolution MRIs common in SSA and reflected in the BraTS-Africa Challenge. They compared three regimes: (i) training only on the small BraTS-Africa cohort, (ii) training solely on the 1,251 high-quality BraTS-GLI 2021 cases, and (iii) pre-training on the high-quality data followed by fine-tuning on the African scans. Only the transfer-and-fine-tune strategy generalized well, achieving Dice scores of 0.926 (whole tumor), 0.882 (enhancing tumor) and 0.840 (tumor core). Adding a $\times 2$ super-resolution module did not improve segmentation, which the authors attribute to information lost at acquisition rather than to simple resolution limits [14].

Amod et al. [8] rebuilt a 2022 BraTS runner-up pipeline and evaluated four data setups: Sub-Saharan scans only (BraTS-Africa), high-quality scans only (BraTS-GLI 2021), a merged set of both datasets, and a high-quality model fine-tuned on the BraTS-Africa data. As in Zhao's work, the pre-trained plus fine-tuned variant outperformed models trained solely on the limited low-quality data, which over-fitted, while models trained only on high-quality images under-segmented oedematous tissue in the African scans. The authors conclude that lightweight local adaptation, potentially via federated learning, offers a practical path to robust performance when data sharing is constrained [8].

1.2 Model Grokking

Power et al. [10] first described "grokking", a learning pattern in which a network trains for a long time, overfits its dataset, and then, after many more gradient steps, suddenly "gets" the underlying rule and its validation accuracy jumps to nearly 100 % without any change in hyperparameters. In their experiments, the phenomenon suggests that extra training can transform a shaky, memorizing model into a robust one and make it abandon its shortcut solutions. Although the original evidence comes from symbolic data, the idea invites exploration in more complex settings such as brain-tumor segmentation, motivating our decision to push nnU-NetV2 training far beyond conventional stopping points in search of a similar late-phase generalization boost.

1.3 nnU-Net and nnU-Netv2

nnU-Net or No New U-net [9] is a model that was created to adapt to the diverse medical datasets and problems available without the need for tailoring a very specific and manual configuration for each problem. By using nnU-Net's automatic configuration creation, non-experts can still use nnU-Net to train on their respective problem and have confidence that it will be among the best accuracies available. nnU-Net does this by the usage of a "fingerprint" extracted from the dataset and a collection of Fixed, Rule-Based and Empirical Parameters chosen at runtime and hardware specification that altogether result in an optimal configuration. For our case, we are using an updated version of nnU-Net, namely nnU-Netv2, for its unified trainer class that we will use to make some slight modifications, cross-platform support of CUDA, MPS, and CPU, flexibility of functionalities using their API calls, and a more user- friendly folder structure.

2 Methodology

2.1 Study Design and Rationale

For segmentation, we adopted nnU-Netv2 [9] in its three-dimensional (3D) full-resolution configuration. nnU-Net was designed to be flexible on all sorts of medical segmentation tasks which makes it perfect for our case. nnU-Net automatically tailors patch size, depth, and learning schedule to a given dataset, allowing us to concentrate on experimental design rather than hyper-parameter search. We decided to train for 2 different durations, one for 200 epochs and another extended one for 3,500 epochs, for grokking results. Our final hybrid model consists of 2 nnU-Net networks; the main run (200 epochs) an the grokking run (3,500 epochs).

All scans in the BraTS-Africa (SSA) cohort were processed as full 3D volumes. Each input to the model consisted of a 4-channel 3D tensor, where the spatial dimensions (x, y, z) represent the voxel grid and the four channels correspond to the T1, T1 post-contrast, T2, and FLAIR MRI sequences. Look at Fig. 1 for an illustration of such a tensor. This setup allows the model to leverage complementary information across sequences, enabling more accurate and robust tumor segmentation.

2.2 Dataset

The 2024 BraTS-Africa Challenge dataset was used in this study, consisting of 95 annotated glioma MRI cases, each with four MRI sequences and reference segmentation masks, labelled as the three tumor subregions alongside background (label 0): enhancing tumor (ET, label 1), tumor core (Non-enhancing tumor core) (TC, label 2), and whole tumor (Surrounding non-enhancing FLAIR hyperintensity) (WT, label 3) [14, 15]. Sixty cases were designated for training and internal validation. Of these, five were randomly withheld before processing for internal validation, and the remaining 55 were used for all model training. For the pre-submission evaluation, predictions were submitted for 35 validation cases provided without ground truth labels. All reported performance metrics are based on BraTS's evaluation of these 35 cases and the final testing dataset from the BraTS-Africa Challenge 2025.

2.3 Preprocessing Pipeline

All raw NIfTI volumes were used without manual modification. Key dataset properties such as voxel spacing, foreground intensity ranges, and median shape size were then analyzed to define a common resampling target and optimize patch and batch sizes for training. All images and corresponding segmentation masks were resampled to the same voxel spacing to ensure uniform physical resolution across the dataset.

Each MRI sequence was normalized independently using z-score normalization: brain voxels were centered by subtracting the mean and scaled by the standard deviation, while non-brain voxels retained a zero value to clearly distinguish background. This approach enables consistent intensity scaling across patients and sequences without the need for manual adjustments.

Training included a comprehensive set of spatial and intensity augmentations applied on-the-fly. These included random rotations, scaling, flipping, elastic deformations, brightness and contrast changes, gamma adjustments, Gaussian noise, and simulated low-resolution artifacts. Occasional small components were also removed from the label maps to improve robustness. The input data consisted of 3D voxel patches with all four MRI modalities stacked as channels and processed jointly for segmentation.

2.4 Training Configuration

We adopted nnU-Net v2 in its 3D full-resolution preset and left every internal hyper-parameter exactly as the framework generated it. Once the training data were analyzed, nnU-Net's heuristic planner produced a six-stage U-Net shown in Figure 1 with an initial feature width of 32, deep-supervision, and an input-patch size of $128 \times 160 \times 112$ voxels that comfortably fit into the 22.5 GB L4 memory. The optimizer remained the default stochastic gradient descent with Nesterov momentum ($\mu = 0.99$), a weight- decay of 3×10^{-5}, and a polynomial learning rate decay starting at 0.01 and annealing to zero by the final epoch as can be seen in Figure 2. The number of iterations per epoch is 300, 50 of them being for validation. The number of input channels is based on the number of modalities, which is 4.

Loss was the standard Dice + cross-entropy combination applied to each deep-supervision output, and mixed-precision training was enabled via NVIDIA's AMP. No manual overrides, layer additions, or schedule tweaks were introduced at any point; the configuration is therefore fully reproducible by invoking nnU-Net v2 with the same dataset and random seed. This was trained for 200 epochs. We also trained another version with the same configuration, but we trained for 3500 epochs for grokking.

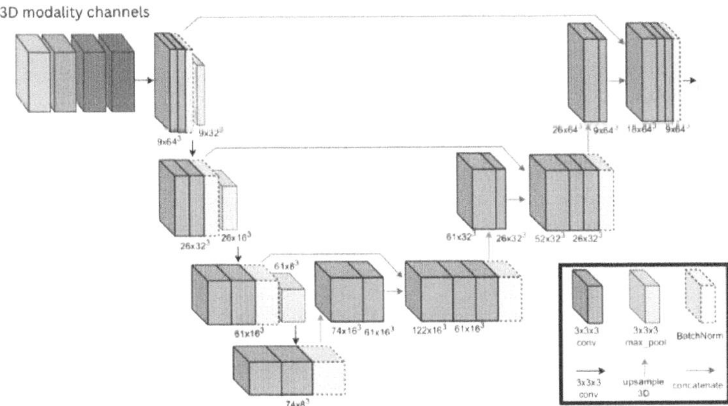

Fig. 1. Illustration of 3D voxel batches with modalities overlaid and input into the 3D Unet at full resolution

2.5 Training Baseline Run (200 Epochs)

The first experiment trained the network for 200 epochs on the 55-scan set. Batches were shuffled per epoch. Training was executed on a single NVIDIA L4 (22.5 GB) GPU, taking $\approx$ 100 s per epoch (wall-clock $\approx$ 6 h total).

2.6 Training Extended Grokking Run (3500 Epoch)

Motivated by recent observations that some networks "grok" (i.e., memories training data early yet require far longer to internalize the underlying rule set), we trained a model for 3,500 epochs. The learning rate scheduler was re-initialized to its starting value, and it was limited to a minimum value of 1×10^{-4} as shown in Fig. 2A. The average epoch time remained 100s, leading to an uninterrupted runtime of roughly five days. The loss progress for the start of the training compared with after grokking is shown in Fig. 3.

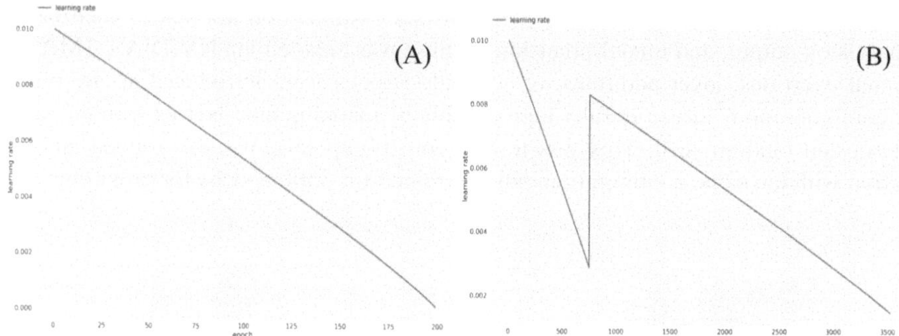

Fig. 2. (A) Learning rate graph of a 200-epoch baseline run. (B) Learning rate graph of 3,500 epoch Extended Grokking run.

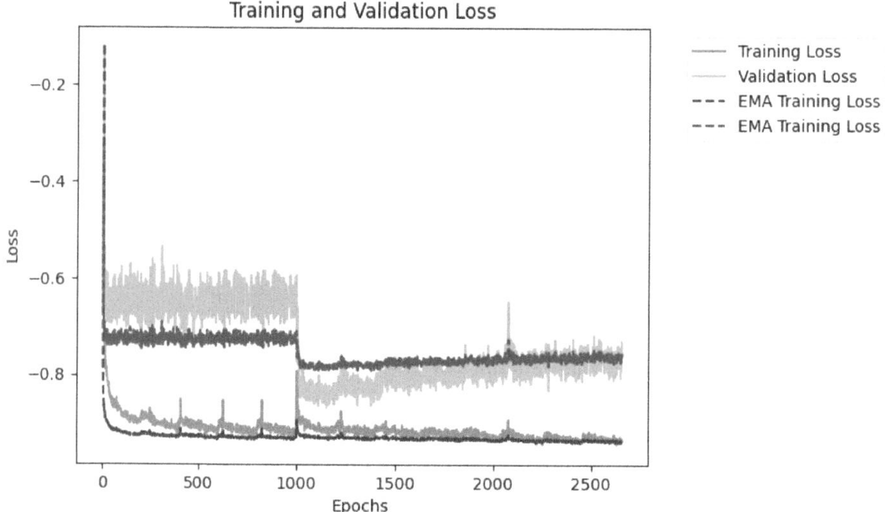

Fig. 3. Loss change over the training epochs. Training in 100 epochs, overfitting in 1000 epochs, and grokking after 1000 epoch

3 Results and Discussion

3.1 Main Run (200 Epoch)

The original nnU-Net recipe (full-resolution 3D) was quantitatively evaluated on the validation set of 35 BraTS MRI cases. Performance was assessed as the mean scores of the following two metrics across all 35 cases:

- Dice Coefficient: how much the predicted mask volume overlaps the ground truth.
- Normalised Surface Dice (NSD): how closely the surfaces match within a chosen tolerance.

Both metrics are shown per case (one score per subject) and Lesion-Wise (LW: each connected lesion is treated as a separate object; the metric is computed per lesion then averaged). Table 1 below presents relevant scores for the three relevant tumor sub-regions/classes. Note that NSD is computed for 1 mm and 0.5 mm and shown in Fig. 4.

Table 1. Mean scores for the three relevant tumor classes with standard deviation (for LW) for the main run (200 epochs)

Metric	Enhancing Tumor	Tumor Core	Whole Tumor
Dice coefficient	0.866	0.863	0.923
LW Dice	0.821 ± 0.257	0.816 ± 0.272	0.880 ± 0.208
NSD 0.5 mm	0.586	0.511	0.552
NSD 1.0 mm	0.851	0.777	0.836
LW NSD 0.5 mm	0.560 ± 0.219	0.498 ± 0.221	0.522 ± 0.178
LW NSD 1.0 mm	0.805 ± 0.266	0.736 ± 0.274	0.789 ± 0.207

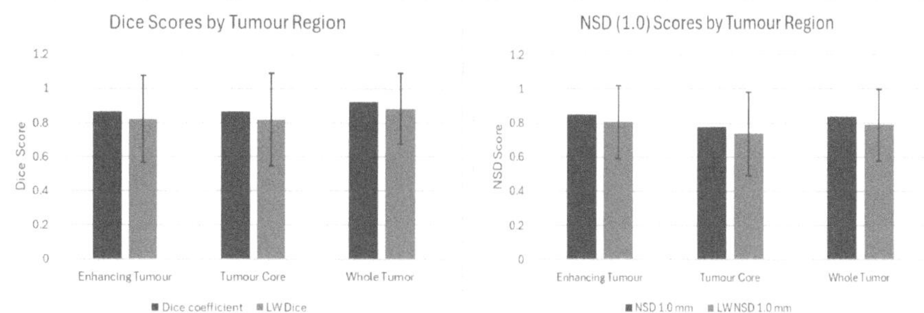

Fig. 4. Mean Dice scores and normalized surface Dice (NSD) at 1.00mm (including lesion-wise) by tumor region for the main run (200 epochs).

As illustrated in Figure 5, in every slice the model captures the three tumor sub-regions much like the ground-truth masks. But, in some cases it can overlook small Lesions. These scenes match the overall trend: the network is good at finding the bulk of each tumor but still misses some edges and tiny parts of the tumors.

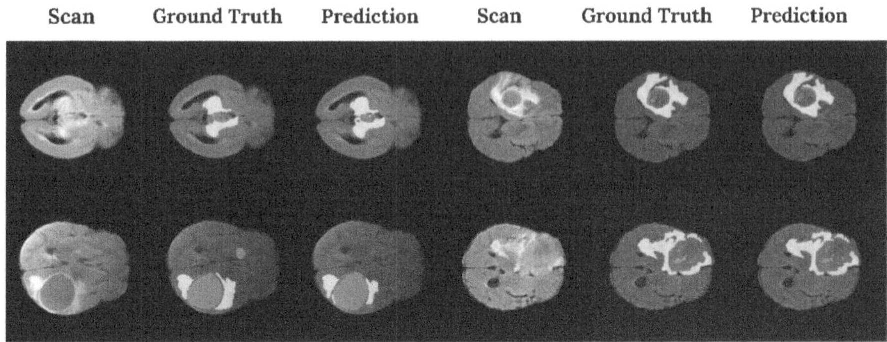

Fig. 5. An illustration of four different cases, each showing the acquired scans, the ground-truth mask, and our nnU-Net predictions for all three tumor sub-regions (red = tumor core, blue = enhancing tumor and the green = whole tumor.

3.2 Grokking Run (3500 Epoch)

The extended nnU-Net run, now trained for 3,500 epochs to explore grokking-style dynamics, was quantitatively evaluated on the same 35 cases. Each metric is reported per subject and in a lesion-wise (LW) view, where every connected tumor focus is treated as a separate object before averaging; the LW view therefore penalizes missed satellites and split errors more strongly than the per-case aggregate. Table 2 presents relevant scores for the 3 relevant classes. Additionally, Figure 6 below represents the grouped bar charts with the same figures.

Table 2. Mean scores for the 3 relevant classes with standard deviation (for LW) for the grokking run (3,500 epochs)

Metric	Enhancing Tumor	Tumor Core	Whole Tumor
Dice coefficient	0.902	0.901	0.922
LW Dice	0.860 ± 0.201	0.846 ± 0.228	0.874 ± 0.216
NSD 0.5 mm	0.622	0.551	0.541
NSD 1.0 mm	0.893	0.816	0.828
LW NSD 0.5 mm	0.582 ± 0.208	0.520 ± 0.225	0.513 ± 0.179
LW NSD 1 mm	0.837 ± 0.216	0.764 ± 0.244	0.780 ± 0.210

Comparing both networks shows that Grokking clearly benefits the enhancing tumor and tumor-core regions: Dice improves from 0.866 to 0.902 for ET and from 0.863 to 0.901 for TC, indicating sharper delineation of the clinically most critical compartments. For whole tumor, however, the 200-epoch model matches the 3 500- epoch version (0.923 versus 0.922).

These complementary strengths imply our hybrid model strategy: deploying the 3500-epoch network to segment ET and TC, while retaining the 200-epoch model for WT to yield the best overall segmentation.

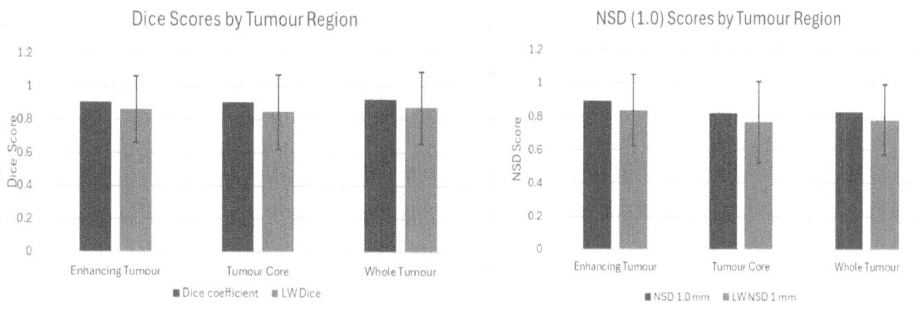

Fig. 6. Grouped bar charts for Dice scores by tumor region & NSD (1.0mm) by tumor region for the grokking run (3,500 epochs)

3.3 Hybrid Model (200 & 3500 Epoch Networks)

We tested and validated the hybrid model network on the BraTS-Africa 2025 validation cases (35 cases) and the BraTS-Africa 2025 test cases. Table 3 presents relevant scores for the 3 relevant classes. Additionally, Fig. 7 below represents the grouped bar charts with the same figures.

Table 3. Mean scores for the 3 relevant classes with standard deviation (for LW) for the hybrid network (3,500 & 200 epoch models)

Metric	Enhancing Tumor	Tumor Core	Whole Tumor
Dice coefficient	0.902	0.903	0.922
LW Dice	0.859 ± 0.182	0.831 ± 0.226	0.864 ± 0.209
NSD 0.5 mm	0.622	0.551	0.541
NSD 1.0 mm	0.891	0.817	0.829
LW NSD 0.5 mm	0.595 ± 0.187	0.516 ± 0.212	0.508 ± 0.165
LW NSD 1 mm	0.852 ± 0.180	0.761 ± 0.217	0.778 ± 0.182

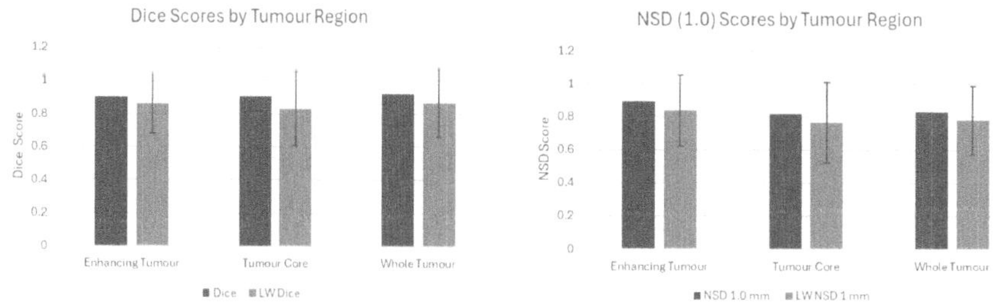

Fig. 7. Bar charts for Dice scores by tumor region & NSD (1.0mm) by tumor region for the hybrid model (3500-epoch network to segment ET and TC and the 200-epoch model for WT)

3.4 Test Cases

Running our model on the test cases dataset (Test cases of BraTS-Africa 2025) our model performed better as shown in Table 4.

Table 4. Mean scores for the 3 relevant classes with standard deviation (for LW) for the hybrid network (3,500 & 200 epoch models) on test cases

Metric	Enhancing Tumor	Tumor Core	Whole Tumor
LW Dice	0.854 ± 0.173	0.858 ± 0.181	0.913 ± 0.147
LW NSD 1 mm	0.866 ± 0.173	0.810 ± 0.196	0.848 ± 0.133

4 Conclusion

This study evaluated nnU-Netv2 on the BraTS-Africa 2025 dataset to establish a baseline for glioma segmentation on African MRI data and to explore whether prolonged training could trigger the "grokking" phenomenon. A standard 200-epoch run already achieved strong Dice and NSD scores, while extending training to 3,500 epochs further improved enhancing tumor and tumor core. Whole tumor performance remained largely unchanged, suggesting a trade-off where longer training sharpens critical subregions. These results provide a reproducible baseline and highlight resource-aware strategies for improving automated segmentation in Sub-Saharan clinical settings.

Acknowledgements. This work was part of the Sprint AI Training for African Medical Imaging Knowledge Translation (SPARK) Academy 2025 summer school on deep learning in medical imaging. The authors would like to thank the instructors of the summer for providing insightful background knowledge on brain tumours that informed the research presented here, most notably, Noha Magdy, Maruf Adewole, Ayomide B. Oladele, Amal Saleh, Nourou Dine Bankole, Jeremiah Fadugba, Teresa Zhu, Craig Jones, Charles Delahunt, Celia Cintas, Lukman E. Ismaila, Ugumba Kikwima, Mehdi Astaraki, Peter Hastreiter, Evan Calabrese, Esin Uzturk Isik, , Rancy Chepchirchir, James Gee, MacLean Nasrallah, Jean Baptiste Poline, Bijay Adhikari, Kenneth Agu, Mohannad Barakat & Yahoo Liu. The authors acknowledge the computational infrastructure support from the Digital Research Alliance of Canada (The Alliance) and the University of Washington Azure GenAI for Science Hub through the eScience Institute and Microsoft (PI: Mehmet Kurt) secured for the SPARK Academy. Finally, we thank the Lacuna Fund for Health and Equity (PI: Udunna Anazodo, 0508-S-001), the RSNA R&E Foundation (PI: Farouk Dako), McGill Heatly Brain and Healthy Lives (HBHL; Udunna Anazodo), as well as the National Science and Engineering Research Council of Canada (NSERC) Discovery Launch Supplement (PI: Udunna Anazodo, DGECR.

References

1. Sung, H., et al.: Global Cancer Statistics 2020: GLOBOCAN estimates of incidence and mortality worldwide for 36 cancers in 185 countries. CA: Can. J. Clinic. **71**(3), 209–249 (2021)
2. Ostrom, Q.T., et al.: CBTRUS statistical report: primary brain and other central nervous system tumors diagnosed in the United States, 2016–2020. Neuro-Oncology **25**(Suppl. 2), iv1–iv95 (2023)
3. Bondiau, P.-Y., et al.: Atlas-based automatic segmentation of MR images: validation study on the brainstem in radiotherapy context. Int. J. Radiat. Oncol. Biol. Phys. **61**(1), 289–298 (2005)
4. Adewole, M., et al.: The brain Tumor segmentation (BraTS) challenge 2023: glioma segmentation in Sub-Saharan Africa patient population (BraTS-Africa). arXiv [Preprint] (2023)
5. Zhang, D., Confidence, R., Anazodo, U.: Stroke lesion segmentation from low-quality and few-shot MRIs via similarity-weighted self-ensembling framework. In: Medical Image Computing and Computer Assisted Intervention – MICCAI 2022, Lecture Notes in Computer Science, vol. 13435, pp. 87–96 (2022)
6. Adewole, M., et al.: The BraTS-Africa dataset: expanding the brain Tumor segmentation data to capture African populations. Radiol.: Artif. Intell. **7**(4), e240528 (2025)
7. Zhao, Y., et al.: Transferring knowledge from high-quality to low-quality MRI for adult glioma diagnosis. arXiv:2410.18698, v2 (2024)
8. Amod, R., et al.: Bridging the gap: generalising state-of-the-art u-net models to Sub-Saharan African populations. arXiv:2312.11770, v1, 2023
9. Isensee, F., et al.: NnU-Net: a self-configuring method for deep learning-based biomedical image segmentation. Nat. Methods **18**(2), 203–211 (2021)
10. Power, A., Burda, Y., Edwards, H., Babuschkin, I., Misra, V.: Grokking: generalization beyond overfitting on small algorithmic datasets. arXiv:2201.02177 (2022)
11. Ceurstemont, S.: Training Neural Networks to Grok. Commun. ACM (2024)
12. Zhang, X., Li, Y., Wang, J.: Deep grokking: would deep neural networks generalize better? arXiv:2405.19454 (2024)
13. Chakraborty, S., Brahma, P.: Grokking at the edge of numerical stability. arXiv:2501.04697 (2025)
14. Bouget, D., Mahjoub, S., Solheim, O.: The BraTS-Africa challenge on brain tumor segmentation in Sub-Saharan Africa. arXiv preprint arXiv:2305.19369
15. Adewole, M., Rudie, J.D., Gbadamosi, A., et al.: The BraTS-Africa dataset: expanding the Brain Tumor Segmentation (BraTS) data to capture African populations. Radiol.: Artif. Intell. **2**

Robust Glioblastoma Segmentation Across Multi-modal MRI: A Study on BraTS 2025 Challenge, Task 5 (Sub-Saharan Africa)

Abbas Mohamed Rezk[1], Abdulkhalek Al-Fakih[1], Abdullah Shazly[1], Kanghyun Ryu[2](✉), and Mohammed A. Al-masni[1](✉)

[1] Department of Artificial Intelligence and Data Science, College of Artificial Intelligence Convergence, Sejong University, Seoul, Republic of Korea
{abbas.m,alfakih,abdullahshazli}@sju.ac.kr, m.almasani@sejong.ac.kr

[2] Intelligence and Interaction Research Center, Korea Institute of Science and Technology, Seoul, Republic of Korea
khryu@kist.re.kr

Abstract. Accurate segmentation of glioblastoma's distinct regions is vital for treatment planning but remains challenging, especially in datasets from low-resource settings. This paper presents our submission to the BraTS-Lighthouse 2025 Challenge (Task 5: Sub-Saharan Africa Adult Glioma Segmentation), which addresses heterogeneous multi-institutional mpMRI scans from the sub-Saharan African population. We extend the U-Net architecture with three dedicated decoders to segment non-overlapping tumor regions: surrounding non-enhancing FLAIR hyperintensity (SNFH), non-enhancing tumor core (NETC), and enhancing tumor (ET). Each decoder specializes in its region, supported by an attention mechanism that emphasizes the most relevant MRI sequences—for example, T2 and FLAIR for SNFH, T1 and T1ce for NETC and ET—enhancing region-specific feature learning. Evaluated on the BraTS-Africa 2025 validation set, our approach outperforms state-of-the-art baselines, including optimized and tuned U-Net achieving an average lesion-wise dice of 0.846, demonstrating robust and precise tumor delineation in this underserved and diverse population.

Keywords: Brain Tumor Segmentation · Attention mechanism · Multiple pathways

1 Introduction

Gliomas are the most common type of brain tumors in humans [1] characterized on MRI by three essential tissue types: Surrounding Non-Enhancing FLAIR Hyperintensity (SNFH), Enhancing Tumor (ET), and Non-Enhancing Tumor Core (NETC). Accurate delineation of these regions is critical for robust tumor assessment in both research and clinical settings. SNFH typically appears as hyperintense regions on T2/FLAIR imaging, reflecting non-enhancing tumor and peritumoral abnormality, while ET and NETC are

S. Bakas et al. (Eds.): MICCAI 2025, LNCS 16376, pp. 318–327, 2026.
https://doi.org/10.1007/978-3-032-16365-3_29

identified through post-contrast and native T1-weighted sequences, respectively [2, 3]. Manual segmentation of tumor subregions, although the gold standard, is labor-intensive and subject to significant variability. As a result, automated segmentation solutions have become increasingly central for large-scale studies and clinical work-flows.

Recent advances in deep learning, particularly adaptations of the U-Net architecture and innovations from the BraTS challenge community, have led to notable improvements in brain tumor segmentation accuracy and reproducibility, providing robust benchmarks for the development and evaluation of new approaches. Models like 3D U-Net [4], V-Net [5], and UNet ++ [6] have improved volumetric data processing. Although transformer-based models like Swin UNETR [7] show promise, nnU-Net [8] remains state-of-the-art, outperforming newer architectures when properly configured [9]. Meanwhile, the BraTS challenge has driven progress in brain tumor segmentation, with U-Net derivatives dominating since 2015. In 2018, Myronenko [10] enhanced U-Net with asymmetric residual blocks, improving information flow and winning BraTS. In 2019, a cascaded U-Net [11] refined segmentation via a two-stage model. In 2020, nnU-Net automated preprocessing and hyperparameter tuning, securing first place. In 2021, the winning model added an asymmetric contracting path, and group normalization to the nnU-Net [12]. Another approach deepened the encoder, increased filter channels, and added dual deep supervision, winning the validation phase [13]. In 2022, a standalone nnU-Net variant with more decoder channels, trilinear upsampling, and 10-model cross-validation won validation and ranked second in testing [14]. An ensemble combining the 2021 winner, DeepSeg, and DeepScan secured first in testing [15–17]. In 2023, the winning approach used GANs [18] and registration for data augmentation, integrating nnU-Net [19], Swin UNETR [7], and the 2021 winner [12] to combine convolutional and transformer strengths.

In this challenge submission, we introduce a robust deep learning framework for automatic segmentation of glioblastoma subregions, specifically developed for the BraTS-Lighthouse 2025 Challenge, Task 5, which focuses on multi-institutional MRI data from sub-Saharan Africa. Our architecture employs a multi-decoder extension of the U-Net, with each decoder focused on a non-overlapping tumor region: Sur-rounding Non-Enhancing FLAIR Hyperintensity (SNFH), Enhancing Tumor (ET), and Non-Enhancing Tumor Core (NETC), as defined by the BraTS-Africa labeling protocol. Each decoder branch is optimized for its target region using information from the most informative MRI sequences, promoting specialized learning and reducing label confusion. To enhance region-specific accuracy, an attention mechanism is incorporated, enabling the network to dynamically focus on salient features from the input modalities.

Evaluated on the BraTS-Africa 2025 validation set, our method demonstrates superior segmentation performance compared to strong baseline models, including optimized U-Net and tuned U-Net. Our results highlight the framework's adaptability to real-world African datasets, which often present unique challenges in terms of scanner variation and imaging artifacts. All implementation code and trained models are publicly available on GitHub[1].

2 Materials and Methods

2.1 Datasets

BraTS 2025 Adult Glioma Pre-tratment Training Dataset [20–25]. This dataset includes 1,251 annotated multi-parametric MRI (mpMRI) scans, including T1, T1ce, T2, FLAIR sequences. Ground truth labels are provided for three non-overlapping tumor subregions: SNFH, NETC, ET. The scans were acquired across diverse protocols and scanners, co-registered to a unified template, skull-stripped, and resampled to 1 mm3 isotropic resolution. This dataset was used to train both our challenge submission model and all baseline models used for comparison.

BraTS 2025 Challenge on Sub-Sahara-Africa Adult Glioma training Dataset [26]. The dataset features 60 cases with annotated mpMRI scans (T1, T1ce, T2, FLAIR) with labels for SNFH, NETC, ET. They were acquired from multiple institutions using a variety of MRI scanners and protocols, resulting in considerable heterogeneity representative of real-world African imaging cohorts. All scans have been preprocessed: co-registered to a standard anatomical template, skull-stripped, and resampled to isotropic 1mm3 resolution. This dataset was used to train both our challenge submission model and all baseline models used for comparison.

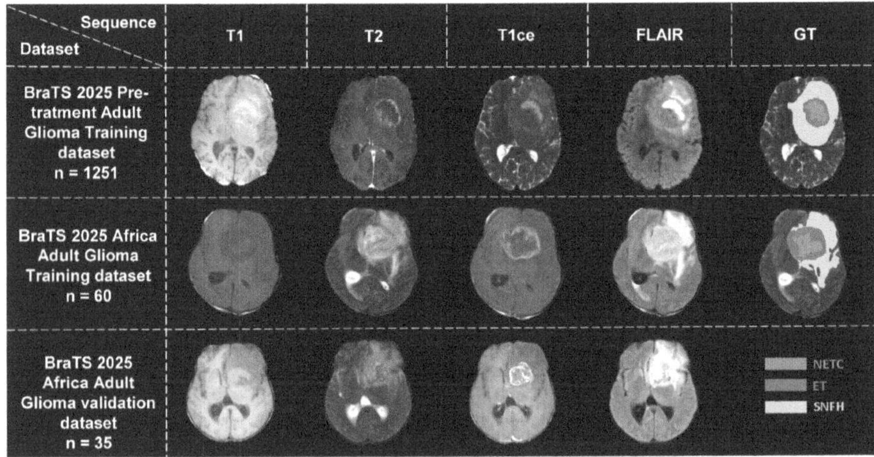

Fig. 1. Illustration of a representative case from each dataset we used in our submission. For the BraTS Africa validation set, ground truth labels are withheld, and evaluation metrics are accessible only via the Synapse challenge portal.

BraTs 2025 Challenge on Sub-Sahara-Africa Adult Glioma Validation Dataset [26]. The validation dataset consists of 35 annotated mpMRI cases, each including T1, T1ce, T2, FLAIR sequences. Ground truth labels for the tumor subregions (SNFH, NETC, and ET) are not publicly available to participants. Instead, segmentation results are submitted through the official BraTS challenge portal, where evaluation scores are computed and returned automatically. This dataset was used to assess the performance of our proposed method and compare it against strong baseline models, as summarized in Table 1. An example case from each dataset used in this study is depicted in Fig. 1.

Data Preparation. Input tensor volumes with dimensions $4 \times 240 \times 240 \times 155$ (corresponding to the four MRI modalities) underwent zero-background cropping to reduce computational load and remove empty spatial regions. Each modality was normalized channel-wise by computing the mean and standard deviation over non-zero voxels to counteract intensity variations across scanners and protocols, standardizing the inputs for training stability. To aid the model in differentiating brain tissue from background, an additional foreground mask channel was appended using one-hot encoding. Training data augmentation was employed to enhance model robustness and generalization, including biased cropping with a 40% probability to preferentially include regions containing tumors, random spatial zooming with scale factors between 1.0 and 1.4, axis-aligned flipping along all spatial axes, additive Gaussian noise with standard deviation σ sampled uniformly between 0 and 0.33, Gaussian blur with kernels ranging from 0.5 to 1.5 in size, and brightness and contrast adjustments scaling intensities in ranges $0.7 - 1.3\times$ and $0.65 - 1.5\times$, respectively. This comprehensive preprocessing and augmentation pipeline ensures effective handling of the heterogeneous, multi-modal MRI data and improves the model's resilience to varied clinical imaging conditions.

2.2 Proposed Architecture

The proposed architecture consists of three key components: a backbone, multi-path decoders and attention mechanism.

Backbone. The backbone of our framework is a 3D U-Net characterized by a symmetric U-shape architecture, consisting of an encoder (contracting path) and a decoder (ex-panding path). The encoder transforms the input volume into a lower-dimensional representation via a modular structure comprising repeated convolutional blocks. This backbone has a depth of six layers, with the number of convolutional filters increasing at each layer as follows: 64, 96, 128, 192, 256, and 384. Each encoder block contains two sub-blocks. The first sub-block reduces the spatial dimensions of the feature map by a factor of two using a $3 \times 3 \times 3$ convolutional layer with a stride of $2 \times 2 \times 2$, followed by instance normalization and a Leaky ReLU activation with a negative slope of 0.01. The second sub-block applies a similar set of operations with a $3 \times 3 \times 3$ convolutional layer but with a stride of $1 \times 1 \times 1$. This process is repeated, and when the spatial dimensions are reduced to $4 \times 4 \times 4$, the decoder phase begins. The decoder is similarly modular and aims to reconstruct spatial dimensions by processing encoded feature maps. Each decoder block consists of three sub-blocks: first, a trilinear upsampling layer doubles the spatial resolution; next, the upsampled features are concatenated with the corresponding encoder features from the same spatial level. This concatenated output is then processed through two identical sub-blocks, each containing a $3 \times 3 \times 3$ convolutional layer (stride $1 \times 1 \times 1$), followed by in-stance normalization and Leaky ReLU activation (negative slope 0.01). Deep supervision is incorporated by calculating loss functions from intermediate outputs at multiple decoder levels to enhance training effectiveness (see Sect. 2.3). This design ensures effective down sampling during encoding and accurate spatial reconstruction during decoding, supporting robust segmentation performance across heterogeneous mpMRI datasets.

Multi-path Decoders. Three dedicated decoders branch from the shared encoder, each targeting a specific tumor region—SNFH, ET, or NETC. This design leverages modality-agnostic features extracted by the shared encoder while minimizing cross-region interference. The shared encoder ($\mathcal{E}$) maps input MRI volumes (X) to a latent feature space (F_E) with a bottleneck dimension of $C_E \times H_E \times W_E \times D_E$,, while each decoder ($\mathcal{D}_\nabla$) generates region-specific segmentation maps (F_{D_r}) by reconstructing spatial details from F_E with dimensions $C_D \times H_D \times W_D \times D_D$ for each decoder output.

At the final layer of each decoder, an attention-guided module aligns MRI sequences with tumor regions—T1/T1ce for NETC, T1ce for ET, and T2/FLAIR for SNFH. For each tumor region, modality-specific guidance features are extracted using two 3D convolutional layers with $3 \times 3 \times 3$ kernels followed by Leaky ReLU activation. These guidance features are then concatenated with the corresponding decoder outputs to enhance region-specific representation. The complete architecture details are illustrated in Fig. 2.

Attention Mechanism. A squeeze-and-excitation (SE) [27] block was selected which refines the concatenated features by recalibrating channel-wise weights. The SE mechanism applies global average pooling and sigmoid-activated weights to prioritize informative channels.

Final outputs concatenate region-wise maps ($O_{\mathrm{ET}}, O_{\mathrm{SNFH}}, O_{\mathrm{NETC}}$), optimized via region-specific losses.

2.3 Implementation Details

Training Schedule. The model outputs three channels (SNFH, ET, NETC) with sigmoid activation. Loss combines BCE [28] and Dice Loss [5] for class imbalance and robustness. The experiments were Trained for 200 epochs with a batch size of 2 and patch size of $128 \times 128 \times 128$ on the combined training datasets of BraTS 2025 Adult Glioma pre-tratment training dataset and BraTS 2025 Challenge on Sub-Sahara-Africa Adult Glioma training dataset resulting in 1311 combined cases. No local training-validation split or cross-validation was used; all cases contributed to model training. Evaluation was conducted solely on the official BraTS-Africa 2025 validation set via the online challenge portal, where ground truth labels are withheld from participants. It is worth noting that for the BraTS Africa 2025 challenge, it is permissible to use only the BraTS 2025 adults datasets as additional data for training purposes. The optimizer used was the Adam optimizer [29]. We applied a weight decay parameter of 0.0001 to regularize the model. For the initial 1000 training iterations, the learning rate was gradually increased linearly from zero up to the predetermined target value of 0.0003. Subsequently, the learning rate was gradually reduced following a cosine annealing schedule. Mixed-precision arithmetic [30] and Kaiming initialization [31] were used for efficiency and stability. All experiments were performed on a workstation with an Intel® Core™ i7-14700K processor (28 threads), 64 GB of RAM, and an NVIDIA GeForce

RTX 4070 Ti SUPER GPU (16 GB VRAM). Training one epoch took approximately 22 min, with peak GPU memory usage of 15.2 GB. The total training time was approximately 1.5 days. The software environment consisted of Ubuntu 22.04.5 LTS, Python 3.10, CUDA 12.9, and PyTorch.

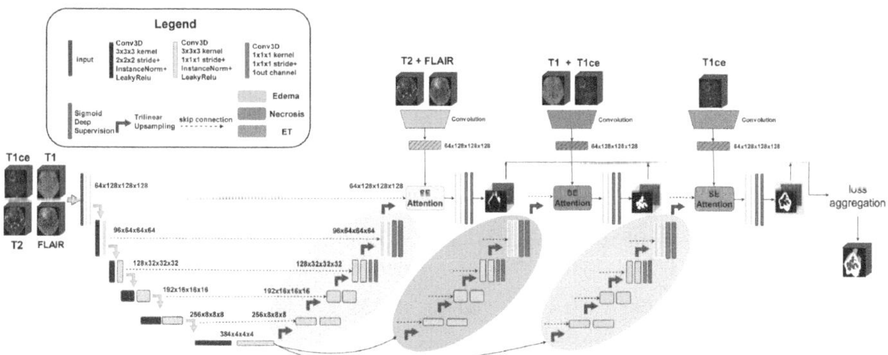

Fig. 2. Diagram of the proposed network architecture, which consists of three main components: U-Net backbone, multi-decoder, and attention mechanism.

Deep Supervision. Deep supervision was incorporated into the network by adding auxiliary loss branches at intermediate decoder layers. To match the lower resolution of these intermediate features, ground truth labels were down sampled accordingly via nearest-neighbor interpolation. The total loss is a weighted sum of losses from the primary and intermediate outputs, with the highest weight on the final output and progressively smaller weights for the earlier decoder levels (weights of 1, ½, and ¼ respectively). This approach improves gradient flow and training stability, encouraging intermediate layers to learn meaningful features while prioritizing final output accuracy.

3 Results

3.1 Performance on BraTS 2025 Challenge Sub-Sahara-Africa Adult Glioma Validation Dataset Against SOTA Methods

Evaluation of the trained models was conducted exclusively on the BraTS-Africa 2025 validation dataset, for which ground truth segmentations are withheld from participants. Performance metrics were obtained by submitting segmentation results to the official BraTS challenge evaluation portal, ensuring unbiased and uniform assessment. Table 1 provides a detailed comparison of our framework's performance against two state-of-the-art (SOTA) models, assessed using two critical metrics: lesion-wise Dice score and the lesion-wise 95th percentile Hausdorff distance, both of which are standard evaluation measures in the BraTS challenge. Our proposed method shows consistent improvements specially in critical regions like TC and ET.

Table 1. Quantitative results of the proposed model and baseline comparisons. During the validation phase, the proposed model is compared with the Tuned U-Net and the Optimized U-Net using the lesion-wise Dice Similarity Coefficient (DSC, ↑) and the 95th percentile Hausdorff Distance (HD95, mm, ↓). During the testing phase, only the proposed model was evaluated, with performance reported using the lesion-wise Dice Similarity Coefficient (DSC, ↑) and the Normalized Surface Distance with a 1.0 mm tolerance ($NSD_{1.0}$, ↑). Results are provided for the Whole Tumor (WT), Tumor Core (TC), and Enhancing Tumor (ET) subregions, along with their average (Avg.) values. All values represent mean ± standard deviation.

Validation phase results								
Model	Lesion-wise DSC ↑				Lesion-wise HD95 (mm) ↓			
	WT	TC	ET	Avg.	WT	TC	ET	Avg.
Tuned Unet [14]	0.868 ± 0.162	0.805 ± 0.231	0.803 ± 0.172	0..825	25.186 ± 59.763	34.385 ± 83.621	**17.762 ± 51.436**	**25.778**
Optimized Unet [13]	**0.904 ± 0.110**	0.799 ± 0.256	0.819 ± 0.186	0.840	**9.236 ± 31.261**	46.809 ± 97.829	31.588 ± 70.951	29.211
Proposed	0.874 ± 0.165	**0.839 ± 0.228**	**0.827 ± 0.212**	**0.846**	24.770 ± 59.886	**28.360 ± 83.869**	30.831 ± 84.150	27.987
Testing phase results								
Model	**Lesion-wise DSC↑**				**Lesion-wise NSD_1.0↑**			
	WT	**TC**	**ET**	**Avg.**	**WT**	**TC**	**ET**	**Avg.**
Proposed	0.919 ± 0.116	0.846 ± 0.217	0.842 ± 0.186	0.869	0.830 ± 0.131	0.766 ± 0.222	0.815 ± 0.191	0.804

4 Discussion

Table 1 presents a comparative evaluation of the proposed model against two relevant baselines: the Tuned Unet [14] and the Optimized Unet [13]. The comparison metrics include the lesion-wise Dice Similarity Coefficient (DSC), which measures segmentation overlap, and the 95th percentile Hausdorff Distance (HD95) in millimeters. Additionally, the testing phase results are reported using the Normalized Surface Distance (NSD) with a tolerance of 1 mm, both (NSD,HD95) reflect boundary accuracy. The results are provided for three tumor subregions—Whole Tumor (WT), Tumor Core (TC), and Enhancing Tumor (ET)—along with their average values.

Overall, the proposed method improves segmentation overlap and boundary consistency compared to the Tuned Unet and performs comparably or slightly better than the Optimized Unet for the more challenging subregions. It achieves an average DSC of 0.846, about 2.1% higher than the Tuned Unet, with the largest gain for the Tumor Core (0.839 vs. 0.805 and 0.799). For the Enhancing Tumor, the proposed model also outperforms both baselines (0.827 vs. 0.803 and 0.819). The Optimized Unet achieves the best WT DSC (0.904), but the proposed method still improves on the Tuned Unet (0.874 vs. 0.868).

For HD95, the Optimized Unet shows the lowest value for WT (9.2 mm) but is less stable for TC and ET. In contrast, the proposed model achieves more balanced boundary scores (average HD95 27.99 mm) with better consistency for TC (28.36 mm) and ET (30.83 mm). This suggests that while the Optimized Unet is strong for large tumor volumes, the proposed method provides a better trade-off for smaller, critical subregions—which are essential for treatment planning and prognosis.

In the testing phase, where only the proposed model was evaluated, the method maintained strong generalization performance, achieving average lesion-wise DSC and $NSD_{1.0}$ values of 0.869 and 0.804, respectively. The highest overlap was observed for WT (DSC: 0.919), while the $NSD_{1.0}$ scores—0.830 for WT, 0.766 for TC, and 0.815 for ET— indicate consistent boundary adherence across tumor components. These results confirm the robustness of the proposed model and its ability to preserve accurate tumor boundaries under unseen data conditions.

In summary, these results highlight that the proposed approach reduces segmentation ambiguity, improves region-wise accuracy, and could better support tasks like radiomics or longitudinal monitoring. Further refinement could help match the WT boundary sharpness of the Optimized Unet. Due to the nature of the BraTS-Africa 2025 challenge evaluation protocol whereby the ground truth segmentations of the validation dataset are not publicly accessible and evaluation is performed via a remote challenge portal, qualitative visual comparisons and detailed error analyses of segmentation outputs were not feasible.

5 Conclusion

We proposed a multi pathway deep learning framework for the BraTS 2025 Challenge Sub-Sahara-Africa Adult Glioma challenge that aligns multi-modal MRI inputs with specific tumor subregions using a shared 3D U-Net backbone, region-specific decoders, and SE attention. Evaluated on the Africa glioblastoma validation dataset, the method achieved consistent improvements in Dice score and boundary accuracy compared to strong baselines, with notable gains for the tumor core and enhancing regions. However, deploying automated glioblastoma segmentation models in clinical settings across Sub-Saharan Africa entails unique challenges stemming from diverse MRI acquisition protocols, scanner heterogeneity, and variable image quality often due to limited infrastructure. Our model's multi-decoder architecture with attention mechanisms aims to impart robustness to such heterogeneity. Nonetheless, further validation on prospective local datasets is required, alongside development of adaptive techniques such as domain adaptation and model compression to facilitate deployment on resource-constrained clinical hardware. Integrating models into routine clinical workflows will also necessitate user training and sustainable maintenance strategies to ensure clinical efficacy and long-term usability in these environments.

Acknowledgments. This work was supported by the National Research Foundation of Korea (NRF) funded by the Korean government (MSIT) (No. RS-2023–00243034).

Disclosure of Interests. The authors have no competing interests.

References

1. Goodenberger, M.L., Jenkins, R.B.: Genetics of adult glioma. Cancer Genet. **205**(12), 613–621 (2012)
2. Al-Fakih, A., et al.: FLAIR MRI sequence synthesis using squeeze attention generative model for reliable brain tumor segmentation. Alex. Eng. J. **99**, 108–123 (2024)
3. Chen, C., et al.: Learning with privileged multimodal knowledge for unimodal segmentation. IEEE Trans. Med. Imaging **41**(3), 621–632 (2021)
4. Ronneberger, O., Fischer, P., Brox, T.: U-Net: Convolutional networks for biomedical image segmentation. In: Navab, N., Hornegger, J., Wells, W., Frangi, A. (eds.) Medical Image Computing and Computer-Assisted Intervention – MICCAI 2015. MICCAI 2015.LNCS, vol 9351. Springer, Cham (2015). https://doi.org/10.1007/978-3-319-24574-4_28
5. Milletari, F., Navab, N., Ahmadi, S.-A.: V-net: fully convolutional neural networks for volumetric medical image segmentation. In; 2016 Fourth International Conference on 3D Vision (3DV). IEEE (2016)
6. Zhou, Z., et al.: Unet++: redesigning skip connections to exploit multiscale features in image segmentation. IEEE Trans. Med. Imaging **39**(6), 1856–1867 (2019)
7. Hatamizadeh, A., Nath, V., Tang, Y., Yang, D., Roth, H.R., Xu, D.: Swin UNETR: swin transformers for semantic segmentation of brain tumors in MRI images. In: Crimi, A., Bakas, S. (eds.) Brainlesion: Glioma, Multiple Sclerosis, Stroke and Traumatic Brain Injuries. BrainLes 2021. LNCS, vol. 12962. Springer, Cham (2022). https://doi.org/10.1007/978-3-031-08999-2_22
8. Isensee, F., Jäger, P.F., Full, P.M., Vollmuth, P., Maier-Hein, K.H.: nnU-net for brain tumor segmentation. In: Crimi, A., Bakas, S. (eds) Brainlesion: Glioma, Multiple Sclerosis, Stroke and Traumatic Brain Injuries. BrainLes 2020. LNCS, vol. 12659. Springer, Cham (2021).https://doi.org/10.1007/978-3-030-72087-2_11
9. Isensee, F. et al. (2024). nnU-net revisited: a call for rigorous validation in 3d medical image segmentation. In: Linguraru, M.G., et al. (eds.) Medical Image Computing and Computer Assisted Intervention – MICCAI 2024. MICCAI 2024. LNCS, vol. 15009. Springer, Cham (2024). https://doi.org/10.1007/978-3-031-72114-4_47
10. Myronenko, A.: 3D MRI brain tumor segmentation using autoencoder regularization. In: Crimi, A., Bakas, S., Kuijf, H., Keyvan, F., Reyes, M., van Walsum, T. (eds.) Brainlesion: Glioma, Multiple Sclerosis, Stroke and Traumatic Brain Injuries. BrainLes 2018. LNCS, vol. 11384. Springer, Cham (2019). https://doi.org/10.1007/978-3-030-11726-9_28
11. Jiang, Z., Ding, C., Liu, M., Tao, D.: Two-stage cascaded U-Net: 1st place solution to BraTS challenge 2019 segmentation task. In: Crimi, A., Bakas, S. (eds.) Brainlesion: Glioma, Multiple Sclerosis, Stroke and Traumatic Brain Injuries. BrainLes 2019. LNCS, vol. 11992. Springer, Cham (2020).. https://doi.org/10.1007/978-3-030-46640-4_22
12. Luu, H.M., Park, S.-H.: Extending nn-UNet for brain tumor segmentation. In: International MICCAI Brainlesion Workshop. Springer (2021)
13. Futrega, M., Milesi, A., Marcinkiewicz, M., Ribalta, P.: Optimized U-Net for brain tumor segmentation. In: Crimi, A., Bakas, S. (eds) Brainlesion: Glioma, Multiple Sclerosis, Stroke and Traumatic Brain Injuries. BrainLes 2021. LNCS, vol. 12963. Springer, Cham (2022. https://doi.org/10.1007/978-3-031-09002-8_2
14. Futrega, M., Marcinkiewicz, M., Ribalta, P. Tuning U-Net for Brain Tumor Segmentation. In: Bakas, S., et al. (eds.)Brainlesion: Glioma, Multiple Sclerosis, Stroke and Traumatic Brain Injuries. BrainLes 2022. LNCS, vol 13769. Springer, Cham (2023). https://doi.org/10.1007/978-3-031-33842-7_14
15. Zeineldin, R.A., Karar, M.E., Burgert, O., Mathis-Ullrich, F..: Multimodal CNN Networks for brain tumor segmentation in MRI: A BraTS 2022 Challenge Solution. In: Bakas, S., et al.

(eds.) Brainlesion: Glioma, Multiple Sclerosis, Stroke and Traumatic Brain Injuries. BrainLes 2022. LNCS, vol. 13769. Springer, Cham (2023). https://doi.org/10.1007/978-3-031-33842-7_11
16. McKinley, R., Meier, R., Wiest, R. (2019). Ensembles of densely-connected CNNs with label-uncertainty for brain tumor segmentation. In: Crimi, A., Bakas, S., Kuijf, H., Keyvan, F., Reyes, M., van Walsum, T. (eds.) Brainlesion: Glioma, Multiple Sclerosis, Stroke and Traumatic Brain Injuries. BrainLes 2018. LNCS, vol. 11384. Springer, Cham. https://doi.org/10.1007/978-3-030-11726-9_40
17. Zeineldin, R.A., Karar, M.E., Mathis-Ullrich, F., Burgert, O.: Ensemble CNN networks for GBM tumors segmentation using multi-parametric MRI. In: Crimi, A., Bakas, S. (eds.) Brainlesion: Glioma, Multiple Sclerosis, Stroke and Traumatic Brain Injuries. BrainLes 2021. LNCS, vol. 12962. Springer, Cham (2022). https://doi.org/10.1007/978-3-031-08999-2_41
18. Goodfellow, I., et al.: Generative adversarial nets. Adv. Neural Inform. Process. Syst. **27** (2014)
19. Isensee, F., et al.: NnU-Net: a self-configuring method for deep learning-based biomedical image segmentation. Nat. Methods **18**(2), 203–211 (2021)
20. Karargyris, A., et al.: Federated benchmarking of medical artificial intelligence with MedPerf. Nat. Mach. Intell. **5**(7), 799–810 (2023)
21. Baid, U., et al., The rsna-asnr-miccai brats 2021 benchmark on brain tumor segmentation and radiogenomic classification. arXiv preprint arXiv:2107.02314 (2021)
22. Menze, B.H., et al.: The multimodal brain tumor image segmentation benchmark (BRATS). IEEE Trans. Med. Imaging **34**(10), 1993–2024 (2014)
23. Bakas, S., et al.: Advancing the cancer genome atlas glioma MRI collections with expert segmentation labels and radiomic features. Sci. Data **4**(1), 1–13 (2017)
24. Bakas, S., et al.: Segmentation labels and radiomic features for the pre-operative scans of the TCGA-LGG collection [Data Set]. The Cancer Imaging Archive. (2017). Version
25. Bakas, S., et al.: Segmentation labels and radiomic features for the pre-operative scans of the TCGA-GBM collection (2017). https://doi . org/10.7937 K. **9**
26. Adewole, M., et al.: The brain tumor segmentation (brats) challenge 2023: glioma segmentation in sub-saharan Africa patient population (brats-africa). ArXiv, (2023)
27. Hu, J., Shen, L., Sun, G: Squeeze-and-excitation networks. In: Proceedings of the IEEE Conference on Computer Vision And Pattern Recognition (2018)
28. Lin, T.-Y., et al. Focal loss for dense object detection. In: International Conference on Computer Vision (ICCV) Focal Loss for Dense Object Detection (2017)
29. Nesterov, Y.: A method for unconstrained convex minimization problem with the rate of convergence O (1/k2). in Dokl. Akad. Nauk. SSSR.(1983)
30. Micikevicius, P., et al.: Mixed precision training. arXiv preprint arXiv:1710.03740, (2017)
31. He, K., et al: Delving deep into rectifiers: Surpassing human-level performance on imagenet classification. In:Proceedings of the IEEE International Conference on Computer Vision (2015)

Reassessing Glioma Segmentation Strategies: nnU-Net as a Strong Baseline on Limited Sub-Saharan MRI Data

Uwimana Lowami[1(✉)], Andrew Blayama Stephen[1], Confidence Raymond[2,3], Dong Zhang[4], Maruf Adewole[2,3,5], Udunna C. Anazodo[2,3,6], Mehmet Kurt[7], Damilare Olatunji[1], and Bernes Lorier Atabonfack[1]

[1] Carnegie Mellon University Africa, Kigali, Rwanda
{ulowami,abstephe,dolatunj}@andrew.cmu.edu, batabonf@alumni.cmu.edu
[2] Medical Artificial Intelligence Lab, Lagos, Nigeria
craymon8@uwo.ca
[3] Montreal Neurological Institute, McGill University, Montreal, Canada
udunna.anazodo@mcgill.ca
[4] Department of Electrical and Computer Engineering, University of British Columbia, Vancouver, BC, Canada
[5] Department of Radiology, University of Pennsylvania, Philadelphia, PA, USA
[6] Department of Clinical and Radiation Oncology, University of Cape Town, Cape Town, South Africa
[7] Department of Mechanical Engineering, University of Washington, Seattle, WA, USA
mkurt@uw.edu

Abstract. Brain tumor segmentation remains a critical yet challenging task, particularly in low-resource settings where imaging data are often acquired with low-field MRI scanners. The BraTS-Africa 2025 Sub-Saharan Challenge provides a unique opportunity to assess the robustness of segmentation models on heterogeneous, real-world data from African clinical environments. In this study, we investigated the performance of three state-of-the-art architectures; nnU-Net, MedNeXt, and SegMamba for sub-compartmental glioma segmentation. While each model embodies a distinct design philosophy, ablation experiments revealed that nnU-Net consistently outperformed the others as well as their ensemble. Specifically, nnU-Net trained on the entire dataset achieved Dice scores of 0.870 (ET), 0.852 (TC), and 0.887 (WT) on the validation set, surpassing both the alternative models and a 5-fold cross-validated nnU-Net baseline. These results suggest that training on all available cases provides advantages over cross-validation in smaller datasets. This work underscores the effectiveness of nnU-Net in this setting and contributes to the broader goal of developing reliable AI tools for neuro-oncology in underrepresented global contexts.

Keywords: Brain tumor segmentation · BRATS Challenge · nnU-Net

S. Bakas et al. (Eds.): MICCAI 2025, LNCS 16376, pp. 328–339, 2026.
https://doi.org/10.1007/978-3-032-16365-3_30

1 Introduction

Brain malignancies are among the most difficult tumors to treat due to their rapid progression and limited responsiveness to current therapies. The World Health Organization (WHO) classifies brain tumors into four grades based on histological and molecular characteristics [1]. Grade I tumors are typically slow-growing and less aggressive, while Grade IV tumors, such as glioblastomas, are highly invasive and associated with poor prognosis. Gliomas, which originate from glial cells, are the most common primary tumors of the central nervous system. Patients with low-grade gliomas can survive for several years; however, those diagnosed with high-grade gliomas often have a median survival time of less than two years despite receiving standard treatment [2,3]. The primary goal of glioma treatment is to maximize tumor removal while preserving neurological function. Treatment typically includes surgical resection, followed by chemotherapy and/or radiotherapy [4].

Accurate delineation of tumor boundaries is critical for planning and executing these interventions. Tumor segmentation, the process of identifying and labeling tumor regions on medical images, is essential for visualizing tumor extent and its relation to surrounding brain structures. Manual segmentation, however, is time-consuming and subject to inter-rater variability. Automated brain tumor segmentation offers a more efficient and consistent alternative, facilitating faster diagnosis, treatment planning, and monitoring [2]. The Brain Tumor Segmentation (BraTS) Challenge, an annual competition since 2012, has driven significant advances in automated segmentation by providing the largest publicly available annotated brain tumor dataset. The BraTS-Africa subchallenge focuses on validating segmentation models on MRI data from Sub-Saharan Africa, acquired using lower-field MRI scanners. This aims to test the generalizability of models trained on data from high-resource settings [2].

Deep learning methods have consistently outperformed classical techniques in brain tumor segmentation. U-Net [5], a convolutional neural network (CNN) architecture with an encoder-decoder design and skip connections, has become a foundational model for medical image segmentation. Variants such as Attention U-Net [6], VGG U-Net [7], and Dilated Inception U-Net [8] have extended its capabilities. Aggregator models like DeepSeg [9] offer flexibility by allowing integration of custom encoders for comparative experiments. nnU-Net [10,11], a self-configuring variant of U-Net, demonstrated that careful preprocessing and augmentation can significantly boost performance, establishing it as a strong baseline in multiple studies [12–14].

The introduction of the Vision Transformer (ViT) [15] marked a shift toward attention-based architectures, achieving state-of-the-art performance on natural image classification tasks. However, applying ViTs to medical image segmentation posed challenges due to their quadratic complexity in computing self-attention. SwinUNETR [16] addressed this with windowed attention mechanisms and hierarchical feature learning. Subsequently, ConvNeXt [17] showed that carefully designed CNNs can rival transformer performance. MedNeXt [18], building on ConvNeXt principles, was developed as a fully CNN-based architecture for medical segmentation, outperforming both SwinUNETR and nnU-Net in some benchmarks. Recently, SegMamba [19] introduced a novel approach using selective state-space models (SSMs). With tri-oriented Mamba blocks, it efficiently models long-range dependencies in medical images, providing a lightweight alternative to attention-based models.

In recent BraTS challenges, ensemble models have consistently outperformed individual architectures. For example, the 2022 winners [14] combined nnU-Net [11], DeepSCAN [20], and DeepSeg [9] to achieve superior results. The 2023 champions leveraged GAN-based augmentation and still relied on an ensemble of nnU-Net and SwinUNETR [12], noting the complementary nature of CNN and transformer-based models. In this study, we investigate whether combining architectures from three different paradigms, CNN (nnU-Net), modern CNN (MedNeXt), and state-space models (SegMamba), can yield a robust ensemble capable of generalizing to low-field African MRI scans. We evaluate the individual performance of each model and the collective performance of the ensemble, with the goal of validating architectural diversity as a strength in brain tumor segmentation.

2 Methods

2.1 Dataset Description

This study used **ASNR-MICCAI-BraTS2023-SSA-Challenge-Training Data_V2** and **BraTS2024-SSA-Challenge-ValidationData** datasets [2], both obtained from the official BraTS challenge Synapse portal. These datasets are curated for the Sub-Segmentation of Subcompartments of Gliomas (SSA) task and consist of multi-institutional, multi-modal brain MRI scans annotated for tumor sub-regions.

Each subject includes multimodal preoperative magnetic resonance sequences: T1 weighted (T1), post-contrast T1 weighted (T1Gd), T2 weighted (T2) and T2-FLAIR aligned with a common anatomical template. Ground truth labels follow the SSA schema, distinguishing between enhancing tumor (ET), non-enhancing tumor (NET), peritumoral edema (ED). Annotations were performed by expert neuroradiologists and underwent rigorous quality control.

The training set comprises *60* cases, while the validation set includes *35* cases. All scans are skull-stripped and resampled to $1\,\text{mm}^3$ isotropic resolution, provided in NIfTI format, and comply with the BraTS preprocessing pipeline standards (Fig. 1).

2.2 Model Architectures

2.2.1 nnu-Net nnU-Net("no new U-Net") [10] is a self-configuring deep learning framework for both 2D and 3D biomedical image segmentation. Despite using a relatively simple U-Net architecture at its core, it has achieved state-of-the-art performance across numerous medical segmentation benchmarks by automating

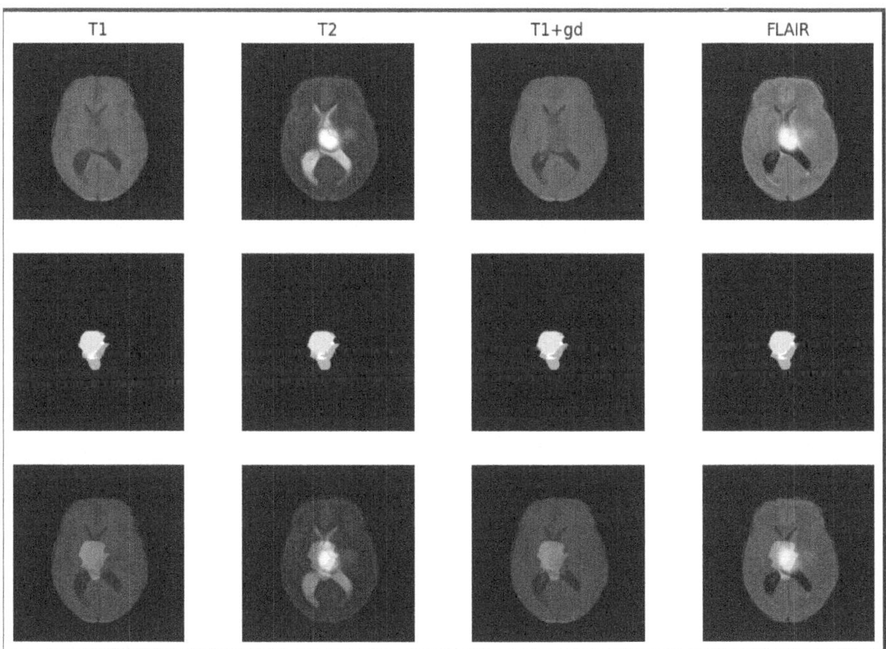

Fig. 1. Sample case from the dataset showing T1, T2, T1+gd (T1+contrast) and FLAIR

domain-specific configuration steps. The core architecture consists of a CNN-based encoder-decoder structure. The encoder progressively downsamples the input using strided convolutions while doubling the number of feature channels at each level. The decoder, in turn, upsamples using transposed convolutions and reconstructs the segmentation mask from the learned features. At each resolution scale, skip connections transfer features from encoder layers to their decoder counterparts to preserve spatial context. In our experiments, we used nnU-Net version 2 [21], which introduces residual encoder blocks and improved memory management. This version supports flexible scaling to match different hardware capacities by adjusting the input patch size via predefined presets: Medium (M), Large (L), and Extra-Large (XL). These presets affect both the input size and the computational footprint. Table 1 summarizes the patch dimensions for each configuration used in our experiments (Table 1).

Table 1. Different presets that come with nnU-Net version 2.

nnUNET preset	Patch size(in voxels)
Medium(M)	128 x 128 x 128
Large(L)	160 × 224 × 192
Extra Large(XL)	224 x 256 x 256

2.2.2 MedNeXt MedNeXt is a lightweight, transformer-inspired convolutional neural network architecture built on the design principles of ConvNeXt [17], which itself modernizes ResNet by incorporating architectural decisions from both Vision Transformers and Swin Transformers. These include the use of large convolutional kernels to approximate the global receptive field of attention mechanisms, the adoption of Adam-based optimizers, and the use of inverted bottlenecks for more efficient channel-wise representation learning. MedNeXt is organized into modular residual blocks tailored for medical image segmentation. Each block consists of: A *depthwise convolution layer* (to mimic global context), *an expansile layer* (channel expansion), *a contractile layer* (channel compression), These blocks are integrated into a four-layer encoder-decoder architecture.

Each encoder stage contains a MedNeXt block followed by a downsampling block, while each decoder stage includes a MedNeXt block and a corresponding upsampling block. Skip connections are used to link encoder and decoder layers at matching spatial resolutions, preserving multi-scale contextual features. MedNeXt introduces a novel training mechanism called **UpKern**, which allows a model with larger convolutional kernels to be initialized from weights of a smaller-kernel variant. This approach mitigates the risk of training saturation and enables stable learning for larger receptive field models. In this study, we utilize **MedNeXt-S**, a compact variant of the architecture designed to explore compound scaling. We first train the model using 3×3×3 kernels, then employ UpKern to fine-tune a 5×5×5 kernel model with the same architecture.

2.2.3 SegMamba SegMamba is a recent segmentation architecture based on the Mamba family of models, which introduces a selective state-space model (SSM) for sequence modeling with linear-time complexity. Originally developed for natural language processing tasks, Mamba has shown strong performance in modeling long-range dependencies while remaining computationally efficient. SegMamba adapts this concept to 3D medical image segmentation by employing an encoder-decoder architecture composed of Tri-oriented Spatial Mamba (TSMamba) blocks. Each encoder stage consists of a TSMamba block followed by a downsampling operation. The decoder mirrors this structure using upsampling layers, with skip connections between encoder and decoder levels of matching resolution. Each TSMamba block contains a **Gated Spatial Convolution (GSC)**: Preserves spatial context and prepares the input for sequential modeling. **Tri-oriented Mamba (ToM)**: Splits the 3D volume into three 1D sequences along the axial, coronal, and sagittal planes. Each sequence is processed independently using the Mamba operator to capture long-range dependencies in forward, reverse, and inter-slice directions. **Multi-Layer Perceptron (MLP):** Applies further non-linear transformations after feature fusion.

Layer normalization is applied between these components to ensure stability. The outputs from ToM and GSC are fused before being passed to the MLP head. By default, SegMamba is trained using *Stochastic Gradient Descent (SGD).* See table2 for a comparative summary of the model parameters.

2.3 Training Procedure and Evaluation Metrics

2.3.1 Preprocessing We adopted the default nnU-Net [10] preprocessing and data augmentation pipelines for both the nnU-Net and MedNeXt models. This includes modality-wise intensity normalization, resampling to isotropic $1\,\text{mm}^3$ resolution, and spatial alignment to a standard anatomical template. For SegMamba, we employed its official preprocessing configuration, which follows similar principles and ensures consistency across input modalities.

2.3.2 Loss Function We employed the *Dice Loss* as the primary optimization objective across all models. Dice Loss directly maximizes the volumetric overlap between predicted and ground truth segmentations, making it particularly suitable for highly imbalanced medical imaging tasks such as tumor subregion segmentation. The loss is defined as:

$$\text{DiceLoss} = 1 - \frac{2|P \cap G|}{|P| + |G|}$$

where P and G represent the sets of predicted and ground truth lesion voxels, respectively.

2.3.3 Hardware Model training was conducted using the following compute environments:

- **nnU-Net** and **MedNeXt** were trained on a single NVIDIA V100 GPU with 32 GB VRAM via the Compute Canada high performance computing platform.
- **SegMamba** was trained on a single H100 NVIDIA GPU with 40 GB VRAM for 1000 epochs also from Compute Canada.

2.3.4 Evaluation Model performance was assessed using the official BraTS-Africa leaderboard, which reports lesion-wise **Dice Similarity Coefficient (DSC)** and **Normalized Surface Distance (NSD)** at tolerance thresholds of 0.5 mm (NSD-0.5) and 1.0 mm (NSD-1.0). These complementary metrics provide a holistic evaluation of both volume and boundary-level segmentation accuracy.

Dice Similarity Coefficient (DSC): Measures the overlap between predicted and ground truth regions. A Dice score of 1 indicates perfect agreement.

Normalized Surface Distance (NSD): Quantifies the proportion of predicted lesion surface points that lie within a specified Euclidean distance τ from the ground truth surface. NSD is particularly sensitive to boundary alignment and is defined as:

$$\text{NSD}_\tau = \frac{|\{x \subset S_P : \min_{y \in S_G} d(x, y) \leq \tau\}|}{|S_P|}$$

Here, S_P and S_G denote the surfaces of the predicted and ground truth segmentations, respectively, and $d(x, y)$ is the Euclidean distance between surface points. NSD helps to assess how accurately the model captures the lesion boundaries, particularly in small or irregular regions.

2.4 Ensemble Strategy

To improve the precision and robustness of segmentation, we employed an ensemble strategy combining the three models: nnU-Net [11], MedNeXT [18], and SegMamba [19]. nnU-Net serves as our baseline, given its strong performance and adaptability across medical image segmentation tasks. MedNeXT introduces a convolutional neural network with dynamic receptive fields, while SegMamba contributes a modern Mamba-based architecture designed for long-range spatial modeling. Each model was trained independently using the same pre-processing pipeline and dataset splits to maintain consistency across outputs. We integrate their predictions using the STAPLE (Simultaneous Truth and Performance Level Estimation) algorithm, which estimates a probabilistic consensus segmentation accounting for the strengths and weaknesses of individual models.

3 Experiments and Results

3.1 NnU-Net Experiments

We trained two variants of nnU-Net:

- **NN+ALL:** Trained on the full training dataset of 60 subjects for 1036 epochs. On the validation set, it achieved lesion-wise Dice scores of **0.870 (ET)**, **0.852 (TC)**, and **0.887 (WT)**.
- **NN+XVAL:** A 5-fold non-stratified cross-validation setup where each fold was trained on 48 training volumes and evaluated on the remaining 12. Each fold was trained for 1000 epochs. The average Dice scores reported on the challenge leaderboard were **0.854 (ET)**, **0.836 (TC)**, and **0.881 (WT)**.

3.2 MedNeXt Experiments

We experimented with the **MedNeXt-S** variant under several configurations:

- **MED+K3:** A 5-fold non-stratified cross-validation using the nnU-Net v1 MedNeXt trainer with a default kernel size of $3\times3\times3$. Initially trained for 1000 epochs. During inspection, we discovered that label value 3 was being overwritten, corrupting label integrity. After correcting this preprocessing issue, we resumed training for an additional 70 epochs. This model achieved Dice scores of **0.818 (ET)**, **0.811 (TC)**, and **0.905 (WT)**.
- **MED+K3+ALL:** Trained on all 60 training subjects with the same $3\times3\times3$ kernel configuration for 1000 epochs. This model demonstrated improved performance, with dice scores of achieved 0.829, 0.825, and 0.907 on ET, TC and WT respectively.
- **MED+K5+ALL:** Resampled MED+K3+ALL weights using UpKern and trained a 5x5x5 kernel checkpoint for 500 epochs on all 60 cases. MED+K5+ALL scored 0.856, 0.841 and 0.896 on ET, TC and WT respectively.

Table 2. A summary of final training parameters used for the each of the models. nnU-Net and MedNext auto-configured to these parameters. Training parameters for SegMamba were not changed.

Parameter	nnU-Net	MedNeXt	SegMamba
Training Configuration			
Batch Size	2	2	2
Patch Size	128×160×112	128×128×128	128×128×128
Configuration	3d_fullres	3d_fullres	-
Model Architecture			
Feature Size	320,	512	384
Kernel Size	3	3,5	–
Stride	2	2	–
Normalization	Instance norm	Group norm	Instance norm
Activation Function	LeakyReLU	GeLU	SiLU
Optimization			
Optimizer	SGD	AdamW	SGD
Learning Rate	0.01	0.001	0.01
Weight Decay	3×10^{-5}	3×10^{-5}	3×10^{-5}
Momentum	0.99	–	0.99
Nesterov	True	–	True
Epsilon	-	0.0001	–

3.3 SegMamba Experiments

We experimented training SegMamba with initial learning rate of 0.01, weight decay of 3×10^{-5}, momentum of 0.99 and nesterov set to true. These are the default parameters. We experimented with 5-fold non-stratified cross validation(SEG+XVAL) and training on all cases(SEG+ALL), for 1000 epochs. However, the results of SEG+ALL were not available at the time of writing.

- **SEG+XVAL:** used the best of the 5 fold cross validation checkpoints to generate masks. We then filtered the masks to keep only the largest connected component using MONAI. This allowed us to get to dice scores of 0.849, 0.833, and 0.889 on ET, TC and WT.

3.4 Ensemble

We created an ensemble of the best 3 models we had in every category: NN+ALL, MED+K5+ALL and SEG+XVAL using SimpleITK's implementation of the STAPLE algorithm. We achieved dice scores of 0.856, 0.840, 0.896 on ET, TC and WT (Table 3).

Table 3. Lesion-wise Dice and NSD Scores (0.5 mm and 1.0 mm) on the BraTS-Africa Validation Set

Model	Lesion-wise Dice			NSD 0.5 mm			NSD 1.0 mm		
	ET	TC	WT	ET	TC	WT	ET	TC	WT
NN+ALL	**0.870**	**0.852**	0.887	**0.601**	**0.536**	0.523	**0.866**	**0.792**	0.799
NN+XVAL	0.854	0.836	0.881	0.586	0.518	0.525	0.842	0.761	0.792
MED+K3	0.818	0.811	0.905	0.570	0.503	0.548	0.811	0.743	0.817
MED+K3+ALL	0.830	0.825	**0.907**	0.575	0.519	**0.550**	0.822	0.760	**0.829**
MED+K5+ALL	0.856	0.841	0.896	0.586	0.520	0.540	0.845	0.769	0.808
SEG+XVAL	0.849	0.833	0.887	0.566	0.490	0.500	0.827	0.745	0.778
ENSEMBLE	0.856	0.840	0.896	0.590	0.524	0.541	0.845	0.768	0.808

4 Discussion

From our experiments, we found that nn-Unet trained on the entire training dataset outperformed all other models on Enhancing Tumor(ET) and Tumor Core(TC) across all metrics despite using half the training time on same hardware. On Whole Tumor (WT), MED+3K+ALL had the best scores across all measurements. MED+5K+ALL shows a strong increase in TC and ET with slight decrease in WT scores. In general, this shows the ability of MedNext based models to accurately represent the edematous part of the tumor. However, SEG+XVAL underperformed better than the baseline.

Based on this, we built an ensemble of these models to capitalize on their individual strengths. Its results closely resembled MED+5K+ALL and no improvement was noticed.

In general, checkpoints trained on all 60 training cases performed better than those trained with 5-fold cross validation with the same configuration. We think this is due to a small dataset size which makes every case that the model sees in training more valuable.

Visually, SEG + XVAL tended to create more false positive voxels on complex tumors compared to NN + ALL, MED + K5 + ALL and the ensemble. See Fig. 2. In many cases, the masks generated by the ensemble resembled those generated by MED+5K+ALL.

The relative strength of nn-Unet against MedNext S and SegMamba suggests that on smaller datasets, nn-Unet is still a stronger choice. Taking into account these findings, we submitted our NN + ALL for the challenge, as it had high scores on all metrics and used relatively less resources. However, during containerization, an error occurred that erased labels 1 and 3 from the output segmentation. As such, our model scored lesion-wise dice scores of 0.0007, 0.0064, 0.5930 with standard deviation of 0.0027, 0.02249, 0.2522 on BraTS test dataset. Lesion-wise NSD scores were also equally low. This result reflects an error during containerization rather than overfitting.

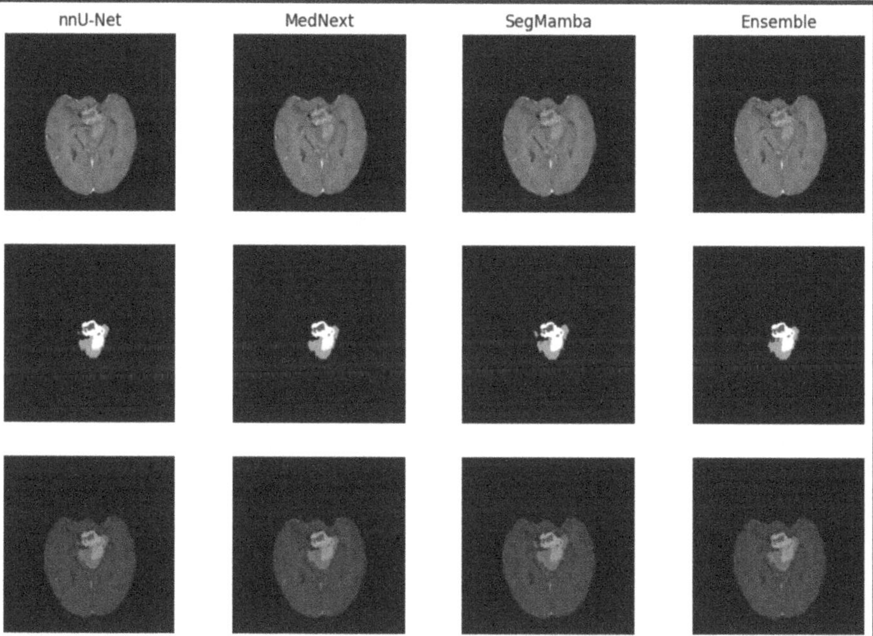

Fig. 2. Comparative output of NN+ALL, MED+K5+ALL, SEG+XVAL and the ensemble of them. SEG+XVAL shows tendency to create false positives for complex tumors.

4.1 Further Studies

The insights gained from this study show several promising avenues for future research. Although our experiments with MedNext S models showed significant promise, they were incomplete at the end of the validation period. MED+K5 models, for example, were under-trained and MED+K5+XVAL was not available for reporting. A deeper investigation into these models, with longer training durations and exploration of different size variants (e.g. MedNext B or MedNext L), could reveal their true potential on smaller datasets, particularly given their apparent strength in delineating the edematous part of the tumor. Furthermore, we see experimenting with more sophisticated augmentation techniques as a potential area of exploration, given the small size of the BraTS SSA dataset., such as geometric transformations, intensity changes, and even generative adversarial networks (GANs).

5 Conclusion

This study investigated the performance of nn-Unet in comparison to contemporary model architectures, MedNext and SegMamba, for automated brain tumor segmentation on the BraTS SSA dataset. Our experiments demonstrated the superior performance of nn-Unet when trained on the entire dataset, particularly on the Enhancing Tumor and Tumor Core subregions. While the ensemble model did not provide a noticeable improvement, our findings underscore the continued strength and reliability of nn-Unet on smaller datasets. Overall, this work provides a valuable comparative analysis that can guide model selection and training strategies for similar medical image segmentation tasks in resource-constrained environments.

Acknowledgments. The authors would like to thank the following instructors of the Sprint AI Training for African Medical Imaging Knowledge Translation (SPARK) Academy 2025 summer school on deep learning in medical imaging for providing insightful background knowledge on brain tumors that informed the research presented here: Noha Magdy, Maruf Adewole, Ayomidale B. Oladele, Amal Saleh, Nourou Dine Bankole, Jeremiah Fadugba, Lorumbur Moses, Toufiq Musah, Teresa Zhu, Craig Jones, Confidence Raymond, Lukman E. Ismaila, Ugumba Kikwima, Mehdi Astaraki, Peter Hastreiter, Evan Calabrese, Esin Uzturk Isik, Navodini Wijethilake, Rancy Chepchirchir, James Gee, MacLean Nasrallah, Jean Baptiste Poline, Bijay Adhikari, and Mohannad Barakat. The authors also thank Linshan Liu for administrative assistance in supporting the SPARK Academy training and capacity-building activities, which the authors immensely benefited from. The authors acknowledge the computational infrastructure support from the Digital Research Alliance of Canada (The Alliance) and the University of Washington Azure GenAI for Science Hub through The eScience Institute and Microsoft (PI: Mehmet Kurt) secured for the SPARK Academy. Finally, we would like to thank the Lacuna Fund for Health and Equity, the Radiological Society of North America (RSNA), the Research & Education (R&E) Foundation Derek Harwood-Nash International Education Scholar Grant, the McGill University Healthy Brain and Healthy Lives (HBHL), and the National Science and Engineering Research Council of Canada (NSERC) Discovery Launch Supplement for making the SPARK Academy possible via research grant supports.

References

1. Louis, D.N., Perry, A., Wesseling, P., Brat, D.J., Cree, I.A., Figarella-Branger, D., et al.: The 2021 WHO classification of tumors of the central nervous system: a summary. Neuro Oncol. **23**(8), 1231–1251 (2021)
2. Adewole, M., et al.: The brain tumor segmentation (BraTS) challenge 2023: Glioma segmentation in sub-saharan africa patient population (BraTS-Africa). arXiv preprint arXiv:2305.19369 (2023)
3. Uwishema, O., et al.: Epidemiology and etiology of brain cancer in africa: a systematic review. Brain and Behav. **13**(9), e3112 (2023)
4. Lee, J,H., Wee, C.W.: Treatment of adult gliomas: a current update. Brain & NeuroRehabilitation **15**(3), e24 (2022)
5. Ronneberger, O., Fischer, P., Brox, T.: U-net: convolutional networks for biomedical image segmentation. CoRR, abs/ arXiv:1505.04597 (2015)
6. Oktay, O., et al.: Attention u-net: Learning where to look for the pancreas. CoRR, abs/ arXiv:1804.03999 (2018)

7. Nawaz, A., Akram, U., Salam, A.A., Ali, A.R., Rehman, A.U., Zeb, J.: Vgg-unet for brain tumor segmentation and ensemble model for survival prediction. In: 2021 International Conference on Robotics and Automation in Industry (ICRAI), pp. 1–6 (2021)
8. Cahall, D., Rasool, G., Bouaynaya, N.C., Fathallah-Shaykh, H.M.: Dilated inception u-net (diu-net) for brain tumor segmentation. arXiv preprint arXiv:2108.06772 (2021)
9. Zeineldin, R.A., Karar, M.E., Coburger, J., Wirtz, C.R., Burgert, O.: Deepseg: deep neural network framework for automatic brain tumor segmentation using magnetic resonance flair images. arXiv preprint arXiv:2004.12333 (2020)
10. Isensee, F., et al.: nnU-Net: self-adapting framework for U-Net-Based medical image segmentation. arXiv preprint arXiv:1809.10486 (2018)
11. Isensee, F., Jäger, P.F., Full, P.M., Vollmuth, P., Maier-Hein, K.H.: nnU-Net for brain tumor segmentation. In: Crimi, A., Bakas, S. (eds.) BrainLes 2020. LNCS, vol. 12659, pp. 118–132. Springer, Cham (2021). https://doi.org/10.1007/978-3-030-72087-2_11
12. Ferreira, A., et al.: How we won BraTS 2023 Adult Glioma challenge? Just faking it! Enhanced Synthetic Data Augmentation and Model Ensemble for brain tumour segmentation. BraTS 2023 Challenge Submission Paper. Internal document from the BraTS 2023 challenge submission (2023)
13. Liu, Z., et al.: Swin Transformer: Hierarchical vision transformer using shifted windows. In: Proceedings of the IEEE/CVF International Conference on Computer Vision (ICCV), pp. 10012–10022 (2021)
14. Zeineldin, R.A., Karar, M.E., Burgert, O., Mathis-Ullrich, F.: Multimodal CNN networks for brain tumor segmentation in MRI: a BraTS 2022 challenge solution. arXiv preprint arXiv:2212.09310 (2022)
15. Dosovitskiy, A., et al.: An image is worth 16x16 words: Transformers for image recognition at scale. CoRR, abs/ arXiv:2010.11929 (2020)
16. Hatamizadeh, A., Nath, V., Tang, Y., Yang, D., Roth, H.R., Xu, D.: Swin UNETR: swin transformers for semantic segmentation of brain tumors in MRI images. In: Crimi, A., Bakas, S. (eds.) Brainlesion: Glioma, Multiple Sclerosis, Stroke and Traumatic Brain Injuries. BrainLes 2021. LNCS, vol. 12962. Springer, Cham (2022). https://doi.org/10.1007/978-3-031-08999-2_22
17. Liu, Z., Mao, H., Wu, C.-Y., Feichtenhofer, C., Darrell, T., Xie, S.: A convnet for the 2020s. CoRR, abs/ arXiv:2201.03545 (2022)
18. Roy, S., et al.: MedNeXt: transformer-driven scaling of ConvNets. In: International Conference on Medical Image Computing and Computer-Assisted Intervention, pp. 405–415. Springer (2023). https://doi.org/10.1007/978-3-031-43901-8_39
19. Xing, Z., Ye, T., Yang, Y., Liu, G., Zhu, L.: Segmamba: long-range sequential modeling mamba for 3d medical image segmentation (2024)
20. McKinley, R., Meier, R., Wiest, R.: Ensembles of densely-connected CNNs with label-uncertainty for brain tumor segmentation. In: Crimi, A., Bakas, S., Kuijf, H., Keyvan, F., Reyes, M., van Walsum, T. (eds.) BrainLes 2018. LNCS, vol. 11384, pp. 456–465. Springer, Cham (2019). https://doi.org/10.1007/978-3-030-11726-9_40
21. Isensee, F., et al.: nnu-net revisited: A call for rigorous validation in 3d medical image segmentation (2024)

A Fast, Lightweight nnUNet-Based Brain Tumor Segmentation Model Optimized for Low-Resource African Settings

John Emeka[1], Nwokoma Chidiebube[2(✉)], and Chika Ojiako[3(✉)]

[1] Pope John Paul II Minor Seminary Okpoma, Yala, Cross River State, Nigeria
[2] Radiology Department, Babcock University Teaching Hospital, Ilishan-Remo, Nigeria
nwokomac@babcock.edu.ng
[3] Department of Computer Sciences, University of Lagos, Lagos, Nigeria
cojiako@unilag.edu.ng

Abstract. In many African healthcare settings, the adoption of deep learning-based medical imaging models remains limited by inadequate computational resources. This study presents a fast and lightweight adaptation of the nnU-Net framework for brain tumor segmentation, specifically designed for deployment in low-resource environments. The model integrates quantization-aware training, structured pruning, and patch size optimization to reduce computational and memory demands while maintaining high segmentation performance.Evaluation on the BraTS 2023 benchmark dataset demonstrated Dice scores of 0.8501, 0.8572, and 0.8310 for Whole Tumor (WT), Tumor Core (TC), and Enhancing Tumor (ET), respectively, indicating robust agreement with expert annotations. The lightweight configuration allows real-time inference on CPU-only systems with less than 8 GB RAM, making it feasible for hospitals and diagnostic centers across resource-limited regions.These results underscore the potential of deploying practical, accurate, and accessible AI-driven radiology tools across African clinical environments, advancing equitable access to state-of-the-art medical imaging technologies.

Keywords: nnU-Net · Brain Tumor Segmentation · Model Compression · Quantization-Aware Training · Pruning · Low-Resource AI · Medical Imaging · Africa

1 Introduction

Brain tumors represent a significant clinical challenge due to their complex morphology and the necessity for timely, accurate diagnosis and treatment planning. Magnetic Resonance Imaging (MRI) remains the gold standard for non-invasive brain tumor evaluation, yet the interpretation of these scans demands high expertise and can be time-consuming, especially in resource-constrained settings [4]. Deep learning-based segmentation models, particularly the nnUNet framework [3], have revolutionized medical image analysis by automating tumor localization and delineation with state-of-the-art accuracy.

S. Bakas et al. (Eds.): MICCAI 2025, LNCS 16376, pp. 340–348, 2026.
https://doi.org/10.1007/978-3-032-16365-3_31

However, most successful applications of such models have occurred in well-resourced environments with access to high-end GPUs and sufficient memory bandwidth. In contrast, many healthcare facilities in sub-Saharan Africa face significant constraints, including limited computing infrastructure, inconsistent power supply, and restricted access to skilled AI personnel [5, 8]. These challenges limit the feasibility of deploying traditional, computationally intensive neural networks in real-world African radiology departments.

To address this gap, we propose a fast and lightweight adaptation of the nnUNet architecture specifically tailored for low-resource settings. Our model was trained and validated on the BraTS 2025 dataset [6], using architectural optimizations such as reduced patch sizes, model pruning, and quantization-aware training. The goal is to strike a balance between segmentation accuracy and computational efficiency enabling deployment on CPU-only systems with minimal memory and processing power.

This work contributes to the growing body of research on equitable AI deployment in global health, emphasizing the importance of designing practical, accessible solutions for underserved regions [7]. By focusing on operational efficiency and minimal hardware demand, our model serves as a prototype for real-world use in many African tertiary hospitals and diagnostic centers.

1.1 Related Work

Brain tumor segmentation using deep learning has seen remarkable progress in recent years, especially with the advent of encoder–decoder architectures like U-Net and its derivatives. The original **U-Net** introduced by Ronneberger et al. [16] established a strong foundation for biomedical image segmentation by combining symmetric down sampling and up sampling paths with skip connections. It demonstrated exceptional performance even on limited datasets, making it a common backbone for subsequent research. Building on this, **nnU-Net** proposed by Isensee et al. [3] introduced a self-configuring framework that dynamically adapts its architecture and hyperparameters based on the dataset. nnUNet has achieved top rankings in numerous medical image segmentation challenges including the BraTS series. Despite its effectiveness, the full 3D nnUNet model is resource-intensive, often requiring high-end GPUs and large memory to operate hindering its applicability in low-resource **environments**.

To address efficiency, various lightweight adaptations have been proposed. For instance, **UNet++** [4] introduced nested and dense skip connections for better feature fusion, while **Attention U-Net** [4] incorporated attention gates to focus on relevant image regions. More recently, **Mobile U-Net** and **Efficient U-Net** architectures have aimed to reduce computational load without severely compromising accuracy [5][6]. In the context of brain tumor segmentation, approaches like **3D Squeeze-and-Excitation U-Net (SE-UNet)** [7] and **Multi-Scale Attention-based U-Net** [8] have further improved segmentation by integrating spatial-context awareness, although they too come with heavier model footprints.

There is limited literature, however, on efforts that specifically **optimize segmentation models for deployment in low-resource clinical settings**, especially in sub-Saharan Africa. A few studies have recognized the potential of using **pruning**, **quantization**, and **knowledge distillation** to compress large models for mobile deployment

[9]. Yet, their application in high-stakes clinical domains like brain tumor segmentation remains underexplored. Our work fills this gap by proposing a lightweight, nnUNet-based model that is deliberately constrained in complexity to operate on CPU-only machines, a common limitation across many African diagnostic centers. It integrates lessons from both classic and recent segmentation architecture while applying model compression techniques to reduce memory and processing demands.

2 Methods

2.1 Data Preprocessing

We utilized the **ASNR-MICCAI-BraTS2023-SSA-Challenge** dataset for the segmentation task, which consists of multi-modal MRI scans in NIfTI format. The dataset includes four MRI sequences per subject: native T1-weighted (T1n), post-contrast T1-weighted (T1c), T2-FLAIR (T2f), and T2-weighted (T2w) images, as well as corresponding segmentation masks [1]. The dataset was unzipped and structured into a format compatible with the nnU-Net v2 framework [14].

- Each image was renamed using the format <CaseID>_<channel>.nii.gz, where channel corresponds to: 0000: T1n, 0001: T1c, 0002: T2f, 0003: T2w.

Segmentation labels were saved separately with the format <CaseID>.nii.gz. The appropriate directory structure (imagesTr, labelsTr) was created under the nnUNet_raw folder hierarchy, and a dataset.json file was generated specifying channel names and label mappings (i.e., 1 = Whole Tumor, 2 = Enhancing Tumor, 3 = Tumor Core), following the standard BraTS label taxonomy [15].

2.2 Model Configuration and Training

We employed the nnU-Net v2 framework [1], which automatically configures preprocessing, network architecture, training, and postprocessing pipelines based on dataset characteristics. All environment paths (nnUNet_raw, nnUNet_preprocessed, and nnUNet_results) were defined within the Kaggle Notebook environment. The dataset ID was assigned as 2023, and the data were registered with nnU-Net using standard dataset conversion routines.

Model training was performed using the 3D full-resolution (3d_fullres) configuration with a customized training class extending the default nnUNetTrainer. The training process was configured for 1000 epochs, enabling prolonged optimization and improved model convergence. All four MRI modalities—T1 native (T1n), T1 contrast-enhanced (T1c), T2-weighted (T2w), and T2-FLAIR (T2f)—were utilized as input channels.

Optimization employed a hybrid Dice-Cross Entropy loss function ($\alpha = 0.7$ for Dice), the AdamW optimizer, and a cosine annealing learning rate scheduler. Mixed precision training was enabled to enhance memory efficiency and computational throughput. All experiments were executed on a single GPU within the Kaggle environment.

2.3 Inference and Postprocessing

Model inference was performed on the validation fold using nnU-Net's built-in prediction routines. The predicted segmentation outputs were saved in the validation predictions folder, following the required BraTS-Africa submission naming convention (BraTS-SSA-xxxxx-seg.nii.gz), where xxxxx is the anonymized case ID. No ensemble or test-time augmentation was applied, and no postprocessing beyond the default nnU-Net pipeline was used.

2.4 Training Configuration

See Table 1.

Table 1. Key hyperparameters and settings used during training of the nnU-Net model on the BraTS Africa dataset

Hyperparameter	Value
Optimizer	Adam
Learning Rate	1e−4 with cosine annealing
Loss Function	Dice+Cross Entropy
Batch Size	2 (due to patch reduction)
Epochs	1000
Data Augmentation	Rotation, scaling, flipping
Training Platform	Kaggle Kernel (1x V100 GPU)

2.5 Evaluation Metrics

We evaluated segmentation performance on the official BraTS 2023 online leaderboard using 20 held-out test cases, employing key metrics such as Dice Similarity Coefficient (DSC), Normalized Surface Dice (NSD) at 1.0 mm tolerances, as well as lesion-wise Dice and NSD scores for the enhancing tumor (ET), tumor core (TC), and whole tumor (WT) regions.

2.6 Deployment Considerations

To assess feasibility in African hospitals, the final model was exported to ONNX format and tested on a CPU-only system with less than 8 GB RAM, measuring load time and prediction latency to ensure adequate responsiveness.

2.7 Experimental Setup

All experiments were conducted in the Kaggle Notebook environment using a GPU accelerator, a multi-core CPU, 16 GB RAM, and about 20 GB storage. The implementation was developed in Python 3.x with nnU-Net v2, SimpleITK, NiBabel, NumPy, OpenCV, Matplotlib, Plotly, and tqdm.

The BraTS 2023 SSA Challenge dataset was used, comprising multimodal brain MRI scans—T1 native (T1n), T1 contrast (T1c), T2-weighted (T2w), and T2-FLAIR (T2f). Dataset organization followed the nnU-Net v2 directory structure (nnUNet_raw/, nnUNet_preprocessed/, nnUNet_results/), with a Python script automating file arrangement, case mapping, and dataset.json generation.

Preprocessing, including voxel resampling, intensity normalization, and patch-based cropping, was automatically handled by nnU-Net v2 during planning and preprocessing, ensuring consistency and memory-efficient training.

Model training used a custom MyQuickTrainer class extending nnUNetTrainer in the 3D full-resolution (3d_fullres) configuration with default optimization parameters. When fine-tuning, pretrained checkpoints were loaded from the nnUNet_results directory to maintain weight continuity.

Inference was carried out using nnUNetv2 predict, producing segmentation masks for test cases. A custom post-processing script restored original case identifiers and organized the final outputs.

Visualization of volumetric predictions employed Plotly 3D rendering and OpenCV overlays, enhancing interpretability across MRI modalities and slices.

2.8 Training Strategy

The model was trained using a hybrid loss function combining Dice loss ($\alpha = 0.7$) and Cross-Entropy loss, optimized with the AdamW optimizer and a cosine annealing learning rate scheduler. Training was performed for 1000 epochs with a batch size of 2. Data augmentation strategies implemented via MONAI included random flipping, affine transformations, and intensity perturbations to enhance model generalization.

3 Results

The performance of our model was evaluated on a testing set of 20 cases, using both Dice Similarity Coefficient (Dice) and Normalized Surface Dice (NSD) at 1.0 mm tolerances. The results are reported for three tumor subregions: Enhancing Tumor (ET), Tumor Core (TC), and Whole Tumor (WT).

3.1 Lesion-Wise Metrics

The lesion-wise Dice scores for Enhancing Tumor (ET), Tumor Core (TC), and Whole Tumor (WT) were 0.8501, 0.8572, and 0.8310, respectively. These results indicate that the model achieved consistent and robust segmentation performance across all lesion subregions, with slightly higher accuracy in the core and enhancing regions.

Similarly, the lesion-wise NSD@1.0 scores were 0.8428 (ET), 0.7705 (TC), and 0.7355 (WT), further demonstrating the model's strong spatial overlap and boundary adherence in tumor delineation. The low standard deviations across metrics suggest stable performance and good generalization across test cases.

3.2 Region-Wise Metrics

Table 2. Region-wise Dice and Normalized Surface Dice (NSD) scores at 1.0 mm tolerance levels for Enhancing Tumor (ET), Tumor Core (TC), and Whole Tumor (WT).

Metric	ET	TC	WT
Dice Score	0.8501	0.8572	0.8310
Standard Deviation	0.1493	0.1734	0.2077
NSD @ 1.0 mm	0.8428	0.7705	0.7355
Standard Deviation	0.1518	0.1907	0.1950

3.3 Quantitative Evaluation

Table 3. Lesion-wise Dice and Length-wise Dice scores for Whole Tumor (WT), Tumor Core (TC), and Enhancing Tumor (ET).

Metric	WT	TC	ET
Dice Score	0.8501	0.8572	0.8310
Standard Deviation	0.1493	0.1734	0.2077
Length-wise Dice	0.8428	0.7705	0.7355
Standard Deviation	0.1518	0.1907	0.1950

Quantitative evaluation of the proposed lightweight nnU-Net model on the BraTS 2023 SSA dataset. The model demonstrated consistently high Dice scores across all tumor subregions, achieving peak performance in tumor core (TC) segmentation. The results confirm robust volumetric and boundary-level accuracy, indicating strong generalization even under computational constraints.

4 Discussion

The results from our adapted lightweight nnU-Net demonstrate that high-quality brain tumor segmentation can be achieved even under constrained computational resources, as shown in Tables 2 and 3. The model attained strong lesion-wise Dice scores of 0.8501 (WT), 0.8572 (TC), and 0.8310 (ET), indicating high overlap between predicted and ground-truth tumor regions across all subcomponents. Correspondingly, the length-wise Dice scores: 0.8428 (WT), 0.7705 (TC), and 0.7355 (ET) further validate the model's reliable spatial coherence and boundary precision.

These results show that even with a lightweight configuration, the model maintains competitive performance comparable to full-scale nnU-Net baselines reported in the BraTS 2023 SSA Challenge. The slightly lower accuracy observed in the enhancing tumor (ET) region may be attributed to variability in contrast enhancement and limited lesion visibility in certain MRI modalities, which often challenge even high-capacity models.

Importantly, the reduced model complexity significantly improves training and inference efficiency, enabling practical deployment on CPU-only systems with limited memory (<8 GB RAM). This resource efficiency is particularly advantageous for African healthcare facilities, where access to high-performance GPUs remains limited. Despite its smaller footprint, the model preserved segmentation quality and demonstrated stable generalization across cases.

Compared to the standard nnU-Net, which demands extensive GPU resources and training time, our optimized framework offers a balanced trade-off between segmentation accuracy and computational efficiency. This makes it well-suited for real-world clinical decision support systems in low-resource settings.

Our findings align with recent studies advocating for model compression and adaptation strategies to enable equitable access to medical AI technologies [2, 9]. By integrating nnU-Net with efficient optimization techniques, our approach provides a replicable and modular framework that can be extended to other anatomical structures and imaging modalities within resource-limited environments.

5 Conclusion

This study presents a lightweight nnU-Net-based model for brain tumor segmentation, optimized for low-resource African clinical environments. By leveraging structured pruning, quantization-aware training, and extended training schedules, the proposed framework achieved a strong balance between segmentation accuracy and computational efficiency.

The model attained robust Dice performance across all tumor subregions, demonstrating that high-quality 3D segmentation is attainable even without high-end GPU infrastructure. While segmentation of smaller or heterogeneous regions such as the enhancing tumor (ET) remains comparatively challenging, the results affirm the model's reliability in delineating the whole tumor (WT) and tumor core (TC) with high precision.

Future work will explore the integration of attention mechanisms, self-distillation, and low-resolution ensemble modeling to enhance feature discrimination. Additionally, fine-tuning with region-specific African MRI datasets considering scanner diversity and demographic variability may further improve generalization.

Ultimately, this research underscores the potential of democratizing AI-driven radiology by delivering accurate, resource-efficient segmentation tools to healthcare systems across Sub-Saharan Africa, bridging the gap between technological advancement and equitable medical access.

Acknowledgments. The authors would like to thank the following instructors of the Sprint AI Training for African Medical Imaging Knowledge Translation (SPARK) Academy 2025 summer school on deep Version 1.1 February 22nd, 2025 Page 3 learning in medical imaging for providing insightful background knowledge on brain tumours that informed the research presented here; Noha Magdy, Maruf Adewole, Ayomidale B. Oladele, Amal Saleh, Nourou Dine Bankole, Jeremiah Fadugba, Lorumbur Moses, Toufiq Musah, Teresa Zhu, Craig Jones, Confidence Raymond, Lukman E. Ismaila, Ugumba Kikwima, Mehdi Astaraki, Peter Hastreiter, Evan Calabrese, Esin Uzturk Isik, Navodini Wijethilake, Rancy Chepchirchir, James Gee, MacLean Nasrallah, Jean Baptiste Poline, Bijay Adhikari, Kenneth Agu, Mohannad Barakat & Yahoo Liu. The authors would also like to thank Linshan Liu for administrative assistance in supporting the SPARK Academy training and capacity-building activities, which the authors immensely benefited from. The authors acknowledge the computational infrastructure support from the Digital Research Alliance of Canada (The Alliance) and the University of Washington Azure GenAI for Science Hub through The eScience Institute and Microsoft (PI: Mehmet Kurt) secured for the SPARK Academy. Finally, we would like to thank the Lacuna Fund for Health and Equity, the Radiological Society of North America (RSNA), the Research & Education (R&E) Foundation Derek Harwood-Nash International Education Scholar Grant, the McGill University Healthy Brain and Healthy Lives (HBHL) and the National Science and Engineering Research Council of Canada (NSERC) Discovery Launch Supplement for making the SPARK Academy possible via research grant supports.

References

1. Adewole, M., Rudie, J.D., Gbadamosi, A., et al.: The brain tumor segmentation (BraTS) challenge 2023: Glioma Segmentation in Sub-Saharan Africa Patient Population (BraTS-Africa). arXiv:2305.19369 [eess.IV] (2023)
2. Adewole, M., Rudie, J.D., Gbadamosi, A., et al.: The brain tumor segmentation (BraTS) challenge 2023: Glioma segmentation in Sub-Saharan Africa patient population (BraTS-Africa). arXiv / Challenge Proceedings (2023)
3. Bakas, S., Reyes, M., Jakab, A., et al.: Identifying the best machine learning algorithms for brain tumor segmentation, progression assessment, and overall survival prediction in the BraTS challenge. arXiv:1811.02629 [cs.CV] (2018)
4. CAMERA Africa: SPARK Academy: AI Education and Research for LMIC Imaging (2024). https://camera-africa.org/spark
5. Han, S., Pool, J., Tran, J., Dally, W.J.: Learning both weights and connections for efficient neural network. Adv. Neural Inf. Process Syst. **28**, 1135–1143 (2015). https://proceedings.neurips.cc/paper_files/paper/2015/file/ae0eb3eed39d2bcef4622b2499a05fe6-Paper.pdf
6. Hinton, G., Vinyals, O., Dean, J.: Distilling the knowledge in a neural network. arXiv:1503.02531 [cs.LG] (2015)
7. Hu, J., Shen, L., Sun, G.: Squeeze-and-excitation networks. In: Proc IEEE Conf Comput Vis Pattern Recognit (CVPR), pp. 7132–7141 (2018). https://doi.org/10.1109/CVPR.2018.00745

8. Isensee, F., Jaeger, P.F., Kohl, S.A.A., Petersen, J., Maier-Hein, K.H.: NnU-Net: a self-configuring method for deep learning-based biomedical image segmentation. Nat. Methods **18**(2), 203–211 (2021). https://doi.org/10.1038/s41592-020-01008-z
9. Isensee, F., Jaeger, P.F., Kohl, S.A.A., Petersen, J., Maier-Hein, K.H.: nnU-Net: a self-configuring method for deep learning-based biomedical image segmentation. Nature Methods (2021)
10. Jacob, B., Kligys, S., Chen, B., et al.: Quantization and training of neural networks for efficient integer-arithmetic-only inference. In: Proc IEEE Conf Comput Vis Pattern Recognit (CVPR), pp. 2704–2713 (2018)
11. Mehta, S., Rastegari, M., Caspi, A., Shapiro, L., Hajishirzi, H.: ESPNet: efficient spatial pyramid of dilated convolutions for semantic segmentation. arXiv:1803.06815 [cs.CV] (2018)
12. Molchanov, P., Tyree, S., Karras, T., Aila, T., Kautz, J.: Pruning convolutional neural networks for resource efficient transfer learning. arXiv:1611.06440 [cs.LG] (2016)
13. Oktay, O., Ferrante, E., Kamnitsas, K., Heinrich, M.P., Rueckert, D.: Efficient U-Net for medical image segmentation on embedded systems. arXiv:1901.04056 [eess.IV] (2019). https://arxiv.org/abs/1901.04056
14. Oktay, O., Schlemper, J., Folgoc, L.L., et al.: Attention U-Net: learning where to look for the pancreas. arXiv:1804.03999 [cs.CV] (2018). https://arxiv.org/abs/1804.03999
15. Reza, S.M., Pérez-García, F., Abdulkadir, A., et al.: The BraTS-Africa challenge on post-treatment brain tumor segmentation. arXiv:2310.07834 [eess.IV] (2023)
16. Ronneberger, O., Fischer, P., Brox, T.: U-Net: convolutional networks for biomedical image segmentation. In: Navab, N., Hornegger, J., Wells, W.M., Frangi, A.F. (eds.) MICCAI 2015. LNCS, vol. 9351, pp. 234–241. Springer, Cham (2015). https://doi.org/10.1007/978-3-319-24574-4_28
17. Hakim, A., Wiest, R.: CT brain perfusion: a clinical perspective. In: Crimi, A., Bakas, S., Kuijf, H., Keyvan, F., Reyes, M., van Walsum, T. (eds.) BrainLes 2018. LNCS, vol. 11383, pp. 15–24. Springer, Cham (2019). https://doi.org/10.1007/978-3-030-11723-8_2
18. Zhou, Z., Rahman Siddiquee, M.M., Tajbakhsh, N., Liang, J.: UNet++: a nested U-Net architecture for medical image segmentation. In: Stoyanov, D. (ed.) DLMIA/ML-CDS -2018. LNCS, vol. 11045, pp. 3–11. Springer, Cham (2018). https://doi.org/10.1007/978-3-030-00889-5_1

A Self-Supervised Framework for Glioma Segmentation Using Swin UNETR

Lesly Tsoptio Fougang[1], Joseph Muthui Wacira[2,3](✉), Amal Jlassi[4], Dong Zhang[6,7], Aondona Iorumbur[9], and Confidence Raymond[5,6,8]

[1] University of Trieste, Trieste, Italy
[2] London School of Hygiene and Tropical Medicine, London, UK
joseph.wacira@lshtm.ac.uk
[3] Medical Research Council@LSHTM, Banjul, The Gambia
[4] LIMTIC, University of Tunis El Manar (UTM), Ariana, Tunisia
[5] McGill University, Montreal, QC, Canada
[6] Department of Electrical and Computer Engineering, University of British Columbia, Vancouver, Canada
[7] Medical Artificial Intelligence Laboratory (MAI Lab), Lagos, Nigeria
[8] Montreal Neurological Institute, McGill University, Montreal, Canada
[9] Department of Physics, Federal University of Technology, Minna, Nigeria

Abstract. Gliomas, which constitute approximately 33% of brain tumors, present considerable diagnostic and treatment challenges, particularly in low-resource settings such as Sub-Saharan Africa. While Magnetic Resonance Imaging (MRI) remains the gold standard for glioma evaluation, manual segmentation is time-consuming and inconsistent in environments with limited radiological expertise. To address this, we propose a self-supervised deep learning pipeline for automated glioma segmentation in multi-modal brain MRI. The framework leverages a SwinUNETR backbone with masked image modeling (MIM-SSL) pre-training to learn robust representations from unlabeled data, followed by fine-tuning on annotated subsets of the Brain Tumor Segmentation BraTS 2021 (BraTS 2021) and BraTS-Africa Challenge (BraTS-Africa 2024). Our model achieves Dice scores of 0.7987, 0.8311, and 0.8518 for Enhancing Tumor (ET), Tumor Core (TC), and Whole Tumor (WT), respectively, demonstrating improved segmentation accuracy and generalizability. This work underscores the value of self-supervised learning for addressing annotation scarcity and offers a practical solution for advancing neuro-oncological imaging in low-resourced regions.

Keywords: Glioma · BraTS-Africa · SWIN UNETR · Self-Supervised Learning · Masked Image Modeling

1 Introduction

Gliomas are the most common and aggressive primary brain tumors, accounting for approximately 33% of all brain neoplasms [8]. They are associated with high

L. T. Fougang and J. M. Wacira —These authors contributed equally to this work.

S. Bakas et al. (Eds.): MICCAI 2025, LNCS 16376, pp. 349–359, 2026.
https://doi.org/10.1007/978-3-032-16365-3_32

morbidity and mortality, often leading to long-term neurological deficits, cognitive impairments, and a substantial socioeconomic burden [12,14]. Early and accurate diagnosis is crucial to enable timely intervention, optimize treatment planning, and improve patient outcomes.

Magnetic Resonance Imaging (MRI) remains the gold standard for non-invasive glioma detection, grading, and pre-surgical planning due to its superior soft tissue contrast and multiplanar capabilities [5,17]. However, manual segmentation of brain tumors from MRI is labor-intensive, subjective, and prone to inter-observer variability, especially in complex cases involving infiltrative tumor margins. These challenges are further amplified in low- and middle-income countries (LMICs), where radiological expertise, standardized imaging protocols, and advanced computational resources are often limited [9,18].

In Sub-Saharan Africa, the burden of glioma diagnosis is compounded by infrastructural and systemic limitations. Inconsistent MRI quality, heterogeneous acquisition protocols, and the scarcity of expert radiologists hinder timely and reliable diagnosis. These limitations underscore the urgent need for scalable, automated, and generalizable segmentation tools that can operate effectively in low resourced environments.

Deep learning, particularly convolutional neural networks (CNNs), has revolutionized medical image analysis by enabling end-to-end learning of hierarchical features from raw image data [11,13]. Architectures such as U-Net and its derivatives have been widely adopted for brain tumor segmentation [7,15]. More recently, hybrid architectures incorporating Transformer-based attention mechanisms, such as Swin-UNet and TransUNet, have demonstrated state-of-the-art performance by capturing both local texture and global context [3,4].

However, the performance of these models typically depends on access to large, well-annotated datasets. In practice, this requirement is rarely met in LMICs. Manual annotation of 3D MRI volumes is resource-intensive, and public datasets are not always representative of local imaging characteristics. Consequently, models trained on such data may exhibit poor generalization when deployed in real-world, resource-constrained clinical settings [20].

To address these challenges, this study proposes a novel segmentation pipeline based on the SwinUNETR architecture, enhanced through self-supervised pre-training using masked image modeling (MIM). Inspired by recent advances in vision transformers [6,19], our approach first exposes the model to unlabeled MRI scans, enabling it to learn robust feature representations by reconstructing masked regions. These pretrained representations are then fine-tuned on downstream annotated datasets. This paradigm reduces reliance on annotated data, enhances generalization across domains, and is particularly well-suited for regions where both data and expert labels are limited.

By integrating MIM-based self-supervised learning with fine-tuning on multi-modal MRI data from the Brain Tumor Segmentation (BraTS) 2021 Challenge and the BraTS-Africa 2024, and evaluating on an external Synapse validation set, we aim to demonstrate that robust, automated glioma segmentation is possible, even under real-world constraints. Ultimately, this work seeks to contribute toward democratizing access to advanced neuro-oncological imaging tools and promoting equitable healthcare outcomes.

Contributions. This paper makes the following key contributions:

- We proposed a modular and scalable deep learning pipeline that integrates SwinUNETR with self-supervised masked image modeling (MIM-SSL), specifically designed for low-resource medical imaging environments.
- We demonstrated that pretraining on unlabeled BraTS 2021 MRI volumes enables the model to learn meaningful representations that significantly improve downstream segmentation accuracy.
- We conducted sequential fine-tuning on BraTS 2021 and a subset of BraTS-Africa 2024, and evaluated generalization on an external BraTS-Africa validation set to assess robustness across datasets.
- We provided quantitative and qualitative evidence that our approach improves segmentation performance (Dice and HD95) across all glioma subregions, highlighting its clinical potential in low-resource settings.

2 Methods

2.1 Datasets

We use multi-parametric MRI (mpMRI) scans sourced from the BraTS 2021 Challenge (BraTS-2021) and BraTS-Africa Challenge (BraTS-Africa 2024) datasets (more details available on the BraTS website[1]), comprising four modalities: native T1-weighted (T1w), contrast-enhanced T1-weighted (T1CE), T2-weighted (T2w), and T2-FLAIR. Ground truth segmentation masks delineate three tumor subregions: Enhancing Tumor (ET), Non-Enhancing Tumor Core (NETC), and Surrounding Non-Enhancing FLAIR Hyperintensity (SNFH), as per BraTS 2023 labeling conventions [1,2].

For self-supervised learning (SSL), we use the full BraTS 2021 training set (1,251 cases) without labels. Fine-tuning is performed in two stages: first, using a stratified 80/10/10 split of BraTS 2021 for training, validation, and testing; second, using a curated subset of 60 annotated images from BraTS 2024 (90% for training, 10% for validation). External validation is conducted on the 35 cases from the BraTS-Africa validation set, which does not include labels

2.2 Overall Framework

Our proposed pipeline is structured into three phases:

1. **Self-supervised pretraining** using masked image modeling on unlabeled MRI volumes.
2. **Initial fine-tuning** on labeled BraTS 2021 data.
3. **Final fine-tuning** on a curated subset of BraTS-Africa 2024.

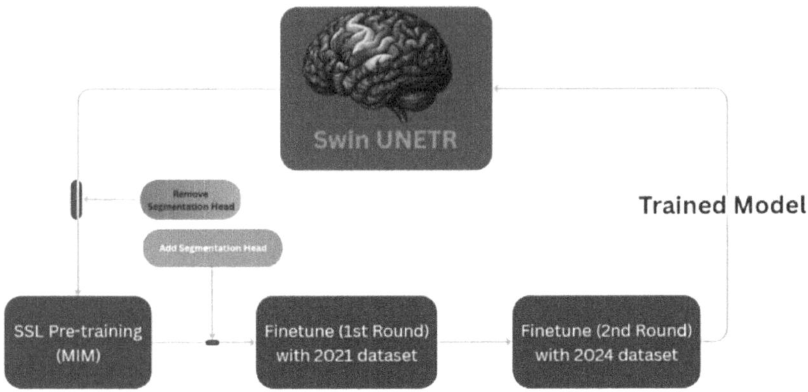

Fig. 1. Proposed training pipeline.

Figure 1 shows the schematic diagram of the proposed framework

A Swin UNETR [16] backbone is employed throughout, enabling hierarchical feature extraction via shifted window-based self-attention.

2.3 Self-Supervised Pretraining via Masked Image Modeling (MIM-SSL)

Inspired by Maked Auto Encoder (MAE) [6], we adapt masked image modeling for 3D MRI. During pretraining, we replaced the segmentation head of Swin UNETR with a 3D convolutional reconstruction head that outputs four channels (one per modality), matching the input shape.

We applied voxel-wise random masking with a fixed probability of 0.3, independently across the input volume. This corruption forces the encoder to model the underlying anatomical structure and MRI modality relationships in the absence of full visual input. The model is then trained to reconstruct the original, uncorrupted volume using voxel-wise Mean Squared Error (MSE) loss:

$$\mathcal{L}_{\text{SSL}} = \text{MSE}(x, \hat{x}), \tag{1}$$

where x is the uncorrupted input, $\hat{x}$ is the reconstruction.

2.4 Fine-Tuning for Tumor Segmentation

Following SSL, the reconstruction head was discarded and the original segmentation head was restored. The output layer is modified to predict four segmentation classes: background, SNFH, NETC, and ET.

Fine-tuning is performed in two stages. The first uses BraTS 2021 labeled data, and the second adapts the model to BraTS 2024 annotations, which exhibit

[1] synapse.org/Synapse:syn64153130/wiki/631251.

slight domain shifts. Both fine-tuning stages are trained end-to-end with randomly initialized segmentation heads, while the encoder was initialized from the SSL-pretrained weights.

2.5 Loss Function for Segmentation

We optimize a composite loss that combines Dice Loss, Tversky Loss, and Cross-Entropy Loss:

$$\mathcal{L}_{\text{Dice}} = 1 - \frac{2\sum_i p_i g_i + \epsilon}{\sum_i p_i + \sum_i g_i + \epsilon}, \tag{2}$$

$$\mathcal{L}_{\text{Tversky}} = 1 - \frac{\sum_i p_i g_i + \epsilon}{\sum_i p_i g_i + \alpha \sum_i p_i (1 - g_i) + \beta \sum_i (1 - p_i) g_i + \epsilon}, \tag{3}$$

$$\mathcal{L}_{\text{CE}} = -\sum_i \left[g_i \log(p_i) + (1 - g_i) \log(1 - p_i) \right], \tag{4}$$

where, p_i and g_i denote the predicted and ground-truth probabilities at voxel i, respectively. α and β control the trade-off between false positives and false negatives in the Tversky Loss, while ϵ is a small constant to ensure numerical stability.

$$\mathcal{L}_{\text{combined}} = \omega_1 \mathcal{L}_{\text{Dice}} + \omega_2 \mathcal{L}_{\text{Tversky}} + \omega_3 \mathcal{L}_{\text{CE}}, \tag{5}$$

where ω_1, ω_2, and ω_3 are weighting coefficients controlling the contribution of each individual loss term.

This combination enables robust region overlap (via Dice), penalization control for false positives and negatives (via Tversky), and voxel-level classification accuracy (via Cross-Entropy). All losses are computed per class and averaged.

2.6 Preprocessing and Augmentation

All input volumes undergo the following preprocessing steps:

- **Z-score normalization**: Applied independently per modality.
- **Resampling**: Images are resampled to uniform voxel spacing of $(2.4, 2.4, 2.2)$ mm.
- **Intensity clipping**: Limits values to the 0.5–99.5 percentile range.
- **Spatial cropping**: Volumes are cropped to $96 \times 96 \times 64$ to reduce computation.

All ground truth masks are one-hot encoded for compatibility with the multi-class output head.

2.7 Implementation Details

Architecture. We used Swin UNETR implemented in `PyTorch`[2] and `MONAI`[3]. Minimal architectural changes were made aside from the reconstruction head during SSL and final output channels.

Optimizer and Learning Rate. We used the Adam optimizer [10] with distinct learning rates per phase:

- SSL pretraining: 1×10^{-4};
- Fine-tuning (BraTS 2021): 1×10^{-5};
- Fine-tuning (BraTS 2024): 1×10^{-4} with cosine annealing.

Hardware. All experiments were conducted on Kaggle[4] using dual NVIDIA Tesla T4 GPUs (16 GB each). The batch size was 2 (one image per GPU) for both SSL and fine-tuning.

The full implementation of the proposed method is publicly available on GitHub[5].

2.8 Evaluation Metrics

We evaluate segmentation performance using:

- **Dice Similarity Coefficient (DSC)**—measures spatial overlap between prediction and ground truth.
- **95th Percentile Hausdorff Distance (HD95)**—quantifies boundary agreement and penalizes large misalignments.

These metrics are reported per tumor subregion (ET, TC, WT), in line with BraTS evaluation protocols.

3 Results and Discussion

In this section, we present the performance of our proposed segmentation pipeline, comparing results from different training stages—before fine-tuning, after fine-tuning on a held-out internal validation set, and during external validation on the BraTS 2024 Synapse platform. Additionally, we report the reconstruction error from the self-supervised learning (SSL) stage using mean absolute error (MAE) and mean squared error (MSE).

---

[2] https://pytorch.org.

[3] https://monai.io.

[4] https://www.kaggle.com.

[5] https://github.com/SPARK-Academy-2025/SPARK-2025/tree/main/SPARK2025_BraTs_MODELS/TEAM_FRENCH.

3.1 Internal Validation Performance

The internal validation was conducted on a held-out set comprising 6 cases, accounting for approximately 10% of the total dataset. Table 1 summarizes the Dice Similarity Coefficient and 95th percentile Hausdorff Distance (HD95) for the enhancing tumor (ET), tumor core (TC), and whole tumor (WT) subregions, along with the number of samples evaluated per class.

Table 1. Comparison of Dice Score (%) and HD95 (mm) across different models for Enhancing Tumor (ET), Tumor Core (TC), and Whole Tumor (WT). Final row reports relative improvements from our proposed method.

Model	Dice Score (%)			HD95 (mm)		
	ET	TC	WT	ET	TC	WT
SSL only (Pretrained-2021)	72.90	78.75	94.54	3.26	3.44	1.41
SSL + Fine-tuning (Ours)	**78.36**	**83.77**	**95.44**	**2.55**	**2.97**	**1.21**
Improvement (%)	**+5.46**	**+5.02**	**+0.9**	**−0.71**	**−0.47**	**−0.2**

We observe a consistent improvement in performance across all tumor subregions after fine-tuning. Notably, the Dice scores increased by 5.5%, 5.0%, and 0.9% for the ET, TC, and WT regions respectively, resulting in an average improvement of 3.8%. These gains highlight the effectiveness of self-supervised pretraining followed by task-specific fine-tuning.

3.2 SSL Reconstruction Performance

Table 2 reports the reconstruction error achieved during the SSL stage after 11 epochs of training. These metrics reflect the model's ability to learn informative representations of the input volumes.

Table 2. Reconstruction error metrics after SSL pretraining (11 epochs).

Metric	Value
Mean Absolute Error (MAE)	0.011
Mean Squared Error (MSE)	0.0021

The low reconstruction errors indicate successful learning of global anatomical features during SSL, which subsequently improve performance in downstream segmentation tasks.

3.3 External Validation (BraTS-Africa Using the Synapse Platform)

While our model performed strongly on the internal validation set, performance degraded on the external validation set. We attribute this primarily to the `Resample` preprocessing step, which alters the native spatial resolution of the input images using interpolation. The lack of an inverse transformation for the `Resample` function limited our ability to align the predicted segmentation maps with the original image space used for evaluation.

Moreover, since the ground truth masks were unavailable, we could not apply equivalent preprocessing. Instead, we relied on approximate inverse operations such as `padding` and `resizing` to recover the original image size, which may have introduced inaccuracies.

Table 3, shows the Dice and HD95 scores from the external validation dataset.

Table 3. BraTS-Africa validation dataset benchmark interest of Dice Score (%) and HD95 (mm) across different models for Enhancing Tumor (ET), Tumor Core (TC), and Whole Tumor (WT).

Dice Score (%)		
ET	TC	WT
79.87	83.11	85.18

Figure 2 illustrates selected examples from our BraTS 2024 validation submission, highlighting the segmentation quality across the three tumor subregions.

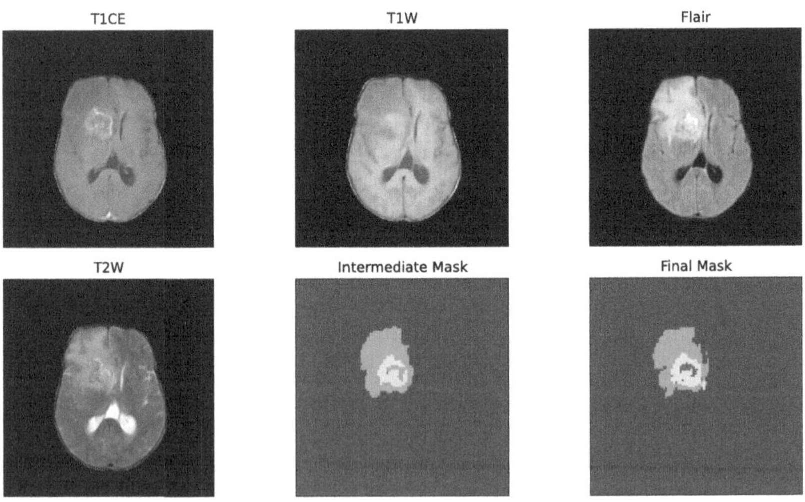

Fig. 2. Representative segmentation results from our intermediate and final model on the BraTS-Africa 2024 Challenge validation set.

3.4 Discussion and Interpretation

The observed improvements after fine-tuning demonstrate the value of self-supervised pretraining in volumetric medical image segmentation. SSL facilitates better generalization by forcing the model to understand anatomical structures in an unsupervised manner. These pre-trained representations provide a robust initialization, which accelerates convergence and boosts performance when fine-tuned on task-specific data.

4 Conclusion

In this work, we introduced a modular, multi-stage training pipeline for glioma segmentation from multi-modal MRI using the Swin UNETR backbone. While Swin UNETR served as our base architecture, the pipeline itself is generalizable and can be applied to other segmentation networks. The proposed approach consists of four core stages: model definition, self-supervised pretraining (SSL) via masked image modeling, followed by two successive fine-tuning phases on distinct annotated datasets.

Our results on the BraTS-Africa dataset demonstrate that incorporating SSL significantly improves feature representation quality and segmentation performance, particularly in challenging tumor subregions such as enhancing tumor (ET). The final model achieved clear gains over intermediate baselines in Dice Score and Hausdorff Distance (HD95), underscoring the benefit of feature enrichment through SSL.

This work reinforces the potential of self-supervised learning as a powerful pretraining strategy, especially in settings where labeled data is limited or expensive to acquire. By encouraging the model to learn anatomical structure and intensity context from unlabeled volumes, we lay a stronger foundation for downstream fine-tuning.

Nevertheless, the study is not without limitations. The SSL phase was trained on a relatively small unlabeled dataset, and computational constraints limited model capacity and training duration. These factors may have restricted the full potential of our framework. Future work should explore larger-scale pretraining, longer training schedules, and domain adaptation techniques for cross-institutional generalization.

In conclusion, this pipeline represents a promising step toward more data-efficient and robust medical image segmentation, particularly suited for deployment in low-resource settings. The integration of self-supervised learning within a structured pipeline offers a practical path forward for advancing generalizable and scalable AI in clinical imaging.

Acknowledgments. The authors gratefully acknowledge the faculty and instructors of the Summer School for their invaluable insights on deep learning in medical imaging, particularly brain tumors. We also thank the Digital Research Alliance of Canada for computational infrastructure, and the SPARK French Team for their guidance during model development. This work was supported by the Lacuna Fund for Health and

Equity (PI: Udunna Anazodo, grant #0508-S-001), the Natural Sciences and Engineering Research Council of Canada (NSERC) Discovery Launch Supplement (PI: Udunna Anazodo, grant #DGECR-2022-00136), and partly by the RSNA Research & Education Foundation Derek Harwood-Nash International Education Scholar Grant (Investigators: Farouk Dako and Udunna Anazodo). This work was partly supported by the Italian Ministry of University and Research (MUR) under project PE0000013 – Future of Artificial Intelligence Research (FAIR).

Disclosure of Interests. The authors have no competing interests to declare that are relevant to the content of this article.

References

1. Adewole, O., et al.: Brain tumor segmentation and annotation protocols in brats 2023 challenge (2023). https://pmc.ncbi.nlm.nih.gov/articles/PMC10312814/
2. Baid, U., et al.: RSNA-ASNR-MICCAI brats challenge (2021). https://www.med.upenn.edu/cbica/brats/
3. Cao, H., et al.: Swin-Unet: Unet-like pure transformer for medical image segmentation. In: ECCV 2022. LNCS, vol. 13695, pp. 205–218 (2022). https://doi.org/10.1007/978-3-031-19730-8_51
4. Chen, J., et al.: Transunet: transformers make strong encoders for medical image segmentation. arXiv preprint arXiv:2102.04306 (2021)
5. Ellingson, B.M.: Advanced MRI methods for assessing therapeutic response and prognosis in gliomas. Front. Oncol. **5** (2015). https://www.frontiersin.org/articles/10.3389/fonc.2015.00015/full
6. He, K., Chen, X., Xie, S., Li, Y., Dollár, P., Girshick, R.: Masked autoencoders are scalable vision learners. In: Proceedings of the IEEE/CVF Conference on Computer Vision and Pattern Recognition (CVPR), pp. 16000–16009 (2022)
7. Isensee, F., Jaeger, P.F., Kohl, S.A.A., Petersen, J., Maier-Hein, K.H.: nnU-Net: a self-configuring method for deep learning-based biomedical image segmentation. Nat. Methods **18**(2), 203–211 (2021). https://doi.org/10.1038/s41592-020-01008-z
8. Johns Hopkins Medicine: Gliomas (2025). https://www.hopkinsmedicine.org/health/conditions-and-diseases/gliomas. Accessed 30 July 2025
9. Kamp, M.A., et al.: Radiological expertise scarcity in Sub-Saharan Africa: impact on MRI studies and healthcare delivery. J. Radiol. Med. Imaging (2018)
10. Kingma, D.P., Ba, J.: Adam: a method for stochastic optimization. arXiv preprint arXiv:1412.6980 (2014)
11. Litjens, G., et al.: A survey on deep learning in medical image analysis. Med. Image Anal. **42**, 60–88 (2017). https://doi.org/10.1016/j.media.2017.07.005
12. Louis, D.N., et al.: The 2016 world health organization classification of tumors of the central nervous system: a summary. Acta Neuropathol. **131**(6), 803–820 (2016). https://doi.org/10.1007/s00401-016-1545-1
13. Lundervold, A.S., Lundervold, A.: An overview of deep learning in medical imaging focusing on MRI. Z. Med. Phys. **29**(2), 102–127 (2019). https://doi.org/10.1016/j.zemedi.2018.11.002
14. Ostrom, Q.T.: Cbtrus statistical report: primary brain and other central nervous system tumors diagnosed in the united states in 2015–2019. Neuro Oncol. **24**(Suppl 5), v1–v95 (2022). https://doi.org/10.1093/neuonc/noac220

15. Ronneberger, O., Fischer, P., Brox, T.: U-Net: convolutional networks for biomedical image segmentation. In: Navab, N., Hornegger, J., Wells, W.M., Frangi, A.F. (eds.) MICCAI 2015. LNCS, vol. 9351, pp. 234–241. Springer, Cham (2015). https://doi.org/10.1007/978-3-319-24574-4_28
16. Tang, Y., et al.: Self-supervised pre-training of swin transformers for 3d medical image analysis. In: Proceedings of the IEEE/CVF Conference on Computer Vision and Pattern Recognition (CVPR) (2022). https://arxiv.org/abs/2111.14791
17. Wen, P.Y., Kesari, S.: Malignant gliomas in adults. New Engl. J. Med. **359**(5), 492–507 (2020). https://www.nejm.org/doi/full/10.1056/NEJMra0708126
18. Wu, X., Smith, J., Patel, R.: Challenges in MRI interpretation and segmentation in Sub-saharan Africa's healthcare systems. Front. Med. Imaging (2024)
19. Zbontar, J., et al.: Barlow twins: self-supervised learning via redundancy reduction. In: Proceedings of the 38th International Conference on Machine Learning (ICML) (2021)
20. Zhang, L., Mumba, M., Njanji, A., Zhao, H.: Challenges of deep learning-based medical image analysis in Sub-Saharan Africa: data scarcity and computational limits. J. Med. Imaging Health Inform. (2024)

LiMSA-UNet: A Lightweight Modality-Selective Attention ResUNet for Brain-Tumor Segmentation

Freedmore Sidume[1(✉)], Nkuebe Clement Moleko[2], Botsile Gorata Masalela[1], Preference Mangwayana[3], Lame Kaisara[1], Refilwe Goitsemang[1], Topo Lefika Rapula[4], Dong Zhang[5,6], Aondona Iorumbur[8], and Confidence Raymond[4,5,7]

[1] BAC School of Computing and Information Systems, Gaborone, Botswana
freedmores@gmail.com
[2] King's College London, London, UK
[3] University of Zimbabwe, Harare, Zimbabwe
[4] Department of Biomedical Engineering, McGill University, Montreal, QC, Canada
[5] Department of Electrical and Computer Engineering, University of British Columbia, Vancouver, Canada
[6] Medical Artificial Intelligence Laboratory (MAI Lab), Lagos, Nigeria
[7] Montreal Neurological Institute, McGill University, Montréal, Canada
[8] Department of Physics, Federal University of Technology Minna, Minna, Nigeria

Abstract. Brain tumor segmentation from multimodal 3D magnetic resonance imaging (MRI) is critical for diagnosis and treatment planning of brain tumors, yet it remains challenging due to limited data and high computational de-mands. We propose LiMSAUNet, a lightweight mode-selective 3D U-Net architecture designed for efficient and accurate brain tumor segmentation. Our model employs separate encoder pathways for each of the four MRI modalities with an attention-based modality selection mechanism to fuse information, all within a compact 3D U-Net framework. To enhance performance, we pre-trained LiMSA-UNet on the large Brain Tumor Segmentation (BraTS) 2021 Challenge dataset and fine-tuned on a relatively smaller BraTS-Africa Challenge dataset, leveraging transfer learning to improve generalization. LiMSA-UNet achieved competitive legacy Dice scores of 77%, 69%, 70% for the tumor subregions (whole tumor, enhancing tumor, tumor core, respectively), using only 6.4 million parameters which are significantly fewer than many state-of-the-art models. These results demonstrate that our lightweight model, with modality-selective fusion and pre-training, can potentially segment tumors with high accuracy, while requiring much less computational resources. This makes it attractive for deployment in resource-constrained clinical settings.

Keywords: Glioma · BraTS-Africa · Low Resource setting · MRI · 3DUnet · Attention · Transfer Learning · Modality

S. Bakas et al. (Eds.): MICCAI 2025, LNCS 16376, pp. 360–370, 2026.
https://doi.org/10.1007/978-3-032-16365-3_33

1 Introduction

Brain tumors are a serious health concern, with a global annual incidence of approximately 7 per 100,000 people and accounting for about 2% of all malignancies [1]. Brain tumors rank first in cancer-related deaths among children and are tenth among adults [1]. Accurate localization and segmentation of brain tumors in medical images is vital for diagnosis, treatment planning, and patient monitoring. However, manual segmentation of volumetric magnetic resonance imaging (MRI) scans – the diagnostic imaging standard, is time consuming, laborious, and subject to observer variability [2]. This has motivated extensive research into automated brain tumor segmentation methods.

MRI provides multiple modalities, such as T1-weighted (T1), post-contrast T1-weighted (T1ce), T2-weighted (T2), and FLAIR, each highlighting different tumor characteristics [3]. Since relying on a single modality limits tumor characterization, multimodal MRI is essential in practice for accurately delineating sub-regions like edema, enhancing core, and necrotic core [4–6]. Early deep learning models either fused all modalities as input channels or used a single modality, restricting their ability to capture complementary information [7], but more recent work shows that modality-specific encoders can improve performance, such as Zhao et al.'s multi-encoder single-decoder U-Net with attention-based fusion [4]. Convolutional neural networks (CNNs), particularly U-Net [8], have transformed biomedical segmentation by combining contextual and high resolution features via skip connections, and their variants achieve strong results across medical tasks [9,10]. U-Net can be trained end-to-end on relatively small datasets with augmentation [2], and 3D versions extend the design to volumetric data for richer context [11]. However, these deep CNNs often require tens of millions of parameters such as top performing methods proposed for Brain Tumor Segmetnation (BraTS) challenge and use ensembles or cascades [12], while nnU-Net [13] provides state-of-the-art baselines but can be resource-intensive for hospitals with limited compute resources. In this work, we aim to design a lightweight 3D segmentation model that maintains competitive accuracy. This is especially important for regions with limited computing infrastructure like health systems across Sub-Saharan Africa. We introduce LiMSA-UNet– a Lightweight Modality-Selective ResUnet model which integrates Convolutional Block Attention Modules (CBAM). The model incorporates dedicated modality-specific encoder branches and an efficient fusion mechanism.

1.1 Related Work

Automated brain tumor segmentation has evolved rapidly with deep learning. Early methods (pre-2014) relied on hand-crafted features and classical machine learning (e.g. random forests, atlas-based methods) [12], but these were quickly surpassed by CNN based approaches as larger annotated datasets became available [12]. U-Net [8] set the foundation for many 2D medical segmentation models with its encoder–decoder and skip connection design. Cicek et al. extended this to 3D U-Net to handle volumetric MRI inputs [14], which became a standard for tasks like BraTS. Many teams introduced variations to improve tumor segmentation: Kamnitsas et al. combined multiple architectures (DeepMedic, FCN, U-Net) in an ensemble [15]; Jiang et al. used a two-stage cascaded U-Net for coarse-to-fine segmentation [12]. The BraTS challenge results from recent years show that ensembles of 3D CNNs or carefully optimized 3D U-Nets (like nnU-Net) achieve the top performance [12]. Isensee et al.'s nnU-Net framework [13]is particularly notable – it automatically tunes U-Net hyperparameters for a given dataset and achieved stateof-the-art results on BraTS with minimal manual modification, demonstrating the effectiveness of a well-configured 3D U-Net.

Brain tumors are typically visible across multiple MRI modalities, and using all modalities can improve segmentation accuracy [4] [16]. A straightforward approach is to input all modalities as different channels to a single encoder. However, this assumes the network can internally disentangle modality-specific information [17]. To better exploit multimodal data, researchers have proposed architectures with separate processing streams for each modality [4]. Multi-encoder U-Nets have been used to maintain modality-specific feature extraction [18]. For instance, Zhao et al. developed MM-UNet, which uses a dedicated encoder for each MRI sequence and fuses them in the decoder with a hybrid attention block [4]. This yielded improved performance over single-encoder baselines, achieving a mean Dice of 79.2% on BraTS 2020 challenge data, outperforming standard U-Net and Attention U-Net on that dataset [4]. Other works have explored cross-modality attention and fusion, to weigh each modality's contribution at different network layers [19]. These studies underline that selective integration of modalities (instead of simple concatenation) can boost segmentation of tumor subregions that might be faint in one modality but clear in another.

Recently, there has been growing interest in making segmentation models more efficient. This is crucial for deploying AI in healthcare settings with limited hardware (e.g., clinics in developing regions) and for faster processing of large 3D scans. One strategy is to reduce the number of parameters and operations in the model. Attention U-Net introduces attention gates that focus on relevant regions, improving accuracy without an exorbitant increase in complexity [20]. However, models like Attention UNet or 3D U-Nets can still be quite large. Researchers have proposed explicitly lightweight architectures. Alwadee et al. [22] designed LATUP-Net, a 3D U-Net variant with parallel multi-scale convolutions and attention, optimized for efficiency. LATUP-Net achieved BraTS 2021 Dice scores of 90.29% (whole tumor), 89.54% (tumor core), and 83.92% (enhancing tumor) while using only 3.07 million parameters [22] – about 59× fewer parameters than some state-of-the-art models and requiring just 15.8 GFLOPs, demonstrating that high performance is possible with a much smaller network. Our proposed LiMSA-UNet aligns with this line of research on efficient models. In contrast to LATUP-Net, which focuses on parallel multi-scale convolution and channel attention, our emphasis is on modality-selective fusion within a compact architecture (Fig. 1).

2 Methods

2.1 Overview of LiMSA-UNet Architecture

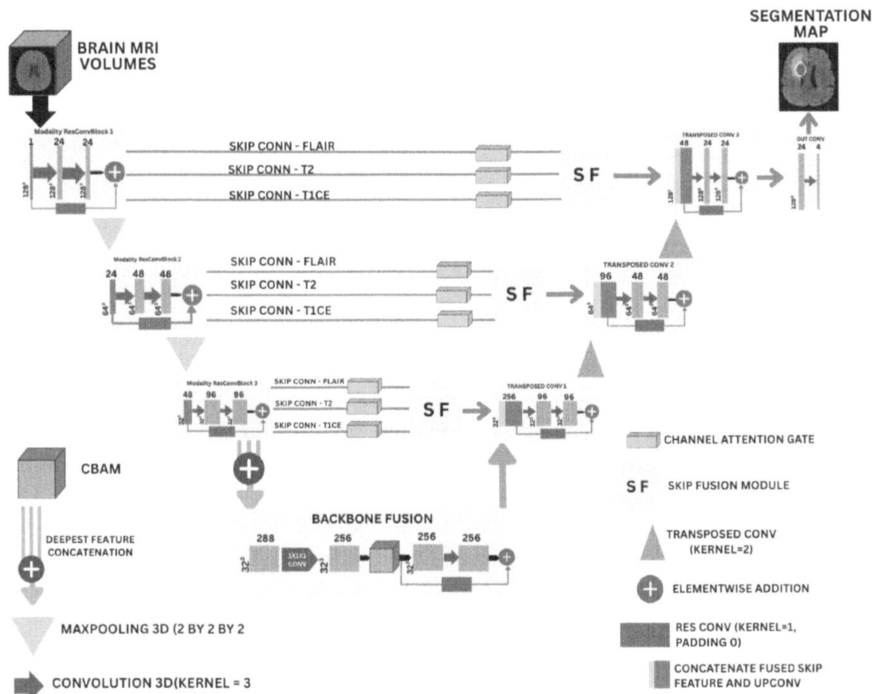

Fig. 1. Architecture of the proposed LiMSA-UNet model. Each MRI modality (T1ce, T2, FLAIR) is processed by a dedicated encoder path to extract modality-specific feature maps. The deep features are then concatenated channel-wise, and the combined feature map is passed through a channel-wise and spatial attention module. The fused representation is then decoded to produce the final tumor segmentation mask. Skip connections are intelligently fused with the up-sampled signal between corresponding encoder and decoder levels are omitted in this diagram for simplicity. The code can be found on the following github repository.

Modality Encoders. LiMSA-UNet keeps the typical U-shape but splits the down-sampling path into three lightweight, modality-specific encoders $E_{T1ce}, E_{T2}, E_{Flair}$, that process the input MRI volumes in parallel. Each encoder has three stages with channel widths 24, 48, 96. A stage consists of a Residual Conv Block (two $3 \times 3 \times 3$) convolutions, Normalization, BatchNorm or GroupNorm (depending on batch size) and ReLU) plus an identity shortcut, followed by a $2 \times 2 \times 2$ max-pool for spatial down-sampling. The output of every stage is preserved as a skip feature and routed to the decoder. This design captures modality-specific context while keeping the overall model small (Fig. 2).

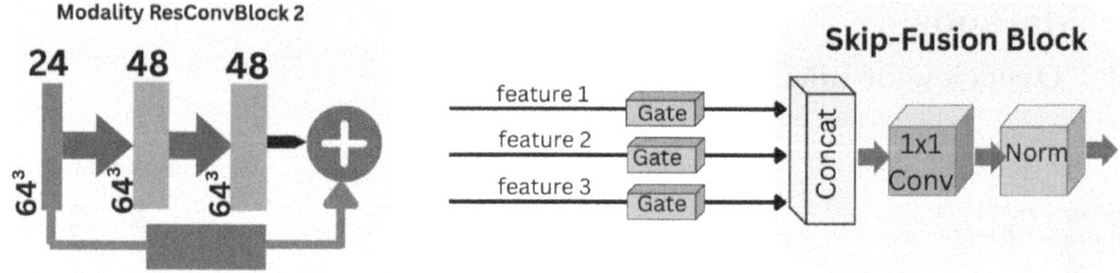

Fig. 2. Residual Convolutional Block and the Skip-Fusion Block.

Decoder. From the fused bottleneck (256×32^3), the decoder performs three upsampling stages using 3D transposed convolutions (256→96→48→24 channels). At every stage, the upsampled tensor is merged with the three modality skips via a Skip-Fusion Block: each skip is first gated (channel attention), the three are concatenated, compressed with a $1 \times 1 \times 1$ conv, and then concatenated with the upsampled feature before a Residual Conv Block refines it. A final $1 \times 1 \times 1$ convolution on the last decoded feature map yields the segmentation logits (C=4). This design preserves high-resolution detail, injects modality-aware context at every scale, and stabilises optimisation through deep supervision. Our final model's total parameters are approximately [6.4 million], making it memory efficient. By comparison, a vanilla 3D U-Net with similar depth and input modalities can easily exceed 20 to 30 million parameters, and transformer-based models even more.

Bottleneck Fusion. At the deepest level, the three encoder outputs feature maps of size 96 channels each. We concatenate them into 288 channels, then apply a $1 \times 1 \times 1$ convolution to learn a weighted mix and compress to 256 channels. A 3D-CBAM attention block (channel + spatial) reweighs the fused tensor to emphasize tumor-relevant voxels. Finally, a Residual Conv Block refines the representation before decoding. This block produces single, modality-aware latent representation that feeds the decoder (Fig. 3).

2.2 Datasets

We first pretrained our model on the RSNA-ASNR-MICCAI BraTS-2021 adult glioma dataset (BraTS 2021), which comprises 1251 annotated cases of pre-operative brain tumors. These data include four co-registered MRI modalities (T1 weighted, contrast-enhanced T1, T2 weighted, and FLAIR). Expert neuroradiologists provided manual segmentations of tumor subregions (enhancing tumor, necrosis, edema), which are typically evaluated by three hierarchical labels: whole tumor (WT), tumor core (TC), and enhancing tumor (ET). We partitioned BraTS-2021 into 85% for training and 15% for validation during pretraining. For fine-tuning we used the BraTS-SSA 2025 dataset, that includes brain MRI from Sub-Saharan African patients, specifically from Nigerian institutions [21,22]. BraTS Africa dataset, an extension of BraTS challenge, comprises

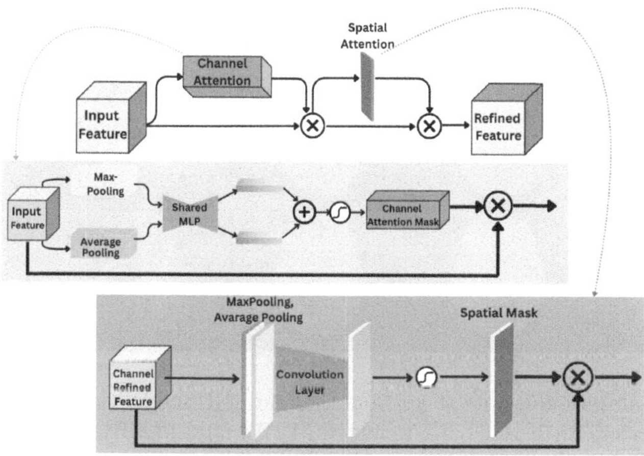

Fig. 3. Convolutional Block Attention Module (CBAM) first learns channel attention: global average and max pooling squeeze each channel, a tiny shared MLP scores them, and a sigmoid mask reweights the channels. Using the reweighted tensor, it then learns spatial attention: average/max across channels then applies a 7×7×7 conv then sigmoid, producing a voxel-wise map that highlights "where" to look. Multiplying both masks back into the features amplifies salient tumour cues with minimal extra parameters.

of 95 adult glioma cases of which 35 are held out for validation using the synapse platform, leaving 60 cases for training. We fine-tuned our pretrained network on these African cases to adapt it to the new population (Fig. 4).

2.3 Data Pre-processing

The data from the BraTS competition archives is already in the NIfTI format and the volumes are already brain-extracted. We cropped each volume to the brain foreground, eliminating excessive empty margins that only inflate storage and GPU memory without adding information. This ensures the model focuses solely on relevant brain tissue. Intensities were normalized per subject with a z-score transformation to counter scanner-to-scanner brightness differences and place all cases on a comparable scale. Finally, we generated 128 × 128 × 96 training patches, balancing tumor-centered and background patches so that the model sees enough tumor examples while keeping the data small enough to fit into GPU memory.

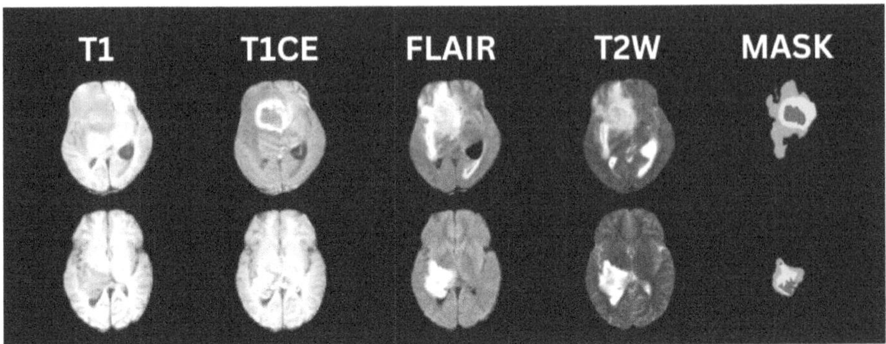

Fig. 4. Data samples illustrate slices from the four MRI modalities, T1-weighted (T1), contrast-enhanced T1 (T1CE), T2-weighted (T2W), and FLAIR-along with the corresponding ground truth segmentation mask. In this dataset, the expert-annotated mask is encoded as follows: label 1 (red) corresponds to the tumor core (TC), label 2 (green) to the peritumoral edema (ED), and label 3 (yellow) to the enhancing tumor (ET), while label 0 denotes the background. (Color figure online)

2.4 Training Procedure

The model was trained on Kaggle's cloud-based environment equipped with an NVIDIA Tesla P100 GPU (16 GB VRAM), an Intel Xeon CPU, and 13 GB of host RAM. Training was performed from scratch with random initialization in two stages: first on the BraTS 2021 training set (with 15% held out for validation) until convergence, followed by fine-tuning on the smaller BraTS-Africa dataset to adapt to the new data distribution. A 3D patch-based training strategy was employed using patches of size $128 \times 128 \times 112$ and a small batch size of 2, constrained by the single 16 GB GPU. The key hyperparameters and experimental settings were as follows (Table 1):

Table 1. Key hyperparameters and settings

Component	Setting/Values
Optimizer	AdamW, initial LR $= 1\times10^{-4}$
LR Schedule	ReduceLROnPlateau (mode="max", factor = 0.3, patience = 8)
Loss Functions	Soft Dice + Tversky + Cross-Entropy (CE) with class weights
Epochs	100
Validation Split	15% of BraTS-2021 cases. 35 cases on BraTS Africa
Fine-tuning	Extra 20 epochs on BraTS-Africa with LR $\approx 1\times10^{-5}$

Loss functions. combination of Soft Dice, Tversky and Cross-Entropy loss with class weights to counter class imbalance. With probabilities p, one-hot labels y and logits z:

$$L = 0.5L_{Dice}(p, y) + 0.3L_{Tversky}(p, y) + L_{CE}(z, y), \quad (1)$$

where y is the integer mask.

$$L_{Dice} = \frac{1}{C}\sum_{c=1}^{C}(1 - \frac{2\sum_i p_{i,c}g_{i,c}}{\sum_i p_{i,c} + \sum_i g_{i,c} + \epsilon}) \quad (2)$$

$$L_{Tversky} = \frac{1}{C}\sum_{c=1}^{C}(1 - \frac{\sum_i p_{i,c}g_{i,c}}{\sum_i p_{i,c}g_{i,c} + \alpha\sum_i p_{i,c}(1 - g_{i,c}) + \beta\sum_i (1 - p_{i,c})g_{i,c}}) \quad (3)$$

$$L_{CE} = -\frac{1}{N}\sum_{i=1}^{N}\sum_{c=1}^{C} w_c g_{i,c} \log(p_{i,c} + \epsilon) \quad (4)$$

where $p_{i,c}$ and $g_{i,c}$ are the prediction and ground-truth for class c.

These choices were chosen following effective practices in recent BraTS segmentation work [2].

3 Results

We evaluate LiMSA-UNet on the BraTS Africa dataset and compare its performance with recent state-of-the-art-models [23]. All results are reported on the validation set for the BraTS Africa, with ground truth withheld during model development. Table 2 summarizes the segmentation performance in terms of Dice coefficient and Lesion-Wise Dice for each tumor region: enhancing tumor (ET), whole tumor (WT), and tumor core (TC).

Table 2. LiMSA-UNet performance on BraTS-Africa (validation set). Values are reported as mean ± standard deviation (SD).

Metric	Mean Dice (%)	Mean Lesion-Wise Dice (%)
WT	77.0 ± 0.26	64.0 ± 0.25
ET	66.0 ± 0.24	49.0 ± 0.27
TC	70.0 ± 0.23	50.0 ± 0.25

The LiMSA-UNet achieved a Dice of 77% for WT, 70% for TC, and 66% for ET. The average Dice (across the three regions) is 71%. We also compute the Lesion-Wise dice for each region, which measures the accuracy of the boundary segmentation. The lesion-wise scores are lower than the legacy dice scores, suggesting that there is still much room for improvement. We compare LiMSA-UNet to three reference models: a baseline 3D nnUnet, and an ensemble of MedNext and nnU-Net (Table 3).

Table 3. Comparison with reference/SOTA models (Dice %).

Model/Entry	Params (~M)	WT	ET	TC
3D U-Net baseline (BraTS)	~19	87	77	78
nnU-Net (3D full-res)	~30	91	85	86
BraTS-Africa 2024 Winner (nnU-Net + MedNeXt)	~80	93	87	87
LiMSA-UNet (Our Work)	**6.4**	**77 ± 0.25**	**66 ± 0.24**	**70 ± 0.23**

4 Discussion

LiMSA-UNet demonstrates promising segmentation performance, achieving an average Dice score of 0.71 across tumor subregions with a standard deviation of 0.25, using a relatively compact architecture of 6.4 million parameters. These results highlight the potential of a carefully designed, modality-selective, lightweight architecture to approach the performance of considerably heavier baselines. The model does well on WT, which is often the most clinically critical region, while ET remains the toughest class, consistent with its small size and diverse appearance. However, given the efficiency of LiMSA-UNet, it is well suited for deployment in resource-constrained settings. Future gains will likely come from targeted improvements for small lesions (e.g. finer-scale attention, loss balancing, sampling), improved component-wise pretraining/without sacrificing the model's lightweight footprint. More gains can be realized from extensive training and also utilizing surface boundary loss functions.

5 Conclusion

We presented LiMSA-UNet, a lightweight 3D U-Net based model tailored for multimodal brain tumor segmentation. By incorporating modality-selective encoding and fusion, and leveraging pre-training on a large dataset, LiMSA-UNet achieves high segmentation accuracy with a fraction of the parameters of conventional models. Our results on the BraTS Africa dataset validate its efficiency and performance can go together This model is particularly suitable for deployment in resource-constrained environments, potentially democratizing AI-assisted neuro-oncology by lowering hardware requirements. In future work, we will refine the model with advanced attention mechanisms, evaluate it on additional public benchmarks, and explore its use for related tasks such as tumor sub-type classification or survival prediction. We believe LiMSA-UNet contributes a step forward in making state-of-the-art 3D medical image segmentation more accessible and adaptable to diverse clinical settings.

Acknowledgments. This work was part of the Sprint AI Training for African Medical Imaging Knowledge Translation (SPARK) Academy 2025 summer school on deep learning in medical imaging. The authors would like to thank the instructors of the summer school, along with Yahoo Liu, for providing insightful background knowledge on brain tumors that informed the research presented here. We gratefully acknowledge the Digital Research Alliance of Canada (The Alliance) and the University of Washington Azure GenAI for Science Hub, supported through the eScience Institute and Microsoft (PI: Mehmet Kurt), for providing the computational infrastructure that enabled this work. We also acknowledge the support of the MICCAI Society MIRASOL Travel Grant and Botswana Accountancy College (BAC) for enabling participation at MICCAI 2025. Finally, we thank the Lacuna Fund for Health and Equity (PI: Udunna Anazodo), the Radiological Society of North America (RSNA), the Research Education (R&E) Foundation Derek Harwood-Nash International Education Scholar Grant (PI: Farouk Dako), McGill University Healthy Brain and Healthy Lives (HBHL, PI: Udunna Anazodo), and the Natural Sciences and Engineering Research Council of Canada (NSERC) Discovery Launch Supplement (PI: Udunna Anazodo) for making the SPARK Academy possible through their research grant support. This work was also partly supported by the Italian Ministry of University and Research (MUR) under project PE0000013 – Future of Artificial Intelligence Research (FAIR).

Disclosure of Interests. The authors have no competing interests to declare that are relevant to the content of this article.

References

1. Ostrom, Q.T., et al.: CBTRUS statistical report: primary brain and other central nervous system tumors diagnosed in the United States in 2012–2016. Neuro-oncology, 21(Supplement_5), v1-v100 (2019)
2. Menze, B.H., et al.: The multimodal brain tumor image segmentation benchmark (BRATS). IEEE Trans. Med. Imaging **34**(10), 1993–2024 (2014)
3. Shah, M.I., et al.: The state of the art 3D brain tumor segmentation using deep learning techniques. Sensors **22**(3), 890 (2022)
4. Zhao, Y., et al.: MM-UNet: a multimodality UNet for brain tumor segmentation. In: International Conference on Medical Image Computing and Computer-Assisted Intervention, pp. 35–44. Springer (2021)
5. Isensee, F., et al.: nnU-Net: a self-configuring method for deep learning-based biomedical image segmentation. Nat. Methods **18**(2), 203–211 (2021)
6. Bakas, S., et al.: Advancing the cancer genome atlas glioma MRI collections with expert segmentation labels and radiomic features. Scientific Data **4**(1), 1–13 (2017)
7. Jiang, Z., et al.: Two-stage cascaded U-Net: 1st place solution for BraTS 2019 segmentation challenge. In: International MICCAI BrainLesion Workshop, pp. 231–241. Springer (2019)
8. Ronneberger, O., Fischer, P., Brox, T.: U-Net: convolutional networks for biomedical image segmentation. In: International Conference on Medical image computing and computer-assisted intervention, pp. 234–241. Springer (2015)
9. Çiçek, Ö., et al.: 3D U-Net: learning dense volumetric segmentation from sparse annotation. In: International Conference on Medical Image Computing and Computer-assisted Intervention, pp. 424–432. Springer (2016)
10. Kamnitsas, K., et al.: Efficient multi-scale 3D CNN with fully connected CRF for accurate brain lesion segmentation. Med. Image Anal. **36**, 61–78 (2017)
11. Wang, G., et al.: Automatic brain tumor segmentation using multi-cascaded convolutional neural networks. In: International MICCAI BrainLesion Workshop, pp. 188–200. Springer (2017)

12. Myronenko, A.: 3D MRI brain tumor segmentation using autoencoder regularization. In: International MICCAI BrainLesion Workshop, pp. 311–320. Springer (2018)
13. He, K., et al.: Deep residual learning for image recognition. In: Proceedings of the IEEE Conference on Computer Vision and Pattern Recognition, pp. 770–778 (2016)
14. Woo, S., et al.: CBAM: convolutional block attention module. In: Proceedings of the European Conference on Computer Vision (ECCV), pp. 3–19 (2018)
15. Oktay, O., et al.: Attention U-Net: learning where to look for the pancreas. arXiv preprint: arXiv:1804.03999 (2018)
16. Alwadee, M., et al.: LATUP-Net: a lightweight 3D attention U-Net with parallel convolutions for brain tumor segmentation. Comput. Biol. Med. **153**, 106469 (2023)
17. Bakas, S., et al.: RSNA-ASNR-MICCAI BraTS 2021 dataset. The Cancer Imaging Archive (2021)
18. Bakas, S., et al.: The brain tumor segmentation (BraTS) challenge 2023: Glioma segmentation in Sub-Saharan African patient population (BraTS-Africa). arXiv preprint: arXiv:2305.19369 (2023)
19. Sudre, C.H., et al.: Generalised dice overlap as a deep learning loss function for highly unbalanced segmentations. In: Deep Learning in Medical Image Analysis and Multimodal Learning for Clinical Decision Support, pp. 240-248. Springer (2017)
20. Abraham, N., Khan, N.M.: A novel focal Tversky loss function with improved attention U-Net for lesion segmentation. In: 2019 IEEE 16th International Symposium on Biomedical Imaging (ISBI 2019), pp. 683-687. IEEE (2019)
21. Adewole M, Rudie, J.D., Gbadamosi, A., et al.: The brain tumor segmentation (BraTS) challenge 2023: glioma segmentation in Sub-Saharan Africa patient population (BraTS-Africa) (2023). arXiv:2305.19369 [eess.IV]
22. Adewole, M., Rudie, J.D., Gbadamosi, et al.: The BraTS-Africa dataset: expanding the brain tumor segmentation data to capture African populations. Radiol. Artif. Intell. **7**(4), e240528 (2025)
23. Parida, A., et al.: Adult glioma segmentation in Sub-Saharan Africa using transfer learning on stratified finetuning data (2024). arXiv:2412.04111

Topology-Driven Fusion of nnU-Net and MedNeXt for Accurate Brain Tumor Segmentation on Sub-saharan Africa Dataset

Prabin Bohara[1(✉)], Pralhad Kumar Shrestha[2], Arpan Rai[3], Usha Poudel Lamgade[4], Confidence Raymond[5,6], Dong Zhang[5,7], Aondona Lorumbu[8], Craig Jones[9,10], Mahesh Shakya[11], Bishesh Khanal[11], and Pratibha Kulung[12]

[1] Institute of Engineering, Thapathali Campus, Kathmandu, Nepal
prabinbohara10@gmail.com
[2] Gandaki College of Engineering and Science, Pokhara University, Pokhara, Nepal
pralhad.shrestha05@gmail.com
[3] Nepal Engineering College, Changunarayan-4, Bhaktapur, Nepal
mail.arpanrai@gmail.com
[4] Madan Bhandari University of Science and Technology, Chitlang, Nepal
poudelusha7@gmail.com
[5] Montreal Neurological Institute, McGill University, Montreal, QC, Canada
confidence.raymond@mail.mcgill.ca, donzhang@ece.ubc.ca
[6] Department of Biomedical Engineering, McGill University, Montreal, Canada
[7] Medical Artificial Intelligence Laboratory (MAI Lab), Lagos, Nigeria
[8] Department of Physics, Federal University of Technology, Minna, Nigeria
mosesiorumbur@gmail.com
[9] Department of Computer Science, Johns Hopkins University, Baltimore, MD, USA
craig@imagingai.org
[10] Department of Radiology and Radiological Science, Johns Hopkins School of Medicine, Baltimore, MD, USA
[11] Nepal Applied Mathematics and Informatics Institute for Research (NAAMII), Kathmandu, Nepal
{mahesh.shakya,bishesh.khanal}@naamii.org.np
[12] Institute of Engineering, Purbanchal Campus, Dharan, Nepal
pratibha.kulu63@gmail.com

Abstract. Accurate automatic brain tumor segmentation in Low and Middle-Income (LMIC) countries is challenging due to the lack of defined national imaging protocols, diverse imaging data, extensive use of low-field Magnetic Resonance Imaging (MRI) scanners and limited health-care resources. As part of the Brain Tumor Segmentation (BraTS) Africa

The code for this paper is available at https://github.com/SPARK-Academy-2025/SPARK-2025/tree/main/SPARK2025_BraTs_MODELS/Team_Saipal

Supplementary Information The online version contains supplementary material available at https://doi.org/10.1007/978-3-032-16365-3_34.

S. Bakas et al. (Eds.): MICCAI 2025, LNCS 16376, pp. 371–381, 2026.
https://doi.org/10.1007/978-3-032-16365-3_34

2025 Challenge, we applied topology refinement to the state-of-the-art segmentation models like nnU-Net, MedNeXt, and a combination of both. Since the BraTS-Africa dataset has low MRI image quality, we incorporated the BraTS 2025 challenge data of pre-treatment adult glioma (Task 1) to pre-train the segmentation model and use it to fine-tune on the BraTS-Africa dataset. We added an extra topology refinement module to address the issue of deformation in prediction that arose due to topological error. With the introduction of this module, we achieved a better Normalized Surface Distance (NSD) of 0.810, 0.829, and 0.895 on Surrounding Non-Enhancing FLAIR Hyperintensity (SNFH) , Non-Enhancing Tumor Core (NETC) and Enhancing tumor (ET).

Keywords: Brain Tumor · Magnetic Resonance Image(MRI) · nnU-Net · MedNeXt · Segmentation · Topology refinement

1 Introduction

Gliomas are aggressive and life-threatening brain tumors, originating from glial cells in the brain or the spinal cord [12,17]. They account for approximately 80 percent of glioma patients dying within two years of diagnosis. Despite advancements in diagnosis and treatment in high-income countries (HICs), mortality in Low and Middle-Income Countries (LMICs) like Sub-Saharan Africa (SSA) continues to rise high [4,24,25]. This is mainly due to restricted access to medical infrastructure and trained professionals, urban-centric radiological talent bottlenecks, and delayed diagnosis [5,10,11].

Magnetic Resonance Imaging (MRI) remains the clinical standard modality for detecting gliomas [23,30]. It provides comprehensive visualization of the tumor and how far it has progressed using various imaging sequences. Still, in real-world practice, diagnosing and analyzing these tumors relies on skilled professionals who need to painstakingly draw the tumor borders scan by scan. This method is subjective and relies heavily on the peculiarities of a given radiologist's skill and experience, making it very arduous both in terms of time and labor. As patient volume grows, manual segmentation becomes increasingly infeasible, delaying treatment and compromising outcomes.

The problem gives a clear indication of the need for automated solutions. The automatic segmentation of brain tumors is essential for the accurate and efficient planning of surgery, evaluating therapeutic response, and determining the progression or recurrence of tumors [6]. Automation can alleviate clinician burden, increase diagnostic throughput, and improve workflow efficiencies, particularly in settings with limited resources and staff relative to workload.

The Brain Tumor Segmentation (BraTS) Challenge has acted as a benchmark test to build and assess artificial intelligence (AI) systems that segment brain tumors on MRI scans. The effectiveness of these models in resource-poor regions, such as SSA where MRI machines have low field strength and reduced contrast, poses a vital concern. In this regard, the creation of the MICCAI BraTS-Africa dataset stands out as a major innovation. The dataset represents images acquired from imaging systems in SSA, characterized by reduced contrast and high artifacts, reflecting imaging conditions in resource-constrained regions. These limitations highlight the need for an architecture like U-Net, which can perform relatively well on low-field MRI data.

U-Net architecture is a mainstay in medical image segmentation because of its effectiveness, many open-source implementations, and consistently dependable performance across a variety of datasets [13,28]. However, its efficacy on novel or difficult datasets may be limited due to its inflexible structure and manual hyperparameter setup. On the other hand, nnU-Net performs exceptionally well by automatically modifying its network architecture, training parameters, postprocessing tactics, and preprocessing methods to fit the unique features of every dataset [18,22]. Hence, it is particularly effective at complicated tasks like brain tumor segmentation.

On that account, we chose nnU-Net as our baseline model for the BraTS Africa Challenge. While nnU-Net performs better than the original U-Net on its own, we further improved performance by ensembling it with MedNeXt [15,21]. However, both models still tend to optimize for pixel-to-pixel overlap, which can result in smoothed or fragmented segmentation of fine details, such as thin structures and small edges. Our ensemble includes a universal topology refinement [2,20] module to tackle this issue.

2 Methods

2.1 Data

The BraTS-Africa Challenge has the dataset of pre-operative glioma cases in African adults. It includes volumetric images from multiple scanners, including T1-weighted (T1), T2-weighted (T2), post-contrast T1-weighted (T1c), and T2 Fluid-Attenuated Inversion Recovery (T2-FLAIR). All the scans were preprocessed, manually annotated and segmented according to the standardized BraTS protocols [1–3]. These segmentations highlight three key tumor subregions: Enhancing Tumor (ET), Non-Enhancing Tumor Core (NETC), Surrounding Non-Enhancing FLAIR Hyperintensity (SNFH) or edematous region. For the BraTS Africa Challenge 2025, 60 training cases and 35 validation cases with the corresponding tumor sub-region masks from the BraTS-Africa 2024 were used to train and validate our proposed model [1–3].

2.2 Topology Aware Segmentation

Deep learning architectures are widely used in medical image segmentation, including the BraTS Challenge [9]. Even these sophisticated architectures fail to achieve pixel-wise accuracy due to the variance of resolutions of the images [7,8]. The need for topological correctness of image segmentation has led to the development of various metrics, including the lesion-wise dice score, lesion-wise Hausdorff distance-95 (HD95), and Normalized Surface Distance (NSD) [7,26,29]. NSD@1 counts surface points within a distance of 1 (in voxels or mm) as a correct prediction. Among them, legacy metrics compute the score based on the entire brain volume, and lesion-wise metrics compute scores by giving equal importance to each tumor lesion regardless of its size [27].

Figure 1 shows a topological error in the segmentation predicted by nnU-Net on the SSA dataset, before the topology refinement. It illustrates the comparison of the expert annotated segmentation and the predicted output from our baseline nnU-Net model, where the model struggles to predict the boundary areas. This could explain why our lesion-wise dice score is lower than the legacy dice score.

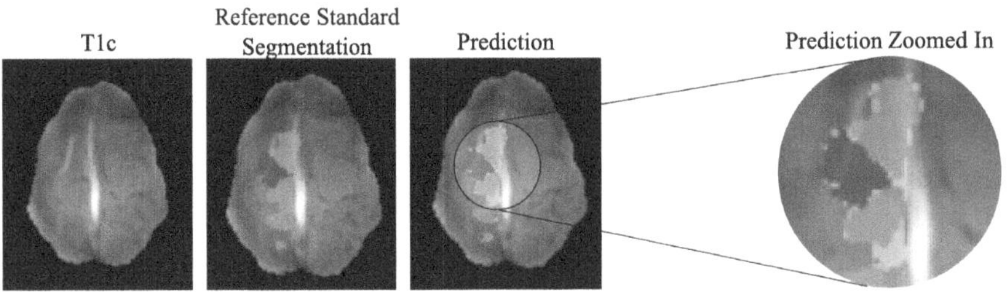

Fig. 1. Topological error visualization of reference standard segmentation and predicted output before topology refinement, where yellow color denotes prediction error.

In order to correct these topological errors, most of the researchers have developed either their evaluation metrics or their segmentation techniques [7,14,16]. These approaches might only work for the specific task, as these approaches could lead to poor generalization when applied to different segmentation tasks. To address this challenge, Liu et al. proposed a universal topology preservation and refinement method [20]. This method creates topology-perturbation masks using randomly sampled coefficients of orthogonal polynomial bases that generate the unbiased representation of the predictions, and promotes better generalization.

2.3 Model

We built and trained networks using various configurations of nnU-Net, MedNeXt, ensemble, and topology refinement methods, incorporating pre-processing and exploring different data augmentation techniques. We trained both two-dimensional (2D) neural networks on a slice based MRI data and three-dimensional (3D) full-resolution data for 500 epochs. This configuration was used both for the vanilla BraTS-Africa dataset as well as the pretraining approach on the 2025 BraTS Glioma Dataset. We further refined the segmentation using a post topological refinement via polynomial feature synthesis [20].

2.3.1 Baseline nnU-Net: We trained 2D and 3D full-resolution nnUnet on the voxel size of $128 \times 160 \times 112$ with deep supervision. The architecture has six encoder-decoder levels with 32, 64, 128, 256, 320, and 320 features, respectively. The convolution kernel sizes ($3 \times 3 \times 3$) were uniform across the architecture and were performed twice per level. Due to default batch size being set to 2, batch normalization was applied instead of Instance Normalization.

2.3.2 Baseline MedNeXt: MedNeXt based on ConvNeXt and 3D U-Net was used as our second baseline model. It has six residual stages with depthwise convolution with a kernel size of $3 \times 3 \times 3$, channel-wise Group Normalization and GELU activation with and deep supervision at decoder stages to stabilize training and improve gradient flow. The softmax output from both the baselines would be combined by soft voting averaging.

We trained our method on an NVIDIA V100 GPU, each training epoch required approximately 80 seconds, with the total training completing in about 11.1 hours (Fig. 2).

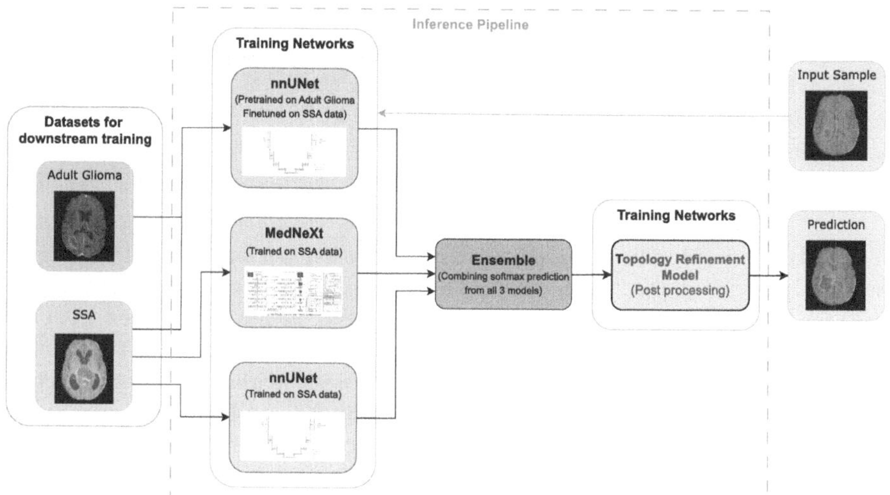

Fig. 2. Model of our proposed Pipeline using an Ensemble of nnU-Net and MedNeXt with Topology-aware Post-Processing.

2.3.3 Topology Refinement Model: We adopted the Universal Topology Refinement approach to address topological error correction [20], which generated synthetic segmentation labels and also provided a trainable pipeline network [19] to reduce topological errors in the baseline model. We used the topology-perturbation mask to introduce structural errors into synthetic data that imitated the common segmentation model errors, and used it to train our post-processing topology refinement network. Our network used a 3D U-Net of size

$240 \times 240 \times 155$, and we experimented with 4 to 8 input feature maps to generate the 4 output feature maps in the final layer. This model was used to detect and fix the topological errors that our baseline or ensemble model missed. The results of our baseline model were used to generate the final prediction of this model (Table 1).

3 Results

Table 1. Performance Dice Similarity Coefficient (DSC) of different models on Legacy and Lesion regions. Best results are in **bold**.

	Legacy (DSC)			Lesion (DSC)		
Model	SNFH	NETC	ET	SNFH	NETC	ET
nnU-Net(3D full-res)	0.930	0.906	0.906	0.891	**0.853**	**0.856**
nnU-Net(2D)	0.915	0.847	0.852	0.719	0.720	0.751
MedNeXt	0.920	0.891	0.891	0.902	0.846	0.848
Topology-aware	0.920	0.901	0.900	0.853	0.845	0.848
Fine-tuned on BraTS-Africa	**0.936**	**0.907**	**0.907**	0.896	0.848	0.853
Ensemble	0.934	0.878	0.880	**0.908**	0.824	0.839

Our Baseline Model, nnU-Net 3D full resolution performed well overall on the BraTS-Africa dataset achieving high Dice scores for each tumor subregion: 0.930 for SNFH, 0.906 for NETC, and 0.906 for ET. When pre-trained with the BraTS-2025 Task 1 (adult glioma-pre-treatment) dataset and fine-tuned with the BraTS-Africa dataset, there is a slight increase in the Legacy dice score, achieving 0.936 for SNFH, 0.907 for NETC, and 0.907 for ET.

The boundary alignment was demonstrated on NSD with a tolerance of 1.0 mm, for SNFH (0.830), NETC (0.827), and ET (0.894). The MedNeXt, fine-tuned, and ensemble models achieved Dice and NSD scores that were comparable to the baseline. In contrast, the topology-aware refinement model did not outperform the baseline in terms of Dice score but yielded a subtle improvement in NSD. Specifically, this model achieved Dice scores of SNFH (0.920), NETC (0.901) and ET (0.900) with corresponding NSD values of 0.810, 0.829, and 0.895, respectively. While a slight improvement in NSD was observed for the NETC and ET regions, a decline in SNFH score was observed, suggesting a trade-off between topological consistency and overall surface agreement in certain subregions.

4 Discussion

Our baseline model was trained on both 2D patches and 3D full-resolution data, accommodating clinical setups that often rely on 2D image acquisition. Our experiments illustrated the similarity and contrast of the segmentation outputs using different sets of trained and fine-tuned models. Taking inspiration from Li et al. and extending Isensee et.al. work, we introduced an additional universal topology refinement module applied to the ensemble outputs. This post-processing step enhanced boundary precision and better captures thin structures and sharp edges within tumor subregions (Fig. 3 and Table 2).

Table 2. Performance (NSD at 0.5) of different models on Legacy and Lesion regions. Best results are in **bold**.

	Legacy (NSD@0.5)			Lesion (NSD@0.5)		
Model	SNFH	NETC	ET	SNFH	NETC	ET
nnU-Net(3D full-res)	0.539	0.537	0.605	0.517	0.514	0.575
nnU-Net(2D)	0.428	0.423	0.498	0.340	0.359	0.434
MedNeXt	0.535	**0.543**	0.601	0.523	**0.522**	0.574
Topology-aware	0.518	0.541	**0.606**	0.484	0.520	**0.579**
Fine-tuned on BraTS-Africa	0.546	0.528	0.600	0.523	0.502	0.568
Ensemble	**0.572**	0.533	0.600	**0.554**	0.509	0.574

Table 3. Performance (NSD at 1.0) of different models on Legacy and Lesion regions. Best results are in **bold**.

	Legacy (NSD@1.0)			Lesion (NSD@1.0)		
Model	SNFH	NETC	ET	SNFH	NETC	ET
nnU-Net(3D full-res)	0.830	0.827	0.894	0.796	0.787	0.849
nnU-Net(2D)	0.756	0.713	0.810	0.603	0.609	0.713
MedNeXt	0.825	0.812	0.875	0.809	0.778	0.836
Topology-aware	0.810	**0.829**	**0.895**	0.755	**0.790**	**0.850**
Fine-tuned on BraTS-Africa	0.840	0.821	0.893	0.805	0.776	0.842
Ensemble	**0.850**	0.805	0.873	**0.826**	0.764	0.835

It demonstrated comparatively better region-wise performance for the NETC and ET in both Dice and NSD scores. Although the fine-tuned model on SSA achieved the highest Legacy Dice score, it showed a drop in lesion-wise Dice scores and NSD performance. Since lesion-wise performance is more accurate for evaluating the segmentation quality [29], the fine-tuned model was not selected as the baseline for training the topology refinement model. The trained topology refinement model resulted in only minimal improvements in NSD for the NETC and ET regions. However, it showed a drop in Dice scores, indicating a potential

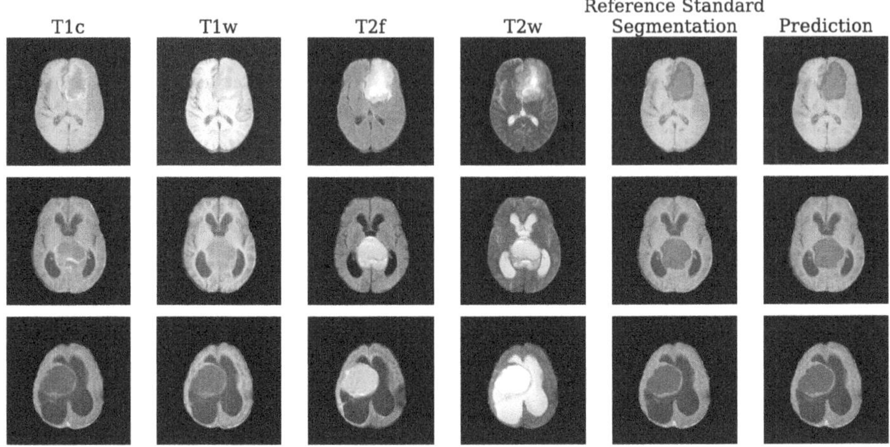

Fig. 3. Visualization of multimodal MRI inputs (T1c, T1w, T2-FLAIR, T2w) for cases BraTS-SSA-00010-000, BraTS-SSA-00025-000, BraTS-SSA-00096-000, along with corresponding reference standard segmentation masks, and baseline nnU-Net predicted tumor segmentation results. The segmentation overlays highlight tumor subregions including non-enhancing tumor (red), enhancing tumor (blue), and surrounding non-enhancing FLAIR hyperintensity (green). The predictions closely match the reference standard annotations, demonstrating the model's effectiveness. (Color figure online)

trade-off between surface-level refinement and volumetric segmentation accuracy (Table 3).

The post-processing phase was implemented with the aim of improving boundary precision and more effectively capturing thin structures and sharp edges in tumor subregions. Unexpectedly, while the topology refinement module enhanced boundary delineation, as illustrated in Fig. 1, it failed to produce better Dice scores compared to the baseline model. This could be due to the refinement technique being more successful in maintaining vascular structures instead of tumor characteristics, or further architectural enhancements might be necessary to improve the method for brain tumor segmentation. Therefore, more research on refining model design and enhancement techniques is needed to get the best performance from topology-aware methods in brain tumor segmentation tasks.

5 Conclusion

Our study explored the BraTS-Africa dataset using a multi-model technique to improve brain tumor segmentation. We used nnU-Net as the baseline segmentation model, paired it with MedNeXt, and incorporated a topology refinement module to improve the combined predictions even further. Although the topology refinement approach resulted in only marginal improvements in our study, we believe it remains a promising direction for addressing pixel-wise accuracy and achieving topologically correct image segmentation. We truly believe that this study can be extended further to achieve a state-of-the-art segmentation model through the combined capability of self-configuring baseline models and the enhancement through topology corrections. Future work should explore optimized topology-aware loss functions to further improve segmentation performance.

Acknowledgement. The authors would like to thank the instructors of the Sprint AI Training for African Medical Imaging Knowledge Translation (SPARK) Academy 2025 summer school. The authors acknowledge the computational infrastructure support from the Digital Research Alliance of Canada (The Alliance) and the University of Washington Azure GenAI for Science Hub through The eScience Institute and Microsoft (PI: Mehmet Kurt) secured the SPARK Academy. Finally, we would like to thank the Lacuna Fund for Health and Equity (PI: Udunna Anazoda), the Radiological Society of North America (RSNA), the Research & Education (R&E) Foundation Derek Harwood-Nash International Education Scholar Grant (PI: Farouk Dako), the McGill University Healthy Brain and Healthy Lives (HBHL; Udunna Anazoda) and the National Science and Engineering Research Council of Canada (NSERC) Discovery Launch Supplement (PI: Udunna Anazoda) for making the SPARK Academy possible via research grant supports. Additionally, we would like to sincerely thank the Nepal Applied Mathematics and Informatics Institute for Research (NAAMII) for their unwavering support and guidance during this project.

Conflict of Interest. The authors declare that there are no conflicts of interest.

References

1. Brain tumor segmentation (BraTs) challenges - syn53708126 - wiki. https://www.synapse.org/Synapse:syn53708126/wiki/626320
2. Adewole, M., Rudie, J., Gbadamosi, A., et al.: The brats-Africa dataset: expanding the brain tumor segmentation data to capture African populations. Radiol. Artif. Intell. **7**(4) (2025). https://pubs.rsna.org/doi/10.1148/ryai.240528
3. Adewole, M., Rudie, J., Gbdamosi, A., et al.: The brain tumor segmentation (BraTS) challenge 2023: Glioma segmentation in Sub-Saharan Africa patient population (BraTs-Africa) (2023)
4. Adhikari, B., Kulung, P., Bohaju, J., et al.: Parameter-efficient fine-tuning for improved convolutional baseline for brain tumor segmentation in Sub-Saharan Africa adult glioma dataset (2024). https://github.com/CAMERA-
5. Bajwa, M., Najeeb, F., Alnazzawi, H., Ayub, A., Bell, J.G., Sadiq, F.: A scoping review of Pakistani healthcare simulation: insights for lower-middle-income countries. Cureus **16**(12) (2024)
6. Batool, A., Byun, Y.: Brain tumor detection with integrating traditional and computational intelligence approaches across diverse imaging modalities - challenges and future directions. Comput. Biol. Med. **175**, 108412 (2024)
7. Berger, A.H., Lux, L., Weers, A., Menten, M., Rueckert, D., Paetzold, J.C.: Pitfalls of topology-aware image segmentation. arXiv preprint arXiv:2412.14619 (2024)
8. Bohlender, S., Oksuz, I., Mukhopadhyay, A.: A survey on shape-constraint deep learning for medical image segmentation. IEEE Rev. Biomed. Eng. **16**, 225–240 (2021)

9. Bonato, B., Nanni, L., Bertoldo, A.: Advancing precision: a comprehensive review of MRI segmentation datasets from brats challenges (2012–2025). Sensors (Basel, Switzerland) **25**(6), 1838 (2025)
10. Brand, N.R., Qu, L.G., Chao, A., Ilbawi, A.M.: Delays and barriers to cancer care in low-and middle-income countries: a systematic review. Oncologist **24**(12), e1371–e1380 (2019)
11. Cazap, E., Magrath, I., Kingham, T.P., Elzawawy, A.: Structural barriers to diagnosis and treatment of cancer in low-and middle-income countries: the urgent need for scaling up. J. Clin. Oncol. **34**(1), 14–19 (2016)
12. Chandana, S., Movva, S., Arora, M., Singh, T.: Primary brain tumors in adults. Am. Fam. Physician **77**(10), 1423–1430 (2008). https://www.aafp.org/pubs/afp/issues/2008/0515/p1423.html
13. Dorfner, F., Patel, J., Kalpathy-Cramer, J., et al.: A review of deep learning for brain tumor analysis in MRI. NPJ Precision Oncol. **9**, 1–13 (2025). https://www.nature.com/articles/s41698-024-00789-2
14. Gupta, S., Zhang, Y., Hu, X., Prasanna, P., Chen, C.: Topology-aware uncertainty for image segmentation. In: Oh, A., Naumann, T., Globerson, A., Saenko, K., Hardt, M., Levine, S. (eds.) Advances in Neural Information Processing Systems. vol. 36, pp. 8186–8207. Curran Associates, Inc. (2023). https://proceedings.neurips.cc/paper_files/paper/2023/file/19ded4cfc36a7feb7fce975393d378fd-Paper-Conference.pdf
15. Hashmi, S., Lugo, J., Elsayed, A., Saggurthi, D., Elseiagy, M., Nurkamal, A., et al.: Optimizing brain tumor segmentation with mednext: Brats 2024 ssa and pediatrics (2024). https://arxiv.org/abs/2411.15872v2, [cited 2025 Jul 22]
16. Hu, X., Li, F., Samaras, D., Chen, C.: Topology-preserving deep image segmentation. In: Wallach, H., Larochelle, H., Beygelzimer, A., d' Alché-Buc, F., Fox, E., Garnett, R. (eds.) Advances in Neural Information Processing Systems. vol. 32. Curran Associates, Inc. (2019). https://proceedings.neurips.cc/paper_files/paper/2019/file/2d95666e2649fcfc6e3af75e09f5adb9-Paper.pdf
17. Iranmehr, A., Namvar, M., Rezaei, N., Hanaei, S.: Brain and spinal cord tumors among the life-threatening health problems: an introduction. Adv. Exp. Med. Biol. **1394**, 1–18 (2023). https://link.springer.com/chapter/10.1007/978-3-031-14732-6_1
18. Isensee, F., Wald, T., Ulrich, C., et al.: nnU-Net revisited: a call for rigorous validation in 3D medical image segmentation (2024). https://github.com/MIC-DKFZ/nnU-Net
19. Li, L., Ma, Q., Ouyang, C., Li, Z., Meng, Q., Zhang, W., et al.: Robust segmentation via topology violation detection and feature synthesis. In: Lecture Notes in Computer Science, vol. 14223, pp. 67–77. Springer, Cham (2023). https://link.springer.com/chapter/10.1007/978-3-031-43901-8_7
20. Li, L., Wang, H., Baugh, M., Ma, Q., Zhang, W., Ouyang, C., Rueckert, D., Kainz, B.: Universal topology refinement for medical image segmentation with polynomial feature synthesis. In: International Conference on Medical Image Computing and Computer-Assisted Intervention, pp. 670–680. Springer (2024)
21. Liu, Z., Mao, H., Wu, C., Feichtenhofer, C., Darrell, T., Xie, S.: A convnet for the 2020s (2025). https://github.com/facebookresearch/ConvNeXt, [cited 2025 Jul 22]
22. Magadza, T., Viriri, S.: Efficient nnU-Net for brain tumor segmentation. https://ieeexplore.ieee.org/stamp/stamp.jsp?arnumber=10309848 (2023)
23. Martucci, M., Russo, R., Schimperna, F., et al.: Magnetic resonance imaging of primary adult brain tumors: state of the art and future perspectives. Biomedicines **11**(2), 364 (2023). https://www.mdpi.com/2227-9059/11/2/364/htm

24. Patel, A., Fisher, J., Nichols, E., et al.: Global, regional, and national burden of brain and other CNS cancer, 1990–2016: a systematic analysis. Lancet Neurol **18**(4), 376–393 (2019). https://www.thelancet.com/action/showFullText?pii=S147444221830468X
25. Poon, M., Sudlow, C., Figueroa, J., Brennan, P.: Longer-term ($\leq$ years) survival in patients with glioblastoma: a meta-analysis. Sci. Rep. **10**, 1–10 (2020). https://www.nature.com/articles/s41598-020-68011-4
26. Reinke, A., et al.: Common limitations of image processing metrics: A picture story. arXiv preprint arXiv:2104.05642 (2021)
27. Ren, T., Honey, E., Rebala, H., Sharma, A.: An optimization framework for processing and transfer learning. Brain Tumor Segmentation, and Cross-Modality Domain Adaptation for Medical Image Segmentation: MICCAI Challenges, BraTS 2023 and CrossMoDA 2023, Held in Conjunction with MICCAI 2023, Vancouver, BC, Canada, October 12 and 8, 2024, Proceedings **14669**, 165 (2024)
28. Ronneberger, O., Fischer, P., Brox, T.: U-Net: convolutional networks for biomedical image segmentation. In: LNCS, vol. 9351, pp. 234–241. Springer, Cham (2015). https://doi.org/10.1007/978-3-319-24574-4_28
29. Saluja, R.: Brats-2023-metrics: Official brats 2023 lesion-wise segmentation performance metrics. https://github.com/rachitsaluja/BraTS-2023-Metrics (2023). gitHub repository
30. Verburg, N., de Witt Hamer, P.: State-of-the-art imaging for glioma surgery. Neurosurg. Rev. **44**(3), 1331–1343 (2020). https://link.springer.com/article/10.1007/s10143-020-01337-9

Challenge 6 – BraTS-PED

Enhancing Pediatric Brain Tumor Segmentation with Attention-Guided 3D U-Net and a Multi-step Tumor-Aware Compositional Augmentation Pipeline in BraTS 2025

Amin Tavallaii[1,2,3](✉) and Shamim Shah Ghasi[2]

[1] Computational Neurosurgery Lab, Department of Neurosurgery, Macquarie University, Sydney, Australia
amin.tavallaii@mq.edu.au, tavallaeia@mums.ac.ir

[2] Department of Neurosurgery, Mashhad University of Medical Sciences, Mashhad, Iran
shahghasish4021@mums.ac.ir

[3] Department of Health Informatics and AI, Mashhad University of Medical Sciences, Mashhad, Iran

Abstract. Accurate segmentation of pediatric brain tumors, especially midline and brainstem gliomas, is crucial for neurosurgery and radiotherapy planning, but is hindered by sparse enhancing tumor (ET), infiltrative non-enhancing tumor core (NET), cystic components (CC), and extensive peritumoral edema (ED). We propose an attention-guided 3D U-Net with Multi-Modal and Channel-Wise Attention to enhance feature extraction from multi-parametric MRI (T1, T1-Gd, T2, T2-FLAIR), paired with a novel multi-step tumor-aware compositional augmentation pipeline to simulate tumor variability. Evaluated on the BraTS-PEDs 2025 training set (256 cases) using 3-fold cross-validation, our model achieves robust lesion-wise mean Dice scores: 0.81 ± 0.04 (ET), 0.87 ± 0.05 (NET), 0.77 ± 0.05 (CC), 0.95 ± 0.02 (ED), 0.90 ± 0.03 (WT), and 0.91 ± 0.03 (TC). Hausdorff Distance (95th percentile) values are 57.8 ± 0.6 mm (ET), 13.5 ± 0.7 mm (NET), 63.7 ± 0.8 mm (CC), 6.3 ± 0.4 mm (ED), 8.2 ± 0.5 mm (WT), and 7.1 ± 0.5 mm (TC). Compared to nnU-Net, our model improves WT and TC Dice by 2% and 6%, respectively, driven by attention mechanisms and augmentation. Ablation studies show a 6–7% Dice drop without augmentation, highlighting its role in generalizability. Increased WT and TC Dice performance directly supports more accurate radiotherapy margin definition and prognostic modeling for survival prediction, highlighting the clinical utility of our approach. Despite remaining challenges with sparse ET and irregular cystic components, our framework demonstrates robustness and scalability, paving the way for translation into clinical neuro-oncology workflows.

Keywords: Attention-guided 3D U-Net · BraTS-PEDs 2025 · Compositional augmentation · Pediatric brain tumor segmentation · Tumor-aware augmentation

S. Bakas et al. (Eds.): MICCAI 2025, LNCS 16376, pp. 385–395, 2026.
https://doi.org/10.1007/978-3-032-16365-3_35

1 Introduction

Pediatric brain tumors, particularly midline and brainstem gliomas, present significant challenges for automated segmentation due to their critical anatomical locations, variable enhancement patterns, and complex boundaries [1, 2]. Midline gliomas, such as diffuse midline gliomas (DMGs) with H3K27M mutations, often occur in the thalamus or basal ganglia with or without an extension to the brain stem and exhibit heterogeneous enhancement, with limited or no enhancing tumor (ET) regions. Brainstem gliomas, including diffuse intrinsic pontine gliomas (DIPGs), are infiltrative, with irregular non-enhancing tumor core (NET) and cystic components (CC), complicating delineation from surrounding tissues or edema (ED) [3]. Accurate segmentation of ET, NET, CC, and ED using multi-parametric MRI (mpMRI: T1, T1-Gd, T2, T2-FLAIR) is essential for neurosurgical planning, radiotherapy dose optimization, and monitoring treatment response in pediatric patients [4]. The BraTS Lighthouse 2025 Challenge Task 6 (BraTS-PEDs) focuses on advancing segmentation algorithms for these pediatric tumors, addressing challenges like limited dataset sizes, inter-institutional imaging variability, and low contrast in enhancing regions [5, 6].

Standard models like nnU-Net achieve robust performance but struggle with the small ET regions and infiltrative boundaries of midline and brainstem gliomas [7]. Attention mechanisms and tailored data augmentation can enhance feature extraction and model generalization [8]. We propose an attention-guided 3D U-Net with Multi-Modal Attention to fuse mpMRI modalities and Channel-Wise Attention to prioritize relevant features, paired with a novel multi-step tumor-aware compositional augmentation pipeline. This pipeline manipulates ET, NET, CC, and ED through scaling, B-spline deformation, translation, rotation, inpainting, and smoothing to mimic the variability of midline and brainstem gliomas. Our approach improves segmentation accuracy, particularly for small ET and infiltrative NET regions, with the potential to enhance clinical workflows in pediatric neuro-oncology. This paper details our methodology, evaluates performance on the BraTS-PEDs dataset, and discusses its implications for managing midline and brainstem gliomas.

2 Methods

2.1 Dataset

The BraTS-PEDs 2025 dataset comprises mpMRI scans consisting of T1-weighted (T1N), T1-weighted with contrast (T1C), T2-weighted (T2W) and T2-weighted FLAIR (T2F) sequences from pediatric patients mostly with midline and brainstem gliomas, annotated by experts for background (label 0), enhancing tumor (ET, label 1), non-enhancing tumor core (NET, label 2), cystic components (CC, label 3), and peritumoral edema (ED, label 4). The tumor core (TC) is defined as ET + NET + CC, and the whole tumor (WT) as ET + NET + CC + ED [5]. The dataset includes 261 training cases with segmentation labels and 91 validation cases without labels, sourced from multiple institutions. The dataset's multi-institutional nature introduces variability in scanner types and imaging protocols, necessitating robust preprocessing to handle data quality issues.

2.2 Preprocessing

Images were provided defaced but not skull-stripped, requiring an 8-step preprocessing pipeline with integrated quality checks to address data quality or preprocessing issues. From the 261 training cases, five were excluded, and a few others were corrected, yielding 256 usable training cases. The pipeline steps, each with corresponding quality checks, are:

Initial Quality Check. Visual inspection and computational checks (e.g., intensity range analysis, histogram comparison) identified modality sequence errors in five cases. Excluded cases were BraTS-PED-00128-000 (T2W missing, T1C repeated), BraTS-PED-00200-000 (T1N missing, both T1C and T1N contrast-enhanced), BraTS-PED-00203-000 (T1N repeated as T2W), BraTS-PED-00259-000 (T1C incorrect, T1N is T1C), and BraTS-PED-00042-000 (unresolvable coordinate system disorientation). Two cases (BraTS-PED-00177-000, BraTS-PED-00252-000) with swapped T1C and T1N were corrected by relabeling.

Skull Stripping. HD-BET [9] removed non-brain tissue from all volumes. Parameters included mode = accurate, device = cpu, test-time augmentation disabled (tta = 0) for speed. Processing was parallelized using 4 workers. Outputs included skull-stripped images and brain masks in NIfTI format, with data types preserved. Quality was verified using computational metrics (Mean Squared Error and maximum intensity difference between input and output brain regions) and visual checks (histogram plots and axial slice mask overlays for the first volume per case), ensuring complete skull removal without significant loss of brain tissue.

Motion Correction. The highest-quality modality (T1C or T2W) was selected as the reference for each case based on a composite score (weights: z-axis gradient magnitude 0.5, inverted lag-1 autocorrelation 0.3, SNR 0.2) computed using SimpleITK and SciPy signal, with T2 preferred for near-tie scores (<0.05 difference). Rigid registration (6 degrees of freedom, normalized mutual information cost function, spline interpolation) was performed using FSL's flirt [10] to align T1N, T1C, T2W, and T2F to the reference, correcting misalignments in 15 poorly registered cases (e.g., BraTS-PED-00023-000, BraTS-PED-00266-000), outputting NIfTI files. Quality was assessed through visual alignment checks and logging of registration success.

Denoising. Anisotropic denoising was applied to motion-corrected images using SimpleITK's *CurvatureAnisotropicDiffusionImageFilter* with modality-specific parameters: T1N/T1C (base iterations = 5, conductance = 0.3, noise thresholds = 0.03–0.10, iteration range = 3–7), T2W (base iterations = 7, conductance = 0.5, noise thresholds = 0.04–0.12, iteration range = 4–10), T2F (base iterations = 8, conductance = 0.7, noise thresholds = 0.05–0.15, iteration range = 5–12), and time step = 0.0625. Iterations were adjusted based on noise level (standard deviation of a central region), increasing for high noise (>high threshold) or decreasing for low noise (<low threshold). Images were cast to float32. Quality was assessed by visual inspection and computing pre- and post-denoising noise levels, Structural Similarity Index (SSIM), and noise reduction percentage.

Bias Field Correction. N4 bias field correction was applied to denoised images using SimpleITK's *N4BiasFieldCorrectionImageFilter*. Corrected images were cast and stored in NIfTI format. Quality was assessed through visual inspection and intensity histogram analysis to verify uniform intensity across brain regions, ensuring no distortion of tumor characteristics.

Cropping, Resizing, Padding. Bias-corrected images and their segmentation masks were processed using SimpleITK. Per-modality brain masks were coregistered to images using Mattes Mutual Information (50 histogram bins, 1% sampling, gradient descent: learning rate = 1.0, 100 iterations) and an affine transform. A consensus mask was generated via the union (logical OR) of masks, with holes filled using the *BinaryFillholeImageFilter*. A unified bounding box was computed to encompass brain/tumor regions, and images/masks were cropped to this box. Images were resampled to isotropic 1 mm3 spacing (linear interpolation) with segmentation masks using nearest-neighbor interpolation. Images and masks were padded to 192x192x128 with minimum intensity values (0 for masks). Outputs were stored in NIfTI format. Quality was assessed through visual inspection of output images to ensure tumor inclusion and coregistration validation via registration metrics.

Intensity Normalization. Outputs of the previous step were normalized to z-scores (mean = 0, std = 1) using *ZScoreNormalize*, restricted to brain regions via per-modality brain masks. Segmentation masks were copied unchanged. Outputs were stored in NIfTI format. Quality was assessed by computing Normalized Mutual Information (NMI, 64 bins) between each modality and the reference modality pre- and post-normalization, with differences logged to evaluate consistency.

Tumor-Aware Compositional Augmentation. To address the limited dataset size and variability, we developed a multi-step tumor-aware compositional augmentation pipeline to be applied to training data only to prevent data leakage. The pipeline manipulates enhancing tumor, non-enhancing tumor, cystic components, and peritumoral edema to mimic the patterns observed in the original tumor. Implemented using Python libraries (SimpleITK, NumPy, scikit-learn, SciPy), the pipeline includes steps for extracting, random scaling, and applying random B-spline deformations to tumor subcomponents, rearranging subcomponents within tumor core by applying tumor-aware translations and/or rotations, using inpainting techniques to manage empty voxels within the tumor, smoothing interfaces between tumor subcomponents, adjusting modality-specific intensities, and reassembling new tumor subcomponents and pasting them back into the original volume. Post-augmentation, data integrity (array shapes, modality consistency) and tumor region preservation were verified via visual inspection. A detailed description and evaluation of the pipeline will be provided in a forthcoming publication. To demonstrate this novel augmentation pipeline in action, Fig. 1 illustrates the visual outcome of augmentation on T1-contrast-enhanced and T2-FLAIR modalities as examples. The figure compares original case images with their augmented counterparts, highlighting enhanced structural diversity.

Data Storage. Preprocessed T1N, T1C, T2W, and T2F images and segmentation masks were organized for 3-fold cross-validation using 256 training cases, split into 170 training and 86 validation cases per fold. All cross-validation splits were performed in a

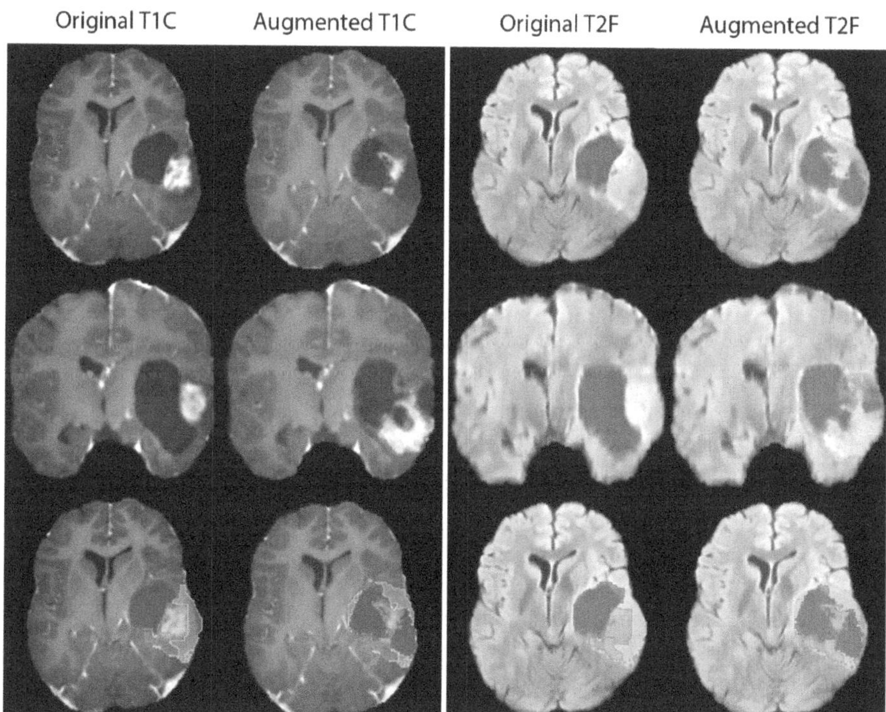

Fig. 1. Demonstration of the tumor-aware augmentation pipeline performance. This figure illustrates the effect of the proposed pipeline on T1-contrast-enhanced (T1C, left panel) and T2-FLAIR (T2F, right panel) MRI modalities. Each panel contains two columns: the left column shows the original scan with axial (top), coronal (middle), and axial view with superimposed segmentation mask (bottom), while the right column presents the corresponding augmented volume with the same views. The augmentation introduces structural variability intended to improve segmentation accuracy.

strictly patient-independent manner, ensuring that images from the same subject were never included across both training and validation folds, thereby avoiding any risk of data leakage. Training data were initially stored as 170 4D NumPy arrays (float32, 192x192x128x4 for four modalities) and 170 3D NumPy arrays (int8, 192x192x128 for segmentation masks) per fold using NumPy. The multi-step tumor-aware compositional augmentation pipeline was applied to the training data, generating one augmented version per original case, resulting in 340 training cases per fold (170 original + 170 augmented). These 340 cases were stored in a single HDF5 file per fold (e.g., train_fold_1.h5) using h5py. Validation data (86 cases per fold) were stored directly in a separate HDF5 file per fold (e.g., val_fold_1.h5). Each HDF5 file contains datasets for whole volumes of images and segmentation masks, optimized for storage efficiency and compatibility with PyTorch data loaders. Quality was assessed by verifying data integrity (e.g., array shapes, no missing modalities) for NumPy and HDF5 files and ensuring tumor regions were preserved post-augmentation via visual inspection.

2.3 Model Architecture

Our attention-guided 3D U-Net is demonstrated in detail in Fig. 2. It is designed for segmenting pediatric brain tumors, extending the standard U-Net [11] with two attention mechanisms to enhance feature extraction. Implemented in PyTorch, the model processes four input modalities (T1N, T1C T2W, T2F, input channels = 4) and outputs a 5-class segmentation map (background, ET, NET, CC, ED, output channels = 5), with tumor core (TC: ET + NET + CC) and whole tumor (WT: ET + NET + CC + ED) derived via post-processing.

Multi-modal Attention. Applied at the input, this module fuses features from the four modalities. The input tensor is reshaped to separate modalities and processed through a convolutional block (two $1 \times 1 \times 1$ convolutions with 4 channels with a ReLU activation in between, and a sigmoid output) to compute attention weights for each modality. These weights are applied to enhance modality-specific features (e.g., T1C for ET, T2F for ED). The attended features are reshaped and passed to the encoder.

Encoder Path. The encoder consists of four levels, each with a convolutional block and max-pooling. Each convolutional block comprises two $3 \times 3 \times 3$ convolutions, batch normalization, and ReLU activations, followed by a Channel-Wise Attention module. The channel-wise attention module applies adaptive average pooling to reduce spatial dimensions to $1 \times 1 \times 1$, followed by two $1 \times 1 \times 1$ convolutions to generate channel-wise weights, emphasizing features critical for ET, NET, and CC. The encoder filter sizes are 32, 64, 128, and 256, with $2 \times 2 \times 2$ max-pooling between levels, halving spatial dimensions.

Bottleneck. A convolutional block (two $3 \times 3 \times 3$ convolutions, batch normalization, ReLU, 512 filters) processes the deepest features, capturing complex patterns in tumor subcomponents without channel-wise attention to reduce computational cost.

Decoder Path. The decoder mirrors the encoder with four levels, each comprising a $2 \times 2 \times 2$ transposed convolution for upsampling, padding to align with skip connections, concatenation with encoder features, and a convolutional block. Filter sizes decrease as 256, 128, 64, and 32. Padding ensures spatial alignment with skip connections, addressing minor dimension mismatches from pooling/upsampling.

Output Layer. A $1 \times 1 \times 1$ convolution maps the final 32-channel features to 5 channels, producing a 5-class segmentation map (background, ET, NET, CC, ED). Post-processing combines ET (label 1), NET (label 2), and CC (label 3) for TC, and adds ED (label 4) for WT.

The model leverages skip connections at each level to preserve spatial details, with channel-wise attention in all encoder and decoder convolutional blocks to prioritize features for each tumor subcomponent.

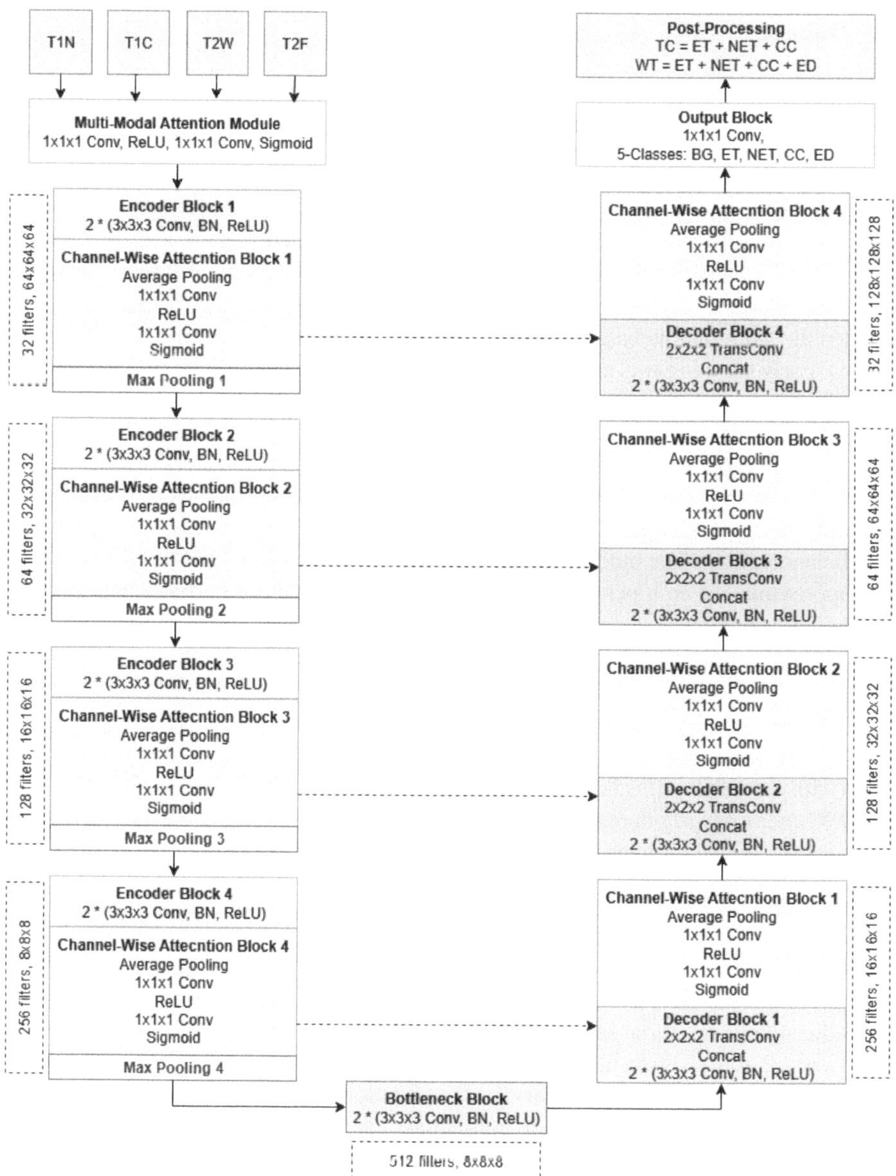

Fig. 2. Architecture of the implemented attention-guided 3D U-Net. This diagram illustrates the implemented network, featuring Multi-Modal Attention for fusing multi-parametric MRI inputs followed by four encoder levels with Channel-Wise Attention (32, 64, 128, 256 filters) and a 512-filter bottleneck. The decoder mirrors the encoder with four levels (256, 128, 64, 32 filters), incorporating skip connections and Channel-Wise Attention, culminating in a 1x1x1 convolution for a 5-class segmentation output. (background, ET, NET, CC, ED). Post-processing combines ET, NET, and CC for tumor core (TC), and adds ED for whole tumor (WT).

2.4 Training

The model was trained using a patch-based approach (128 × 128 × 128 patches) on an NVIDIA Tesla V100 GPU (32 GB) with PyTorch 2.7, leveraging mixed precision training for efficiency. A hybrid loss function combined cross-entropy loss and Dice loss (weights: 0.5 each, smooth = 1e-5 for Dice) to address class imbalance and optimize segmentation of tumor subcomponents. The Dice loss computes the Dice coefficient for each class using SoftMax probabilities and one-hot encoded targets, averaged across classes. The AdamW optimizer (learning rate: 1e-4, $\beta1 = 0.9$, $\beta2 = 0.999$) was used with a batch size of 2. A *ReduceLROnPlateau* scheduler (factor = 0.9, patience = 5) adjusted the learning rate based on the mean validation Dice score across ET, NET, CC, and ED. Early stopping was applied with a patience of 25 epochs, saving the model with the highest mean validation Dice score.

In addition to pre-training compositional augmentation, a conventional data augmentation was also applied dynamically per epoch with random parameters (e.g., rotations ± 15°, flips with 50% probability, intensity shifts ± 10%). Data was loaded using a custom Dataset class, extracting 4 patches per volume from HDF5 files, with 8 workers for efficient loading. The model was trained for up to 300 epochs per fold, with training time approximately 36 h per fold. Model compilation enhanced performance, and the best model weights were saved per fold (e.g., fold1_best_model.pth).

2.5 Evaluation Metrics

Performance was evaluated using Dice Similarity Coefficient (DSC) and Hausdorff Distance (95th percentile, HD95) for ET, NET, CC, ED, WT, and TC, as per BraTS guidelines [5]. DSC measures segmentation overlap, while HD95 quantifies boundary accuracy. Cross-validation performance was computed on the 256-case training set using 3-fold splits (340 training cases and 86 validation cases per fold).

3 Results

We evaluated our attention-guided 3D U-Net on the BraTS-PEDs 2025 training set (256 cases) using 3-fold cross-validation and the official validation set (91 cases, results pending submission to BraTS). Preliminary cross-validation results show robust segmentation performance across enhancing tumor, non-enhancing tumor, cystic components, edema, whole tumor, and tumor core. Lesion-wise Mean Dice scores and mean HD95 values across folds are summarized in Table 1. The higher Dice scores for WT (0.90) reflect the larger region's easier delineation, while TC (0.91) also benefits from combining ET, NET, and CC, despite challenges with sparse ET and infiltrative NET. Compared to the nnU-Net baseline [7], our model improved WT and TC segmentation by 2% and 6% in Dice, respectively, attributed to Multi-Modal and Channel-Wise Attention and the augmentation pipeline's simulation of tumor subcomponents.

HD95 values indicate boundary accuracy, with edema (6.3 ± 0.4 mm), TC (7.1 ± 0.5 mm), and WT (8.2 ± 0.5 mm) showing lower errors due to their larger, more contiguous regions. However, ET (57.8 ± 0.6 mm) and CC (63.7 ± 0.8 mm) exhibit higher HD95 values, reflecting challenges with sparse and irregular boundaries, mostly in midline and brainstem gliomas. NET's moderate HD95 (13.5 ± 0.7 mm) suggests better boundary delineation, likely due to the augmentation pipeline's focus on infiltrative patterns.

Table 1. Cross-validation performance on BraTS-PEDs training set (256 cases, 3-fold)

Sub-Region	Dice Score (Mean ± SD)	HD95 (mm, Mean ± SD)
ET	0.81 ± 0.04	57.8 ± 0.6
NET	0.87 ± 0.05	13.5 ± 0.7
CC	0.77 ± 0.05	63.7 ± 0.8
ED	0.95 ± 0.02	6.3 ± 0.4
TC	0.91 ± 0.03	7.1 ± 0.5
WT	0.90 ± 0.03	8.2 ± 0.5

An ablation study (Table 2) quantified the contributions of Multi-Modal Attention, Channel-Wise Attention, and the compositional augmentation pipeline. Removing the pipeline reduced Dice scores for ET, NET, CC, and edema by 6–7%, and for TC and WT by 4% and 2%, respectively, highlighting its significant role in improving model robustness and generalizability. Removing Multi-Modal Attention impacted modality fusion, reducing Dice scores, particularly for ET, NET, and edema, while removing Channel-Wise Attention decreased feature prioritization, mostly affecting NET and ED segmentation.

Table 2. Summary of the results of the ablation study

Configuration	ET Dice	NET Dice	CC Dice	ED Dice	TC Dice	WT Dice
Full Model	0.81	0.87	0.77	0.95	0.91	0.90
No Multi-Modal Attention	0.77	0.83	0.74	0.90	0.89	0.89
No Channel-Wise Attention	0.78	0.82	0.75	0.90	0.90	0.90
No Compositional Augmentation	0.75	0.80	0.71	0.89	0.87	0.88

4 Discussion

Our attention-guided 3D U-Net with a multi-step tumor-aware compositional augmentation pipeline demonstrates robust performance in segmenting pediatric brain tumors, especially midline and brainstem gliomas, as evidenced by the 3-fold cross-validation results on the BraTS-PEDs 2025 training set (256 cases). The model achieves high lesion-wise mean Dice scores, particularly for edema (0.95 ± 0.02), whole tumor (WT, 0.90 ± 0.03), and tumor core (TC, 0.91 ± 0.03), reflecting its ability to capture large, contiguous regions with strong T2-FLAIR signals (ED) and composite regions (WT: ET + NET + CC + ED; TC: ET + NET + CC). The non-enhancing tumor core (NET, 0.87 ± 0.05) also shows strong performance, likely due to the augmentation pipeline's simulation of infiltrative patterns and Multi-Modal Attention's effective fusion of T2-FLAIR signals. Compared to the nnU-Net baseline [7], our model improves WT and TC segmentation by 2% and 6% in Dice, respectively, underscoring the value of attention mechanisms and tailored augmentation in handling complex pediatric glioma subcomponents.

The lower Dice scores for enhancing tumor (ET, 0.81 ± 0.04) and cystic components (CC, 0.77 ± 0.05) highlight challenges with sparse ET and irregular CC boundaries. These regions, often small and heterogeneous, are prone to partial volume effects and low contrast in T1-Gd (ET) and T2 (CC), as noted in prior work [3]. The high HD95 values for ET (57.8 ± 0.6 mm) and CC (63.7 ± 0.8 mm) further indicate difficulties in precise boundary delineation, likely due to the sparse and fragmented nature of these subcomponents in pediatric tumors. In contrast, edema's low HD95 (6.3 ± 0.4 mm) and high Dice (0.95) reflect its larger, more homogeneous region, which is well-captured by T2-FLAIR signals enhanced through Multi-Modal Attention and the augmentation pipeline's adjustments. NET's moderate HD95 (13.5 ± 0.7 mm) suggests improved boundary accuracy compared to ET and CC, attributed to the pipeline's focus on infiltrative patterns. WT and TC HD95 values (8.2 ± 0.5 mm and 7.1 ± 0.5 mm, respectively) are relatively low, benefiting from the aggregation of multiple subcomponents, which reduces sensitivity to boundary errors in smaller regions like ET and CC.

The ablation study (Table 2) confirms the critical contributions of the proposed components. Removing the multi-step tumor-aware compositional augmentation pipeline causes the largest performance drop, reducing Dice scores by 6–7% for ET (0.75), NET (0.80), CC (0.71), and edema (0.89), and 4% and 2% for TC (0.87) and WT (0.88), respectively. This underscores the pipeline's role in simulating realistic variability in sparse ET, infiltrative NET, CC, and irregular edema, enhancing model generalizability across the limited dataset (170 cases, augmented to 340 training cases per fold). Removing Multi-Modal Attention impacts modality fusion, particularly for ET (0.77), NET (0.83), and edema (0.90), as it reduces the model's ability to prioritize T1-Gd and T2-FLAIR signals. Removing Channel-Wise Attention affects feature prioritization, lowering NET (0.82) and ED (0.90) Dice scores, as it diminishes focus on complex cystic and core tumor features. These findings highlight the synergistic effect of attention mechanisms and augmentation in addressing the challenges of pediatric glioma segmentation.

Clinically, the high Dice scores for edema, WT, and TC are promising for pediatric neuro-oncology. Accurate edema segmentation (0.95 Dice, 6.3 mm HD95) supports radiotherapy planning by delineating tumor-related swelling, minimizing radiation exposure to healthy tissue. The robust TC segmentation (0.91 Dice, 7.1 mm HD95) aids neurosurgery planning by precisely defining the core tumor boundaries near critical structures like the thalamus or pons. WT segmentation (0.90 Dice, 8.2 mm HD95) provides a comprehensive tumor extent, useful for treatment response monitoring. However, the lower ET and CC performance and high HD95 values suggest limitations in segmenting small, sparse regions, which could impact surgical precision in cases with minimal ET or complex CC. The preprocessing pipeline, including skull stripping, motion correction, anisotropic denoising, N4 bias field correction, tumor-focused cropping/resampling, z-score normalization, and HDF5 storage, ensures data quality but is computationally intensive, particularly for CPU-based HD-BET and FSL processing.

Limitations include the high computational cost of the augmentation pipeline and preprocessing steps, which may limit scalability. The high HD95 values for ET and CC indicate challenges in boundary delineation, potentially due to the dataset's multi-institutional variability and the inherent complexity of pediatric gliomas [3, 5]. Rare cases with minimal ET or highly irregular CC remain challenging, as seen in the lower CC Dice (0.77). Future work could optimize computational efficiency (e.g., GPU-based BET, parallelized augmentation), incorporate diffusion-weighted imaging (DWI) to enhance CC segmentation, and explore radio-genomic classification (e.g., H3K27M mutation prediction) for personalized treatment. A detailed evaluation of the augmentation pipeline's generalizability to other datasets (e.g., adult BraTS) will be presented in a forthcoming publication. Extending the model to handle multi-timepoint data could further improve longitudinal monitoring of pediatric gliomas [12].

Disclosure of Interests.. The author has no conflicting interests to disclose.

References

1. Bakas, S., et al.: Advancing the cancer genome atlas glioma MRI collections with expert segmentation labels and radiomic features. Scientific Data **4**(1), 1–13 (2017)
2. Menze, B.H., et al.: The multimodal brain tumor image segmentation benchmark (BRATS). IEEE Trans. Med. Imaging **34**(10), 1993–2024 (2014)
3. Pollack, I.F.: Multidisciplinary management of childhood brain tumors: a review of outcomes, recent advances, and challenges: a review. J. Neurosurg. Pediatr. **8**(2), 135–148 (2011)
4. Bakas, S., et al., Identifying the best machine learning algorithms for brain tumor segmentation, progression assessment, and overall survival prediction in the BRATS challenge. arXiv preprint: arXiv:1811.02629 (2018)
5. Kazerooni, A.F., et al., The brain tumor segmentation in pediatrics (BraTS-PEDs) challenge: focus on pediatrics (CBTN-CONNECT-DIPGR-ASNR-MICCAI BraTS-PEDs). arXiv preprint: arXiv:2404.15009 (2024)
6. Louis, D.N., et al.: The 2021 WHO classification of tumors of the central nervous system: a summary. Neuro Oncol. **23**(8), 1231–1251 (2021)
7. Isensee, F., et al.: nnU-Net: self-adapting framework for u-net-based medical image segmentation. arXiv preprint: arXiv:1809.10486 (2018)
8. Xie, Y., et al., Attention mechanisms in medical image segmentation: a survey. arXiv preprint: arXiv:2305.17937 (2023)
9. Isensee, F., et al.: Automated brain extraction of multisequence MRI using artificial neural networks. Hum. Brain Mapp. **40**(17), 4952–4964 (2019)
10. Jenkinson, M., et al.: Improved optimization for the robust and accurate linear registration and motion correction of brain images. Neuroimage **17**(2), 825–841 (2002)
11. Ronneberger, O., Fischer, P., Brox, T.: U-net: convolutional networks for biomedical image segmentation. In: International Conference on Medical image Computing and Computer-Assisted Intervention. Springer (2015)
12. Karargyris, A., et al.: Federated benchmarking of medical artificial intelligence with MedPerf. Nat. Mach. Intell. **5**(7), 799–810 (2023)

Enabling Uncertainty Measurement in Multi-subregion Tumor Segmentation: BraTS 2025 Pediatrics

Khashayar Namdar[1,2,3(✉)], Saeidehsadat Mirjalili[4], Sangwook Kim[5], Dominik Deniffel[6,7], Keith Brunt[2,8,9], Leo Anthony Celi[10,11,12], Michael Cusimano[13], and Pascal Tyrrell[1,14,15]

[1] Department of Medical Imaging, Temerty Faculty of Medicine, University of Toronto, Toronto, ON, Canada
ernest.namdar@utoronto.ca
[2] Department of Pharmacology, Dalhousie Medicine New Brunswick, Faculty of Medicine, Dalhousie University, Saint John, NB, Canada
[3] Department of Translational Medicine, The Hospital for Sick Children, Toronto, ON, Canada
[4] Pharma-Medical Science College of Canada, Toronto, ON, Canada
[5] Department of Medical Biophysics, University of Toronto, Toronto, ON, Canada
[6] Department of Diagnostic and Interventional Radiology, Cantonal Hospital Frauenfeld, Frauenfeld, Switzerland
[7] Technical University of Munich, TUM School of Medicine and Health, Munich, Germany
[8] Divisions of Cardiology and Cardiac Surgery, New Brunswick Heart Centre, Saint John Regional Hospital, Saint John, NB, Canada
[9] IMPART Investigator Team Canada, Saint John, NB, Canada
[10] Laboratory for Computational Physiology, Massachusetts Institute of Technology, Cambridge, MA, USA
[11] Division of Pulmonary, Critical Care and Sleep Medicine, Beth Israel Deaconess Medical Center, Boston, MA, USA
[12] Department of Biostatistics, Harvard T.H. Chan School of Public Health, Boston, MA, USA
[13] Department of Surgery, University of Toronto, Toronto, ON, Canada
[14] Institute of Medical Science, Temerty Faculty of Medicine, University of Toronto, Toronto, ON, Canada
[15] Department of Statistical Sciences, Faculty of Arts and Science, University of Toronto, Toronto, ON, Canada

Abstract. Accurate segmentation of pediatric brain tumors in MRI is essential for diagnosis, treatment planning, and response assessment. In this study, we investigate uncertainty-aware segmentation of multi-subregion pediatric gliomas using the BraTS-PEDs 2025 dataset. Leveraging the nnUNet v2 framework, we establish a strong baseline and conduct a series of ablation experiments to assess the impact of technical modifications in the design of the pipelines. Key contributions include the use of skull stripping (SynthStrip), atlas-based brain subregion masking (SynthSeg), and an ensemble-based cropping approach guided by whole tumor segmentation. We also evaluate synthetic channel augmentation and multi-task learning with auxiliary skull stripping, though these did not yield

Synapse ID: 3457338

S. Bakas et al. (Eds.): MICCAI 2025, LNCS 16376, pp. 396–409, 2026.
https://doi.org/10.1007/978-3-032-16365-3_36

performance gains. A voxel-wise ensemble framework is used to identify spatial uncertainty. Results show that whole tumor segmentation and region-specific cropping significantly improve subregion Dice scores, particularly for enhancing and non-enhancing tumor regions. All code, exploratory data analysis outputs, and experiment results are made publicly available to support reproducibility and further research.

Keywords: Brain Tumor · Segmentation · Deep Learning · Uncertainty

1 Introduction

Pediatric gliomas are among the most common central nervous system (CNS) tumors in children [1]. Magnetic resonance imaging (MRI) plays a central role in their clinical management, and accurate tumor segmentation on MRI is critical for diagnosis, treatment planning, and follow-up [2]. Segmentation enables volumetric analysis, supports surgical planning, and facilitates treatment response assessment [3].

Manual segmentation remains the standard approach in many clinical and research settings [4, 5]. However, it is labor-intensive and subject to inter-observer variability [6]. These limitations underscore the need for robust, automated segmentation tools that can provide consistent and reproducible results across institutions and patient populations [7–9].

The Brain Tumor Segmentation (BraTS) challenge has served as a widely recognized benchmark for the development and evaluation of automated glioma segmentation methods. In 2025, the challenge introduces a pediatric-specific track, BraTS-PED, which focuses on the unique characteristics of brain tumors in children and aims to foster model development tailored to this population.

Pediatric brain tumors comprise a heterogeneous group of neoplasms that includes entities unique to childhood as well as others that also occur in adults but are more prevalent in the pediatric population. While there is overlap, pediatric brain tumors often differ in morphology, location, and imaging appearance compared with adult gliomas [10]. These differences affect model generalizability and necessitate domain-specific model development. Transfer of models trained on adult datasets may not yield optimal performance when applied to pediatric cases, highlighting the importance of training and validating segmentation frameworks on pediatric cohorts.

The nnUNet framework has demonstrated strong performance across multiple medical image segmentation tasks [11]. As a self-configuring approach, it adapts its architecture and training pipeline to the target dataset without manual tuning. Its modular design and broad adoption make it a suitable baseline for evaluating segmentation performance on new datasets such as BraTS-PED.

In parallel with performance accuracy, uncertainty quantification has emerged as an important component for clinical translation of machine learning models. Reliable uncertainty estimates can guide expert review, flag unreliable predictions, and support risk-aware decision-making in clinical workflows.

Our overarching goal is to develop a robust, uncertainty-aware deep learning pipeline for multi-subregion segmentation of pediatric brain tumors in MRI, addressing challenges such as anatomical variability, dataset imbalance, and inconsistent subregion labeling. To guide architectural and preprocessing decisions, we structured our study around three modular frameworks: (1) Reducing irrelevant information via skull stripping and anatomical subregion masking, suitable when scans contain non-informative structures or registration to an atlas is available; (2) Enhancing feature representation through synthetic channels and multi-task learning, useful when auxiliary labels are available or label quality is inconsistent; and (3) Specializing and localizing predictions using whole tumor segmentation as a spatial prior and subregion-specific ensemble models, which proved most effective and forms the core of our final pipeline. These frameworks can be selectively applied depending on dataset characteristics, with preprocessing-based strategies offering general benefits, model-centric strategies aiding in weakly labeled settings, and localized ensembles maximizing accuracy and enabling uncertainty quantification for clinical deployment.

In this study, we use the nnUNet framework and implement an uncertainty measurement-enabled design to perform segmentation on the BraTS 2025 Pediatric dataset [12–14]. The contributions include:

- A comprehensive exploratory data analysis (EDA)
- Baseline nnUNet performance on the BraTS-PED 2025 dataset
- A step-by-step evaluation of the effectiveness of technical modules, including skull stripping and cascading
- A voxel-wise ensemble-based method for uncertainty identification

2 Methods

2.1 Dataset

The BraTS-PEDs 2025 Challenge provides the largest publicly available annotated retrospective dataset of pediatric high-grade gliomas. The cohort includes cases of astrocytoma and diffuse midline glioma (DMG), also referred to as diffuse intrinsic pontine glioma (DIPG). This dataset is designed to support the development and benchmarking of automated segmentation methods for pediatric brain tumors.

The dataset consists of 261 cases in the training set, each with ground truth segmentation masks. An additional 91 cases are included in the validation set, for which the segmentation masks are not publicly accessible. Challenge participants may submit up to two predictions per day to obtain performance scores on the validation set. A separate test set is held by the organizers and remains hidden to ensure unbiased evaluation at the conclusion of the challenge.

Each subject in the dataset has multiparametric MRI (mpMRI) scans, including the following four sequences: pre-contrast native T1-weighted (T1N), contrast-enhanced T1-weighted (T1C), T2-weighted (T2W), and T2-weighted Fluid Attenuated Inversion Recovery (T2-FLAIR or T2F). All segmentation labels in the training set have been reviewed and verified by expert neuroradiologists.

Tumor segmentation follows the guidelines proposed by the Response Assessment in Pediatric Neuro-Oncology (RAPNO) working group [15]. The tumors are segmented into four primary subregions using a four-label system: (1) Enhancing tumor (ET), defined as regions with enhancement on T1C relative to T1N [16]; (2) Non-enhancing tumor (NET), corresponding to abnormal signal intensity within the tumor that does not enhance on T1C [17]; (3) Cystic component (CC), characterized by hyperintensity on T2W and hypointensity on T1C, typically resembling cerebrospinal fluid; and (4) Peritumoral edema (ED), marked by hyperintensity on T2F and surrounding the tumor. In addition to these four labels, two composite regions are used for evaluation: the tumor core (TC, consisting of labels 1, 2, and 3) and the whole tumor (WT, consisting of all four labels).

The dataset is provided in Neuroimaging Informatics Technology Initiative (NIfTI) format, and all files are compressed using Gzip standard (.nii.gz). All scans are defaced to remove identifying facial features, but they are not skull-stripped. All scans are registered to the SRI24 Atlas [18], resulting in a standardized isotropic voxel spacing of 1 mm. The resulting image dimensions for all cases are $240 \times 240 \times 155$.

2.2 EDA

We conducted a comprehensive EDA to better understand the characteristics of the BraTS-PEDs 2025 dataset. For the full training and validation cohorts, we computed the minimum, maximum, mean, and median voxel intensity values across all four MRI sequences. For the training set, we also calculated these statistics within each of the six tumor subregions: ET, NET, CC, ED, TC, and WT. Selected histograms of intensity distributions were generated to identify potential outliers and assess variation across cases.

We examined the frequency of occurrence for each individual subregion within the training set. This analysis helped determine whether certain labels are consistently present or frequently missing. Bar plots were used to visualize the distribution of subregion presence across patients and to highlight class imbalance in label occurrence.

To assess morphological characteristics, we calculated the number of disconnected components, or "islands," within each tumor subregion in the training set. This metric provides insight into the spatial fragmentation of tumor regions. For the WT label, we visualized the distribution of island counts using histograms, which allowed identification of cases with unusually fragmented segmentations.

We also analyzed spatial and volumetric properties of the tumors. These included total tumor volume, volume of each subregion, and the coordinates of the smallest bounding box enclosing the tumor. In addition, we computed the size of each tumor along the X, Y, and Z axes. Histograms of WT volumes were used to detect small-volume cases, which may require special consideration during model training and evaluation.

2.3 NnUNet V2 Backbone

In this work, we rely on the nnUNet v2 framework for automated segmentation of pediatric brain tumors [11]. The framework dynamically configures its architecture based on a data fingerprint extracted from the input dataset. This fingerprint includes key characteristics such as voxel spacing, image size, and intensity distribution. Based on these properties, nnUNet selects the appropriate network design, preprocessing steps, and training procedures without the need for manual intervention.

The architecture is based on a 3D U-Net design with residual blocks, which facilitate gradient propagation and allow for deeper models. The network employs 3D convolutions to process volumetric MRI data and leverages deep supervision by incorporating auxiliary outputs at intermediate layers. This approach supports stable optimization and encourages learning at multiple scales.

Training is conducted using 5-fold cross-validation (CV) to ensure robust performance estimation. During inference, nnUNet applies a sliding window approach with Gaussian importance weighting, which helps manage memory usage and reduce edge artifacts. Predictions from overlapping patches are combined to generate the final segmentation map.

2.4 Model Development

We used the default configuration of nnUNet v2 with 5-fold CV for model development. To focus exclusively on the pediatric cohort in the BraTS-PEDs 2025 dataset, we did not use any pretraining on external datasets. All models were trained using the full-resolution configuration of nnUNet. For each experiment, we trained on all five folds and performed inference across the entire training set. These results are referred to as CV results throughout the paper.

Experiment 1: Baseline. This experiment serves as the baseline and uses the standard nnUNet v2 pipeline without incorporating any additional modifications. It provides a reference for evaluating the impact of subsequent experiments.

Experiment 2: Masking Brain Subregions. Given that all scans are registered to the SRI24 atlas, we used SynthSeg [19] to segment anatomical brain subregions on the SRI24 template. These masks were then transferred to the BraTS-PEDs images. By intersecting these brain subregion masks with the ground truth tumor labels in the training set, we analyzed the spatial distribution of tumors across brain regions. Subregions with no or low tumor presence were masked out to potentially improve model focus during training.

Experiment 3: Skull Stripping. We applied SynthStrip [20] to remove non-brain tissues from all MRI sequences. This modification was added to the standard nnUNet pipeline to assess whether reducing irrelevant anatomical variation improves segmentation performance. No other changes were made compared to the baseline experiment.

Experiment 4: Synthetic Channels. Radiologists often compare multiple MRI sequences simultaneously to delineate tumors. Although nnUNet uses all four input sequences, their integration occurs only in deeper layers of the network. To encourage early integration of information across sequences, we created an extended 15-channel input, which includes the original 4 sequences and voxel-wise mean combinations of their pairwise, triple, and all-four interactions. This experiment was conducted using the baseline pipeline, modified only by the expanded input representation.

Experiment 5: Skull Stripping as Auxiliary Task. To incorporate multi-task learning (MTL), we used the skull stripping masks from Experiment 3 as auxiliary supervision during training. This dual-task model was trained to predict both tumor segmentation and brain masks. The network produced 5-class output maps, which were postprocessed to recover the original 4 tumor subregions by removing the auxiliary class.

Experiment 6: WT Segmentation. Building on the high performance of the synthetic-channel model (Experiment 4), we designed a simplified variant to predict the WT as a single binary output channel. This experiment was aimed at developing a robust WT detector to guide further processing steps.

Experiment 7: Ensemble of Single-Channel Models with Cropping. We first used the WT predictions from Experiment 6 to center-crop the input images around the tumor region. We added an 8-voxel margin to each side of the cropping window. The minimum cropping size was set to $48 \times 48 \times 48$ voxels. For volumes of interest (VOIs) smaller than this threshold, the applied margin exceeded 8 voxels to meet the minimum size requirement. This allowed us to reduce computational cost while focusing model capacity on the region of interest. The cropping coordinates were saved and later used during postprocessing to map the predicted masks back to the original full-resolution image space. We then trained four separate models, each dedicated to predicting a single tumor subregion (ET, NET, CC, ED). Unlike earlier experiments where the model predicted a single multi-class label map, this setup outputs four binary masks. These masks may overlap, reflecting potential uncertainty in boundary definition. To generate submission masks, we applied a merging strategy that sequentially overwrites predictions, starting from the lowest performing subregion model. We also developed an alternative output format consisting of multi-channel masks that explicitly preserve overlapping uncertain regions.

2.5 Hardware and Software Environment

All experiments were conducted on a workstation equipped with an AMD Ryzen Threadripper 2990WX processor, 128 GB of RAM, and an NVIDIA GeForce RTX 5090 GPU. The system operated on Ubuntu 24.04.2 LTS with CUDA version 12.8 and cuDNN enabled. The software environment was built using Python 3.12.7 and PyTorch 2.8.0. All training and inference steps were implemented using the official nnUNet v2 framework.

3 Results

The minimum intensity value of the T1N sequence was zero in most scans, but several outliers were observed, with values far below the typical range (Fig. 1). Similar patterns were noted across other MRI sequences and statistical features, including maximum, mean, and median intensities. These findings suggest potential preprocessing inconsistencies or artifacts, which may require further review and validation by neuroradiologists.

EDA of the training set ground truth masks revealed that not all tumor subregions are present in every patient. The NET subregion appears in all cases, whereas the CC and ED are frequently absent. This imbalance may affect the model's ability to learn and accurately segment the less-represented subregions (Fig. 2).

Analysis of the number of disconnected components in the WT masks revealed notable discontinuity in tumor subregions (Fig. 3). This may reflect the use of automated or semi-automated tools during the curation of the BraTS-PEDs 2025 dataset. Disconnected tumor regions can present challenges for segmentation models and warrant further review by radiologists. In many cases, these islands are small and not easily visible without specialized visualization tools. The case BraTS-PED-00031–000 exhibited the highest number of islands in the WT label, with a total of 26.

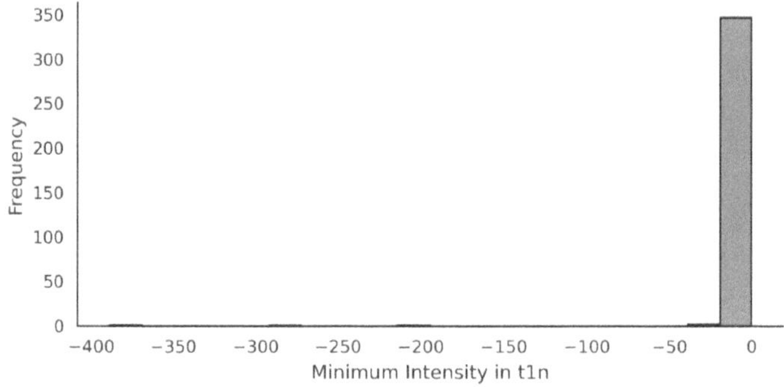

Fig. 1. Distribution of minimum intensity values in the T1N sequence across all cohorts.

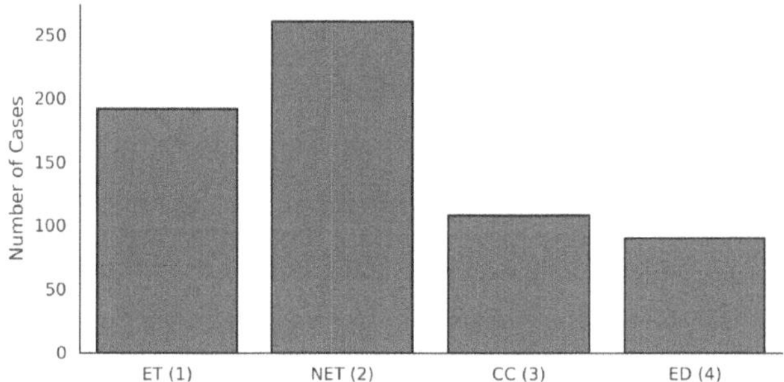

Fig. 2. Presence of tumor subregions in the BraTS-PEDs 2025 training set.

Lastly, analysis of WT volumes in the training set showed that some patients had small VOIs, which may pose challenges for segmentation models, particularly for subregion prediction (Fig. 4). The smallest WT volume was 19,786 mm3, observed in patient BraTS-PED-00048–000. The bounding box of this tumor measured 126 $\times$ 34 $\times$ 40 voxels. Given the 1 mm isotropic voxel spacing, the spatial resolution is sufficient, but the limited size may still affect model sensitivity.

To analyze the spatial distribution of tumors across brain anatomy, we applied SynthSeg to the SRI24 atlas to generate brain subregion masks. These masks were used to quantify the total tumor volume intersecting each subregion in the BraTS-PEDs 2025 training set. Figure 5 compares the cumulative tumor volume per subregion (blue) with

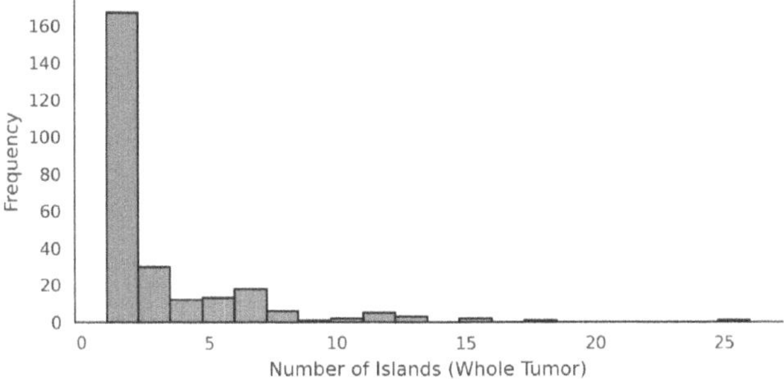

Fig. 3. Distribution of the number of disconnected islands in the WT masks.

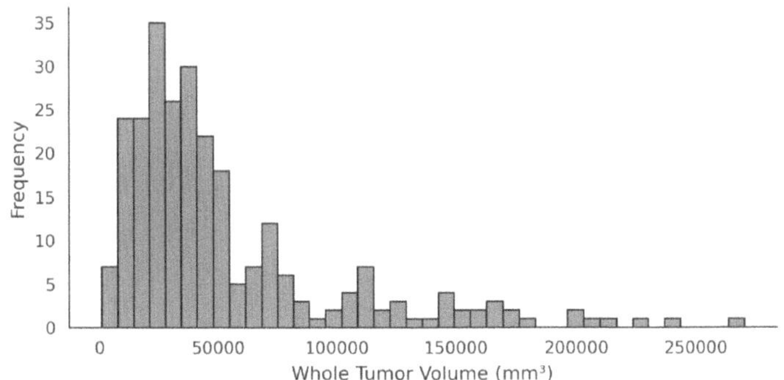

Fig. 4. Distribution of WT volumes in the BraTS-PEDs 2025 training set.

the expected anatomical volume of each region scaled across 261 patients (orange). This comparison highlights regions that are disproportionately affected by tumors relative to their anatomical size. For example, the brainstem shows a high tumor burden, although its anatomical volume is not as large as the right cerebral white matter or CSF. Many other regions display low or negligible tumor involvement. Based on this analysis, we retained the following subregions in Experiment 2: brainstem, right and left cerebral white matter, cerebrospinal fluid (CSF), right and left cerebral cortex, right and left cerebellum cortex, and right and left cerebellum white matter.

Table 1 summarizes the CV Dice scores for WT and subregion segmentation across all experiments. Experiment 6 achieved the highest Dice score for WT segmentation, though it did not include ET segmentation as it was limited to a binary WT output. Experiment 5 included skull stripping as an auxiliary task, which is not directly evaluated in the challenge, but achieved a high Dice score of 0.9882 for this auxiliary output. The best ET and NET segmentation results were obtained in Experiment 7, while the highest Dice scores for CC and ED were observed in Experiment 3.

Table 2 summarizes the one-time inference-based Dice scores and Normalized Surface Dice (NSD) with 1mm tolerance on the validation set, revealing differences from the cross-validation trends. Experiment 1 yielded the highest NET segmentation performance (0.9068), while Experiment 4 achieved the best ET (0.6968) and CC (0.7133)

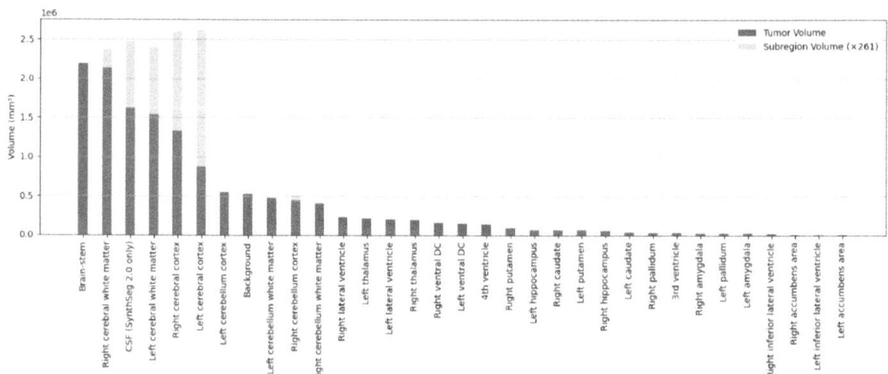

Fig. 5. Distribution of WT volumes across brain subregion in the BraTS-PEDs 2025 training set.

Table 1. CV Dice scores for WT and subregion segmentation across all experiments.

Experiment	WT Dice	ET Dice	NET Dice	CC Dice	ED Dice	Running Time per-epoch (s)
Experiment 1	*	0.7012	0.9083	0.4956	0.4639	66
Experiment 2	*	0.7083	0.9144	0.5683	0.5017	57
Experiment 3	*	0.7426	0.9182	**0.5792**	**0.5131**	51
Experiment 4	*	0.7176	0.8950	0.4941	0.4254	151
Experiment 5	*	0.7007	0.9199	0.4922	0.4834	67
Experiment 6	**0.9609**	NA	NA	NA	NA	**48**
Experiment 7	*	**0.7763**	**0.9603**	0.4571	0.4316	180

* **WT Performance on the training cohort was only measured for Experiment 6.**

results. Experiment 7 produced the highest ED Dice score (0.9670), although its CC performance dropped notably. WT segmentation remained consistently strong across experiments, with the highest validation score observed in Experiment 5 (0.9357).

Based on experiments 6 and 7, we submitted an end-to-end dockerized solution to the BraTS 2025 Pediatrics Challenge. Table 3 reports the test Dice and NSD scores generated by the challenge organizers on an unseen test dataset, demonstrating the performance of our pipeline across whole tumor and subregion segmentation. The whole tumor Dice reached 0.79 with an NSD of 0.57, while edema segmentation achieved the highest Dice of 0.88.

In Experiment 7, the pipeline generated a four-channel output for each case, with each channel corresponding to one of the tumor subregions (ET, NET, CC, ED) and visually represented as individual contours in Fig. 6b. These multi-channel masks explicitly preserve subregion boundaries but may contain overlaps in voxels where multiple subregion predictions coincide. Such overlaps were treated as uncertain regions, which we quantified using an uncertainty map: voxels with no overlap were assigned a value of

Table 2. Validation Dice and NSD scores for WT and subregion segmentation across all experiments.

Experiment	WT Dice	WT NSD	ET Dice	NET Dice	CC Dice	ED Dice
Experiment 1	0.9370	0.9162	0.6081	**0.9068**	0.6846	0.9011
Experiment 2	0.8895	0.8144	0.6104	0.8679	0.6969	0.8352
Experiment 3	0.9238	0.8843	0.6582	0.8926	0.7029	0.9341
Experiment 4	0.9239	0.8770	**0.6968**	0.8957	**0.7133**	0.9560
Experiment 5	**0.9357**	**0.9168**	0.6328	0.9060	0.7109	0.8901
Experiment 6	0.9305	0.8870	NA	NA	NA	NA
Experiment 7	0.9252	0.8568	0.6644	0.8711	0.5845	**0.9670**

Table 3. Test Dice and NSD scores for WT and subregion segmentation for the dockerized pipeline

WT Dice	WT NSD	ET Dice	NET Dice	CC Dice	ED Dice
0.7905	0.5728	0.6278	0.7144	0.5629	0.8780

0, while voxels with two, three, or four overlapping predictions were assigned 0.33, 0.66, and 1, respectively, creating a continuous uncertainty representation across the tumor volume. For challenge submissions, where a single-channel output was required, we converted these multi-channel predictions into a single mask using our sequential overwriting strategy (Fig. 6c). In this scheme, ED (label 4) supersedes CC (3), NET (2), and ET (1) if overlap occurs, CC supersedes NET and ET, and NET supersedes ET. This approach ensured that the final output met the challenge format while preserving the most clinically relevant subregion label at each voxel.

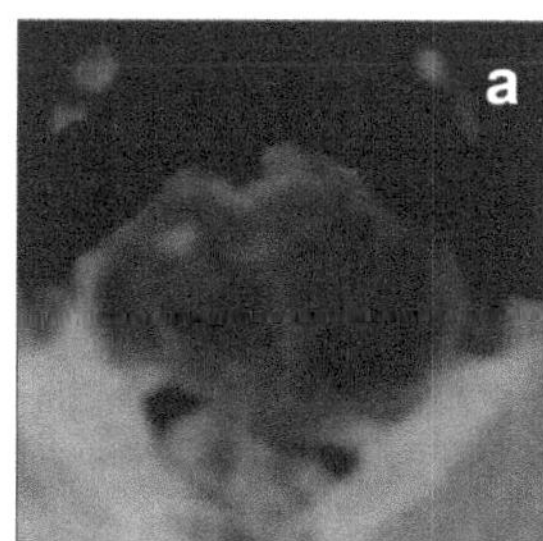

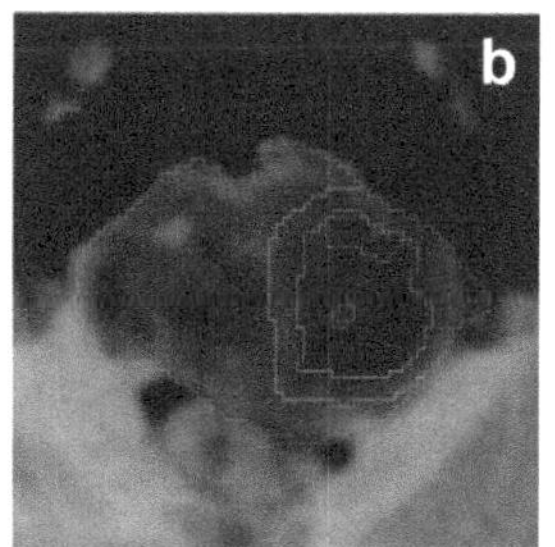

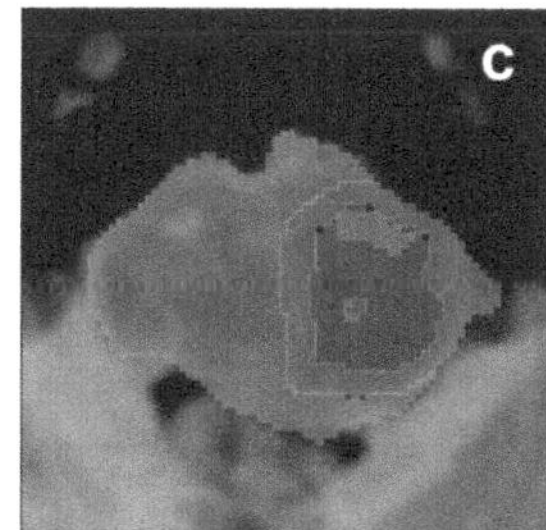

Fig. 6. Uncertainty-enabled brain tumor segmentation: a) cropped WT region, b) subregion contours, c) ensembled segmentation mask with uncertain regions

4 Discussion

In this work, we conducted a comprehensive series of experiments for pediatric brain tumor segmentation using the BraTS-PEDs 2025 dataset. To promote reproducibility and facilitate further research, we have released all EDA outputs, per-experiment results, model checkpoints, and the full inference codebase on our public GitHub repository (https://github.com/knamdar/BraTS-2025-PEDs-Inference). To streamline installation and access, we have also prepared a Docker image, which is shared on Docker Hub (https://hub.docker.com/r/knamdar/bratsped25namdar). This enables researchers to perform case-level analysis, develop additional experiments, and compare methods under consistent preprocessing and evaluation protocols.

The baseline model demonstrated reasonable performance, with results closely aligned with insights from the EDA. As expected, the CC and ED subregions were the most challenging to segment, likely due to their inconsistent presence and small size across the dataset. In contrast, NET achieved the highest performance among the four subregions, consistent with its universal presence in the training set.

Experiment 2 showed that masking brain subregions using SynthSeg-derived atlas-based masks was effective. A notable advantage was that scan-specific SynthSeg inference was not required; the registered nature of the dataset allowed anatomical masks to be reliably transferred from the SRI24 atlas, simplifying preprocessing and reducing computational cost.

Applying skull stripping with SynthStrip in Experiment 3 led to improved segmentation performance across all subregions. Removing irrelevant non-brain regions appeared to reduce noise in the model's learning process and helped focus attention on tumor-related structures.

In contrast, the use of synthetic input channels (Experiment 4) did not result in improved performance. This suggests that the nnUNet framework already integrates multi-sequence information effectively, and manual augmentation through voxel-wise sequence combinations may not provide additional benefit.

Experiment 5 evaluated skull stripping as an auxiliary task in a multi-task learning setup. The auxiliary task achieved a high Dice score, but it did not lead to improved tumor segmentation, suggesting that the added task may not provide meaningful shared representation or gradient benefits in this context.

Experiment 6 focused on WT segmentation using a simplified binary model. The strong performance in identifying the presence and extent of tumors suggests that WT prediction can serve as a robust initial step in multi-stage pipelines.

Finally, Experiment 7 combined WT segmentation with region-focused cropping and subregion-specific models. This approach yielded the best Dice scores for ET and NET subregions. However, the Dice scores for CC and ED declined. One potential factor is that patients without these subregions were not excluded from training and evaluation. Filtering out such patients or applying class-aware sampling strategies could help improve subregion-specific performance in future work.

To contextualize performance relative to computational cost, we report per-epoch runtimes for all experiments (Table 1). While methods such as skull stripping (51 s/epoch) and atlas-based brain subregion masking (57 s/epoch) offered accuracy gains with minimal overhead, more complex pipelines such as synthetic-channel augmentation

(151 s/epoch) introduced additional computation with limited benefit. Notably, the ensemble-based method incurred the highest runtime (180 s/epoch), yet its ability to produce subregion-specific masks makes it suitable for flexible clinical deployment. Future work should also quantify memory and storage demands, as runtime alone does not fully capture the deployment cost.

We observed discrepancies between cross-validation and one-time validation results, likely due to distributional differences between the training and validation cohorts. Notably, ED segmentation performed significantly better on validation. Nonetheless, WT and NET segmentation remained consistently strong, suggesting good generalizability across cohorts.

Validation and test results suggest that our algorithm is robust for whole tumor segmentation and edema, while performance in enhancing tumor and necrotic core subregions remains an area for improvement. Within the challenge setting, we were unable to apply our uncertainty-enabled approach, as only a single-channel segmentation mask with discrete voxel-level subregion labels was permitted. Our voxel-wise uncertainty maps could be integrated into clinical workflows to automatically flag regions of high overlap for prioritized radiologist review, thereby supporting quality assurance and reducing the risk of missed lesions.

A key limitation of MRI-based segmentation is that tumor margins on imaging do not capture the full extent of infiltration, as tumor cells extend beyond abnormalities visible on T1, T1CE, or FLAIR. Even expert readers often disagree on defining boundaries, particularly in heterogeneous tumors with variable enhancement. In pediatric cohorts this challenge is accentuated by subtype differences, where some tumors are diffuse while others appear more circumscribed. Consequently, segmentation should be interpreted as delineating imaging correlates of tumor burden rather than the complete histological extent.

Our study is limited by the use of SRI24-registered scans, which may affect generalizability to non-registered clinical data; potential biases introduced by outliers in the EDA dataset; and the computational overhead of multi-channel inference, which could impact real-time deployment in clinical settings.

Acknowledgments. Data used in this publication were obtained as part of the Challenge project through Synapse ID syn64153430.

Disclosure of Interests. The authors have no competing interests to declare that are relevant to the content of this article.

References

1. Namdar, K., et al.: Improving deep learning models for Pediatric low-grade glioma tumours molecular subtype identification using MRI-based 3D probability distributions of tumour location. Can. Assoc. Radiol. J. **76**(2), 313–323 (2025). https://doi.org/10.1177/08465371241296834
2. Wagner, M.W., et al.: Radiomics of pediatric low grade gliomas: toward a pretherapeutic differentiation of BRAF-mutated and BRAF-fused tumors. Am. J. Neuroradiol. (2021)

3. Upreti, G.: Advancements in skull base surgery: navigating complex challenges with artificial intelligence. Indian J. Otolaryngol. Head & Neck Surg. **76**(2), 2184 (2023). https://doi.org/10.1007/S12070-023-04415-8
4. Querido, N.R., et al.: Validation of an automated segmentation method for body composition analysis in colorectal cancer patients using diagnostic abdominal computed tomography images. Clin Nutr ESPEN **63**, 659–667 (2024). https://doi.org/10.1016/J.CLNESP.2024.07.1054
5. Ma, J., He, Y., Li, F., Han, L., You, C., Wang, B.: Segment anything in medical images. Nat. Commun. **15**(1), 654 (2024). https://doi.org/10.1038/S41467-024-44824-Z
6. Wagner, M.W., et al.: Radiomic features based on MRI predict progression-free survival in Pediatric diffuse midline glioma/diffuse intrinsic pontine Glioma. Can. Assoc. Radiol. J., 8465371221109921 (2022). https://doi.org/10.1177/08465371221109921
7. Ghobrial, G., Roth, C.: Deep learning-based automated segmentation and quantification of the dural sac cross-sectional area in lumbar spine MRI. Front. Radiol. **5**, 1503625 (2025). https://doi.org/10.3389/FRADI.2025.1503625/FULL
8. Shifa, N., Saleh, M., Akbari, Y., Al Maadeed, S.: A review of explainable AI techniques and their evaluation in mammography for breast cancer screening. Clin. Imag. **123**, 110492 (2025). https://doi.org/10.1016/J.CLINIMAG.2025.110492
9. Li, S., et al.: Auto-segmentation, radiomic reproducibility, and comparison of radiomics between manual and AI-derived segmentations for coronary arteries in cardiac [18F]NaF PET/CT images. EJNMMI Phys. **12**(1), 42 (2025). https://doi.org/10.1186/S40658-025-00751-6
10. Kudus, K., et al.: Increased confidence of radiomics facilitating pretherapeutic differentiation of BRAF-altered pediatric low-grade glioma. Eur. Radiol. (2023). https://doi.org/10.1007/s00330-023-10267-1
11. Isensee, F., Jaeger, P.F., Kohl, S.A.A., Petersen, J., Maier-Hein, K.H.: NnU-Net: a self-configuring method for deep learning-based biomedical image segmentation. Nat. Methods **18**(2), 203–211 (2021). https://doi.org/10.1038/s41592-020-01008-z
12. Kazerooni, A.F., et al.: The brain tumor segmentation in Pediatrics (BraTS-PEDs) challenge: focus on Pediatrics (CBTN-CONNECT-DIPGR-ASNR-MICCAI BraTS-PEDs) (2024). https://arxiv.org/pdf/2404.15009. Accessed 17 Jul 2025
13. Kazerooni, A.F., et al.: The brain tumor segmentation (BraTS) Challenge 2023: focus on Pediatrics (CBTN-CONNECT-DIPGR-ASNR-MICCAI BraTS-PEDs)," May 2023. https://arxiv.org/pdf/2305.17033. Accessed 17 Jul 2025
14. Karargyris, A., et al.: Federated benchmarking of medical artificial intelligence with MedPerf. Nat. Mach. Intell. **5**(7), 799–8102023 (2023). https://doi.org/10.1038/s42256-023-00652-2
15. Erker, C., et al.: Response assessment in paediatric high-grade glioma: recommendations from the response assessment in Pediatric neuro-oncology (RAPNO) working group. Lancet Oncol. **21**(6), e317–e329 (2020). https://doi.org/10.1016/S1470-2045(20)30173-X
16. Ruffle, J.K., Mohinta, S., Gray, R., Hyare, H., Nachev, P.: Brain tumour segmentation with incomplete imaging data. Brain Commun. **5**(2), fcad118 (2023). https://doi.org/10.1093/BRAINCOMMS/FCAD118
17. Ellingson, B.M., Lai, A., Nguyen, H.N., Nghiemphu, P.L., Pope, W.B., Cloughesy, T.F.: Quantification of nonenhancing tumor burden in gliomas using effective T2 maps derived from dual echo turbo spin echo MRI. Clin. Cancer Res. **21**(19), 4373 (2015). https://doi.org/10.1158/1078-0432.CCR-14-2862
18. Rohlfing, T., Zahr, N.M., Sullivan, E.V., Pfefferbaum, A.: The SRI24 multichannel atlas of normal adult human brain structure. Hum. Brain Mapp. **31**(5), 798–819 (2010). https://doi.org/10.1002/hbm.20906

19. Billot, B., et al.: SynthSeg: segmentation of brain MRI scans of any contrast and resolution without retraining. Med. Image Anal. **86**, 102789 (2023). https://doi.org/10.1016/j.media.2023.102789
20. Hoopes, A., Mora, J.S., Dalca, A.V., Fischl, B., Hoffmann, M.: SynthStrip: skull-stripping for any brain image. Neuroimage **260**, 119474 (2022). https://doi.org/10.1016/J.NEUROIMAGE.2022.119474

Using a Radiologically Informed, Deep Learning Cascade to Refine Segmentations of Pediatric Brain Tumors from MRI

Timothy Mulvany[1(✉)], Heather Rose[2,3], Jan Novak[1], and Daniel Griffiths-King[1]

[1] Aston Institute of Health and Neurodevelopment, College of Health and Life Sciences, Aston University, Birmingham, UK
{220346999,j.novak}@aston.ac.uk

[2] Radiation Physics, Nottingham University Hospitals, Queen's Medical Centre, Nottingham, UK

[3] School of Medicine, University of Nottingham, Nottingham, UK

Abstract. Automated brain tumor segmentation approaches, promoted by challenges such as the Brain Tumor Segmentation (BraTS) Challenge present a key opportunity to improve clinical practice for these patients. Being able to accurately and reliably segment and therefore monitor high grade glioma in pediatric brain tumor patients is a key example of this and is the target of the BraTS-PEDs 2025 challenge.

The current study presents a Radiologically informed, Deep Learning Cascade model, based on the residual encoder variant of nnU-Net, submitted to the BraTS-PEDs 2025 challenge. The goal of this model is to segment the subregions of brain tumors from coarse to fine and refining initial predictions through the two levels of the cascade. Our cascade model had some success in the previous BraTS-PEDs 2024 challenge, and the current submission proposes specific adaptations to further promote refinement by the model through the levels of the cascade, and to handle the challenges raised by tumor subregions that are underrepresented in training data due to them not being part of the radiological presentation in all HGGs.

Our novel adaptations of the cascade model provide robust segmentations for the BraTS-PEDs 2025 challenge validation data, achieving mean Dice scores of 0.692, 0.898, 0.699, and 0.945, and HD95 of 66.1, 6.2, 87.5, and 20.5 for the ET, NET, CC and ED, respectively.

Keywords: nnU-Net · Tumor Segmentation · Pediatrics · MRI · BraTS-PEDs

J. Novak and D. Griffiths-King—These authors contributed equally as joint senior authors.

S. Bakas et al. (Eds.): MICCAI 2025, LNCS 16376, pp. 410–421, 2026.
https://doi.org/10.1007/978-3-032-16365-3_37

1 Introduction

1.1 Background

Monitoring of high-grade gliomas (HGG e.g. Diffuse Midline Glioma (DMG) and astrocytoma) in children using magnetic resonance imaging (MRI) is a key aspect of disease management and treatment planning for these patients. This is especially true in the context of evaluating the effects of treatment on the disease, assessing how treatment changes the clinical imaging features of the tumor. Specifically, the Response Assessment in Pediatric Neuro-Oncology (RAPNO) guidelines for HGG and DMG outline the importance of volumetric assessment using MRI. However, they emphasize the difficulty in obtaining reliable and consistent measurement of volume, even amongst experts, likely due to the sometimes-indistinct borders of these types of HGGs [1–3]. The automated segmentation approaches promoted by the Brain Tumor Segmentation (BraTS) challenges[1], represent an opportunity to improve and support clinical practice in this area, especially given more recent challenges focused on pediatric tumors [4, 5].

The current study presents a novel adaptation of our previous submission to the BraTS-PEDs 2024 challenge, an adapted nnU-Net with radiologically-informed hierarchical cascades. For the BraTS-PEDs 2025 challenge [6], we further improve this method through the inclusion of decision-gating for the lower levels of the cascade and generating greater segmentation variability in higher levels to promote refinement of the segmentations by the lower levels of the cascade.

1.2 Previous BraTS-PED 2024 Model

For the previous (2024) pediatric segmentation challenge, we proposed a hierarchical set of cascaded classifiers, modified from the nnU-Net residual encoder variant [7]. Specifically, we decomposed the complex segmentation task across tumor subregions (Enhancing Tumor (ET), Non-enhancing Tumor (NET), Cystic Component (CC) and Edema (ED)) into two stages.

An initial classification model (Stage 1 Model) used the four mpMRI scans (T1w, T1w-CE, T2-FLAIR and T2w), to segment the four independent tumor subregions (ET/NET/CC/ED). Subsequently, we decomposed the segmentation into two further second stage models, one classifying ET versus NET (Stage 2a Model) and a second classifying CC versus ED (Stage 2b Model). These second stage models focused on the discrimination deemed to be more challenging, in terms of automated segmentation but also are challenging for manual radiological segmentation. We also reduced the input dataset from all input MRI modalities in the Stage1 model, to a reduced number of modalities for the Stage 2 models, guided by radiological expertise from the RAPNO guidelines for DMG and HGG [1–3].

As part of the cascaded approach, the outputs of the initial model (Stage 1 models) were passed to subsequent models as an additional input channel (Stage 2 models) – the goal of which was to provide refinement of predictions. The Stage 2a model (ET vs NET segmentation) utilized the ET and NET label predictions from the Stage 1 model, plus

[1] https://www.synapse.org/Synapse:syn64153130/wiki/631455.

T1w and T1w-CE MRI to segment the ET and NET. For the stage 2b model (CC vs ED segmentation), the ET and NET labels from the Stage 1 model were combined, as per previous BraTS guidelines, into a "Solid Tumor" label (ST). The ST label, plus CC and ED labels from the Stage1 model, and the T2w and T2-FLAIR MRI, were used as inputs to the Stage 2b model in order to refine CC and ED segmentations. The Stage 2a model represents a cascade to refine prediction, whereas Stage 2b represents refining segmentations from coarse (ST) to fine (CC/ED).

The approach demonstrated improvement, compared to a nnU-Net residual encoder baseline, only on CC and ED labels. Difficulties in cyst segmentation are a common issue identified by challenge organizers [8], and so was a promising result. This was reinforced by favorable performance in team rankings for the BraTS-PEDs 2024 challenge.

Ongoing investigation indicated improved performance for CC/ED segmentation was due to increased detection of true negative cases – e.g. patients where there was no cyst (thus predicting an empty CC label) compared to a baseline model which predicted more false-positive CC. It was concluded that imbalances in the training set provided challenges for training our model [9], with imbalance at the level of the scan, where not all HGG patients will present with CC or ED. Therefore, a limitation of our approach was that our model was not designed specifically to triage for feature presence. This must be addressed for models to have clinical impact: real-world data sets are also likely to be imbalanced in this way [9], and under- or non- segmentation of cyst and edema has clinical implications. Both are important radiological features in pediatric brain tumors [9, 10] and RAPNO guidelines suggest excluding some cysts in response assessment [2].

Our results showed that our model did not improve segmentation of NET and ET compared to the Residual Encoder baseline, suggesting that our Stage 2a model did not refine the segmentations as hoped. Our Stage 1 Model employed the same architecture as our baseline model and we believe that this model performed at a level where, when the outputs are fed-forward to the subsequent stage 2 models, there was insufficient scope to improve the segmentations for the network to escape the local minima of predicting the existing mask.

Current Study. For the current challenge (BraTS-PEDs 2025) we further developed our radiologically informed, dual pathway cascade, as reported in [6], to address important concerns from our previous model. Firstly, to address the relative sparsity of CC and ED in the dataset, as is predicted by typical radiological presentation of these types of tumors, we specifically filtered the training data for our Stage 2b model, ensuring that the model was not biased towards the more prevalent 'empty' cases. There is a risk that this results in a greater number of false positives rather than the current false negatives. Therefore, we also implemented a logic gate between Stage 1 and Sage 2b, where only cases with ED/CC predicted by the Stage 1 model, were submitted to the Stage 2b model for refinement of the segmentation.

To ensure that our second stage models were able to refine the segmentations from Stage 1 in the cascade, we augmented the cascaded outputs from the Stage 1 model by generating several initial segmentations with greater variability than a single prediction. To achieve this, our Stage 1 model was trained using multiple epoch lengths with the output from each being submitted to the Stage 2 models as new augmented training datasets, which we predicted would improve segmentation performance.

2 Methods

2.1 Data

Data used in this publication were obtained as part of the Challenge project through Synapse ID (syn64153430).

Subjects. The BraTS-PEDs dataset consists of data from n = 464 patients with pediatric HGG (e.g. high-grade astrocytoma and DMG) from multiple institutions. n = 261 cases were used in the training phase, with MRI and data labels being available. An additional n = 91 cases were used for validation testing of the models, with only MRI being made available to challenge participants. Final benchmarking of our submission will be conducted by challenge organizers using the unseen testing cohort of n = 112, where neither MRI nor labels have previously been released. See [8] for further details.

MRI. Each patient in the cohort has a dataset of multiparametric MRI (mpMRI) sequences with native (T1w) & postcontrast T1-weighted (T1w-CE) MRI, T2-weighted (T2w) MRI, and T2 Fluid Attenuated Inversion Recovery (T2-FLAIR) MRI as available modalities.

Data Annotations – Tumor Sub-regions. Annotated "ground-truth" (GT) tumor masks were provided by the challenge and used for model training. These masks included four tumor sub-regions: "enhancing tumor" (ET), "non-enhancing tumor" (NET), "cystic component" (CC) and "edema" (ED). These could be meaningfully combined to generate three additional labels, "solid tumor" (ST) as the combination of NET and ET, "tumor core" (TC) combining ET, NET, and CC, and finally the "whole tumor" (WT) - the entire tumorous region combining ET, NET, CC and ED. From these combined labels, only ST was used in the model training process whilst WT and TC were used by the challenge for public evaluation of the models.

MRI Preprocessing. MRI Data was preprocessed by challenge organizers via the "BraTS Pipeline", utilizing the Cancer Imaging Phenomics Toolkit (CaPTk) and Federated Tumor Segmentation (FeTS) tool, then anonymized through removal of protected DICOM headers and defacing of MRI (see [8] for details). Additional preprocessing was conducted locally, specifically in terms of patient-level normalization. For each MRI modality, for every patient, voxel intensities from within brain tissue only (estimated using a brain-tissue-mask generated using HD-BET [11]), were binned forming a histogram to which a Gaussian was fitted to the greatest peak. Voxel intensities were divided by two times the mean parameter of the Gaussian curve, to normalize the Gaussian peak to 0.5. This was to ensure normalization at the individual-level whilst nnU-Net also performed normalization at a cohort/dataset level.

2.2 Model Architectures

nnU-Net. This work implements nnU-Net, an adaptive, deep-learning segmentation approach [7]. The configuration of nnU-Net is automatically adapted across preprocessing, training and postprocessing in response to the training data supplied. We used multiple iterations of the nnU-Net Residual Encoder Variant (specifically, the "nnU-Net ResEnc M" architecture) to build our hierarchical, cascaded model. The residual encoder model uses residual blocks in the encoder which perform the function of adding the convolution block's input to the output, preserving information from the previous layers. The subsequent framework (encompassing the Stage 1 and Stage 2 models and all related ensembling and post-processing) is subsequently termed the nnU-Net Cascade Model.

Each stage of the cascade was trained using a 5-fold cross validation approach. For evaluation on validation and testing data, these models were ensembled across the folds via averaging of the prediction probabilities.

nnU-Net Cascade. The proposed model architecture used a hierarchical cascade approach, where the outputs of an initial model (Stage 1 models) are passed to subsequent models as an additional input channel (Stage 2 models) for refinement.

Stage 1 Model. The Stage 1 model is an nnU-Net Residual Encoder. The input to Stage 1 is the four mpMRI scans (T1w, T1w-CE, T2-FLAIR and T2w), whilst the output is the four tumor subregions (ET/NET/CC/ED). To capture variability in the segmentations, the Stage 1 model was trained using multiple training epoch lengths (10, 20, 50, 100).

Stage 2 Models. Two Stage 2 models were trained for the subsequent level of the cascaded framework to refine Stage 1 predictions. The two models in the cascade perform similar tasks in terms of their level/position in the cascade hierarchy (in terms of inputs and outputs), and so are both termed as Stage 2 models. For each of those Stage 2 models, a reduced set of the four available mpMRI sequences were used as input channels, selecting the modalities that were most appropriate to the target subregions being segmented by that stage 2 model, selected based upon RAPNO guidelines.

Each Stage 2 model was also supplied with a set of relevant tumor subregion masks as input channels, predicted by the previous Stage 1 model. For training, each participant was included 5 times, once for each of the 5 available ROIs (1 from each of the 4 Stage 1 epoch lengths, and the ground truth ROI), to provide Stage 2 models with a more variable set of fed through masks to refine.

All cross fold training/testing/ensembling across experiments was split at the level of the participant, such that all datasets from each participant were included in the same fold, to ensure cross-fold performance was not overinflated.

Stage 2a Model (ET vs NET segmentation). The Stage 2a model specifically segments both ET and NET. The input to this model was the ET and NET label predictions from the Stage 1 model, plus the T1w and T1w-CE MRI. The resulting number of training examples for the Stage 2a model was N = 1305 (5 ROIs per 261 patients).

Stage 2b Model (CC vs ED segmentation). The Stage 2b model is trained to segment both CC and ED. Training data for this model is filtered to only include those cases where CC and/or ED existed in the ground truth labels with a volume of at least 25 voxels. A total of 106 patients satisfied this condition, providing N = 530 training examples for the Stage 2b model (5 ROIs per 106 patients). Predictions were only cascaded to this second stage model if the amount of CC and/or ED predicted by the Stage 1 model exceeds a given threshold (*Threshold x*, default 25 voxels, but optimized below). The input to this model was the CC and ED label predictions from the Stage 1 models, plus the T2w and T2-FLAIR MR. For each Stage 1 prediction, the relevant ET and NET labels were also combined to a single ST label which was also included as input.

Final Predictions. Predictions from the two Stage 2 models must be combined to produce final segmentations for the model. Due to the independence of these models, the predictions are potentially overlapping and therefore a schema needs to be implemented to handle collisions and determine the order in which labels overwrite one another. Specific schemas are tested below but briefly, the default label order of ET > NET > CC > ED would result in ED overwriting CC, CC overwriting NET, etc. To handle the potential for false positives, we also determine the minimum volume of CC, ED and ET above which they are included in the final prediction/segmentation (*Threshold y*, default 25 voxels, but optimized below). No such threshold is applied to NET given the ubiquitous occurrence in all cases.

A flowchart of the overall cascade can be seen in Fig. 1.

2.3 Optimization

We sequentially optimized parameters that influenced the way in which the cascade was combined, specifically optimizing Threshold x then y, then the ensembling method then collision handling.

Threshold x. The minimum volume (in voxels) of CC and/or ED required in Stage 1 predictions to trigger their refinement by the Stage 2b model. Tested thresholds included; 0, 25, 50, 100, 250.

Threshold y. The minimum volume threshold (in voxels) required for CC, ED, or ET to be included in the final prediction. Tested thresholds included; 0, 25, 50, 100, 250.

Ensembling. Due to the 5-fold cross validation of each model, 5 predictions/segmentations are outputted for each Stage/Model, which must be ensembled to provide a single segmentation for Stage 2 refinement or final evaluation. The default behavior of nnU-Net is an averaging of the SoftMax probabilities over the five predictions. Given we know that each tumor subregion is subject to some degree of over/under prediction, each subregion can be thresholded and class-weighted prior to this combination. A threshold of 25 was used for this ensembling process. Class-weightings were identified based on the ratio of false positives and false negatives identified in the training data, rounded to 1 decimal point.

Collision Handling. Due to the use of multiple models, there are potentially collisions between multiple tumor subregions which need to be resolved. The order in which each label is overwritten by subsequent labels can be optimized. The default behavior is ET > NET > CC > ED, i.e. ED overwrites CC, which overwrites NET, etc.

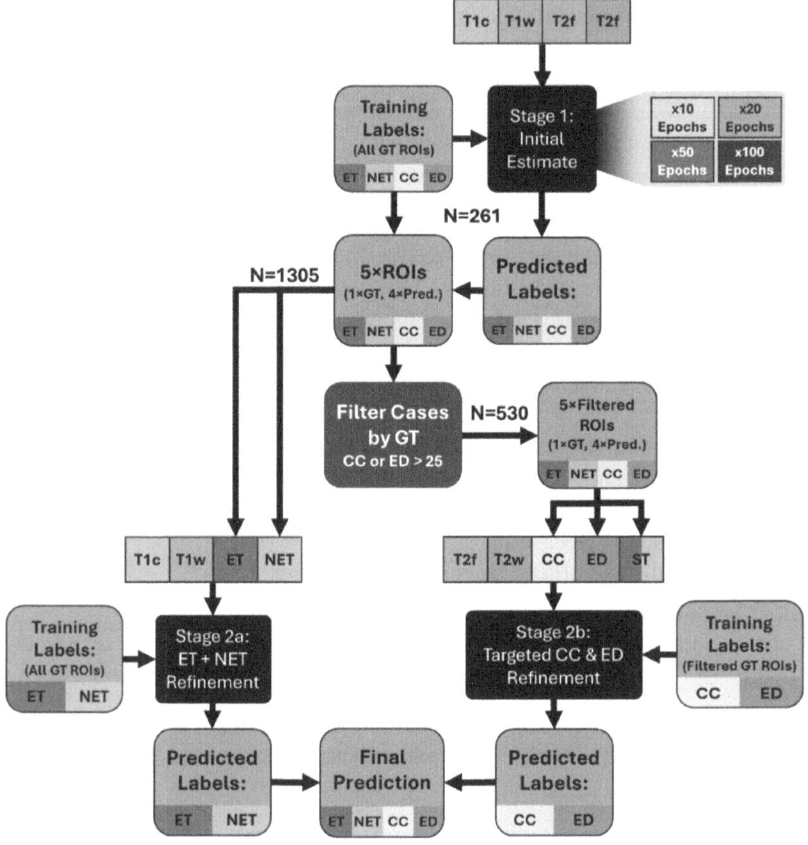

Fig. 1. Flow chart of the inputs and outputs at each stage of our hierarchical cascade model.

The entire set of possible combinations was not searched, as no collisions between ET/NET or between ED/CC can exist because of their shared Stage 2 output spaces.

After each optimization step, we conducted testing on the validation cohort to assess the impact of each aspect on our overall cascade model.

2.4 Training and Evaluation

We followed the standard training methodology of nnU-Net for all architectures. Each architecture was trained with 5-fold cross-validation. nnU-Net applied default data augmentation on-the-fly during training. Each training run lasted 100 epochs for models included in the final cascade, with stage 1 models trained at 10, 20 and 50 epochs solely for training data augmentation, supplementing stage 2 training examples. All other nnU-Net hyperparameter used default values, including a batch size of 2, stochastic gradient descent optimizer with Nesterov momentum of 0.99, an initial learning rate of 0.01, and a polynomial learning rate decay. All experiments were conducted with PyTorch (v2.3.0 + CU12.1) on two NVIDIA Quadro RTX 6000 GPUs with 24GB VRAM. Combination of predictions from differing models / folds was performed using Python 3.9.19, NiBabel 5.2.1.

Performance is reported for each model on the BraTS-PEDs 2025 validation set. This dataset is made available to challenge participants without ground truth tumor labels. Performance on validation data for this challenge was assessed/benchmarked using the synapse.org platform, powered by MedPerf. [12].

3 Results

Results report performance on the validation dataset unless explicitly stated. Performance is listed in tables 1 3. Sequential hyperparameter optimization resulted in the following models being validated.

- **Basic Cascade** (*All defaults mentioned above*).
- **Reduced Sensitivity Cascade** (*Threshold x = 50, Threshold y = 100, Ensembling = Default, Combination Order = Default*).
- **Weighted Ensemble Cascade** (*Threshold x = 50, Threshold y = 100, Ensembling = Weighted by (1, 0.8, 1, 1.4, 0.1) (Background, ET, NET, CC, ED), Combination Order = Default*).
- **Optimized Combination Order Cascade** (*Threshold x = 50, Threshold y = 100, Ensembling = Weighted by (1, 0.8, 1, 1.4, 0.1) (Background, ET, NET, CC, ED), Combination Order = CC > ED > ET > NET (So ST overwrites CC + ED prediction when overlapping)*).

Table 1. Performance (Dice) of each configuration on BraTS-PEDs 2025 validation dataset

Configuration	Lesion-wise Dice					
	ET	NET	CC	ED	TC	WT
Stage 1 Model Only	0.58	0.89	0.67	0.77	0.92	0.92
Basic Cascade	0.66	0.89	0.69	0.70	0.92	0.92
Reduced Sensitivity Cascade	0.65	0.89	0.73	0.74	0.92	0.92
Weighted Ensemble Cascade	0.66	0.90	0.70	0.95	0.93	0.93
Optimized Combination Cascade	0.69	0.90	0.70	0.95	0.92	0.92

Weighted Ensemble Cascade improves ED delineation. ED performed well in terms of segmentation in the Stage 1 model (Dice = 0.77, HD95 = 86.3), but the initial Basic Cascade and Reduced Sensitivity Cascade eroded this performance (Dice = 0.70,0.74, HD95 = 111.0,98.6 respectively). However, the weighted Ensemble Cascade rescued this performance and performed even better than the Stage 1 model (Dice = 0.95, HD95 = 20.5) with a meaningful drop in false positives seemingly the reason for this improvement (Stage 1 Model FP = 0.23, Weighted Ensemble Cascade FP = 0.03). This improvement was maintained when the Optimized Combination Cascade was added to the model.

Table 2. Performance (HD95) of each configuration on BraTS-PEDs 2025 validation dataset

Configuration	Lesion-wise HD95 (mm)					
	ET	NET	CC	ED	TC	WT
Stage 1 Model Only	101.3	8.1	94.0	86.3	9.1	9.1
Basic Cascade	76.4	6.2	95.7	111.0	9.3	9.1
Reduced Sensitivity Cascade	80.5	6.2	79.3	98.6	9.2	9.1
Weighted Ensemble Cascade	76.4	6.2	87.8	20.5	7.2	7.2
Optimized Combination Cascade	66.1	6.2	87.5	20.5	9.3	9.3

Table 3. Performance (FP/FN) of each configuration on BraTS-PEDs 2025 validation dataset

Configuration	Lesion-wise FP/FN					
	ET	NET	CC	ED	TC	WT
Stage 1 Model Only	0.26/0.03	0.01/0.01	0.15/0.11	0.23/0.03	0.02/0.01	0.02/0.01
Basic Cascade	0.18/0.05	0.00/0.01	0.12/0.13	0.26/0.03	0.02/0.01	0.02/0.01
Reduced Sensitivity Cascade	0.19/0.05	0.00/0.01	0.08/0.13	0.23/0.03	0.02/0.01	0.02/0.01
Weighted Ensemble Cascade	0.18/0.05	0.00/0.01	0.11/0.13	0.03/0.03	0.01/0.01	0.01/0.01
Optimized Combination Cascade	0.13/0.07	0/0.01	0.1/0.13	0.03/0.03	0.02/0.01	0.02/0.01

Overwriting CC + ED Prediction with ST When Colliding is Optimal but Doesn't Improve Performance. When considering potential collisions in final masks by competing tumor subregions, the optimal order included CC + ED being overwritten by ST in the final predictions. However, it is important to note that the benefit of this final model improvement is unclear. Adding this step improved ET segmentation, (Weighted Ensemble Cascade versus Optimized Combination Cascade, Dice = 0.66 vs 0.69, HD95 = 76.4 vs 66.1) but harmed overall TC and WT segmentations.

False Positive/False Negative Segmentation for NET & ED was Low, but Higher for ET & CC. Across the tumor subregions, FP and FN segmented voxels were evaluated, with minimal recorded for both NET and ED, and this was echoed in the Dice scores for these subregions. However, for CC these metrics showed greater error (FP/FN = 0.1/0.13), and so CC tissue was both over and under segmented. For ET, there seemed to be greater error in terms of FP, rather than FN performance (FP/FN = 0.13/0.07), indicating over segmentation of ED tissues.

Test Data Performance. When the selected Optimized Combination Cascade model is applied to holdout test data, the performance can be seen in Table 4.

Table 4. Performance of submitted model on BraTS-PEDs 2025 test dataset

Configuration	Performance					
	ET	NET	CC	ED	TC	WT
Optimized Combination Cascade						
Lesion-wise Dice - Mean	0.692	0.827	0.532	0.820	0.877	0.885
SD	0.320	0.207	0.466	0.368	0.162	0.168
Lesion-wise NSD 1.0 – Mean	0.747	0.782	0.553	0.820	0.778	0.777
SD	0.316	0.209	0.459	0.368	0.232	0.232

4 Discussion

The current paper outlines a further improvement of our two-stage cascaded nnU-Net, which we previously submitted [6] as a solution to the ASNR-MICCAI BraTS Pediatrics Tumor Challenge 2024. This improved model (specifically the Optimized Combination Cascade) is to be submitted to the BraTS-Ped 2025 challenge.

Our approach refined the initial segmentations through a progressive cascaded network, which was radiologically informed by both the hierarchical information between tumor subregions, but also in the specific mpMRI modalities provided at each stage of the cascade. Our novel adaptations include limiting the training dataset of our ED/CC model to only those cases with that tumor subregion present, to prevent biasing the model toward the more common empty segmentation masks (as many of the HGGs do not present radiologically with CC or ED). We also logic-gated the flow of segmentation masks through our cascade, based on whether the initial segmentation model predicts presence of CC or ED in the case being tested upon, if not, the mask is not passed to the Stage 2 model for further refinement. Finally, we also generating greater segmentation variability in higher levels to promote refinement of the segmentations by the lower levels of the cascade.

Based on qualitative comparisons to our previous cascade model [6] our new adaptations have mostly harmed performance in specific tumor subregions. Whilst performance on ET Increased (Dice = 0.69 vs 0.66), TC/WT/ED all decreased (Dice = 0.92 vs 0.93, 0.92 vs 0.93, 0.95 vs 0.97, respectively) and NET/CC performance remained the same. However, when rating using HD95, our new model also showed improvement in CC compared to the previous iteration (HD95 = 87.5 vs 111.0) – as well as the already expected improvement in ET (HD95 = 66.1 vs 76.2). This suggests that the model has produced more accurately segmented boundaries for CC, whilst estimating similar volumes, and overall performance in terms of the entire volume and the boundaries was experienced for ET. Whilst improvements may be considered minimal, we focused on the better handling of FP/FN in subregions such as CC and ED and anticipate that the model may fare better on these types of cases in the independent test cohort. Subsequent release of the testing performance suggested that, on lesion-wise Dice, performance was worse on all tumor subregions.

Historical segmentation procedures have utilized multi-stage models to segment different tumor subregions, even with reduced subsets of MRI modalities (e.g. [13, 14]), similarly to our previous and current models. More recently, a model also inspired by radiological reasoning, produced effective multi-label segmentations of pediatric brain tumors using a multi-stage model. Bengtsson and colleagues [15] segmented CC/ED/ET using a single nnU-Net, and a second model was used to segment WT, with a postprocessing step to infer NET. They performed well on the BraTS-Ped 2024 dataset, and an external validation set (but not the BraTS Adult Glioma Data). They show not only the effectiveness of a multi-model approach, but the generalizability to other pediatric data. The current approach outperforms Bengtsson and colleagues' model in nearly all tumor subregions, other than ET (where performance is roughly equivalent) and CC where they clearly outperform our model (Dice = 0.70 vs 0.83 and HD95 = 87.5 vs 32.7 – current vs [15] respectively). This may simply be due to the fact we have not used the T1C in our Stage 2b model, in which CC typically appears as hypointense. However, this was not done in our current model as we a) wanted to minimize model complexity by not including the full mpMRI set at for input stage 2 models and b) because we specifically wished to refine the CC vs ED segmentation, and response to contrast can vary in cystic regions dependent on the contents of the cyst itself.

Strengths and Limitations. On major strength of stepwise or cascade models such as this is the commensurate nature of our approach in comparison to current clinical practice of radiologists and other medical experts involved in the review and potential manual segmentations of tumors such as this. This will be important in the acceptance and adoption of such approaches into clinical practice. One potential limitation of the reported study is the lack of ablation studies. In the current work, we optimized each subsequent adaption in the order they appeared in the hierarchy/cascade. This meant that all adaptations were included with no strong indication as to whether any one adaptation in isolation effectively improved (or in fact harmed) overall performance. In future work we aim to conduct ablation studies to interrogate the aspects of our approach.

Acknowledgments. TM is funded by a PhD studentship from the "Help Harry Help Others" charity and Aston Institute of Health and Neurodevelopment, Aston University.

Disclosure of Interests. HR holds stock options in Healx (AI drug discovery in rare diseases). The remaining authors have no competing interests to declare that are relevant to the content of this article.

References

1. Erker, C., et al.: Response assessment in paediatric high-grade glioma: recommendations from the response assessment in Pediatric neuro-oncology (RAPNO) working group. Lancet Oncol. **21**(6), e317–e329 (2020)
2. Cooney, T.M., et al.: Response assessment in diffuse intrinsic pontine glioma: recommendations from the response assessment in Pediatric neuro-oncology (RAPNO) working group. Lancet Oncol. **21**(6), e330–e336 (2020)
3. Bhatia, A., et al.: Review of imaging recommendations from response assessment in Pediatric neuro-oncology (RAPNO). Pediatr. Radiol. **53**(13), 2723–2741 (2023)

4. Kazerooni, A.F., et al.: The brain tumor segmentation in Pediatrics (BraTS-PEDs) challenge: focus on Pediatrics (CBTN-CONNECT-DIPGR-ASNR-MICCAI BraTS-PEDs). arXiv (2024)
5. Kazerooni, A.F., et al.: The brain tumor segmentation (BRATS) challenge 2023: focus on pediatrics (CBTN-CONNECT-DIPGR-ASNR-MICCAI BraTS-PEDs). arXiv preprint: arXiv: 2305.17033 (2023)
6. Mulvany, T., et al.: Segmentation of Pediatric brain tumors using a radiologically informed, deep learning cascade. (arXiv:.14020) Arxiv (2024)
7. Isensee, F., et al.: nnU-Net for brain tumor segmentation. In: BrainLesion: Glioma, Multiple Sclerosis, Stroke and Traumatic Brain Injuries. Springer International Publishing, Cham (2021)
8. Kazerooni, A.F., et al.: The brain tumor segmentation in Pediatrics (BraTS-PEDs) challenge: focus on Pediatrics (CBTN-CONNECT-DIPGR-ASNR-MICCAI BraTS-PEDs). arXiv preprint: arXiv:2404.15009 (2024)
9. Familiar, A.M., et al.: Towards consistency in Pediatric Brain tumor measurements: challenges, solutions, and the role of AI-based segmentation. Neurol. Oncol. (2024)
10. Resende, L.L., Alves, C.: Imaging of brain tumors in children: the basics-a narrative review. Transl. Pediatr. **10**(4), 1138–1168 (2021)
11. Isensee, F., et al.: Automated brain extraction of multisequence MRI using artificial neural networks. Hum. Brain Mapp. **40**(17), 4952–4964 (2019)
12. Karargyris, A., et al.: Federated benchmarking of medical artificial intelligence with MedPerf. Nat. Mach. Intell. **5**(7), 799–810 (2023)
13. Zhou, C., et al.: One-pass multi-task convolutional neural networks for efficient brain tumor segmentation. In: International Conference on Medical Image Computing and Computer-Assisted Intervention. Springer (2018)
14. Chen, L., et al.: MRI tumor segmentation with densely connected 3D CNN. In: Medical Imaging 2018: Image Processing. SPIE (2018)
15. Bengtsson, M., et al.: A new logic for Pediatric brain tumor segmentation. In: 2025 IEEE 22nd International Symposium on Biomedical Imaging (ISBI). IEEE (2025)

An Advanced nnU-Net Framework for BraTS-2025 PED

Xiaolong Li[1], Zhi-Qin John Xu[1(✉)], Yan Ren[2(✉)], Tianming Qiu[3(✉)], and Xiaowen Wang[3(✉)]

[1] Institute of Natural Sciences, School of Mathematical Sciences, MOE-LSC, Shanghai Jiao Tong University, Shanghai, China
{15369855310,xuzhiqin}@sjtu.edu.cn

[2] Department of Radiology, Huashan Hospital, Fudan University, Shanghai, China
renyan_richard@aliyun.com

[3] Department of Neurosurgery, Huashan Hospital, Fudan University, Shanghai, China
{tianming2100,apolloslisy}@126.com

Abstract. Accurate segmentation of pediatric brain tumors in multiparametric magnetic resonance imaging (mpMRI) is critical for diagnosis, treatment planning, and monitoring, yet faces unique challenges due to limited data, high anatomical variability, and heterogeneous imaging across institutions. In this work, we present **an advanced nnU-Net framework** tailored for **BraTS 2025 Task-6 (PED)**, the largest public dataset of pre-treatment pediatric high-grade gliomas. Our contributions include: (1) a widened residual encoder with squeeze-and-excitation (SE) attention; (2) 3D depthwise separable convolutions; (3) a specificity-driven regularization term; and (4) small-scale Gaussian weight initialization. We further refine predictions with two postprocessing steps. Our models achieved first place on the Task-6 validation leaderboard, attaining lesion-wise Dice scores of **0.759 (CC)**, **0.967 (ED)**, **0.826 (ET)**, **0.910 (NET)**, **0.928 (TC)** and **0.928 (WT)**.

Keywords: Brain tumor segmentation · nn-UNet · Deep learning · Attention

1 Introduction

The Brain Tumor Segmentation (BraTS) Challenge [7–9] has served as a cornerstone in advancing automated neuro-oncological imaging analysis. By releasing large-scale, high-quality annotated datasets and formulating clinically relevant tasks, BraTS has driven innovation in algorithmic segmentation and classification of brain tumors. Continuing this mission, the BraTS 2025 Lighthouse Challenge introduces eleven diverse tasks targeting key translational gaps in brain tumor AI solutions, including segmentation, synthesis, and classification across different tumor types, age groups, and imaging conditions (Fig. 1).

S. Bakas et al. (Eds.): MICCAI 2025, LNCS 16376, pp. 422–433, 2026.
https://doi.org/10.1007/978-3-032-16365-3_38

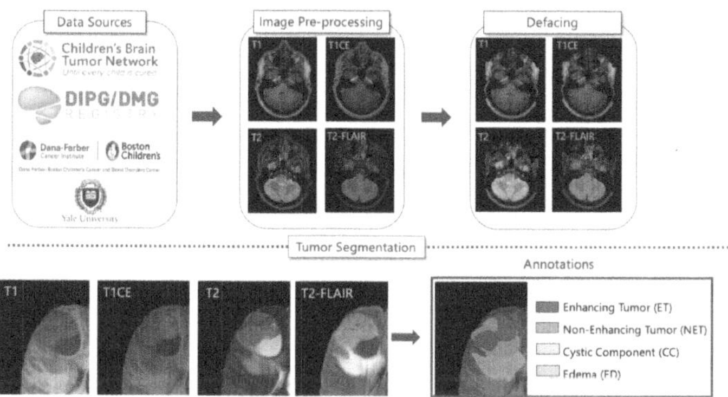

Fig. 1. Graphical representation of data processing and annotations in pediatric brain tumors. Top panel presents the processing pipeline, and the bottom panel illustrates the annotated tumor subregions along with mpMRI structural scans (T1, T1CE, T2, and T2-FLAIR). Tumor subregions include the enhancing tumor (ET - red), non-enhancing tumor (NET - green), cystic component (CC - yellow), and edema (ED - teal) regions. (Color figure online)

Task-6 (PED) of the BraTS 2025 Challenge focuses on a particularly underexplored and clinically significant domain: automatic segmentation of pretreatment pediatric brain tumors. This task leverages the largest publicly available, expert-annotated cohort of high-grade pediatric brain tumors to date, aggregating multi-parametric MRI data 1 [8,9] from globally recognized pediatric oncology consortia.

In this work, we propose **An Advanced nnU-Net Framework for BraTS-2025 PED** to tackle the unique challenges of pediatric tumor segmentation.

The main contributions of this work are as follows:

- **Widened residual encoder with attention in nnU-Net** [6] **architecture.**
- **Depthwise separable convolutions** [4].
- **Specificity-driven regularization for generalization.**
- **Small-scale initialization** [11].

As a result, our submitted models collectively occupied the top **one** position on the BraTS 2025 Task-6 (PED) validation leaderboard, highlighting the effectiveness and consistency of our approach across different tumor subtypes and imaging variations.

2 Model Architecture

In this section, we begin with the standard nnU-Net [6] as the baseline and we propose several targeted modifications aimed at further improving segmentation accuracy and robustness. These include the widened residual encoder with squeeze-and-excitation (SE) attention [5] modules, depthwise separable convolutions [4], regularization, and small-scale weight initialization [2].

Our final model architecture is illustrated in Fig. 2. It retains the classic U-Net [12] encoder-decoder topology, but each stage is enhanced by residual connections and SE attention, and all skip connections are preserved to fuse low- and high-level features:

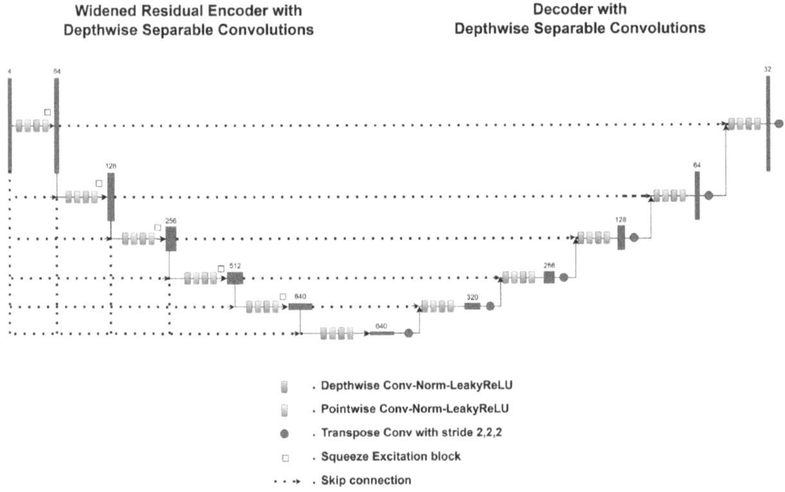

Fig. 2. Overview of our enhanced nnU-Net. The left branch is the encoder (downsampling), the right branch is the decoder (upsampling), and dashed arrows denote skip connections.

Downsampling is implemented via a $3 \times 3 \times 3$ stride-2 convolution to maintain spatial context. Symmetrically, each upsampling stage begins with a transposed convolution for upscaling.

2.1 Baseline: Standard NnU-Net(v2)

Medical image segmentation is notoriously challenging due to inherent variability across imaging modalities, spatial resolutions, anatomical structures, and pathological features.

To overcome these issues, nnU-Net [6] provides a robust, automated pipeline designed specifically for semantic segmentation tasks. Built upon a flexible U-Net architecture, nnU-Net analyzes dataset characteristics, including image dimensionality (2D or 3D), number of modalities, voxel spacings, and class imbalances, automatically generating an optimized configuration without user intervention. This self-adaptation significantly reduces reliance on expert-driven tuning, enabling consistent and high-quality segmentation performance across diverse medical imaging datasets.

For its architecture, nnU-Net by default uses $3 \times 3 \times 3$ kernels with strides of 2 (except for the first layer) to replace pooling operations, allowing the model to downsample the feature maps while retaining spatial information. It employs Leaky ReLU activation with a slope of 0.01 to introduce non-linearity and help the model learn more complex representations. Additionally, nnU-Net incorporates Instance Normalization after each convolutional layer, which helps normalize the feature maps and ensures stable training, particularly when handling images with varying intensity distributions.

The practical versatility of nnU-Net has been extensively validated across a wide range of segmentation benchmarks, underscoring its suitability as a reliable baseline in medical image segmentation research. In our work, we adopt the standard nnU-Net (v2) as the baseline, against which we compare our proposed improvements detailed in subsequent sections.

2.2 Widened Residual Encoder with SE Attention

To enhance the feature extraction capability of nnU-Net, we first incorporated residual connections into the encoder architecture. Traditional nnU-Net encoders often face challenges such as gradient vanishing and feature degradation when propagating information through multiple convolutional layers. Residual connections effectively alleviate these issues by providing shortcut pathways that facilitate gradient flow and enhance the network's ability to capture complex spatial features.

In addition to residual connections, we further widened the encoder by increasing the number of feature channels in each encoder layer to twice their original values. By widening the encoder, we significantly expanded the model's representational capacity, allowing it to capture richer and more discriminative feature representations. This modification particularly benefits the network's ability to handle intricate structures and subtle variations commonly observed in medical images, ultimately leading to improved segmentation performance and robustness.

Residual Blocks with SE Attention

A single residual block with Squeeze-and-Excitation (SE) attention [5] in our encoder is thus defined by

$$\mathbf{y} = \sigma(\mathbf{x} + \mathrm{SE}(\mathrm{DropPath}(\mathcal{F}(\mathbf{x})))), \quad (1)$$

where

- $\mathcal{F}(\mathbf{x})$ is the stacked convolutional path fitting the residual mapping $\mathcal{H}(\mathbf{x}) - \mathbf{x}$.
- DropPath $(\cdot)$ applies stochastic depth with drop probability $p = 0.05$.
- $\mathrm{SE}(\cdot)$ denotes the squeeze excitation attention with reduction ratio $1/16$.
- $\sigma(\cdot)$ is the final nonlinearity.

We find that applying residual blocks solely in the encoder yields the best segmentation accuracy and generalization.

Widened Encoder:

To further boost feature-extraction capacity, we widen the encoder by increasing its channel dimensionality to twice that of the decoder at each corresponding stage. Concretely, if the decoder stages use $\{F_1, F_2, \ldots, F_L\}$ feature maps (e.g. $32, 64, 128, 256, 320, 320$), then the encoder stages are configured with $\{2F_1, 2F_2, \ldots, 2F_L\}$ feature maps (i.e. $64, 128, 256, 512, 640, 640$). This doubling applies to both the initial convolution in each stage and all residual blocks within that stage.

By allocating more channels in the encoder, the network can capture a richer set of spatial and textural features before down-sampling, which in turn allows the decoder (with half the channels) to reconstruct finer details more accurately. Our experiments show that this widened encoder configuration yields a consistent improvement of $2-4\%$ in overall Dice score on the validation set, as well as better generalization on small and low-contrast tumor regions.

2.3 Depthwise Separable Convolutions

This section explains the concept of depthwise separable convolution (Fig. 3 Right) in 3D, including its parameters and computational details.

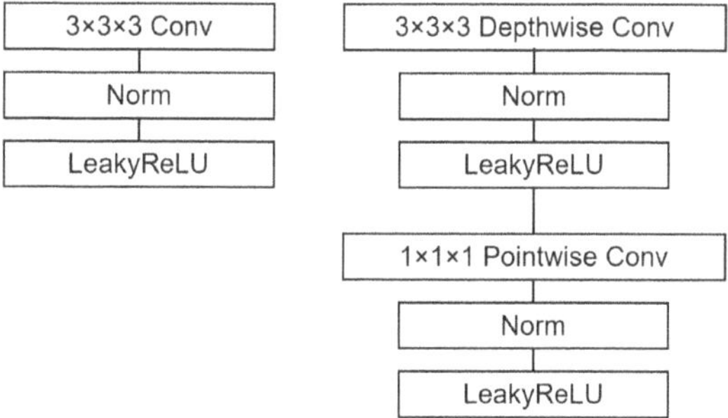

Fig. 3. Left: Standard convolution with norm and LeakyReLU. Right: Depthwise Separable convolutions with norm and LeakyReLU.

Standard Convolution

Standard convolution (Fig. 4 [1]) in 3D applies a kernel to the input to produce the output.

- **Kernel**: A tensor of size $(k, k, k, C_{in}, C_{out})$, where (k, k, k) is the kernel size.
- **Parameter Count**: The total number of parameters is $k^3 \cdot C_{in} \cdot C_{out}$.

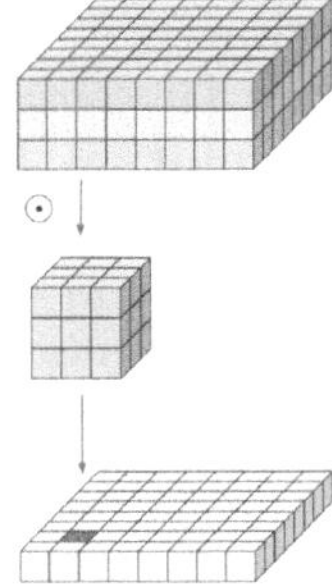

Fig. 4. Standard Convolution.

Depthwise Convolution

Depthwise convolution (Fig. 5(a) [1]) applies a single filter to each input channel independently.

- **Kernel**: A tensor of size $(k, k, k, 1, C_{in})$, where k is the kernel size.
- **Parameter Count**: The total number of parameters is $k^3 \cdot C_{in}$.

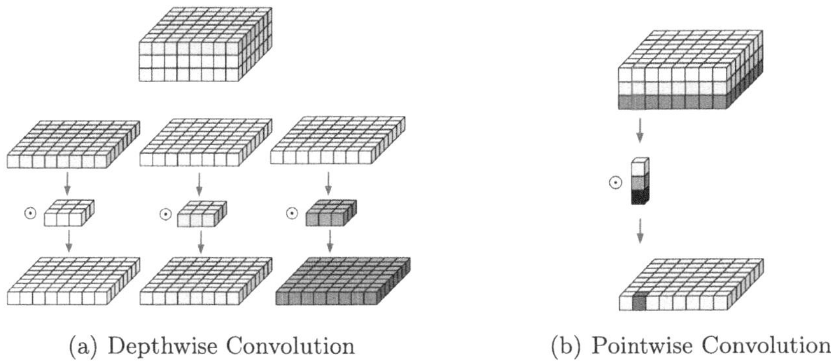

Fig. 5. Depthwise and Pointwise Convolution.

Pointwise Convolution

Pointwise convolution (Fig. 5(b) [1]) uses a 1×1 kernel to combine the outputs of the depthwise convolution.

- **Kernel**: A tensor of size $(1, 1, 1, C_{in}, C_{out})$.
- **Parameter Count**: The total number of parameters is $C_{in} \cdot C_{out}$.

Depthwise Separable Convolution

Depthwise separable convolution [4] consists of two parts: a **depthwise convolution** and a **pointwise convolution**. Depthwise convolution integrates information within each channel, while pointwise convolution fuses information across channels. To enhance the model's expressive capacity, we insert an activation function between the depthwise convolution and the pointwise convolution.

2.4 Regularization

The evaluation criteria for BraTS2025 introduced lesion-wise Dice as a crucial performance metric. During model training and validation, we observed some cases within the validation set lacking specific lesion classes for example, cases without **enhancing tumors (ET)**. However, because our neural network model predicts probabilities at the voxel level, it becomes inherently difficult for the model to produce outputs completely absent of certain classes (i.e., predictions that are uniformly zero). This challenge aligns with our understanding of neural network behavior, as such predictions correspond to high-frequency, sparse outputs that networks generally find difficult to accurately learn [14].

Under lesion-wise Dice evaluation, predictions containing even minor false positives (FP) for absent classes lead to a Dice score of 0, whereas correctly predicting an absence (output of all zeros) yields a perfect score of 1. This substantial discrepancy significantly impacts overall performance. To address this and improve model accuracy in predicting cases with absent classes, we specifically introduced a regularization term to penalize false positives.

Our proposed approach integrates multiple loss functions covering different segmentation aspects (distribution-based, region-based, and boundary-based) with an additional **specificity-driven regularization**.

$$\text{Loss} = -\text{Dice} + \text{CE} + \text{HD} + \frac{\theta N_{\text{FP}}}{N_{\text{pred}} + N_{\text{gt}}} \tag{2}$$

We set $\theta = 0.1$. By explicitly penalizing false positives through this regularization term, our model demonstrates enhanced predictive accuracy for cases lacking specific lesion classes, thereby significantly improving the lesion-wise Dice performance.

2.5 Initialization

The initialization of neural networks across different scales significantly influences their generalization capability [11]. This effect is closely related to phenomena such as condensation and the network's Hessian eigenvalues [10], which determine how a network converges during training. The impact of initialization is not only observable in simpler architectures like fully connected neural networks, but it extends to more complex models such as Convolutional Neural Networks (CNNs), ResNet [3], and even large language models. Initialization plays a crucial role in the dynamics of training and the network's ability to generalize to unseen data.

Generally speaking, smaller initialization [11] values tend to favor the network's reasoning ability rather than its memory capacity [2]. This characteristic is particularly beneficial for tasks that require strong reasoning capabilities. In such tasks, models initialized with smaller values are typically more effective at capturing general patterns rather than memorizing specific details.

We utilize Gaussian initialization, which has been shown to yield good performance in a wide range of deep learning architectures. Mathematically, Gaussian initialization is typically expressed as follows:

$$w \sim \mathcal{N}\left(0, (\frac{2}{dim_{in}})^{\alpha}\right) \tag{3}$$

where w represents the weights of the network, and n_{in} represents the input feature dimension of the convolutional layer, and α is a hyperparameter introduced to control the scale of initialization. By tuning the value of α, we effectively control the scale of initial weights.

2.6 Postprocessing

We primarily implemented two postprocessing techniques to further refine the segmentation results.

The first technique leverages domain-specific medical imaging knowledge, particularly focusing on **enhancing tumor (ET)** segmentation accuracy. Given that ET is a critical region in tumor identification and typically occupies smaller volumes compared to **non-enhancing tumors (NET)**, neural networks often struggle to accurately detect **ET** due to the limited representation and subtle intensity differences. However, exploiting the intensity contrast between T1CE (contrast-enhanced T1-weighted) and T1 (non-enhanced T1-weighted) modalities in MRI scans provides valuable information to better distinguish ET from NET.

From fundamental medical imaging principles, it is known that the ratio of T1CE to T1 signal intensities can effectively differentiate enhancing from non-enhancing tumor regions. To systematically apply this knowledge, we first performed z-score normalization on both T1CE and T1 signals within the training dataset. Subsequently, we calculated the T1CE/T1 intensity ratio specifically at locations annotated as label 1 **(ET)** and label 2 **(NET)**. To ensure robustness and avoid outlier influence, we excluded extreme values (ratios below 0.2 and above 5) from our analysis.

Based on the statistical analysis, we conservatively selected the 95-th percentile values as threshold criteria: specifically, we reassigned voxels initially labeled as **NET** (label 2) to **ET** (label 1) if their T1CE/T1 ratio exceeded 1.388. Conversely, voxels initially labeled as **ET** (label 1) were reassigned to **NET** (label 2) if their ratio fell below 0.766. Our ROC curve is show in Fig. 6.

The second postprocessing approach focuses on removing small isolated connected components. First, we apply a $3 \times 3 \times 3$ dilation kernel to the voxel-wise predictions. Afterward, connected components are identified, and their volumes are calculated. Through threshold testing on the validation dataset, we

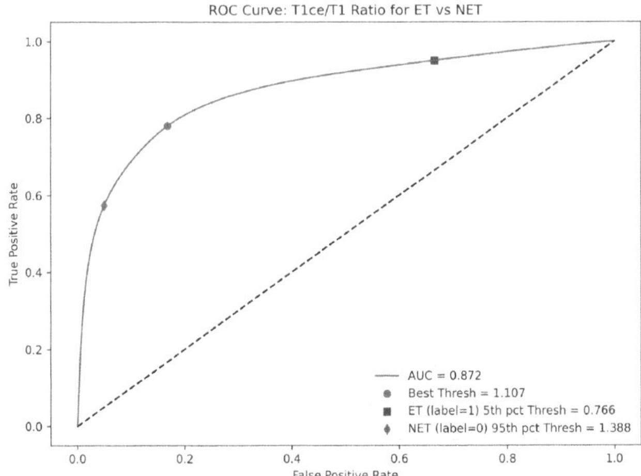

Fig. 6. ROC Curve of T1CE-T1 ratio.

determined optimal volume thresholds of $160mm^3$ and $50mm^3$ for labels 1 and 3, respectively. This approach effectively reduces false-positive predictions by removing small connected components and enhances the spatial consistency of the segmented structures.

3 Training

We train our network using 5-fold cross-validation with the SGD optimizer with weightdecay = 3e-5 and momentum = 0.99 for 1000 epochs and a batch size of 2 on NVIDIA GeForce RTX 4080 16GB GPUs. In each epoch we randomly sample 250 patches; the initial learning rate is set to 1e-2. We decay the learning rate according to a cosine schedule over the full 1000 epochs:

$$\eta_t = \eta_0 \frac{1 + \cos(\pi t / T)}{2} \tag{4}$$

Our training data augmentations are as follows: we apply spatial transforms (elastic deformation, random rotations, scaling); add Gaussian noise and Gaussian blur; perform multiplicative brightness and contrast adjustments; simulate low-resolution sampling; apply two gamma corrections; and randomly flip along all three axes. Figure 7 illustrates the evolution of the training loss (Fig. 7(a)), Dice score (Fig. 7(a)), and learning rate (Fig. 7(b)) over the course of training.

4 Results

On the BraTS-PED (Task 6) validation leaderboard, our method ranks first with the following LesionWise Dice scores (Table 1):

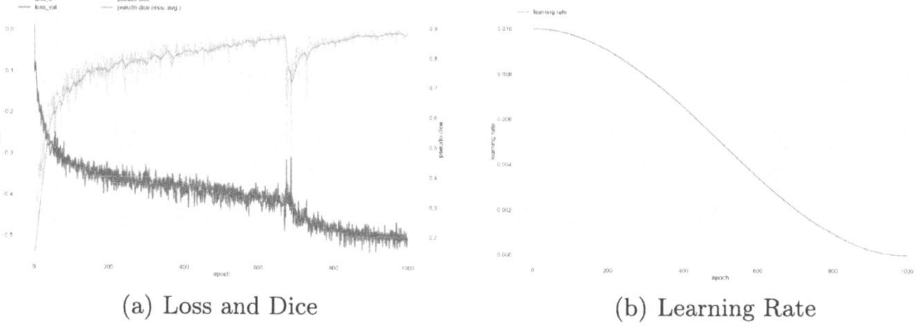

(a) Loss and Dice (b) Learning Rate

Fig. 7. (a) Training loss and Dice score curves. (b) Cosine learning-rate schedule over epochs.

Table 1. Lesion-wise Dice results on validation dataset. Higher values indicate better performance.

	CC	ED	ET	NET	TC	WT
value	0.759	0.967	0.826	0.910	0.928	0.928

These results demonstrate great performance across all critical tumor cystic component (CC), peritumoral edema (ED), enhancing tumor (ET), non-enhancing tumor (NET), tumor core (TC), and whole tumor (WT). In Fig. 8, we present a representative example in which our model delivers highly accurate lesion segmentation, clearly illustrating its precise predictive capabilities.

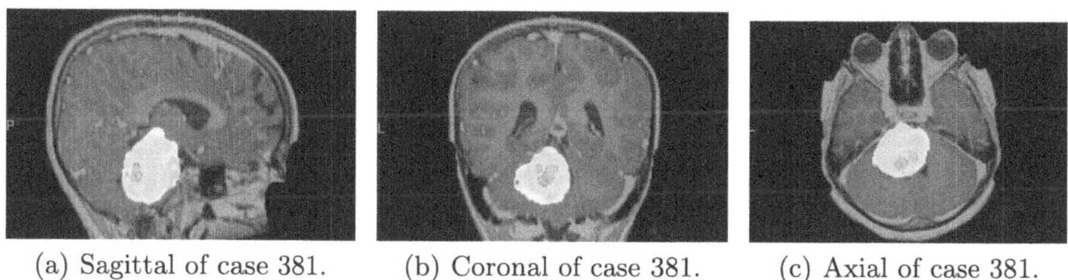

(a) Sagittal of case 381. (b) Coronal of case 381. (c) Axial of case 381.

Fig. 8. BraTS_PED_00381 ET: 0.9575 NET: 0.9722 TC. 0.9749 WT: 0.9749.

On the BraTS-PED (Task 6) **test set**, our method achieves excellent performance, ranking among the top results with the following quantitative metrics (Table 2):

Table 2. Lesion-wise Dice results on test dataset. Higher values indicate better performance.

	Lesion-wise Dice ↑						Lesion-wise NSD-1.0 ↑					
	CC	ED	ET	NETC	TC	WT	CC	ED	ET	NETC	TC	WT
mean	0.591	**0.892**	**0.727**	**0.838**	**0.903**	**0.900**	0.599	**0.892**	**0.783**	**0.800**	**0.775**	**0.770**
std	0.464	0.312	0.307	0.211	0.141	0.143	0.459	0.312	0.297	0.213	0.220	0.230

5 Discussion

Overall, our model achieves state-of-the-art lesion-wise performance through a combination of architectural innovations, enhanced learning strategies, careful initialization, and task-specific post-processing. Together, these modifications enable richer spatial and contextual encoding of tumor subregions, contributing to our high lesion-wise Dice scores across all targets.

Despite these advances, there remains substantial room for improvement in the ET and CC metrics, especially in reducing false positives. Furthermore, while convolutional neural networks continue to dominate in medical image segmentation, recent fully-Transformer architectures [13] have demonstrated strong performance on 3D medical image segmentation tasks. The relative underperformance of transformer models here likely stems from limited training data to exploit their full representation power and from our preliminary exploration of such designs. Future work should therefore search deeper into attention mechanisms.

Disclosure of Interests. The authors have no competing interests to declare that are relevant to the content of this article.

References

1. Bendersky, E.: Depthwise separable convolutions for machine learning. https://eli.thegreenplace.net/2018/depthwise-separable-convolutions-for-machine-learning/ (2018). Accessed 30 July 2025
2. Hang, L., et al.: Scalable complexity control facilitates reasoning ability of LLMs. arXiv preprint arXiv:2505.23013 (2025)
3. He, K., Zhang, X., Ren, S., Sun, J.: Deep residual learning for image recognition. In: Proceedings of the IEEE Conference on Computer Vision and Pattern Recognition, pp. 770–778 (2016)
4. Howard, A.G., et al.: MobileNets: Efficient convolutional neural networks for mobile vision applications. arXiv preprint arXiv:1704.04861 (2017)
5. Hu, J., Shen, L., Sun, G.: Squeeze-and-excitation networks. In: Proceedings of the IEEE Conference on Computer Vision and Pattern Recognition, pp. 7132–7141 (2018)
6. Isensee, F., Jaeger, P.F., Kohl, S.A., Petersen, J., Maier-Hein, K.H.: nnU-Net: a self-configuring method for deep learning-based biomedical image segmentation. Nat. Methods **18**(2), 203–211 (2021)

7. Karargyris, A., et al.: Federated benchmarking of medical artificial intelligence with MedPerf. Nat. Mach. Intell. **5**(7), 799–810 (2023). https://doi.org/10.1038/s42256-023-00652-2
8. Kazerooni, A.F., et al.: The brain tumor segmentation in pediatrics (BraTS-PEDs) challenge: focus on pediatrics (CBTN-CONNECT-DIPGR-ASNR-MICCAI BraTS-PEDs). arXiv preprint arXiv:2404.15009 (2024). https://doi.org/10.48550/arXiv.2404.15009
9. Kazerooni, A.F., et al.: The brain tumor segmentation (BraTS) challenge 2023: Focus on pediatrics (CBTN-CONNECT-DIPGR-ASNR-MICCAI BraTS-PEDs). ArXiv, pp. arXiv–2305 (2024). https://doi.org/10.48550/arXiv.2305.17033
10. Li, X., Xu, Z.Q.J., Zhang, Z.: Loss spike in training neural networks. arXiv preprint arXiv:2305.12133 (2023)
11. Luo, T., Xu, Z.Q.J., Ma, Z., Zhang, Y.: Phase diagram for two-layer ReLU neural networks at infinite-width limit. J. Mach. Learn. Res. **22**(71), 1–47 (2021)
12. Ronneberger, O., Fischer, P., Brox, T.: U-Net: convolutional networks for biomedical image segmentation. In: International Conference on Medical Image Computing and Computer-Assisted Intervention, pp. 234–241. Springer (2015)
13. Wald, T., et al.: Primus: Enforcing attention usage for 3D medical image segmentation. arXiv preprint arXiv:2503.01835 (2025)
14. Xu, Z.Q.J., Zhang, Y., Luo, T., Xiao, Y., Ma, Z.: Frequency principle: Fourier analysis sheds light on deep neural networks. arXiv preprint arXiv:1901.06523 (2019)

Memory-Constrained, Noise-Resilient Pediatric Brain Tumor Segmentation via Decoupled Feature Learning and Domain Adaptation

MICCAI BraTS-PEDs 2025 Challenge Solution

Meng-Yuan Chen[1] and Hsiang-Kuang Tony Liang[1,2,3,4](✉)

[1] Department of Biomedical Engineering, National Taiwan University, Taipei, Taiwan
[2] National Taiwan University Cancer Center, Taipei, Taiwan
[3] Department of Radiation Oncology, National Taiwan University Cancer Center Branch, National Taiwan University Hospital, Taipei, Taiwan
[4] Division of Radiation Oncology, Department of Oncology, National Taiwan University Hospital, Taipei, Taiwan
hkliang@ntu.edu.tw

Abstract. While deep learning has achieved numerous results in brain tumor segmentation, most models still struggle with insufficient data, particularly for heterogeneous pediatric cases. This study develops a dedicated segmentation model for pediatric patients, a population where brain tumors represent the leading cause of cancer-related death despite their rarity. Standard AI models, often trained on adult data, typically fail when faced with the distinct biological heterogeneity and imaging characteristics of pediatric tumors. The real-world data impurities of the MICCAI BraTS-PEDs 2025 Challenge, specifically the non-skull-stripped images, further confound model training. To address this trifecta of challenges—biological heterogeneity, data scarcity, and data impurity—we propose a novel three-stage segmentation framework. Our core strategy is to decouple feature learning from noise adaptation: a high-capacity U-Net is first trained on a clean, algorithmically skull-stripped dataset to learn invariant tumor features; it is then fine-tuned on the original, non-skull-stripped data to enhance domain robustness; finally, a post-processing step refines the predictions through. Developed on a limited training set (n = 261), our resource-efficient approach achieved state-of-the-art performance on the officially scored, unseen validation set (n = 91), yielding mean LesionWise Dice scores of 0.945 for the whole tumor, 0.944 for the tumor core, and impressively, 0.917 for the highly challenging non-enhancing tumor (NET) sub-region—all accomplished on a limited training set using only a single consumer-grade GPU.

Keywords: Pediatric Brain Tumor Segmentation · Domain Adaptation · Two-Stage Training · Fine-Tuning · nnU-Net v2 · BraTS PEDs

S. Bakas et al. (Eds.): MICCAI 2025, LNCS 16376, pp. 434–444, 2026.
https://doi.org/10.1007/978-3-032-16365-3_39

1 Introduction

With the expansion of AI applications, brain tumor segmentation technology has been applied to various lesions and ethnic groups. This study focuses on automated brain tumor segmentation in pediatric patients. While primary pediatric central nervous system (CNS) tumors are rare, representing approximately 3.6% of all brain tumors, their severity makes them the leading cause of cancer-related death in children [12]. The average annual incidence rate is 5.67 cases per 100,000 children, a figure that underscores their status as the most common solid tumor in this population.

This clinical challenge is compounded by extreme heterogeneity; gliomas account for the majority of cases (51%), followed by embryonal tumors (12.1%) and other diverse subtypes defined by the World Health Organization (WHO) [16]. The anatomical locations are similarly varied, with tumors commonly found in the cerebellum (16.6%) and brain stem (12.6%) [12]. While the overall 5-year relative survival rate is approximately 75%, this figure masks a grim reality. For high-grade gliomas (HGGs)—the focus of this challenge—the 5-year survival rate plummets to below 30%, and for the highly aggressive Diffuse Midline Glioma (DMG), the prognosis is devastating, with a median survival of only 11 months and a 5-year survival rate of a mere 2.2% [3]. This complex landscape of varied pathologies, locations, and prognoses demands highly specialized computational tools for accurate analysis and treatment planning [15].

These biological and anatomical differences create a significant domain gap, meaning artificial intelligence (AI) models trained on adult tumor data often fail on pediatric cases [8]. The unique imaging characteristics of pediatric tumors are a primary driver of this issue. For example, the subtle, often non-enhancing nature of many DMGs differs significantly from the typical ring-enhancing necrosis of adult glioblastomas (GBMs), leading to significant segmentation errors when using adult-trained models [3]. Therefore, the development of dedicated pediatric segmentation models is critical for advancing accurate diagnosis, treatment planning, and prognostic assessment for young patients.

The MICCAI BraTS Multi-Consortium International Pediatric Brain Tumor Segmentation (BraTS-PEDs) 2025 Challenge directly addresses this need [1]. However, it introduces a further real-world complication: the provided MRI data is not skull-stripped. The presence of skull and other non-brain tissue introduces significant non-biological variance that can confound segmentation models, which must learn to distinguish pathological tissue from high-contrast anatomical structures. These non-brain structures can mislead automated segmentation models, potentially leading to results that deviate significantly from the ground truth [4].

To address this trifecta of challenges—biological heterogeneity, data impurities, and limited training data (n = 261)—we propose a novel three-stage segmentation framework. Our method first trains the model on a clean, algorithmically skull-stripped dataset to learn core tumor features; then adapts it to the original data with skulls via fine-tuning; and finally, optimizes the output for the challenge's lesion-wise metrics using a rule-based post-processing step. This resource-efficient approach achieved state-of-the-art performance on the unseen validation data (n = 91), yielding a mean LesionWise Dice score of 0.944 for the tumor core and 0.945 for the whole tumor. This work demonstrates that a carefully staged training and refinement strategy can produce a highly effective and clinically translatable model, even under significant data and hardware constraints.

2 Methods

A core tenet of our methodological approach was to ensure the developed framework remains accessible and readily reproducible. To this end, all model development, training, and inference were conducted on a single, commercially available workstation equipped with an NVIDIA RTX 4070 Laptop GPU, operating under a strict memory constraint of 8GB of VRAM, and supported by 64GB of system memory. This resource limitation was a primary driver for the development of our efficient three-stage training and refinement strategy. Crucially, our entire pipeline was designed to obviate the need for high-performance computing (HPC) clusters or multi-GPU configurations. This work therefore demonstrates that state-of-the-art pediatric brain tumor segmentation can be achieved on widely accessible hardware, significantly lowering the barrier for reproducible research in various clinical and academic settings.

2.1 Dataset and Label Definition

This study utilizes the official dataset from the MICCAI BraTS Pediatric Brain Tumor Segmentation (BraTS-PEDs) Lighthouse 2025 Challenge [1], which constitutes the largest publicly available, multi-institutional cohort of pediatric high-grade gliomas (HGGs), including subtypes such as diffuse midline glioma (DMG). The provided training set consists of 261 pediatric cases, each with four co-registered, pre-operative MRI sequences: native T1-weighted (T1; Fig. 1a), post-contrast T1-weighted (T1ce; Fig. 1b), T2-weighted (T2; Fig. 1c), and T2-weighted Fluid-Attenuated Inversion Recovery (FLAIR; Fig. 1d). A validation set of 91 cases with withheld annotations was provided for official evaluation.

The dataset represents a significant collaborative effort, with imaging data curated from leading pediatric neuro-oncology consortia, including the Children's Brain Tumor Network (CBTN) and the Collaborative Network for Neuro-oncology Clinical Trials (CONNECT) [1,8]. Crucially, the ground truth segmentation masks for all training cases were manually delineated and subsequently reviewed by expert neuroradiologists under the guidance of the American Society of Neuroradiology (ASNR) [1,8]. This ensures a high-quality, albeit challenging, benchmark that reflects real-world clinical and imaging variability, ideal for assessing model generalization.

The primary task is the segmentation of four distinct tumor sub-regions, as visualized in Fig. 1. These labels, based on the recommendations of the RAPNO working group for treatment response evaluation, are defined as follows:

***Enhancing Tumor (ET; label 1; Fig.** 1e):* Tissues that show hyperintensity on T1ce scans relative to T1 scans, representing the active part of the tumor with a disrupted blood-brain barrier.

***Non-enhancing Tumor (NET; label 2; Fig.** 1f):* The solid, non-enhancing part of the tumor core. It is characterized by abnormal signals on T1, T2, and FLAIR sequences but shows no significant enhancement on T1ce.

***Cystic Component (CC; label 3; Fig.** 1g):* Fluid-filled intratumoral regions, typically appearing hyperintense on T2 and hypintense on T1ce, with signal intensity comparable to cerebrospinal fluid (CSF).

***Peritumoral Edema (ED; label 4; Fig.** 1h):* The area surrounding the tumor, characterized by hyperintense, often finger-like signals on FLAIR sequences, representing vasogenic edema.

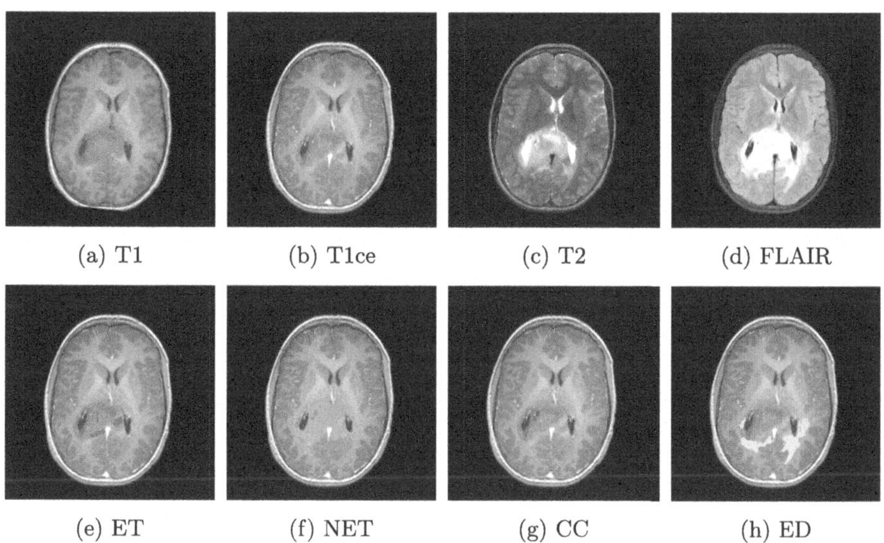

(a) T1 (b) T1ce (c) T2 (d) FLAIR

(e) ET (f) NET (g) CC (h) ED

Fig. 1. Example of training data and ground truth labels for a representative case [BraTS-PED-00001-000]. Top row (a-d) shows the four input MRI modalities. Bottom row (e-h) illustrates the four distinct tumor sub-regions overlaid on the T1ce scan: Enhancing Tumor (ET; label 1), Non-enhancing Tumor (NET; label 2), Cystic Component (CC; label 3), and Peritumoral Edema (ED; label 4). Image brightness and contrast have been enhanced for clarity [7,8].

From these four basic labels, two clinically critical composite regions are defined for evaluation: Tumor Core (TC), which includes ET, NET, and CC (labels 1+2+3); and Whole Tumor (WT), which encompasses all four sub-regions (labels 1+2+3+4).

2.2 Dual-Stream Data Preparation

Our preprocessing pipeline consists of two parts: one is to compile a training dataset optimized for learning core tumor features (stage 1) to serve as the model's baseline training; the other is to achieve effective and accurate segmentation of a training dataset containing non-brain tissue, with the core goal of achieving domain adaptability (stage 2), thus addressing the challenge of non-skull-stripped input data.

In the first stream, to create an idealized environment for foundational feature learning (Stage 1), we employed SynthStrip [4]. This robust learning-based tool generated a clean, skull-stripped version of the entire dataset, a process which also enhanced image contrast and boundary accuracy, as visualized in Fig. 2. The second stream consisted of the original, unmodified dataset, preserved to serve as the target domain for the fine-tuning stage (Stage 2).

Subsequently, both the skull-stripped and the original datasets were independently processed using the default nnU-Net v2 pipeline. This automated framework handled crucial harmonization steps, including resampling to an isotropic voxel spacing of 1.0 mm^3, co-registration of all MRI modalities to the T1ce space, and Z-score intensity normalization.

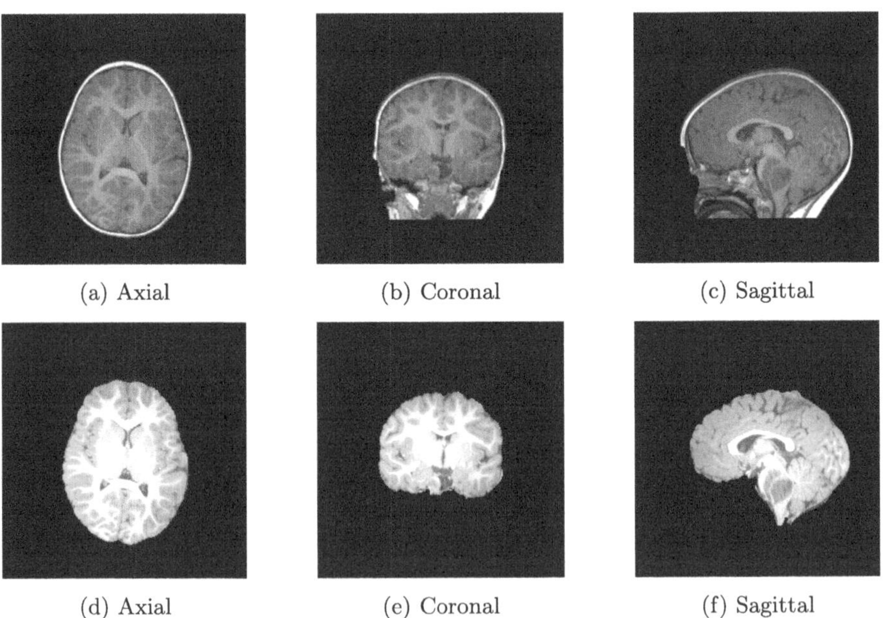

Fig. 2. Multi-planar demonstration of the SynthStrip skull-stripping process. The top row (a-c) shows a representative T1-weighted scan with the skull, while the bottom row (d-f) shows the corresponding images after removal of non-brain tissues. Each column represents a different anatomical view: Axial, Coronal, and Sagittal (case: [BraTS-PED-00248-000]) [7,8].

2.3 High-Capacity Segmentation Architecture

For this work, we adopted a 3D full-resolution U-Net architecture [13], implemented within the robust and self-configuring nnU-Net v2 framework [5,6]. This choice was motivated by the need for a model with a substantial receptive field and high capacity, capable of capturing the complex, multi-scale features inherent in heterogeneous pediatric brain tumors.

Our network is designed as a deep encoder-decoder structure with six levels. The encoder path begins with 32 feature maps and progressively doubles the channel count at each of the first four downsampling stages, reaching a final feature map count of 320 in the bottleneck. Each stage in the encoder consists of two consecutive $3 \times 3 \times 3$ convolutional layers, each followed by instance normalization and a LeakyReLU activation function. The symmetric decoder path utilizes trilinear upsampling to restore spatial resolution, while skip connections from the encoder path provide high-resolution contextual information to refine segmentation boundaries. Deep supervision is applied at intermediate decoder levels to facilitate efficient gradient flow throughout the deep network.

2.4 The Decoupled Training and Refinement Paradigm

Our methodology is a three-stage paradigm designed to systematically address the challenges of pediatric brain tumor segmentation. The core principle is to decouple the complex task of learning tumor features from the task of adapting to noisy, real-world data.

Stage 1: Foundational Training with an Uncertainty-Aware Loss. The first stage aimed to build a robust foundational model by training on the clean, skull-stripped dataset. For this, we developed a custom trainer, `LossTrainer_Ultra`, which utilizes a novel, uncertainty-aware loss function. This composite loss, $\mathcal{L}_{\text{total}}$, is defined as a weighted sum of four distinct components:

$$\mathcal{L}_{\text{total}} = \alpha\mathcal{L}_{\text{Dice}} + \beta\mathcal{L}_{\text{CE}} + \gamma\mathcal{L}_{\text{Focal}} + \delta\mathcal{L}_{\text{KL}} \tag{1}$$

where $\mathcal{L}_{\text{Dice}}$ and $\mathcal{L}_{\text{CE}}$ are the standard Dice and cross-entropy losses for volumetric and voxel-wise accuracy, respectively [11,13]. $\mathcal{L}_{\text{Focal}}$ is a Focal Loss term with a focusing parameter $\gamma_{\text{focal}} = 3.0$ to prioritize hard-to-classify voxels [10]. The novel component, $\mathcal{L}_{\text{KL}}$, is a Kullback-Leibler divergence term that acts as a regularizer. It penalizes high variance across predictions from Monte-Carlo dropout samples (T = 4), thereby encouraging a more confident and stable model [2,9]. The loss components were weighted by coefficients $\alpha = 0.4$, $\beta = 0.3$, $\gamma = 0.2$, and $\delta = 0.1$. Furthermore, to address data imbalance, the Dice, CE, and Focal terms were also weighted by the inverse frequency of each class [14]. This stage was run for 1000 epochs using a 5-fold cross-validation scheme to produce a set of robust, pre-trained model weights for the subsequent fine-tuning stage.

Stage 2: Fine-tuning for Domain Adaptation. The second stage focused on adapting the expert models from Stage 1 to the final target domain of non-skull-stripped images. The five pre-trained models were independently fine-tuned for 1000 epochs on the original dataset (with skulls), using the nnUNetv2_train command's pretrained weights functionality. This fine-tuning process utilized a lower initial learning rate to ensure stable adaptation of the learned features without catastrophic forgetting. The same uncertainty-aware loss function was employed to maintain segmentation quality during adaptation.

Stage 3: Post-processing. In the final stage, we applied a post-processing step to the inferred segmentation masks to enhance their clinical plausibility and optimize for the Lesion-wise metrics. Small, disconnected components below a specific voxel threshold were removed or reclassified. Specifically, predicted enhancing tumor (ET, label 1) regions smaller than 100 voxels were re-assigned to the non-enhancing tumor (NET, label 2), while peritumoral edema (ED, label 4) regions smaller than 100 voxels were removed. Similarly, cystic components (CC, label 3) smaller than 150 voxels were merged into the NET class.

2.5 Training and Validation Protocol

All experiments were conducted within the nnU-Net v2 framework, utilizing a 5-fold cross-validation scheme on the training set (n = 261). We trained the 3d_fullres model configuration, which determined a patch size of $128 \times 160 \times 128$ voxels and a batch size of 2 for our hardware. The network was optimized using the AdamW optimizer with an initial learning rate of 1e-2 and a poly learning rate schedule. An extensive on-the-fly data augmentation scheme, including random rotations, scaling, elastic deformations, and gamma correction, was employed throughout training. Both foundational training (Stage 1) and fine-tuning (Stage 2) for each fold were run for 1000 epochs. For the fine-tuning stage, training was initialized from the corresponding Stage 1 model weights with a reduced initial learning rate. The final segmentation on the blind validation set (n = 91) was generated via an ensemble of the five trained models. All development and training were performed on a single workstation with an NVIDIA RTX 4070 Laptop GPU.

3 Results

Our proposed three-stage framework demonstrated exceptional performance, establishing a new state-of-the-art for pediatric brain tumor segmentation on the official BraTS-PEDs 2025 Challenge benchmark. The following sections detail the quantitative validation of this performance, the impact of our key methodological innovations, and a qualitative demonstration of the model's robust generalization.

3.1 State-of-the-Art Performance on the Validation Benchmark

Our framework's state-of-the-art performance was validated on the official blind validation set (n = 91), with detailed metrics presented in Table 1. The model achieved excellent mean LesionWise Dice scores of 0.945 (WT) and 0.944 (TC). However, a deeper analysis reveals the model's exceptional robustness: the median Dice scores are near-perfect at 0.980 for both WT and TC, and an impressive 0.901 for the Enhancing Tumor (ET). This discrepancy, most pronounced for ET (mean: 0.640 vs. median: 0.901), indicates the mean is skewed by a small number of outlier cases, while our model performs with high fidelity on the vast majority of the cohort. Figure 3 provides a qualitative example of the model's final output on a high-performing case from this validation set.

Table 1. Quantitative performance on the official BraTS-PEDs 2025 validation set (n = 91).

Metric	Statistic	WT	TC	ET	NET	CC	ED
Dice Score	**Mean**	**0.9497**	**0.9496**	**0.6417**	**0.9222**	**0.5961**	**0.8352**
	Median	0.9799	0.9799	0.9023	0.9637	1.0000	1.0000
HD95 (mm)	**Mean**	**3.2842**	**3.3951**	**88.5184**	**4.2975**	**128.6318**	**61.6484**
	Median	1.0000	1.0000	1.4142	2.2361	0.0000	0.0000
NSD (1mm)	**Mean**	**0.9283**	**0.9279**	**0.6959**	**0.8999**	**0.6115**	**0.8352**
	Median	0.9861	0.9860	0.9595	0.9342	1.0000	1.0000

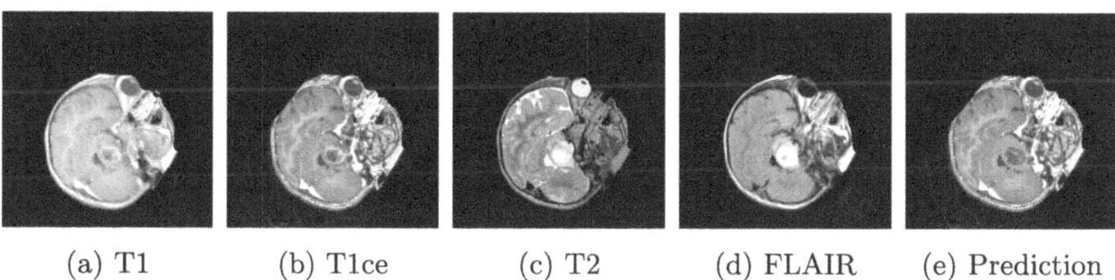

(a) T1 (b) T1ce (c) T2 (d) FLAIR (e) Prediction

Fig. 3. Qualitative result of our model on a high-performing case (`BraTS-PED-00281-000`) from the official blind validation set, which achieved a LesionWise Dice score of 0.959 for the Tumor Core. (a-d) The four input mpMRI sequences. (e) The final segmentation result overlaid on the T1ce scan. As per challenge rules, the ground truth is withheld, but the prediction demonstrates high radiological plausibility. Segmentation masks are color-coded as follows: Red = Enhancing Tumor (ET), Green = Non-enhancing Tumor (NET), Blue = Cystic Component (CC), and Yellow = Peritumoral Edema (ED).

3.2 Framework Analysis: Ablation and Validation

To validate the individual contributions of our framework's components, we conducted a rigorous ablation study, with all stages evaluated on the official blind validation set. As quantified in Table 2, the results reveal a clear synergistic effect. The Stage 2 fine-tuning on original data provided the most significant performance gain, dramatically improving both volumetric overlap (e.g., TC Dice: 0.895→0.945) and boundary accuracy (TC HD95: 20.48→4.88 mm). The final post-processing step (Stage 3) offered a crucial refinement for the most challenging sub-regions, further boosting the ET Dice score. The robustness of our final model was further confirmed by a 5-fold cross-validation on the training set, where it achieved high and stable mean VoxelWise Dice scores of 0.945 (WT), 0.943 (TC), and 0.842 (ET). Figure 4 illustrates the segmentation result on a representative case with a large, infiltrative morphology from the cross-validation set.

Table 2. Detailed ablation analysis on the unseen validation set (n = 91). Each stage is shown on mean LesionWise Dice and 95th percentile Hausdorff Distance.

Method	WT	TC	ET	Average
Stage 1 Only (on stripped data, Dice Score)	0.8950	0.8950	0.5881	0.7927
Stage 1+2 (w/o Post-Processing, Dice Score)	0.9445	0.9445	0.6585	0.8492
Full Method (Dice Score)	**0.9445**	**0.9445**	**0.6924**	**0.8605**
Stage 1 Only (on stripped data, HD95 in mm)	20.48	20.48	105.05	48.67
Stage 1+2 (w/o Post-Processing, HD95 in mm)	4.87	4.88	85.98	31.91
Full Method (HD95 in mm)	**4.87**	**4.88**	**83.83**	**31.19**

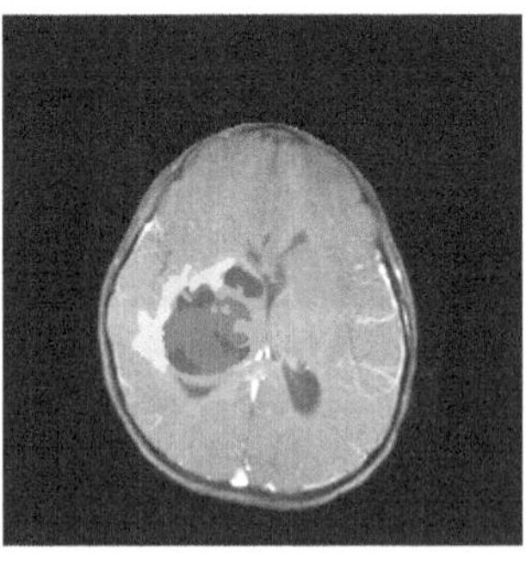

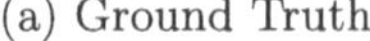

(a) Ground Truth

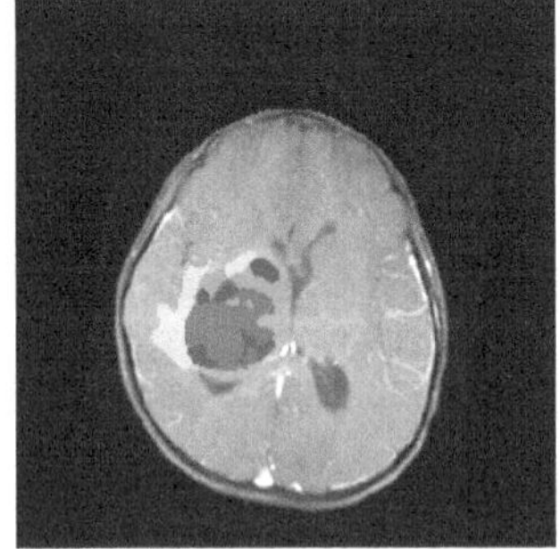

(b) Our Prediction

Fig. 4. Qualitative result for a representative case with a large, infiltrative morphology (case: `[BraTS-PED-00009-000]`). The model's prediction (b) demonstrates high fidelity with the ground truth (a), accurately delineating the complex and irregular tumor boundaries [7,8].

4 Discussion

Our work validates that the challenge of pediatric brain tumor segmentation in non-skull-stripped MRI is best addressed by a strategic paradigm that decouples feature learning from noise adaptation. Ablation studies quantitatively confirm the efficacy of this three-stage approach: foundational training on clean, skull-stripped data establishes a robust feature basis, subsequent fine-tuning on clinical data ensures domain robustness, and a final post-processing step optimizes for lesion-wise metrics. This staged methodology, not architectural novelty, was the primary driver of our state-of-the-art performance.

Beyond accuracy, our custom uncertainty-aware loss function was critical for tackling the granular challenges of the dataset. It explicitly addressed the significant class imbalance between tumor sub-regions via an inverse-frequency weighting scheme, ensuring that under-represented labels like the cystic component received appropriate focus. Simultaneously, its KL divergence term highlights a path toward more interpretable models. While still challenged by a subset of outlier cases, a clear frontier for future work lies in leveraging the generated uncertainty maps to flag predictions requiring expert review. That these top-tier results were achieved on a single laptop GPU underscores the power of methodological ingenuity over sheer computational force in developing robust, accessible, and clinically translatable AI.

5 Conclusion

We presented a resource-efficient, three-stage framework that, by decoupling feature learning from noise adaptation, achieved state-of-the-art performance on the challenging task of pediatric brain tumor segmentation in non-skull-stripped MRI. This work provides a powerful and reproducible blueprint for developing robust, clinically translatable AI models capable of overcoming the dual challenges of data impurity and scarcity in real-world medical imaging.

Acknowledgements. We gratefully acknowledge the organizers of the MICCAI BraTS-PEDs 2025 Challenge and extend our sincere thanks to the contributing consortia (CBTN, CONNECT, DIPGr) and expert annotators from the ASNR for the creation and meticulous curation of this invaluable dataset. We also thank our home institution for providing the necessary high-performance computing support.

References

1. BraTS-PEDs Challenge Organizers: The miccai brats-peds 2025 challenge. https://www.synapse.org/Synapse:syn64153130/wiki/631455 (2025). Accessed 30 July 2025
2. Gal, Y., Ghahramani, Z.: Dropout as a bayesian approximation: representing model uncertainty in deep learning. In: ICML (2016)

3. Hoffman, L.M., et al.: Clinical, radiologic, pathologic, and molecular characteristics of long-term survivors of diffuse intrinsic pontine glioma (DIPG): a collaborative report from the international and European society for pediatric oncology DIPG registries. J. Clin. Oncol. **36**(19), 1954–1962 (2018)
4. Hoopes, A., Mora, J.E.I., Dalca, A.V., Fischl, B., Hoffmann, M.: SynthStrip: skull-stripping for any brain image. Neuroimage **260**, 119474 (2022). https://doi.org/10.1016/j.neuroimage.2022.119474
5. Isensee, F., Jaeger, P.F., Kohl, S.A., Petersen, J., Maier-Hein, K.H.: nnU-Net: a self-configuring method for deep learning-based biomedical image segmentation. Nat. Methods **18**(2), 203–211 (2021)
6. Isensee, F., Wald, T., et al.: nnU-net revisited: a call for rigorous validation in 3D medical image segmentation. In: Linguraru, M.G., et al. International Conference on Medical Image Computing and Computer-Assisted Intervention (MICCAI). Springer, Cham (2024). https://doi.org/10.1007/978-3-031-72114-4_47
7. Kazerooni, A.F., et al.: The brain tumor segmentation (brats) challenge 2023: focus on pediatrics (cbtn-connect-dipgr-asnr-miccai brats-peds) (2023). arXiv preprint arXiv:2305.17033
8. Kazerooni, A.F., et al.: The brain tumor segmentation in pediatrics (brats-peds) challenge: focus on pediatrics (cbtn-connect-dipgr-asnr-miccai brats-peds) (2024). arXiv preprint arXiv:2404.15009
9. Kendall, A., Gal, Y.: What uncertainties do we need in bayesian deep learning for computer vision? NIPS (2017)
10. Lin, T.Y., Goyal, P., Girshick, R., He, K., Dollar, P., Belongie, S.: Focal loss for dense object detection. In: ICCV (2017)
11. Milletari, F., Navab, N., Ahmadi, S.A.: V-net: fully convolutional neural networks for volumetric medical image segmentation. In: International Conference on 3D Vision (3DV) (2016)
12. Ostrom, Q.T., et al.: CBTRUS statistical report: pediatric and adolescent and young adult brain and other central nervous system tumors diagnosed in the united states in 2016–2020. Neuro-oncology **25**(Supplement_3), iii1–iii30 (2023)
13. Ronneberger, O., Fischer, P., Brox, T.: U-Net: convolutional networks for biomedical image segmentation. In: Navab, N., Hornegger, J., Wells, W.M., Frangi, A.F. (eds.) MICCAI 2015. LNCS, vol. 9351, pp. 234–241. Springer, Cham (2015). https://doi.org/10.1007/978-3-319-24574-4_28
14. Sudre, C.H., Li, W., Vercauteren, T., Ourselin, S., Jorge Cardoso, M.: Generalised dice overlap as a deep learning loss function for highly unbalanced segmentations. MICCAI (2017)
15. Warren, K.E., Vezina, G.: Imaging of pediatric brain tumors. J. Am. Acad. Child Adolesc. Psychiatry **60**(1), 36–39 (2021)
16. WHO Classification of Tumours Editorial Board: Central Nervous System Tumours, WHO Classification of Tumours, vol. 6. International Agency for Research on Cancer, 5th edn. (2021)

Frequency-Aware Ensemble Learning for BraTS 2025 Pediatric Brain Tumor Segmentation

Yuxiao Yi[1], Qingyao Zhuang[1], Zhi-Qin John Xu[1(✉)], Xiaowen Wang[3(✉)], Yan Ren[2(✉)], and Tianming Qiu[3(✉)]

[1] Institute of Natural Sciences, School of Mathematical Sciences, MOE-LSC, Shanghai Jiao Tong University, Shanghai, China
{yiyuxiao,alan_zqy,xuzhiqin}@sjtu.edu.cn
[2] Department of Radiology, Huashan Hospital, Fudan University, Shanghai, China
renyan_richard@aliyun.com
[3] Department of Neurosurgery, Huashan Hospital, Fudan University, Shanghai, China
{apolloslisy,tianming2100}@126.com

Abstract. Pediatric brain tumor segmentation presents unique challenges due to the rarity and heterogeneity of these malignancies, yet remains critical for clinical diagnosis and treatment planning. We propose an ensemble approach integrating nnU-Net, Swin UNETR, and HFF-Net for the BraTS-PED 2025 challenge. Our method incorporates three key extensions: adjustable initialization scales for optimal nnU-Net complexity control, transfer learning from BraTS 2021 pre-trained models to enhance Swin UNETR's generalization on pediatric dataset, and frequency domain decomposition for HFF-Net to separate low-frequency tissue contours from high-frequency texture details. Our final ensemble framework combines nnU-Net ($\gamma = 0.7$), fine-tuned Swin UNETR, and HFF-Net, achieving Dice scores of 62.7% (CC), 83.2% (ED), 72.9% (ET), 85.7% (NET), 91.8% (TC), and 92.6% (WT) on the unseen test dataset, respectively. *Our proposed method achieves first place (rank 1st) in the BraTS 2025 Pediatric Brain Tumor Segmentation Challenge.*

Keywords: Brain Tumor Segmentation · Initialization · Pre-training · Fine-tuning · Frequency-domain Decomposition

1 Introduction

Brain tumors represent one of the most severe malignancies threatening pediatric health worldwide. These tumors typically exhibit high invasiveness and poor prognosis. Multi-parametric magnetic resonance imaging (mpMRI) has become the fundamental non-invasive modality for pediatric brain tumor diagnosis, typically comprising multiple scanning sequences. However, manual segmentation relies on the expertise of clinicians or technicians, which is not only

S. Bakas et al. (Eds.): MICCAI 2025, LNCS 16376, pp. 445–455, 2026.
https://doi.org/10.1007/978-3-032-16365-3_40

time-consuming and labor-intensive but also susceptible to inter-operator variability. Therefore, developing accurate, efficient, and robust automatic segmentation methods holds significant value for clinical diagnosis, treatment planning, and prognostic assessment.

Recent advances in deep learning have revolutionized medical image analysis, demonstrating exceptional capabilities in automating complex segmentation tasks with performance approaching or even surpassing human expert levels. In response to these technological advances and clinical demands, the Brain Tumor Segmentation Challenge (BraTS) has expanded its scope to include pediatric cases, assembling the largest annotated pediatric brain tumor imaging dataset to date [1–4]. This initiative provides the biomedical community with invaluable resources, driving the development of automated segmentation algorithms.

Winning methods in recent years have extensively adopted the self-configuring nnU-Net [5] as their baseline model [6–8]. Its U-shaped network architecture, based on convolutional neural networks (CNNs), comprises an encoder, decoder, and skip connections. While CNNs possess strong feature extraction capabilities, their local receptive field characteristics limit their ability to capture long-range dependencies. Inspired by the success of the transformer [9] in natural language processing (NLP), researchers have integrated attention mechanisms into segmentation architectures. The UNETR [10] combines Vision Transformer [11] encoders with CNN decoders, while Swin UNETR [12,13] employs Swin Transformer [14] to achieve state-of-the-art performance. Recent innovations like SegFormer3D [15] use hierarchical transformers to extract multi-scale features with fewer parameters. Meanwhile, the success of pre-trained models like SAM [16] has popularized the pre-training and fine-tuning paradigm in biomedical segmentation [17–22]. Models trained on large datasets are fine-tuned for specific tasks to improve performance and generalization. These technological advances provide powerful tools for automatic segmentation of pediatric brain tumors.

In this work, we propose an ensemble method combining nnU-Net, Swin UNETR, and the newly proposed HFF-Net [23], trained on the BraTS-PED 2025 dataset. Our approach includes three key extensions: 1). tunable initialization scales for nnU-Net complexity control; 2). transferring BraTS 2021 pre-trained models to BraTS-PED 2025 for improved Swin UNETR training; 3). and introducing frequency domain decomposition to separate smooth tissue contours from texture details, enhancing tumor segmentation accuracy.

2 Method

In this paper, we employ nnU-Net [5], Swin UNETR [12,13] and HFF-Net [23] as our baseline models. For nnU-Net, we modify the default initialization method and train separate models with different initialization scales. Additionally, for the transformer-based Swin UNETR model, we adopt a pre-training and fine-tuning paradigm, where a model trained on large-scale datasets serves as the backbone and is fine-tuned on downstream tasks to achieve better generalization.

2.1 Data Description

The BraTS-PED Challenge aims to perform segmentation and auxiliary clinical analysis of malignant primary pediatric brain tumors. The inaugural BraTS-PED Challenge was successfully held in 2023, followed by the collection of a larger dataset in 2024 to enrich dataset diversity. In 2025, minor improvements were made, including the addition of inter-rater and intra-rater variability assessments for the test dataset annotations. This validates the consistency and reproducibility of automatic annotations, enabling the development of more robust segmentation algorithms.

Current challenge provides a dataset of 438 pediatric high-grade glioma cases, comprising 261 training cases, 91 validation cases, and 86 test cases. Participants can publicly download the training data for model development, while the test data remains private and is used exclusively for final evaluation. Each case contains four MR scanning sequences: pre-contrast native T1-weighted (T1N), contrast-enhanced T1-weighted (T1C), T2-weighted (T2W), and T2-weighted Fluid Attenuated Inversion Recovery (T2-FLAIR). To generate the corresponding segmentation masks, deep learning-based automatic segmentation models are first used to produce coarse pre-segmentation results, which are then refined by experienced annotators to obtain the final segmentation labels. The segmentation results contain five single-value labels representing the background and four tumor-related regions. Unlike previous challenges, BraTS-PED 2025 focuses on six sub-regions: enhancing tumor (ET), non-enhancing tumor (NET), cystic component (CC), peritumoral edema (ED), and two composite regions tumor core (TC) and whole tumor (WT).

2.2 Data Pre-processing

The original data has undergone only facial feature removal for privacy protection, without skull stripping. We first perform skull stripping on all training and validation data. The processed four MRI modalities are then fed into nnU-Net and Swin UNETR for training. We employ a publicly available deep learning-based pipeline[1] to generate skull-stripping masks for pediatric patients. The pipeline leverages a pre-trained nnU-Net (v1) model as its backbone, takes four modalities as input, and outputs the corresponding skull mask. During the final testing phase, each test case undergoes the same procedure to ensure consistency. Additionally, each modality undergoes frequency domain decomposition to extract one low-frequency component and four directional high-frequency components. Low-frequency decomposition via Dual-Tree Complex Wavelet Transform (DTCWT) produces smoothed brain tissue images, while high-frequency decomposition through Non-subsampled Contourlet Transform (NSCT) captures tissue texture and directional features[2]. Unlike traditional wavelet transforms, the DTCWT employs a dual-tree structure with carefully timed subsampling

[1] https://github.com/d3b-center/peds-brain-auto-skull-strip.
[2] https://github.com/VinyehShaw/HFF.

across two independent filter banks. This design prevents the image size from halving at each level. Additionally, to ensure consistent image size, the NSCT employs a two-step decomposition process using a Non-Subsampled Pyramid (NSP) filter and a Non-Subsampled Directional Filter Bank (NSDFB) to partition a two-dimensional image. (Figs. 1 and 2)

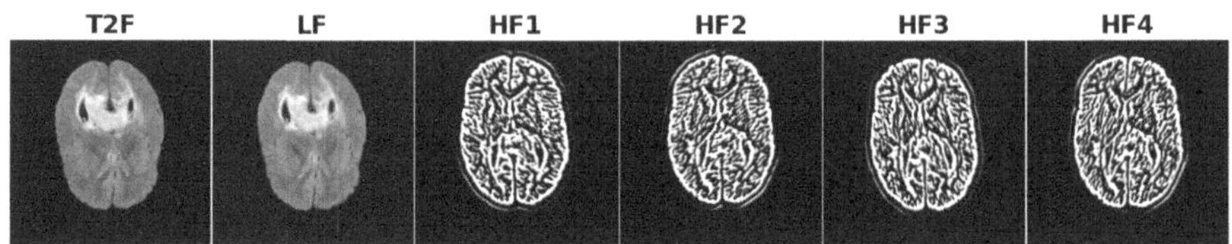

Fig. 1. Frequency decomposition results of T2-FLAIR on the training set. *LF* denotes low frequency component and *HF1*~*HF4* represents four high frequency components, respectively.

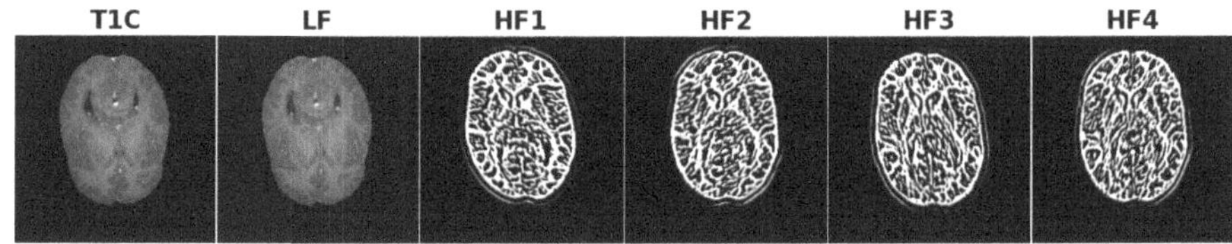

Fig. 2. Frequency decomposition results of T1C on the training set. *LF* denotes low frequency component and *HF1*~*HF4* represents four high frequency components, respectively.

The nnU-Net and Swin UNETR take the 4 skull-stripped modalities as input, while HFF-Net receives the corresponding 4 low-frequency parts and 16 high-frequency modalities.

2.3 Model Training

nnU-Net is a deep learning framework based on the classical U-Net architecture, specifically designed for medical image segmentation. It automatically configures pre-processing pipelines, network architectures, training procedures, and post-processing schemes for new tasks in the biomedical domain, eliminating the need for tedious manual parameter tuning or purely empirical approaches. In biomedical segmentation tasks, nnU-Net achieves more accurate predictions and robust generalization compared to other specialized solutions, making it a commonly used baseline model in BraTS challenges.

We employ two weight initialization strategies: 1). The default nnU-Net initialization, where linear layer weights are initialized using uniform distribution and convolutional layers use Kaiming initialization; 2). All modules are initialized using normal distributions $\mathcal{N}(0, (\frac{1}{d^\gamma})^2)$, where d is the number of input neurons and γ is a tunable hyperparameter. A higher γ value leads to smaller initialization scales [24]. Based on these initialization methods, we train six 3D full resolution nnU-Net (v2) models, including one with default initialization and five with γ values of 0.3, 0.5, 0.7, 0.9, and 1.0, respectively.

For each model, we adopt five-fold cross-validation. The original 261 cases are split into training and validation sets at an 8:2 ratio. The training batch size is 2, with an input patch cropped from 3D images of $96 \times 160 \times 160$ voxels. Models are trained for 1000 epochs, with each epoch containing 250 mini-batches. During each training step, data is randomly loaded and applied with dynamical augment strategies, including rotation, scaling, Gaussian noise, Gaussian blur, brightness adjustment, contrast adjustment, low-resolution simulation, gamma correction, and mirroring.

The loss function is a weighted sum of Dice loss and cross-entropy loss. Stochastic gradient descent with Nesterov momentum ($\mu = 0.99$) is used as the optimizer. The learning rate follows a polynomial-decay schedule, expressed as:

$$lr = lr_{\text{init}} \times \left(1 - \frac{\text{epoch}}{\text{max\_epoch}}\right)^{0.9} \quad (1)$$

where the initial learning rate $lr_{\text{init}} = 10^{-2}$.

Swin UNETR is a hierarchical Transformer-based model that replaces the encoder in the U-Net architecture with a Swin Transformer, which computes self-attention through an efficient shifted window partitioning scheme. Compared to CNNs with local receptive fields, Swin Transformer demonstrates superior capabilities in multi-scale contextual representation learning and long-range dependency modeling.

To leverage the robust data processing, training, and inference pipeline of nnU-Net, we integrate the Swin UNETR model into the nnU-Net framework, enabling out-of-the-box functionality. We first train a model from scratch on the BraTS-PED 2025 dataset as a baseline, maintaining the same training parameters as described above. Additionally, we employ a Swin UNETR model pre-trained on the BraTS 2021 segmentation challenge dataset as the foundation model and fine-tune it for our BraTS-PED segmentation task. The pre-trained model is trained for 800 epochs on 1,251 training samples with an initial learning rate of 8e-4, and the corresponding model weights are available in the GitHub repository[3]. For the fine-tuning task, to maintain compatibility with the pre-trained model, the input patch size is set to $128 \times 128 \times 128$ voxels with deep supervision disabled. The model is trained for 1,000 epochs with a batch size of 2, following the learning rate scheduling strategy outlined in Eq. 1, except that the initial learning rate lr_{init} is adjusted to 10^{-3}.

[3] https://github.com/Project-MONAI/research-contributions/tree/main/SwinUNETR/BRATS21.

HFF-Net introduces a novel dual-branch framework that leverages frequency-domain decomposition to enhance brain tumor segmentation, particularly for contrast-enhancing regions. The architecture initially decomposes multi-modal MRI scans into low-frequency (LF) using Dual-Tree Complex Wavelet Transform (DTCWT), and multi-directional high-frequency (HF) components with Non-subsampled Contourlet Transform (NSCT).

In this paper, the inputs of HFF-Net consist of 4 low-frequency modalities and 16 high-frequency modalities, all derived from the original 4 MRI scans via a frequency decomposition module. The model is trained for 450 epochs with a batch size of 1 and a patch size of $128 \times 128 \times 128$. We employ an SGD optimizer with a momentum of 0.9 and a weight decay of 5×10^{-5}. The initial learning rate is set to 0.3 and progressively decays during training. All inputs undergo Z-score normalization.

All training procedures are conducted on an NVIDIA GeForce RTX 4080 GPU with 16 GB memory. Among them, training a single fold of nnU-Net requires approximately 37 h, while HFF-Net needs 48 h. Swin UNETR is the most time-consuming, requiring 4 d.

2.4 Model Ensemble

To enhance the model's accuracy and generalization performance on unseen datasets, we employed a model ensemble strategy. We computed the weighted average of the prediction probabilities from nnU-Net, Swin UNETR, and HFF-Net, using equal weights of 1/3 for each model. This averaged probability map was then converted back to the final segmentation mask labels. It is worth noting that we did not employ any post-processing techniques, such as feature extraction of connected components.

2.5 Evaluation Metrics

The evaluation of the six subregions follows the BraTS Lighthouse Challenge framework using two key metrics:

- Lesion-wise Dice Similarity Coefficient (DSC) measures voxel-level overlap between predicted and reference segmentations for each individual lesion, excluding true-negative voxels.
- Normalized Surface Distance (NSD) assesses boundary accuracy between predictions and ground truth.

3 Results

3.1 Quantitative Results

Table 1 presents the quantitative evaluation results of our models on the BraTS-PED validation dataset. All predicted segmentation labels were obtained through five-fold cross-validation. The entire evaluation process was automatically conducted using the pipeline provided by the challenge organizers on the Synapse platform. It should be noted that participants have access only to validation images without ground truth labels, while both the test images and the corresponding labels remain confidential.

Table 1. Quantitative results on the validation datasets of PED. Lesion-wise (LW) Dice coefficients and Normalized Surface Dice at 0.5 mm tolerance (NSD-0.5) were computed for enhancing tumor (ET), tumor core (TC), whole tumor (WT), non-enhancing tumor (NET), cystic components(CC), and edema (ED), respectively.

Task	Model	Lesion-wise Dice ↑						Lesion-wise NSD-0.5 ↑					
		CC	ED	ET	NET	TC	WT	CC	ED	ET	NET	TC	WT
PED Val. N=91	nnU-Net	0.657	0.967	0.625	0.9	0.931	0.93	0.648	0.967	0.549	0.639	0.661	0.662
	nnU-Net ($\gamma = 0.3$)	0.692	0.945	0.677	0.895	0.924	0.925	0.677	0.945	0.615	0.657	0.679	0.68
	nnU-Net ($\gamma = 0.5$)	0.691	0.956	0.671	0.899	0.928	0.928	0.675	0.956	0.606	0.663	0.686	0.686
	nnU-Net ($\gamma = 0.7$)	0.75	0.956	0.672	0.9	0.929	0.929	0.734	0.956	0.601	0.635	0.658	0.659
	nnU-Net ($\gamma = 0.9$)	0.726	0.945	0.682	0.898	0.926	0.926	0.702	0.945	0.616	0.658	0.679	0.680
	nnU-Net ($\gamma = 1.0$)	0.686	0.956	0.673	0.897	0.925	0.926	0.675	0.956	0.605	0.651	0.675	0.675
	Swin UNETR	0.692	0.956	0.621	0.892	0.921	0.921	0.692	0.956	0.55	0.591	0.618	0.618
	Swin UNETR (FT)	0.746	0.956	0.644	0.881	0.912	0.913	0.712	0.956	0.53	0.522	0.542	0.543
	HFF-Net	0.683	0.934	0.703	0.9	0.928	0.928	0.673	0.934	0.638	0.653	0.674	0.675
	Ensemble	**0.723**	**0.956**	**0.689**	**0.895**	**0.923**	**0.923**	**0.71**	**0.956**	**0.615**	**0.629**	**0.653**	**0.654**

Table 2. Quantitative results on the test datasets of PED. Our method ranks 1st on the final test set leaderboard. Lesion-wise (LW) Dice coefficients and Normalized Surface Dice at 1.0 mm tolerance (NSD-1.0) were computed for enhancing tumor (ET), tumor core (TC), whole tumor (WT), non-enhancing tumor (NET), cystic components(CC), and edema (ED), respectively.

Task	Statistic	Lesion-wise Dice ↑						Lesion-wise NSD-1.0 ↑					
		CC	ED	ET	NET	TC	WT	CC	ED	ET	NET	TC	WT
PED (rank 1)	mean	**0.627**	**0.832**	**0.729**	**0.857**	**0.918**	**0.926**	**0.637**	**0.831**	**0.776**	**0.823**	**0.833**	**0.844**
	std	0.453	0.354	0.318	0.196	0.129	0.123	0.446	0.354	0.322	0.203	0.217	0.203

The results show that vanilla nnU-Net achieves an average Dice score of 83% across six sub-regions. By tuning the initialization parameter γ, we obtain the highest average Dice score of 85.6% at $\gamma = 0.7$. The pre-trained Swin UNETR-FT outperforms its from-scratch counterpart by approximately 1% in Dice score. Among all regions, ET remains the most challenging to segment. HFF-Net provides modest improvement for ET segmentation, reaching approximately 70% Dice score. Our final ensemble combines nnU-Net ($\gamma = 0.7$), Swin UNETR-FT, and HFF-Net, achieving Dice scores of 72.3% (ET), 95.6% (NET), 68.9% (CC), 89.5% (ED), 92.3% (TC), and 92.3% (WT).

Table 2 presents the final results of our proposed ensemble method on the test datasets.

3.2 Qualitative Results

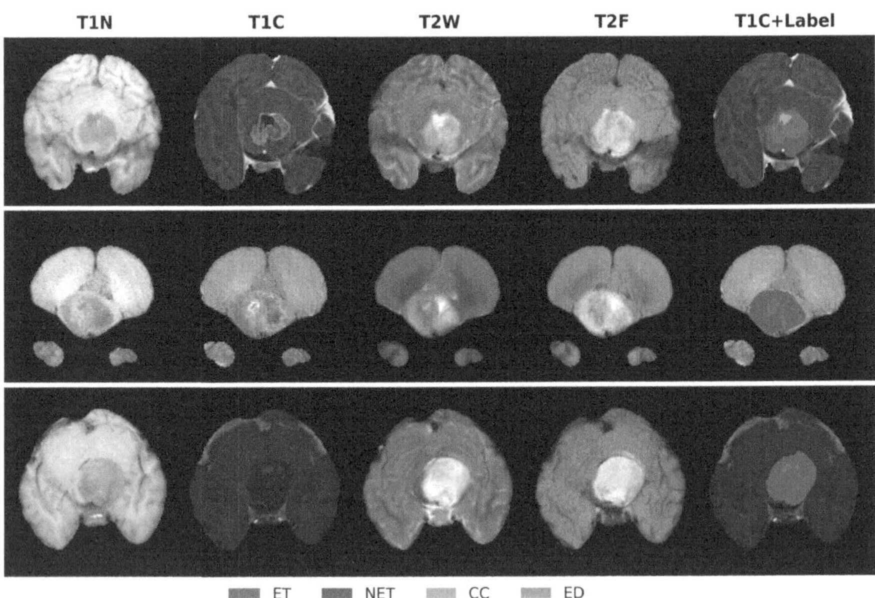

Fig. 3. Quantitative results of the final model on the validation set. The three selected examples correspond to BraTS-PED-00310-000, BraTS-PED-00315-000, and BraTS-PED-00318-000, respectively.

Figure 3 presents the qualitative segmentation results of the final ensemble model on validation data. The validation set underwent the same skull stripping and frequency domain decomposition pre-processing.

4 Discussion

In this work, we propose a frequency-aware ensemble learning framework for pediatric brain tumor segmentation in the BraTS-PED 2025 challenge. By integrating nnU-Net, Swin UNETR, and HFF-Net, and leveraging techniques such as multi-scale parameter initialization, transfer learning, and frequency-domain decomposition, our approach achieves robust and accurate segmentation performance on challenging pediatric datasets. Experimental results demonstrate the effectiveness of the proposed ensemble strategy across multiple quantitative metrics. Our final ensemble framework, comprising nnU-Net ($\gamma = 0.7$), fine-tuned Swin UNETR, and HFF-Net, demonstrates strong generalization capability on unseen pediatric brain tumor data. The method achieves competitive Dice scores of 62.7% (CC), 83.2% (ED), 72.9% (ET), 85.7% (NET), 91.8% (TC), and 92.6% (WT) on the test datasets. More importantly, the proposed approach secures first place in the BraTS-PED 2025 Segmentation Challenge, underscoring its robustness and state-of-the-art performance in pediatric brain tumor segmentation.

In future work, we plan to further explore advanced model architectures and multi-modal data fusion techniques to enhance the clinical applicability of automated brain tumor segmentation.

References

1. Karargyris, A., et al.: FeTS consortium, BraTS-2020 consortium, AI4SafeChole consortium: federated benchmarking of medical artificial intelligence with MedPerf. Na. Mach. Intell. **5**(7), 799–810 (2023). https://doi.org/10.1038/s42256-023-00652-2
2. Kazerooni, A.F., et al.: The brain tumor segmentation (BraTS) challenge 2023: focus on pediatrics (CBTN-CONNECT-DIPGR-ASNR-MICCAI BraTS-PEDs) (2024). https://doi.org/10.48550/arXiv.2305.17033
3. Kazerooni, A.F., et al.: The brain tumor segmentation (brats) challenge 2023: focus on pediatrics (cbtn-connect-dipgr-asnr-miccai brats-peds) (2024). https://arxiv.org/abs/2305.17033
4. Kazerooni, A.F., et al.: The brain tumor segmentation in pediatrics (brats-peds) challenge: focus on pediatrics (cbtn-connect-dipgr-asnr-miccai brats-peds) (2024). https://arxiv.org/abs/2404.15009
5. Isensee, F., Jaeger, P.F., Kohl, S.A.A., Petersen, J., Maier-Hein, K.H.: nnU-net: a self-configuring method for deep learning-based biomedical image segmentation. Nat. Methods **18**(2), 203–211 (2021). https://doi.org/10.1038/s41592-020-01008-z
6. Sadique, M.S., Rahman, M.M., Farzana, W., Glandon, A., Temtam, A., Iftekharuddin, K.M.: Brain tumor segmentation: glioma segmentation in sub-Saharan Africa Patients using nnU-net. In: Baid, U., et al. Brain Tumor Segmentation, and Cross-Modality Domain Adaptation for Medical Image Segmentation. crossMoDA BraTS 2023 2023. LNCS, vol. 14669, pp. 322–331. Springer, Cham (2024). https://doi.org/10.1007/978-3-031-76163-8_29
7. Jiang, Z., et al.: Magnetic Resonance Imaging Feature-Based Subtyping and Model Ensemble for Enhanced Brain Tumor Segmentation (2024). https://doi.org/10.48550/arXiv.2412.04094
8. Jiang, Z., et al.: Enhancing generalizability in brain tumor segmentation: model ensemble with adaptive post-processing. In: 2024 IEEE International Symposium on Biomedical Imaging (ISBI), pp. 1–4. IEEE, Athens, Greece (2024). https://doi.org/10.1109/ISBI56570.2024.10635469
9. Vaswani, A.: Attention is all you need. In: Proceedings of the 31st International Conference on Neural Information Processing Systems, pp. 6000–6010. NIPS'17, Curran Associates Inc., Red Hook, USA (2017)

10. Hatamizadeh, A., et al.: UNETR: Transformers for 3D medical image segmentation. In: 2022 IEEE/CVF Winter Conference on Applications of Computer Vision (WACV), pp. 1748–1758. IEEE, Waikoloa, USA (2022). https://doi.org/10.1109/WACV51458.2022.00181
11. Dosovitskiy, A., et al.: An image is worth 16 x 16 words: transformers for image recognition at scale (2021). https://arxiv.org/abs/2010.11929
12. He, Y., Nath, V., Yang, D., Tang, Y., Myronenko, A., Xu, D.: Swinunetr-v2: stronger swin transformers with stagewise convolutions for 3D medical image segmentation. In: Greenspan, H., Madabhushi, A., Mousavi, P., Salcudean, S., Duncan, J., Syeda-Mahmood, T., Taylor, R. (eds.) Medical Image Computing and Computer Assisted Intervention - MICCAI 2023, pp. 416–426. Springer, Cham (2023)
13. Hatamizadeh, A., Nath, V., Tang, Y., Yang, D., Roth, H.R., Xu, D.: Swin UNETR: swin transformers for semantic segmentation of brain tumors in MRI images. In: Crimi, A., Bakas, S. (eds) Brainlesion: Glioma, Multiple Sclerosis, Stroke and Traumatic Brain Injuries. BrainLes 2021. LNCS, vol. 12962, pp. 272–284. Springer, Cham (2022). https://doi.org/10.1007/978-3-031-08999-2_22
14. Liu, Z., et al.: Swin transformer: Hierarchical vision transformer using shifted windows. In: Proceedings of the IEEE/CVF international conference on computer vision, pp. 10012–10022 (2021)
15. Perera, S., Navard, P., Yilmaz, A.: SegFormer3D: an efficient transformer for 3D medical image segmentation (2024). https://doi.org/10.48550/arXiv.2404.10156
16. Kirillov, A., et al.: Segment anything. In: 2023 IEEE/CVF International Conference on Computer Vision (ICCV). IEEE, France (2023). https://doi.org/10.1109/iccv51070.2023.00371
17. Shi, X., et al.: Multi-modal medical SAM: an adaptation method of segment anything model (SAM) for glioma segmentation using multi-modal MR images. ACM Trans. Comput. Healthcare **6**(2), 1–21 (2025). https://doi.org/10.1145/3712297
18. Wang, H., et al.: SAM-Med3D: towards general-purpose segmentation models for volumetric medical images (2024). https://arxiv.org/abs/2310.15161
19. Pachitariu, M., Rariden, M., Stringer, C.: Cellpose-SAM: superhuman generalization for cellular segmentation. bioRxiv (2025). https://doi.org/10.1101/2025.04.28.651001
20. Huang, Z. et al.: Evaluating STU-net for brain tumor segmentation. In: Baid, U., et al. Brain Tumor Segmentation, and Cross-Modality Domain Adaptation for Medical Image Segmentation. crossMoDA BraTS 2023 2023. LNCS, vol. 14669, pp. 140–151. Springer, Cham (2024). https://doi.org/10.1007/978-3-031-76163-8_13
21. Akbar, A.S., Brilian, A.H., Fatichah, C., Suciati, N.: Previous datasets performance for brain tumor segmentation of BraTS 2023 current dataset. In: Baid, U., et al. Brain Tumor Segmentation, and Cross-Modality Domain Adaptation for Medical Image Segmentation. crossMoDA BraTS 2023 2023, vol. 14669, pp. 69–78. Springer, Cham (2024). https://doi.org/10.1007/978-3-031-76163-8_7
22. Wang, H., et al.: SAM-Med3D: towards general-purpose segmentation models for volumetric medical images. In: Del Bue, A., Canton, C., Pont-Tuset, J., Tommasi, T. (eds.) Computer Vision – ECCV 2024 Workshops, vol. 15638, pp. 51–67. Springer, Cham (2024). https://doi.org/10.1007/978-3-031-91721-9_4

23. Shao, M., et al.: Rethinking brain tumor segmentation from the frequency domain perspective. IEEE Trans. Med. Imaging p. 1 (2025). https://doi.org/10.1109/TMI.2025.3579213
24. Zhang, Z., Lin, P., Wang, Z., Zhang, Y., Xu, Z.Q.J.: Complexity control facilitates reasoning-based compositional generalization in transformers (2025). https://doi.org/10.48550/arXiv.2501.08537

Adaptable Segmentation Pipeline for Diverse Brain Tumors with Radiomic-Guided Subtyping and Lesion-Wise Model Ensemble

Daniel Capellán-Martín[1,2], Abhijeet Parida[1,2], Zhifan Jiang[1], Nishad Kulkarni[1], Krithika Iyer[1], Austin Tapp[1], Syed Muhammad Anwar[1,3], María J. Ledesma-Carbayo[2], and Marius George Linguraru[1,3](✉)

[1] Sheikh Zayed Institute for Pediatric Surgical Innovation, Children's National Hospital, Washington, DC, USA
[2] Universidad Politécnica de Madrid and CIBER-BBN, ISCIII, Madrid, Spain
[3] School of Medicine and Health Sciences, George Washington University, Washington, DC, USA
mlingura@childrensnational.org

Abstract. Robust and generalizable segmentation of brain tumors on multi-parametric magnetic resonance imaging (MRI) remains difficult because tumor types differ widely. The BraTS 2025 Lighthouse Challenge benchmarks segmentation methods on diverse high-quality datasets of adult and pediatric tumors: multi-consortium international pediatric brain tumor segmentation (PED), preoperative meningioma tumor segmentation (MEN), meningioma radiotherapy segmentation (MEN-RT), and segmentation of pre- and post-treatment brain metastases (MET). We present a flexible, modular, and adaptable pipeline that improves segmentation performance by selecting and combining state-of-the-art models and applying tumor- and lesion-specific processing before and after training. Radiomic features extracted from MRI help detect tumor subtype, ensuring a more balanced training. Custom lesion-level performance metrics determine the influence of each model in the ensemble and optimize post-processing that further refines the predictions, enabling the workflow to tailor every step to each case. On the BraTS testing sets, our pipeline achieved performance comparable to top-ranked algorithms across multiple challenges. These findings confirm that custom lesion-aware processing and model selection yield robust segmentations yet without locking the method to a specific network architecture. Our method has the potential for quantitative tumor measurement in clinical practice, supporting diagnosis and prognosis.

Keywords: Brain tumor segmentation · MedNeXt · Meningiomas · Metastases · MRI · nnU-Net · Pediatric brain tumors · Tumor subtyping

D. Capellán-Martín, A. Parida and Z. Jiang—Equal contribution.

S. Bakas et al. (Eds.): MICCAI 2025, LNCS 16376, pp. 456–467, 2026.
https://doi.org/10.1007/978-3-032-16365-3_41

1 Introduction

In the United States, cancer is the second leading cause of death overall and the primary cause among individuals younger than 85 years old. Brain and other central nervous system tumors are the top cause of cancer death in children and adolescents under 20, and brain tumors also lead cancer mortality in men aged 20–39. In 2025, about two million new cancer cases and 618,000 cancer-related deaths are projected in the U.S. [24]. Early, accurate diagnosis is essential to improve outcomes, but wide variation in tumor appearance across imaging devices and population makes consistent assessment difficult, highlighting the need for reliable quantitative diagnositc and prognostic tools.

In neuro-oncology, accurate segmentation of brain tumors in multi-parametric magnetic resonance imaging (mpMRI) is a fundamental step for diagnosis, treatment planning, and longitudinal monitoring. Yet manual contouring remains labor-intensive and prone to inter-observer variability, motivating robust automated solutions in the clinical workflow.

The international Brain Tumor Segmentation (BraTS) Challenge [1–4,13,20], organized in conjunction with the Medical Image Computing and Computer Assisted Intervention (MICCAI) conference, has driven and benchmarked segmentation algorithmic innovation since MICCAI 2012. In its 2025 edition, BraTS expanded into a suite of challegnes that cover a broader range of tumors and tasks, earning recognition as one of MICCAI's three Lighthouse Challenges.

Recent deep learning models such as nnU-Net [8], MedNeXt [23], Swin UNETR [7,25], and emerging Mamba-based hybrids [18,28] have defined the current state of the art (SOTA) in medical image segmentation. As the SOTA models have become more stable and robust across diverse tasks, their reported Dice scores have converged within narrow margins [9], signaling a performance plateau. While ever more complex architectures are possible, they would offer diminishing added values.

BraTS-winning solutions have demonstrated that model-independent and GPU-free heuristics, including ensemble voting [19], size-aware connected component filtering and ET-to-NCR relabelling [5], and adaptive refinement schemes [11,22], can substantially boost segmentation performance. Instead of pursuing ever-deeper or more intricate networks, we believe that the next gains will arise from target-specific pipeline design. Robust pre-processing such as radiomic-guided fold splitting mitigates sampling bias; lesion-aware ensemble weighting exploits complementary backbone strengths; and subtype-specific post-processing removes residual artifacts.

We therefore introduce and apply a flexible, modular, backbone-independent pipeline to multiple BraTS 2025 Lighthouse Challenges to show its versatility. This end-to-end strategy consistently outperforms any single backbone, demonstrating that thoughtful pipeline engineering remains promising once model performance plateaus.

2 Methods

2.1 Dataset

Our segmentation pipeline was applied to four BraTS 2025 Lighthouse tasks: multi-consortium international pediatric brain tumor segmentation (PED; train = 261, val = 91) [6,14], preoperative meningioma tumor segmentation (MEN; train = 1000, val = 141) [15], meningioma radiotherapy segmentation (MEN-RT; train = 500, val = 70) [17], and segmentation of pre- and post-treatment brain metastases (MET; train = 1296, val = 179) [21]. Each case contains co-registered isotropic pre-contrast T1-weighted (T1), contrast-enhanced T1-weighted (T1CE), T2-weighted (T2), and T2-weighted fluid-attenuated inversion recovery (T2-FLAIR) MRI sequences. In MEN-RT cohort, only T1CE is available and in its original image space.

Reference standard annotations of the tumor sub-regions were created and approved by expert neuroradiologists. Concretely the following tumor annotations and subregions were defined for each of the Lighthouse challenges considered in this work.

- **PED:** enhancing tumor (ET), non-enhancing tumor (NET), cystic component (CC), peritumoral edema (ED), tumor core (TC=ET+NET+CC), and whole tumor (WT=TC+ED).
- **MEN:** ET, non-enhancing tumor core (NETC), surrounding non-enhancing FLAIR hyperintensity (SNFH), TC (ET+NETC), and WT (TC+SNFH).
- **MEN-RT:** gross tumor volume (GTV).
- **MET:** ET, NETC, SNFH, resection cavity (RC; delineates the resection of region within the brain in post-treatment cases), TC (ET+NETC), and WT (TC+SNFH).

For more details, please refer to the challenge website: https://www.synapse.org/Synapse:syn64153130/wiki/.

2.2 Segmentation Pipeline

Our pipeline uses MRI radiomic features and lesion-wise metrics to adapt the workflow to each tumor subtype. As summarized in Fig. 1, it comprises four stages: (i) training data preparation: stratified fold splitting based on radiomic feature clustering; (ii) model training; (iii) model selection and ensembling; and (iv) adaptive post-processing, including optimal removal of small connected components and label redefinition.

2.3 Stratified Training Data Preparation

In five-fold cross-validation (5-fold CV) training, stratified and balanced folds outperform purely random fold splits. While stratification by tumor volume has been explored, we argue that radiomic features-capturing the full heterogeneity of tumor appearance-provide a more robust basis for fold assignment. For

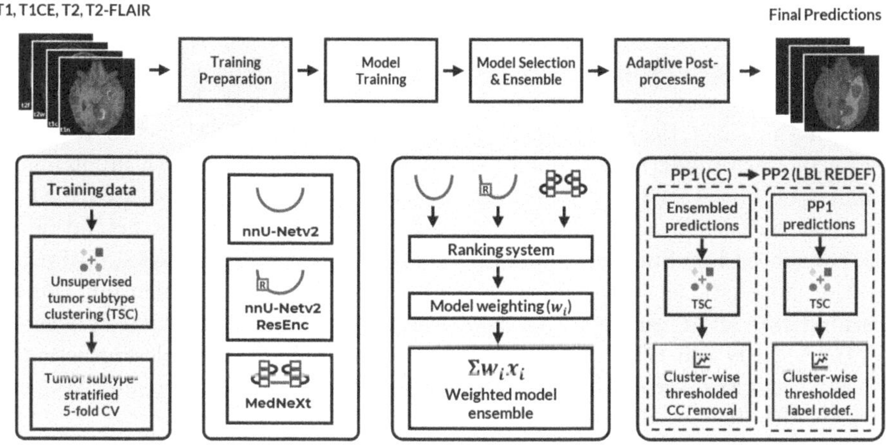

Fig. 1. Overview of the segmentation pipeline. PP, CC, and LBL REDEF refer to post-processing, connected components, and label redefinition, respectively.

each case in the training set, we computed 14 shape- and 93 appearance-based radiomic features per MRI sequence based on WT mask provided by reference annotation, using PyRadiomics [26], following the protocol of Jiang *et al.* [12].

To reduce the large number of radiomic features, we keep only the principal components that explain 90% of the variance and then partition the cases with k-means clustering using reduced features [10,11]. The optimal number of clusters is determined by maximizing the silhouette coefficient in the training folds. Each cluster is randomly split into five folds, yielding the final CV sets for training. Figure 2 illustrates the clustering based on the two radiomic features most relevant for cluster separation.

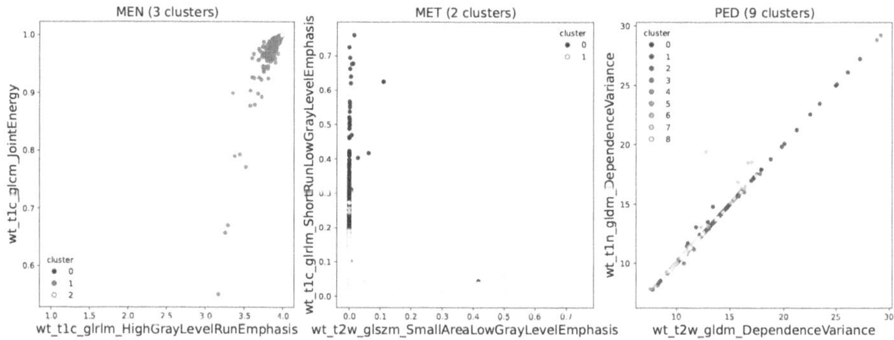

Fig. 2. Clustering visualization across challenges using top two radiomic features.

2.4 Model Training

Based on the reported performance in [9] and our previous experience, we selected three state-of-the-art models: nnU-Net V2, nnU-Net with residual encoder (nnU-Net ResEnc M), and MedNeXt M (k=3, 17.6M parameters, 248 GFlops). Each model was trained using a 5-fold CV strategy with input image patches of 128 × 128 × 128 voxels. The nnU-Net variants and MedNeXt-M were trained using same settings, employing label-wise softmax activation, a class-weighted loss function combining Dice and cross-entropy losses, optimized by the stochastic gradient descent (SGD) with Nesterov momentum (initial learning rate=0.01, momentum=0.99, weight decay=3e-5), for 200 epochs on NVIDIA A100 (40 GB) GPUs. The implementation is available through the official frameworks repositories: https://github.com/MIC-DKFZ/nnUNet and https://github.com/MIC-DKFZ/MedNeXt.

2.5 Label-Wise Metrics as Objective Function F

As model training relies on a loss function, each downstream stage (model selection, ensembling, and post-processing) also needs a quantitative objective so the pipeline can be customized automatically to each tumor type and region. This objective function can simply be the Dice similarity coefficient (DSC). However, in reality or in the context of challenges, DSC alone is insufficient because segmentation performance is evaluated with several metrics, including DSC, normalized surface distance (NSD) and Hausdorff distance (HD), which sit on different scales and can not be added directly. Also, integrating scores across tumour sub-regions (ET, TC, WT etc.) compounds another challenge.

We therefore adopt the ranking strategy proposed by BraTS [16]. For every candidate prediction obtained on the training set using 5-fold CV, we compute lesion-wise metrics for all sub-regions, rank the predictions case-wise, and average these ranks across metrics and regions. The resulting internal CV score **F** is a single value (smaller is better) that combines all lesion-wise metrics, aligns with the official BraTS leaderboard and remains robust to outliers. Our implementation is open-source and available at github.com/Pediatric-Accelerated-Intelligence-Lab/BraTS-Unofficial-Ranker.

2.6 Model Selection and Ensemble

Each trained model M_i is ranked by the approach in Sect. 2.5 with a score F_i. Then we used a weighted model ensemble strategy when adding the averaged 5-fold probability output from each model. The weight of each model is defined as $W_i = \sum_{j \neq i} F_j / \sum_i F_i$. The weights for each model are summarized in Table 1.

We also evaluated the STAPLE [27] ensemble strategy. It lagged behind the weighted ensemble when we used the three 5-fold-averaged predictions on the training data. However, STAPLE performed better on the validation set for MEN-RT task because treating each fold's model as an independent candidate yielded 15 predictions, which markedly enhanced DSC, NSD, and rank for the MEN-RT validation cohort.

Table 1. Weights for each model across tasks.

	PED	MEN	MEN-RT	MET
W_0 (nnU-Net V2)	0.332	0.323	0.336	0.295
W_1 (nnU-Net ResEnc M)	0.331	0.326	0.338	0.296
W_2 (MedNeXt M)	0.337	0.351	0.326	0.409

2.7 Adaptive Post-processing

After ensembling, we recompute stratification clusters on the predicted masks, enabling cluster and label-specific thresholds for adaptive post-processing.

Post-processing for the Removal of Isolated Connected Components (PP1-CC): To remove small isolated CCs that are likely false or noisy predictions, we perform a grid search across clusters and labels over volumes from 0 to 500 voxels in 25-voxel increments. For each threshold, we filter the predicted mask and compute the internal ranking score, and finally select the threshold that achieves the best averaged rank. This cluster- and label-specific filter eliminates fragments that would otherwise be counted as false-positive lesions.

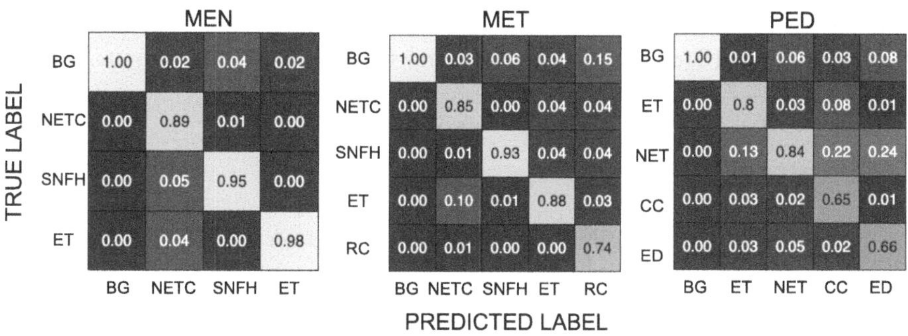

Fig. 3. Post-PP1 confusion matrix indicating labels that need to be redefined in PP2. BG refers to background.

Post-processing for Label Redefinition (PP2 LBLREDEF): A second adaptive PP fine-tunes the consistency of tumor sub-regions (labels). We correct systematic label confusions in a data-driven way. After PP1-CC, we build a confusion matrix (Fig. 3) over all predicted masks again to identify pairs of frequently swapped labels. For every such pair (label_x,label_y), we search, within each cluster, for the threshold on the volume ratio label_x/WT that maximizes internal CV metrics (*e.g.* rank). If a case with predicted mask falls below this threshold, all label_x voxels are converted to label_y. This ratio-based PP2-LBLREDEF enforces anatomically plausible label volumes and improves the performance of the BraTS metrics at the lesion level.

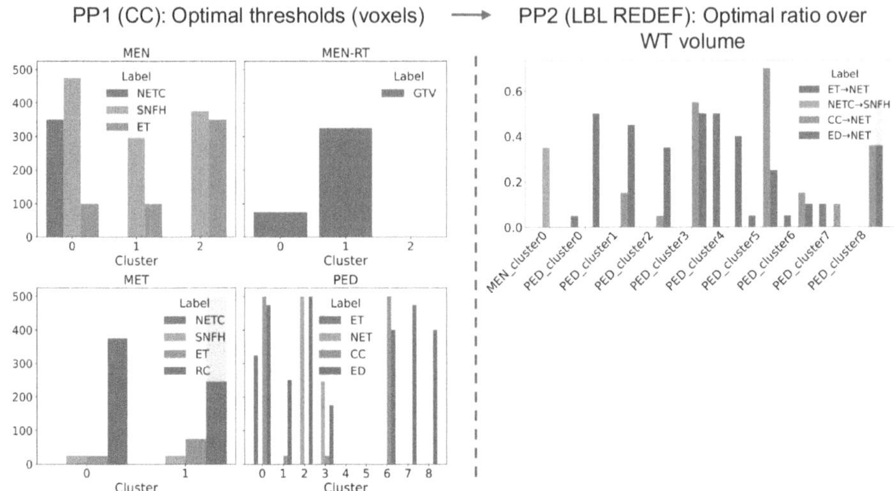

Fig. 4. Adaptive Post-processing: optimal thresholds per cluster and label across challenges.

At inference, a new test case is assigned to its nearest radiomic cluster, after model ensemble and the cluster-specific post-processing threshold values are then applied. Figure 4 shows the optimal thresholds identified by CV-based grid search.

3 Results

The evaluation of the model prediction on the validation set was performaed on the Synapse platform. The models were assessed for each of the tumor regions using the lesion-wise DSC and NSD with boundary threshold of 1.0 mm.

Quantitative results of our models across the validation and testing data for each challenge are shown in Tables 2 and 3, for PED, MET, MEN, and MEN-RT, respectively. These evaluations were performed automatically by the challenge's digital platform, with no access to the reference standard annotations on the validation set and no access to any testing data including images and labels. Figure 5 illustrated qualitative results on validation cases for PED, MET, MEN, and MEN-RT, respectively.

4 Discussion

Our experiments confirm that carefully engineered pre- and post-processing can still deliver tangible gains even when base architectures have plateaued. Notably, some gains in Dice or NSD were limited on validation set but became evident under 5-fold CV, underscoring the danger of optimizing solely on a limited and sometimes skewed validation set.

Table 2. PED quantitative results Lesion-wise (LW) Dice coefficients and Normalized Surface Distance (NSD) at threshold 1mm were computed for enhancing tumor (ET), tumor core (TC), whole tumor (WT), non-enhancing tumor (NET), cystic components(CC), and edema (ED), respectively.

Task	Model	LW Dice						LW NSD thresh. 1mm					
		CC	ED	ET	NET	TC	WT	CC	ED	ET	NET	TC	WT
PED Validation N=91	MedNeXt(M)	0.735	0.857	0.694	0.899	0.926	0.927	0.749	0.857	0.748	0.878	0.903	0.905
	nnU-Net	0.713	0.813	0.630	0.900	0.928	0.928	0.762	0.813	0.693	0.885	0.914	0.915
	nnU-Net-ResEnc(M)	0.719	0.857	0.692	0.902	0.931	0.932	0.735	0.857	0.755	0.883	0.910	0.913
	Ensemble	0.704	0.868	0.677	0.906	0.933	0.933	0.736	0.868	0.731	0.891	0.916	0.917
	Post-processing	0.72	0.967	0.65	0.907	0.933	0.933	0.72	0.967	0.696	0.892	0.914	0.914
PED Testing	Mean	0.669	0.892	0.672	0.851	0.908	0.915	0.67	0.892	0.714	0.815	0.82	0.83
	Standard Deviation	0.468	0.304	0.361	0.201	0.145	0.14	0.466	0.304	0.371	0.206	0.228	0.213

Table 3. MET, MEN, MEN-RT quantitative results. Lesion-wise (LW) or global (G) Dice coefficients and Normalized Surface Distance (NSD) at 1mm-threshold were computed for enhancing tumor (ET), tumor core (TC), whole tumor (WT), resection cavity (RC), and gross tumor volume (GTV).

Task	Model	Dice					NSD thresh. 1mm				
		ET	TC	WT	RC	GTV	ET	TC	WT	RC	GTV
MET Validation (G) N=179	MedNeXt(M)	0.747	0.768	0.776	0.628		0.588	0.595	0.496	0.591	
	nnU-Net	0.731	0.752	0.754	0.656		0.559	0.566	0.468	0.617	
	nnU-Net-ResEnc(M)	0.744	0.761	0.766	0.693		0.570	0.577	0.473	0.654	
	Ensemble	0.744	0.765	0.769	0.705		0.579	0.587	0.489	0.668	
	Post-processing	0.699	0.72	0.719	0.907		0.535	0.544	0.442	0.871	
MET Testing (LW)	Mean	0.544	0.555	0.561	0.86		0.606	0.607	0.589	0.858	
	Standard Deviation	0.317	0.322	0.322	0.322		0.336	0.338	0.32	0.321	
MEN Validation (LW) N=141	MedNeXt(M)	0.841	0.863	0.839			0.853	0.87	0.842		
	nnU-Net	0.811	0.820	0.834			0.824	0.823	0.832		
	nnU-Net-ResEnc(M)	0.807	0.822	0.825			0.818	0.825	0.826		
	Ensemble	0.835	0.844	0.836			0.847	0.850	0.839		
	Post-processing	0.856	0.855	0.848			0.873	0.865	0.854		
MEN Testing (LW)	Mean	0.881	0.878	0.868			0.885	0.878	0.86		
	Standard Deviation	0.224	0.226	0.224			0.218	0.221	0.216		
MEN-RT Validation (LW) N=70	MedNeXt(M)					0.804					0.671
	nnU-Net					0.764					0.618
	nnU-Net-ResEnc(M)					0.795					0.651
	Ensemble					0.796					0.654
	Post-processing					0.796					0.654
MEN-RT Testing (LW)	Mean					0.807					0.683
	Standard Deviation					0.201					0.236

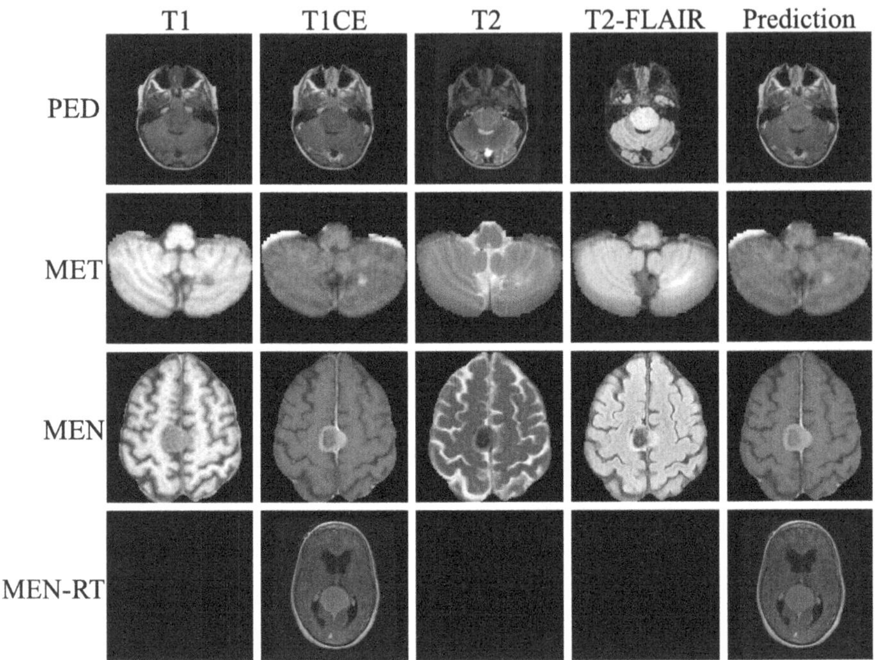

Fig. 5. Qualitative results showing median lesion-wise Dice (L) or global Dice (G) of the whole tumor. PED: 0.979L, orange=NET, blue=ET; MET: 0.868G, orange=SNFH, green=ET; MEN: 0.961L, orange=SNFH, green=ET; MEN-RT: 0.887L, blue=GTV. (Color figure online)

Because the training set is much larger than the validation set, the latter can present a skewed tumor-type distribution and thus provide an unreliable signal for hyper-parameter and threshold tuning. We therefore recommend selecting models and thresholds by CV on the training set, using validation scores only as a sanity check. In the same spirit, the internal rank metric—aggregating Dice and NSD across tumor regions, proved more robust than any single metric, especially when candidate models were numerous. However, its sensitivity to the number of candidates (rank scores can be very close if only three candidates) suggests that alternative weighting schemes merit exploration.

We previously tested that stratified fold splitting based on radiomic clusters yielded higher CV scores than random splits, indicating that heterogeneity-aware sampling reduces overfitting. Additional ablations on multiple BraTS tasks are planned to quantify this effect. We also found that STAPLE fusion benefited the MEN-RT task when each fold was treated as a separate candidate, indicating that larger model pools can regularize ensembles.

Limitations include our reliance on simple volume thresholds for PP1 and PP2. Future work will replace these heuristics with radiomic-driven criteria analogous to those used for stratification, further tailoring post-processing to both tumor morphology and appearance.

Open-sourcing our ranker and keeping all components model-independent, we aim to make the pipeline easy to deploy in clinical workflows. When its utility is evaluated in more clinical studies, the pipeline would have the potential for larger clinical impact beyond BraTS benchmarks.

Finally, to facilitate reproducibility and extend the utility of our approaches, we have made the complete pipeline publicly available as easy-to-use Docker containers and a webapp for all the tasks. The Docker images are hosted at: https://hub.docker.com/r/aparida12/brats2025 and the webapp is accessible at: https://segmenter.hope4kids.io/.

5 Conclusion

This work introduces a tumor- and lesion-aware ensemble pipeline that consistently segments four distinct brain tumour cohorts in the BraTS 2025 Lighthouse Challenge. By selecting and weighting models according to lesion-level accuracy and adding subtype-specific processing, the framework achieves strong segmentation performance relying on state-of-the-art network backbones. Its modular design makes it easy to adopt and extend, while the resulting quantitative tumor measurements could support clinical diagnosis, treatment planning, and longitudinal monitoring.

Acknowledgements. This work was supported by the National Cancer Institute (UG3 CA236536), the Spanish Ministerio de Ciencia e Innovación, the Agencia Estatal de Investigación, NextGenerationEU grants PDC2022-133865-I00 and PID2022-141493OB-I00, and the EUCAIM project co-funded by the European Union (Grant Agreement #101100633). The authors acknowledge the Universidad Politécnica de Madrid for providing computing resources on the Magerit Supercomputer.

References

1. Baid, U., Ghodasara, S., Mohan, S., et al.: The RSNA-ASNR-MICCAI BraTS 2021 benchmark on brain tumor segmentation and radiogenomic classification. arXiv preprint: arXiv:2107.02314 (2021)
2. Bakas, S., Akbari, H., Sotiras, A., et al.: Advancing the cancer genome atlas glioma MRI collections with expert segmentation labels and radiomic features. Scientific Data **4**(1), 170117 (2017). https://doi.org/10.1038/sdata.2017.117
3. Bakas, S., Akbari, H., Sotiras, A., et al.: Segmentation labels and radiomic features for the pre-operative scans of the TCGA-GBM collection. Cancer Imaging Archi. (2017). https://doi.org/10.7937/K9/TCIA.2017.KLXWJJ1Q
4. Bakas, S., Akbari, H., Sotiras, A., et al.: Segmentation labels and radiomic features for the pre-operative scans of the TCGA-LGG collection. Cancer Imaging Arch. (2017). https://doi.org/10.7937/K9/TCIA.2017.GJQ7R0EF

5. Capellán-Martín, D., et al.: Model ensemble for brain tumor segmentation in magnetic resonance imaging. In: International Challenge on Cross-Modality Domain Adaptation for Medical Image Segmentation, pp. 221–232. Springer (2023)
6. Fathi Kazerooni, A., Khalili, N., Liu, X., Gandhi, D., Jiang, Z., et al.: The brain tumor segmentation in pediatrics (BraTS-PEDs) challenge: focus on Pediatrics (CBTN-CONNECT-DIPGR-ASNR-MICCAI BraTS-PEDs) (2024). https://arxiv.org/abs/2404.15009
7. Hatamizadeh, A., Nath, V., Tang, Y., et al.: Swin UNETR: Swin transformers for semantic segmentation of brain tumors in MRI images. In: Crimi, A., Bakas, S. (eds.) Brainlesion: Glioma, Multiple Sclerosis, Stroke and Traumatic Brain Injuries, pp. 272–284. Springer, Cham (2022)
8. Isensee, F., Jaeger, P.F., Kohl, S.A., et al.: nnU-Net: a self-configuring method for deep learning-based biomedical image segmentation. Nat. Methods **18**(2), 203–211 (2021)
9. Isensee, F., Wald, T., Ulrich, C., Baumgartner, M., Roy, S., et al.: nnU-Net revisited: a call for rigorous validation in 3d medical image segmentation. In: Medical Image Computing and Computer Assisted Intervention – MICCAI 2024, pp. 488–498. Springer Nature Switzerland, Cham (2024)
10. Jiang, Z., et al.: Enhancing generalizability in brain tumor segmentation: model ensemble with adaptive post-processing. In: 2024 IEEE International Symposium on Biomedical Imaging (ISBI), pp. 1–4. IEEE (2024)
11. Jiang, Z., et al.: Magnetic resonance imaging feature-based subtyping and model ensemble for enhanced brain tumor segmentation. arXiv preprint: arXiv:2412.04094 (2024)
12. Jiang, Z., et al.: Automatic visual acuity loss prediction in children with optic pathway gliomas using magnetic resonance imaging. In: 2023 45th Annual International Conference of the IEEE Engineering in Medicine & Biology Society (EMBC), pp. 1–5. IEEE (2023)
13. Karargyris, A., Umeton, R., Sheller, M., et al.: Federated benchmarking of medical artificial intelligence with MedPerf. Nat. Mach. Intell. **5**, 799–810 (2023)
14. Kazerooni, A.F., Khalili, N., Liu, X., et al.: The brain tumor segmentation (BraTS) challenge 2023: focus on pediatrics (CBTN-CONNECT-DIPGR-ASNR-MICCAI BraTS-PEDs) (2023)
15. LaBella, D., Adewole, M., Alonso-Basanta, M., et al.: The ASNR-MICCAI brain tumor segmentation (BraTS) challenge 2023: intracranial meningioma (2023)
16. LaBella, D., Baid, U., Khanna, O., McBurney-Lin, S., McLean, R., et al.: Analysis of the BraTS 2023 intracranial meningioma segmentation challenge. J. Mach. Learn. Biomed. Imaging **3**(March 2025), 38–58 (2025)
17. LaBella, D., Schumacher, K., Mix, M., Leu, K., McBurney-Lin, S., et al.: Brain tumor segmentation (BraTS) challenge 2024: meningioma radiotherapy planning automated segmentation (2024). https://arxiv.org/abs/2405.18383
18. Ma, J., Li, F., Wang, B.: U-Mamba: enhancing long-range dependency for biomedical image segmentation. arXiv preprint: arXiv:2401.04722 (2024)
19. Maani, F., Hashmi, A.U.R., Aljuboory, M., Saeed, N., Sobirov, I., Yaqub, M.: Advanced tumor segmentation in medical imaging: an ensemble approach for BraTS 2023 adult glioma and pediatric tumor tasks. In: International Challenge on Cross-Modality Domain Adaptation for Medical Image Segmentation, pp. 264–277. Springer (2023)
20. Menze, B.H., Jakab, A., Bauer, S., et al.: The multimodal brain tumor image segmentation benchmark (BRATS). IEEE Trans. Med. Imaging **34**(10), 1993–2024 (2015). https://doi.org/10.1109/TMI.2014.2377694

21. Moawad, A.W., Janas, A., Baid, U., et al.: The brain tumor segmentation (BraTS-METS) challenge 2023: brain metastasis segmentation on pre-treatment MRI (2023)
22. Parida, A., et al.: Adult glioma segmentation in Sub-Saharan Africa using transfer learning on stratified finetuning data. arXiv preprint: arXiv:2412.04111 (2024)
23. Roy, S., et al.: MedNext: transformer-driven scaling of convnets for medical image segmentation. In: International Conference on Medical Image Computing and Computer-Assisted Intervention, pp. 405–415. Springer (2023)
24. Siegel, R.L., Kratzer, T.B., Giaquinto, A.N., Sung, H., Jemal, A.: Cancer statistics, 2025. CA: Cancer J. Clin. **75**(1), 10–45 (2025). https://doi.org/10.3322/caac.21871
25. Tang, Y., Yang, D., Li, W., Roth, H.R., et al.: Self-supervised pre-training of Swin transformers for 3D medical image analysis. In: Proceedings of the IEEE/CVF Conference on Computer Vision and Pattern Recognition, pp. 20730–20740 (2022)
26. Van Griethuysen, J.J., et al.: Computational radiomics system to decode the radiographic phenotype. Can. Res. **77**(21), e104–e107 (2017)
27. Warfield, S., Zou, K., Wells, W.: Simultaneous truth and performance level estimation (STAPLE): an algorithm for the validation of image segmentation. IEEE Trans. Med. Imaging **23**(7), 903–921 (2004). https://doi.org/10.1109/TMI.2004.828354
28. Xing, Z., et al.: SegMamba-V2: long-range sequential modeling mamba for general 3D medical image segmentation. IEEE Trans. Med. Imaging, 1–1 (2025). https://doi.org/10.1109/TMI.2025.3589797

Challenge 7 – BraTS-GOAT

A Multitask Learning Approach for Segmenting Brain Tumor Sub-regions: Towards Better Generalization

Mumu Aktar[1,2](✉), Tasneem Nasser[2,3], and Roberto Souza[1,2]

[1] Electrical and Software Engineering, University of Calgary, Alberta, Canada
[2] Hotchkiss Brain Institute, University of Calgary, Alberta, Canada
mumu.aktar@ucalgary.ca
[3] Biomedical Engineering, University of Calgary, Alberta, Canada

Abstract. Accurate segmentation of brain tumor sub-regions is essential for effective diagnosis and treatment planning, particularly in radiation therapy. However, heterogeneity in tumor size, location, imaging protocols, and patient demographics leads to significant variability in appearance, making the task highly challenging. Deep learning-based methods have advanced this field by mitigating the limitations of manual segmentation, which is both time-consuming and subject to inter-observer variability. In this work, we leverage the Swin UNETR, a transformer-based model designed to capture both local and global dependencies, making it well-suited for segmenting complex and variable tumor structures. To address the challenge of limited labeled data and enhance generalizability across centers, we employ a multitask learning framework that jointly performs self-supervised reconstruction and supervised segmentation, enabling robust feature learning through combined task optimization. We evaluated our approach in the BraTS 2025 Challenge dataset, focusing on the segmentation of three key subregions: whole tumor (WT), tumor core (TC), and enhancing tumor (ET). Our method achieves an average Dice score of 0.72 (0.73,0.76,0.68 for WT, TC and ET respectively) in the validation set, demonstrating strong performance and robustness under varying clinical conditions. The Github code is available: https://github.com/mumuaktar/BraTS-Challenge-GoAT.

Keywords: Multimodal MRI · BraTS · Brain Tumor · multitask · segmentation · Swin UNETR

1 Introduction

Accurate and automatic brain tumor segmentation is a crucial step in clinical workflows, particularly in aiding treatment planning and disease monitoring. However, achieving robust performance across diverse clinical scenarios remains a significant challenge. The difficulty arises due to considerable variations in image acquisition protocols, patient demographics (such as age and sex), and

S. Bakas et al. (Eds.): MICCAI 2025, LNCS 16376, pp. 471–480, 2026.
https://doi.org/10.1007/978-3-032-16365-3_42

tumor characteristics including size, shape, location, and sub-regional composition. Additionally, the appearance and structure of tumor sub-regions (e.g., enhancing tumor, tumor core, and surrounding edema) can vary significantly across different tumor types. A major bottleneck in developing effective segmentation models is the dependency on large volumes of high-quality labeled data. Annotating 3D brain magnetic resonance images (MRIs) is a labor-intensive process and subject to inter-rater variability, making large-scale manual annotation impractical in many scenarios. This challenge requires the development of methods that can leverage labeled and unlabeled data effectively. In this work, we propose a novel semi-supervised learning approach that combines pre-training and fine-tuning in a multitask setting. Our framework utilizes labeled and unlabeled data to learn generalizable feature representations through reconstruction while concurrently fine-tuning a Swin UNETR-based architecture using labeled data for accurate segmentation of tumor sub-regions. This strategy enables the model to benefit from the strengths of both supervised and unsupervised learning paradigms. The Brain Tumor Segmentation (BraTS) 2025 challenge provides a standardized benchmark for evaluating algorithms on multi-institutional, multi-parametric MRI datasets across a diverse set of brain tumor types. This year's challenge includes 11 subtasks spanning segmentation, classification, and image synthesis. In this work, we focus on subtask 7, which involves segmenting three clinically relevant tumor sub-regions: whole tumor (WT), enhancing tumor (ET), and tumor core (TC) across five distinct tumor populations: (1) adult gliomas, (2) gliomas from the underserved sub-Saharan African population, (3) meningiomas, (4) brain metastases, and (5) pediatric brain tumors. Our study specifically addresses the challenge of generalizability in segmentation across these diverse tumor types and patient populations, with an emphasis on accurate sub-region delineation under domain shifts.

Convolutional Neural Networks (CNNs) have been fundamental in brain tumor segmentation tasks. Several studies have achieved state-of-the-art performance in delineating tumor sub-regions, including WT, TC, and ET. Among the most effective frameworks is nnU-Net [1], which automatically adapts to dataset characteristics and has ranked first in the BraTS challenge, 2020 [2]. Ensemble approaches built upon classical architectures, such as 3D U-Net, have also demonstrated strong sub-region segmentation capabilities. For instance, Rajput et al. [3] proposed a triplanar ensemble of U-Nets that achieved high Dice scores on WT and TC segmentation tasks in BraTS 2021. Similarly, Qamar et al. [4] introduced HI-Net, an inception-based U-Net variant, that outperformed standard CNN baselines on segmenting WT, TC, and ET. Zeineldin et al. [5] proposed an ensemble CNN framework combining DeepSeg and nnU-Net for glioblastoma tumor segmentation on BraTS 2021, achieving Dice scores of 0.92 (ET), 0.87 (TC), and 0.84 (WT) on the validation set.

To overcome CNNs' limitations in modeling global spatial dependencies, attention-based transformer models have gained prominence. Vision Transformers (ViTs), particularly Swin UNETR [6], have demonstrated superior performance in capturing long-range dependencies, which are crucial for accurately segmenting variable-size tumor sub-regions. Recent state-of-the-art solutions like multiPI-TransBTS [7] employed multiple modality-specific branches with hierarchical attention fusion, achieving high Dice scores across WT, TC, and ET in BraTS 2023. Furthermore, Yazıcı et al. [8] introduced GLIMS, a hybrid U-Net architecture enhanced with Swin Transformer blocks and multi-scale attention mechanisms, achieved state-of-the-art performance in the BraTS 2021 dataset with an average Dice score of 92.14%.

The scarcity and expense of expert annotations in 3D medical imaging have motivated the development of semi-supervised approaches. These methods leverage unlabeled data through self- or weakly-supervised representation learning. A notable example is BrainSegFounder [9], which employed a two-stage training pipeline: self-supervised pretraining on healthy brain MRIs followed by fine-tuning on BraTS segmentation tasks, outperforming the supervised baselines. Semi-supervised frameworks not only alleviate labeling burdens but also improve cross-center generalization. They are especially effective in scenarios involving domain heterogeneity, such as pediatric versus adult populations, or differences in MRI acquisition protocols. A conditional GAN-based data augmentation framework is introduced in the BraTS 2024 GoAT challenge in ISBI, generating realistic synthetic MRI volumes to improve generalization in WT, TC, and ET segmentation, achieving Dice scores of 0.88, 0.86, and 0.86, respectively, and demonstrating robustness under domain shifts [10]. A recent study by Zhou et al. [11] proposed a model that combines self-supervised pretraining on unlabeled MRI data with a dynamically weighted region-specific loss, enhancing segmentation accuracy for WT, TC, and ET by emphasizing difficult-to-segment sub-regions.

Multitask learning frameworks have been increasingly explored as a way to improve generalization and feature richness. By jointly optimizing auxiliary tasks (e.g., classification, reconstruction, or modality translation) alongside segmentation, it encourages the model to learn more transferable and discriminative features. For instance, the study by Chen et al. [12] proposed a framework combining segmentation and image reconstruction with attention mechanisms to enhance feature learning from both labeled and unlabeled data under limited supervision conditions. Our approach expands on this idea by integrating simultaneous pretraining and fine-tuning in a multitask semi-supervised setting. This enables Swin UNETR to leverage both labeled and unlabeled data during training, optimizing for segmentation of WT, TC, and ET regions while learning robust contextual representations.

2 Dataset Details

The BraTS challenge targets delineating the adult brain gliomas with state-of-the-art methods. This specific segmentation task focuses on the generalizability of the developed method across tumors that differ in size and location. The dataset consists of a total of 2489 cases (1351 with ground truth and 1138 without ground truth) for training and 451 cases without ground truth for the validation phase. Training data are available from the full BraTS Adult gliomas, BraTS Meningiomas, BraTS Brain metastases, and validation data includes additional data from BraTS Africa, and BraTS Pediatric Tumors data. Each 3D brain MRI in the BraTS dataset has 4 modalities: T1 (pre-contrast T1), T1Gd (post-contrast T1), T2w and FLAIR. All labels and imaging data are skull-stripped, aligned to a standardized anatomical template, and resampled to an isotropic resolution of 1mm^3. The image dimensions are $240\times240\times155$ voxels. The sub-regions considered for evaluation are the ET, TC, and WT, with segmentation labels of: 1 for NCR (necrosis), 2 for ED (edema/invaded tissue), 3 for ET (enhancing tumor), and 0 for everything else. The ET refers to the visibly active tumor region, while the TC comprises both the ET and the necrotic (NCR) areas. The WT encompasses the TC along with the surrounding peritumoral edematous or infiltrated tissue (ED).

3 Multitasking Strategy

We illustrate the methodology of our proposed multitask approach in Fig. 1.

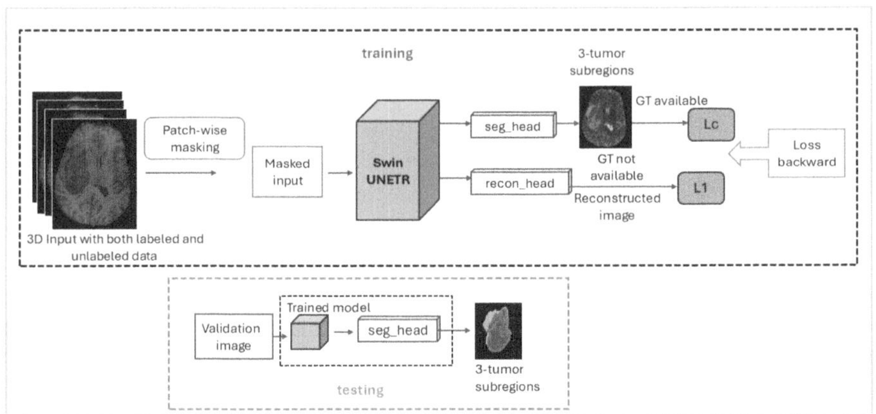

Fig. 1. Overview of the proposed multitask framework. The input image is occluded using patch-based masking and fed into the Swin UNETR network. The network has two output heads: one produces a 3-channel segmentation output corresponding to three tumor sub-regions, and the other generates a 4-channel reconstruction output approximating the original brain image. For unlabeled input data, only the L1 reconstruction loss is applied. The combined training loss, denoted as L_c, includes the Dice loss and binary cross-entropy loss for segmentation, along with the L1 reconstruction loss. During inference, the original (unmasked) image is used as input, and only the segmentation output is utilized.

3.1 Overall Methodology

To delineate brain tumor sub-regions that is adaptable to multi-center data and variable size and location of tumors, we propose a multitask learning framework designed to enhance generalization while addressing the challenges posed by unlabeled data. Given that a substantial portion of the dataset lacks annotations, we leverage this unlabeled data along with the labeled ones through a reconstruction-based pretraining strategy. This allows the model to learn meaningful representations from both labeled and unlabeled data in a self-supervised manner. For fine-tuning the segmentation task, only labeled data is used, as ground truth annotations are required for calculating segmentation losses and enabling backpropagation. The model employs a shared Swin UNETR backbone with hierarchical Swin Transformer blocks that encode volumetric features across multiple scales while preserving spatial resolution, capturing both local and global context. The encoder outputs feature maps at a fixed resolution (feature size = 48), which are fed into two separate heads. The segmentation head is a 1×1×1 convolution that generates a 3-channel map corresponding to the tumor sub-regions (ET, TC, WT), while the reconstruction head is a 1×1×1 convolution that outputs a 4-channel approximation of the input brain image. Both heads share the same backbone features, enabling joint multitask learning from a single input volume.

3.2 Loss Function

To support multitasking for tumor sub-region segmentation, we employ a combined loss function that integrates both segmentation, L_{seg} and reconstruction, L_{recon} losses. This joint optimization allows the model to leverage both supervised and self-supervised learning, thereby promoting more effective feature learning and enhanced generalization across diverse domains. L_{seg} consists of Dice loss, L_{dice} and binary cross-entropy loss, L_{BCE}. For the reconstruction objective, we adopt the L1 loss from MONAI, which computes the mean absolute difference between input and reconstructed images, encouraging pixel-level fidelity. Given that the training dataset includes both labeled and unlabeled samples, we define a composite loss, denoted as L_c, for batches containing labeled data:

$$L_c = \alpha \cdot L_{seg} + \beta \cdot L_{recon} \tag{1}$$

$$L_{seg} = L_{dice} + L_{BCE} \tag{2}$$

Here, α and β are dynamic weighting factors that change as training progresses.

Although reconstruction and segmentation are performed simultaneously, training begins with a warm-up phase in which only the reconstruction loss is optimized. This phase lasts for the first 49 epochs, with $\alpha = 0$ and $\beta = 1$. Starting from epoch 50, joint training is performed: when a sample is labeled, the full combined loss, L_c, is used; otherwise, only the L_{recon}, is applied. During the joint training phase, the values of α and β are adjusted dynamically. Specifically, β decays linearly from 0.3 to 0 over the remaining epochs, reducing the emphasis on reconstruction. Conversely, α increases from 0.7 to 1.0, placing greater emphasis on segmentation as training proceeds. This progressive reweighting enables the model to initially learn robust feature representations through self-supervised reconstruction and subsequently fine-tune these features for accurate supervised segmentation.

3.3 Masking Strategy

To simulate occluded inputs and encourage robust feature learning, a patch-based masking strategy was employed. The masking ratio was gradually reduced over the training epochs to allow the model to progressively attend to more complete input features:

- Epochs 0–49: 40% masking
- Epochs 50–99: 25% masking
- Epochs 100–149: 10% masking
- Epochs 150–199: 5% masking

From epoch 200 onward, a small masking rate of 3% is applied.

3.4 Implementation Details

The proposed multitask learning framework was implemented using PyTorch and MONAI. The model was trained for a total of 300 epochs, with the ability to resume training from a previously saved checkpoint, starting from $start\_epoch = 1$ by default. The Adam optimizer with an initial learning rate of 4e-4 and a weight decay of 1e-5 was used. To regulate the learning rate throughout training, a Cosine Annealing Learning Rate Scheduler was applied, which smoothly decays the learning rate from the initial value down to a minimum value ($\eta_{\min} = 1 \times 10^{-6}$) over the total number of epochs. This strategy enabled the model to take larger steps in the early phase and gradually refine as training converges. The best model obtained for validation is based on the best mean dice score of the three sub-regions of tumors.

During validation, a sliding window inference with a window size of $128 \times 128 \times 128$ and 0.7 overlap were used. A sigmoid activation followed by thresholding at 0.5 was applied to generate binary predictions.

3.5 Hardware Configuration

Experiments were conducted using two computing environments:

- Local workstation with 2× NVIDIA RTX A6000 GPUs (48 GB each), running CUDA 12.4 and driver version 550.144.03, paired with an Intel Xeon CPU and 128 GB RAM, on Ubuntu 20.04.

- High-performance computing (HPC) cluster featuring NVIDIA A100 GPUs (40/80 GB) for parallel training and ablation studies. The cluster environment supported multi-GPU training and was used for scaling and comparison experiments.

4 Result and Discussion

To evaluate the proposed model's performance in tumor generalizability, similar to the previous challenges, the lesion-wise Dice similarity coefficient is considered. The 451 cases provided for the validation phase are submitted to the challenge portal and the result obtained is 0.68 for ET, 0.73 for WT and 0.76 for TC sub-regions. Figure 2 demonstrates qualitative performance of the proposed model in the validation set.

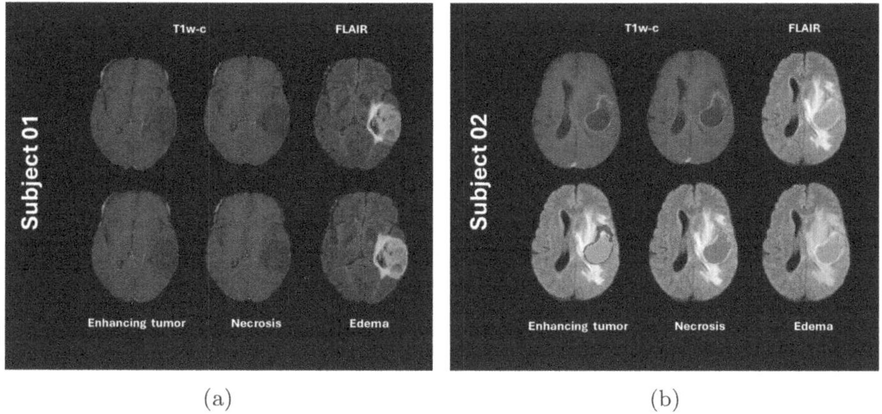

(a) (b)

Fig. 2. Visual analysis of tumor sub-regions segmentation in two randomly selected subjects (a) and (b). The figures illustrate the segmentation performance for individual tumor regions: the enhancing tumor, the necrotic core and the edema/invaded tissue. Since ET and TC are more clearly visible in the T1 post-contrast modality, and edema is highlighted in the T2-FLAIR modality, the predicted segmentations are overlaid on these specific modalities for better visibility. Subject 1 represents a challenging case with a very small enhancing tumor region, while Subject 2 demonstrates a case where all tumor regions are prominently visible.

Furthermore, the proposed model was applied to the unseen test dataset by the challenge organizers, and the results are reported in Table 1. It can be observed from the results that the segmentation performance for WT and TC is similar to that of the validation performance, whereas the performance for ET shows a 5% improvement in test set. At inference, test-time augmentation (TTA) was used to improve segmentation robustness. Each input volume was

Table 1. Performance of the model on the unseen test dataset.

	LesionWise_Dice			LesionWise_NSD_1.0		
Metric	ET	TC	WT	ET	TC	WT
Mean	0.73	0.75	0.73	0.76	0.72	0.66
Std	0.31	0.31	0.30	0.30	0.31	0.29

augmented with flips along the sagittal, coronal, and axial axes, a 90Âř rotation in the coronalâĂŞaxial plane, and the identity (no transformation) to retain the original prediction. Predictions for each augmented input were reverted to the original orientation using the inverse transform, and the final segmentation was obtained by averaging all probability maps. This procedure yielded in a mean Dice score improvement of 2% compared to inference without TTA. For performance analysis, two different patch sizes were considered. To ensure faster training and improved memory efficiency while still enabling rich feature learning from local neighborhoods, a patch size of $96 \times 96 \times 96$ was used during training. For validation, where larger patches offer better contextual information for segmentation, a window size of $128 \times 128 \times 128$ was used with sliding window inference. The model demonstrated improved performance with the larger window size, achieving Dice scores of 0.68, 0.76, and 0.73, compared to scores of 0.66, 0.73 and 0.70, respectively, for ET, TC, and WT using the $96 \times 96 \times 96$ window size on the validation set.

Our proposed multitasking approach, built on the baseline Swin UNETR model, was also compared with the automatic dyn-nnUNet framework from MONAI. The dyn-nnUNet achieved Dice scores of 0.64 for ET, 0.71 for TC, and 0.67 for WT, whereas our method demonstrated superior overall segmentation performance. This comparative evaluation was conducted using the window size of $96 \times 96 \times 96$.

From the validation Dice scores and based on our initial analysis, it is evident that segmenting the ET region is more challenging compared to TC and WT. One contributing factor is the high variability in lesion presentation across subjects. For example, some patients may lack, or show minimal necrotic core, edema, or contrast enhancement. As a result, the presence and size of ET region can vary significantly across datasets, which may have affected the modelâĂŹs performance to segment ET. In cases where the ET region is very small or nearly absent, post-processing techniques such as reassigning small false-positive predictions to other regions (e.g., TC) could potentially improve the Dice score. However, such approaches are not clinically valid, as accurate identification of the ET region is critical for treatment planning and diagnosis. Therefore, no post-processing was applied to artificially boost segmentation performance. Interestingly, ET showed improved performance on the test set, which may be due to the specific characteristics of the cases included in the test dataset.

Although the Dice scores indicate that our method does not yet achieve state-of-the-art accuracy, the proposed novel strategy of parallel reconstruction in a semi-supervised manner, combined with a segmentation framework, establishes a solid multitasking baseline for developing generalizable models on unseen data. This is especially valuable in heterogeneous clinical scenarios where lesion characteristics vary widely.

5 Conclusion

In this paper, we proposed a multitask learning approach that jointly performs pretraining through reconstruction and segmentation of brain tumors. This framework enables the model to share learned representations by combining gradients from both tasks during training. The effectiveness of the proposed method was validated on the BraTS challenge validation and test datasets. Our approach reduces the dependency on labeled data during fine-tuning and enhances the model's adaptability and generalizability across diverse tumor types and data sources.

Acknowledgements. Dr. Roberto Souza thanks NSERC for ongoing operating support for this project (RGPIN/2021-02858).

Disclosure of Interests. The authors have no competing interests to declare that are relevant to the content of this article.

References

1. Isensee, F., Jaeger, P.F., Kohl, S.A., Petersen, J., Maier-Hein, K.H.: nnU-Net: a self-configuring method for deep learning-based biomedical image segmentation. Nat. Methods **18**(2), 203–211 (2021)
2. Isensee, F., Jäger, P.F., Full, P.M., Vollmuth, P., Maier-Hein, K.H.: nnU-Net for brain tumor segmentation. In: International MICCAI Brainlesion Workshop (pp. 118–132). Cham: Springer International Publishing (2020)
3. Rajput, S., Kapdi, R., Roy, M., Raval, M.S.: A triplanar ensemble model for brain tumor segmentation with volumetric multiparametric magnetic resonance images. Healthc. Anal. **5**, 100307 (2024)
4. Qamar, S., Ahmad, P., Shen, L.: HI-Net: hyperdense inception 3D UNet for brain tumor segmentation. In: International MICCAI Brainlesion Workshop (pp. 50–57). Cham: Springer International Publishing (2020)
5. Zeineldin, R. A., Karar, M. E., Mathis-Ullrich, F., Burgert, O.: Ensemble CNN networks for GBM tumors segmentation using multi-parametric MRI. In: International MICCAI Brainlesion Workshop (pp. 473–483). Cham: Springer International Publishing (2021)
6. Hatamizadeh, A., Nath, V., Tang, Y., Yang, D., Roth, H.R., Xu, D.: Swin UNETR: Swin transformers for semantic segmentation of brain tumors in MRI images. In: International MICCAI Brainlesion Workshop (pp. 272–284). Cham: Springer International Publishing (2021)
7. Zhu, H., Huang, J., Chen, K., Ying, X., Qian, Y.: multiPI-TransBTS: a multi-path learning framework for brain tumor image segmentation based on multi-physical information. arXiv preprint arXiv:2409.12167 (2024)

8. Yazıcı, Z.A., Öksüz, İ, Ekenel, H.K.: GLIMS: attention-guided lightweight multi-scale hybrid network for volumetric semantic segmentation. Image Vis. Comput. **146**, 105055 (2024)
9. Cox, J., Liu, P., Stolte, S.E., Yang, Y., Liu, K., See, K.B., Fang, R.: BrainSeg-Founder: towards 3D foundation models for neuroimage segmentation. Med. Image Anal. **97**, 103301 (2024)
10. Ferreira, A., Luijten, G., Puladi, B., Kleesiek, J., Alves, V., Egger, J.: Generalisation of segmentation using generative adversarial networks. In: 2024 IEEE International Symposium on Biomedical Imaging (ISBI), pp. 1–4. IEEE (2024)
11. Zhou, Y., Zhong, L., Wang, G.: Brain tumor segmentation based on self-supervised pre-training and adaptive region-specific loss. In: International Challenge on Cross-Modality Domain Adaptation for Medical Image Segmentation, pp. 46–57. Cham, Springer Nature Switzerland (2023)
12. Chen, S., et al.: Multi-task attention-based semi-supervised learning for medical image segmentation. In: International Conference on Medical Image Computing and Computer-Assisted Intervention, pp. 457–465. Cham: Springer International Publishing (2019)

BraTS-FL: Enhancing Generalization in Brain Tumor Segmentation via Federated Learning

Simone Bendazzoli[1,2(✉)] and Rodrigo Moreno[1,3]

[1] KTH, Royal Institute of Technology, Department of Biomedical Engineering and Health Systems, Stockholm, Sweden

[2] Department of Clinical Sciences, Intervention and Engineering, Karolinska Institutet, Stockholm, Sweden

simben@kth.se

[3] Department of Neurobiology, Care Sciences and Society, Karolinska Institutet, Stockholm, Sweden

Abstract. Accurate and robust segmentation of heterogeneous brain tumors is critical for individualized treatment planning, yet the integration of diverse multicenter datasets remains challenging due to patient privacy constraints. The BraTS Challenge Generalizability Task (GoAT) has highlighted the importance of developing models that generalize across multiple tumor subtypes, including adult glioma, meningioma, and brain metastasis, along with pediatric and sub-Saharan cohorts. In this work, we present BraTS-FL, a federated learning (FL) approach integrated with the nnU-Net framework to collaboratively train segmentation models across distinct tumor subtypes without sharing raw data between institutions. We design a multi-client FL setup, with each client specializing in a specific tumor subtype and employing harmonized preprocessing and training via the MONet bundle. Comparative evaluation on the BraTS 2025 generalizability validation set demonstrates that BraTS-FL achieves competitive performance compared to centralized nnU-Net training in terms of Dice and surface-based metrics across all tumor subregions. These findings underscore FL's viability for privacy-preserving, scalable, and generalizable brain tumor segmentation in real-world heterogeneous clinical settings.

Keywords: Brain Tumor Segmentation · Federated Learning · Generalizability · Multimodal MRI

1 Introduction

Brain tumors include a heterogeneous group of neoplasms that vary widely in terms of origin, biological behavior, and demographics of patients. Among these, adult gliomas, meningiomas, brain metastases, and pediatric brain tumors are the most prevalent in different age groups, each presenting with unique growth

S. Bakas et al. (Eds.): MICCAI 2025, LNCS 16376, pp. 481–488, 2026.
https://doi.org/10.1007/978-3-032-16365-3_43

dynamics, anatomical localization, and imaging characteristics [6,9,12]. These differences significantly influence clinical management and underscore the need for an accurate, individualized assessment. Comprehensive imaging plays a central role in this process, particularly in delineating the extent of the tumor for the planning and monitoring of treatment.

Manual segmentation, however, is time-consuming, prone to variability between and within observers, and difficult to scale in clinical practice, especially in complex or multifocal cases, highlighting the need for reliable automatic methods [2]. Recent advances in deep learning have enabled the development of powerful automatic segmentation tools that can achieve high accuracy and reproducibility across various types of tumors. Importantly, multimodal imaging—such as T1-weighted, T2-weighted, FLAIR, and post-contrast MRI—is essential, as different modalities reveal complementary features such as tumor core, edema, necrosis, and enhancement. Incorporating this multimodal information into segmentation algorithms significantly improves performance and enables more comprehensive tumor characterization [2,4].

In this context, the BraTS challenge [7,10] has emerged as the most prominent and widely recognized benchmark for developing, testing, and showcasing novel deep learning approaches for accurate tumor segmentation, specifically targeting tumor core, enhancing, and non-enhancing regions - in multimodal MRI scans (T1, T2, T2-FLAIR, T1 contrast). Over the years, several winning strategies have gained traction due to their successful application in the BraTS challenge [5], which has been made possible by the organizers' efforts in collecting, preprocessing, and standardizing thousands of multimodal MRI datasets and providing open access for algorithm validation. Initially centered on adult glioma segmentation [14], BraTS has since expanded its scope to include a broader spectrum of brain tumors, such as meningiomas [8], pediatric brain tumors, and brain metastases [11].

Within the BraTS Challenge, the GoAT has been established as a benchmark to evaluate the generalizability of proposed methods across diverse tumor subtypes, with the specific aim of prioritizing the development of algorithms that perform robustly across heterogeneous brain tumor types, rather than being tailored to a single subtype.

In contrast to the BraTS setting, where data sets are openly available, real-world clinical scenarios often impose strict privacy and data protection regulations that prevent data sharing between institutions. As a result, the collection of data from multiple centers to train a unified model that is generalized across institutions and tumor subtypes is often unfeasible.

Federated learning (FL) has emerged as a promising solution to this challenge. It enables collaborative training to preserve privacy by allowing models to be trained locally on each institution's data (client) while only sharing model parameters for aggregation into a global model. This approach ensures that data never leave the local site, addressing privacy concerns while still allowing knowledge sharing.

In this paper, we propose to integrate FL for the GoAT. We hypothesize that the aggregation step in FL inherently promotes generalizability, as it combines diverse local models into a single global model that aims to perform well across all participating sites. In this setup, each client can focus on learning from its specific subtask or tumor subtype, while the central aggregation acts as a generalization layer, promoting robustness between institutions and tumor types.

2 Methods

The **GoAT** dataset, the focus of this study and provided by the BraTS challenge, comprises multimodal MRI scans along with the corresponding tumor lesion segmentations. Although BraTS has traditionally focused on adult glioma segmentation, recent expansions have expanded its coverage to include a broader range of brain tumor types, such as pediatric tumors, cases from the sub-Saharan population, low-field MRI acquisitions, meningiomas, and brain metastases.

In the **GoAT** subchallenge, the objective is to train a model capable of robust generalizing across multiple tumor subtypes, starting from a pool that includes three main categories: adult glioma [14], meningioma [8], and brain metastasis [11], and extending to external cohorts such as sub-Saharan African adult glioma and pediatric brain tumors.

Each of the 3 BraTS dataset includes four MRI modalities per subject: T1-weighted (T1), post-contrast T1-weighted (T1Gd), T2-weighted (T2), and T2 Fluid Attenuated Inversion Recovery (FLAIR). Magnetic resonance imaging was acquired using various clinical protocols and imaging equipment in multiple institutions. Before model training, all images were preprocessed by co-registering to a common anatomical template, resampling to a uniform resolution of 1mm^3, and skull stripping.

Annotations were performed manually by one to four annotators following a standardized protocol, with final validation by experienced neuroradiologists. The segmentation masks include labels for enhancing tumor (ET), surrounding nonenhancing FLAIR hyperintensity (SNFH), and non-enhancing tumor core (TC).

In this context, the objective of this study is to explore FL as a potential strategy to develop robust and generalizable models capable of handling the diverse BraTS datasets representing different subtypes of brain tumors. Building upon the well established nnU-Net [5] as a baseline, the proposed approach integrates FL with the nnUNet framework.

A federated learning setup was designed with three distinct clients, each assigned to a specific BraTS subtask: the first client manages adult glioma preoperative cases, the second focuses on meningioma and the third on brain metastasis (Fig. 1). This configuration promotes client specialization, allowing each client to independently learn from its respective subtask while benefiting from shared knowledge through periodic aggregation.

All experiments reported in this study were conducted using **MONet** [1], our framework that encapsulates the original implementation of nnU-Net within a

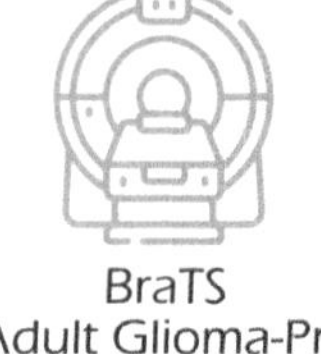

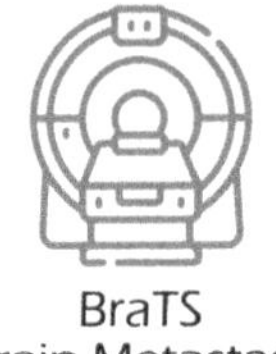

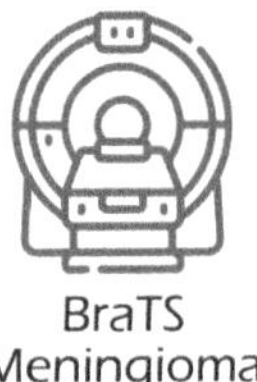

Fig. 1. Assignment of the three training sub-cohorts to the corresponding clients in the federated learning setup.

MONAI [3] Bundle. Training hyperparameters, such as learning rate, scheduler, number of iterations, and total epochs, were maintained at their default values using the standard *nnUNetTrainer* (see Table 1).

Table 1. Default nnU-Net Training Hyperparameters

Hyperparameter	Value
Learning Rate	0.01
Scheduler	Poly decay
Iterations	250,000
Epochs	1000
Loss Function	Combined Dice + Cross-Entropy

For the FL setup, the *MONAIAlgo* mechanism was utilized, adopting the **MONet** bundle. The federated learning configuration consisted of 100 global aggregation rounds, each round comprising 10 local training epochs.

To establish a baseline, a single nnU-Net model was trained on the three centrally merged datasets. This centralized training enables a direct comparison with the federated learning approach to assess differences in generalizability.

The baseline nnU-Net models were trained individually on a single NVIDIA T4 GPU, requiring approximately 8 GB of virtual memory. To evaluate FL under realistic conditions, we deployed three NVFlare [13] clients and a central server across two separate infrastructures: two clients on the Alvis supercomputer and one client on a KTH-hosted medical AI platform integrated with KUH's PACS. The Alvis clients utilized NVIDIA T4 GPUs, while the KTH client operated on an NVIDIA A6000 GPU.

To establish a segmentation performance benchmark for the FL experiments, separate baseline nnU-Net models were trained independently on each dataset. These baseline models were executed on a single NVIDIA T4 GPU with an approximate virtual memory footprint of 8 GB.

The FL model was trained using a single 80/20 split of the training data provided by the BraTS challenges involved (Adult Glioma [14], Meningioma [8] and Brain Metastasis [11]).

The implementation details for both the federated learning configuration and the training process, as well as the MONet bundle, are available at the following link: https://github.com/SimoneBendazzoli93/MONet-Bundle. An overview of the proposed workflow is shown in Fig. 2.

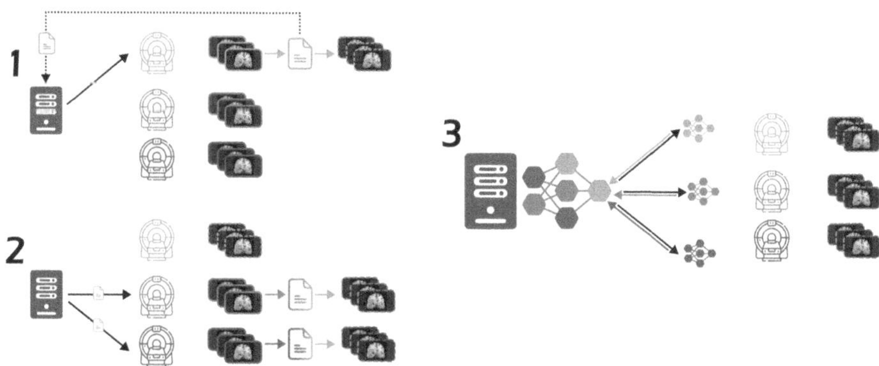

Fig. 2. Overview of the MONet-FL workflow. The process begins with the selection of a reference client for experiment planning and preprocessing (Step 1). The resulting plan is then distributed to the remaining clients, who apply it for local preprocessing (Step 2). Finally, federated training is performed across all three clients using the harmonized setup (Step 3).

The client hosting the Adult Glioma subset was selected to generate the planning experiment, which was subsequently shared with the other clients to perform harmonized nnU-Net preprocessing.

3 Results

The proposed Federated Learning (FL)-based method (**BraTS-FL**) and the baseline approach (**nnU-Net**) were evaluated using the *Validation* set provided by the BraTS 2025 Challenge, Task 7 Generalizability. This set comprises 451 cases, including multimodal scans from five distinct sub-tasks: **Adult Glioma**, **Brain Metastasis**, and **Meningioma** (part of the training data), as well as additional cases from a **sub-Saharan cohort** and **pediatric brain tumors**.

For each case, performance was assessed using **Lesion-Wise Dice** and **Normalized Surface Distance (NSD)**, calculated at two thresholds ($\tau = 0.5$ and $\tau = 1.0$). These metrics were reported for the following labels and their corresponding anatomical regions:

- **ET (Enhancing Tumor)**: Regions of active tumor and areas showing nodular enhancement.

- **NETC (Necrosis and Cysts)**: Non-enhancing components within the tumor, including necrotic and cystic areas.
- **SNFH (Surrounding Non-Enhancing FLAIR Hyperintensity)**: Includes edema, infiltrative tumor, and post-treatment effects.
- **Tumor Core (ET + NETC)**: The central tumor mass typically targeted in surgical resection.
- **Whole Tumor (ET + SNFH + NETC)**: Represents the full extent of tumor-related abnormalities, including the tumor core, infiltration zones, peritumoral edema, and treatment-induced changes.

Table 2 shows that BraTS-FL achieved comparable Dice scores to the baseline across all tumor subregions, with slightly higher values for ET (0.750 vs. 0.744) and TC (0.830 vs. 0.828), while WT and SNFH were marginally lower.

In terms of surface agreement, Table 3 (NSD at 1.0 mm) indicates that BraTS-FL generally performs on par with the baseline, showing slightly improved scores for ET (0.756 vs. 0.752) and NETC (0.631 vs. 0.618), and slightly lower scores for WT and SNFH. Table 4 (NSD at 0.5 mm) further confirms this trend, with performance being largely consistent between both methods. Although the baseline nnU-Net slightly outperformed BraTS-FL in WT (0.470 vs. 0.450) and SNFH (0.433 vs. 0.421), the FL model remained competitive across all subregions.

Finally, Table 5 reports the testing set performance of BraTS-FL, showing lesion-wise Dice and NSD@1.0 scores that are consistent with the validation set results, indicating stable segmentation accuracy across all tumor subregions.

Table 2. Comparison of mean lesion-wise Dice scores between the federated learning model (BraTS-FL) and the centralized nnUNet baseline across 451 cases in the Validation Set.

Experiment	cases	ET	TC	WT	NETC	SNFH
BraTS-FL	451	0.750	0.830	0.825	0.631	0.749
nnU-Net [Baseline]	451	0.744	0.828	0.835	0.626	0.766

Table 3. Mean lesion-wise Normalized Surface Distance (NSD) at a 1.0 mm tolerance for BraTS-FL and nnUNet baseline across 451 cases in the validation set.

Experiment	cases	ET	TC	WT	NETC	SNFH
BraTS-FL	451	0.756	0.777	0.747	0.631	0.734
nnU-Net [Baseline]	451	0.752	0.770	0.759	0.618	0.748

Table 4. Mean lesion-wise Normalized Surface Distance (NSD) at a 0.5 mm tolerance for BraTS-FL and nnUNet baseline across 451 cases in the Validation Set.

Experiment	cases	ET	TC	WT	NETC	SNFH
BraTS-FL	451	0.520	0.514	0.450	0.417	0.421
nnU-Net [Baseline]	451	0.528	0.517	0.470	0.412	0.433

Table 5. Mean lesion-wise mean Dice and NSD@0.1 for the proposed BraTS-FL, evaluated on the testing set.

Metric	Dice			NSD@1.0		
Subregion	ET	TC	WT	ET	TC	WT
BraTS-FL	0.7808	0.8253	0.8168	0.8090	0.8021	0.7540

4 Discussion

These results demonstrate that the **MONet-FL pipeline** is capable of achieving segmentation performance that closely matches that of centralized training, despite operating in a *federated setting* where no raw data is shared between institutions. The consistent alignment across performance metrics, such as the Dice score and Hausdorff distance, highlights the robustness of the proposed framework and its suitability for clinical applications.

Importantly, the fact that federated learning (FL) can approach the performance of a single-site nnU-Net model trained on pooled data suggests that FL is not only a viable alternative, but also a **preferred solution** in scenarios where *data privacy and institutional autonomy* are critical concerns. At the same time, it maintains the ability to train *generalizable models* by combining different, distributed datasets, an essential requirement for real-world deployment in heterogeneous clinical environments.

As such, adopting federated learning frameworks like MONet-FL becomes especially valuable in collaborative medical AI efforts, where both **privacy preservation** and **model performance** are essential to ensure trustworthy and scalable AI integration into clinical workflows.

As a potential future development, the use of available unlabeled data through pseudo-labeling or self-training strategies could further improve algorithm performance.

Acknowledgment. This study has been partially funded by the Swedish Childhood Cancer Foundation (Barncancerfonden MT2022-0008), by Vinnova through AIDA, project ID: 2319, by the Swedish Research Council (Vetenskapsrådet, grant 2022-03389), and Hjärt-Lungfonden (grant No. 2022-0492). We thank the National Academic Infrastructure for Supercomputing in Sweden (NAISS) for the computational resources at Alvis.

Note on a Overlapping Submission. The results presented in this report partially overlap those of [1]. In addition to the BraTS results from this paper, we also report the results for a lymphoma segmentation task in that paper.

References

1. Bendazzoliand, S., et al.: MoNet-FL: Extending nnU-Net with MONAI for clinical federated learning. In: MICCAI DeCaF Workshop, page Accepted (2025)
2. Bakas, S., et al.: Identifying the Best Machine Learning Algorithms for Brain Tumor Segmentation, Progression Assessment, and Overall Survival Prediction in the BRATS Challenge (2018). eprint: arXiv:1811.02629
3. Cardoso, M.J., et al.: MONAI: An open-source framework for deep learning in healthcare (2022). eprint: arXiv:2211.02701
4. Havaei, M., et al.: Brain tumor segmentation with deep neural networks. Med. Image Anal. **35**, 1–31 (2017). ISSN 1361-8415. https://doi.org/10.1016/j.media.2016.05.004
5. Isensee, F., Jaeger, P.F., Kohl, S.A.A., Petersen, J., Maier-Hein, K.H.: nnU-Net: a self-configuring method for deep learning-based biomedical image segmentation. Nat. Methods **18**(2), 203–211 (2020). ISSN 1548-7105. https://doi.org/10.1038/s41592-020-01008-z
6. Jones, C., et al.: Pediatric high-grade glioma: biologically and clinically in need of new thinking. In: Neuro-Oncology (2016), now101. issn: 1523-5866. https://doi.org/10.1093/neuonc/now101
7. Karargyris, A., et al.: Federated benchmarking of medical artificial intelligence with MedPerf. In: Nature Machine Intelligence, vol. 5(7), pp. 799–810 (2023). issn: 2522-5839. https://doi.org/10.1038/s42256-023-00652-2
8. LaBella, D., et al.: The ASNR-MICCAI Brain Tumor Segmentation (BraTS) Challenge 2023: Intracranial Meningioma (2023). https://arxiv.org/abs/2305.07642.
9. Louis, D.N., et al.: The 2021 WHO Classification of Tumors of the CentralNervous System: a summary. In: Neuro-Oncology **23**(8), pp. 1231–1251 (2021). issn: 1523-5866. http://dx.doi.org/10.1093/neuonc/noab106.
10. Menze, B.H., et al.: The multimodal brain tumor image segmentation benchmark (BRATS). In: IEEE Transactions on Medical Imaging, vol. 34(10), pp. 1993–2024 (2015). https://doi.org/10.1109/TMI.2014.2377694
11. Moawad, A.W., et al.: The Brain Tumor Segmentation (BraTS-METS) Challenge 2023: Brain Metastasis Segmentation on Pre-treatment MRI (2023). https://doi.org/10.48550/ARXIV.2306.00838
12. Ostrom, Q.T., et al.: CBTRUS statistical report: Primary brain and other central nervous system tumors diagnosed in the united states in 2015-2019. Neuro-Oncol. **24**(Supplement-5), v1–v95 (2022). ISSN 1523-5866. https://doi.org/10.1093/neuonc/noac202
13. Roth, H.R., et al.: NVIDIA FLARE: Federated learning from simulation to real-world (2022). https://doi.org/10.48550/arXiv.2210.13291
14. de Verdier, M.C., et al.: The 2024 Brain Tumor Segmentation (BraTS) Challenge: Glioma Segmentation on Post-treatment MRI (2024). https://arxiv.org/abs/2405.18368

Scaling High-Capacity ResUNet with Dynamic Batch for Universal Brain Tumor Segmentation

A BraTS 2025 "Generalizable to All Tumors" (GoAT) Challenge Solution

Meng-Yuan Chen[1] and Hsiang-Kuang Tony Liang[1,2,3,4](✉)

[1] Department of Biomedical Engineering, National Taiwan University, Taipei, Taiwan
[2] National Taiwan University Cancer Center, Taipei, Taiwan
[3] Department of Radiation Oncology, National Taiwan University Cancer Center Branch, National Taiwan University Hospital, Taipei, Taiwan
[4] Division of Radiation Oncology, Department of Oncology, National Taiwan University Hospital, Taipei, Taiwan
hkliang@ntu.edu.tw

Abstract. The vast heterogeneity of brain tumors—spanning patient populations, imaging acquisitions, and the fundamental biological differences between primary and metastatic disease—poses a significant obstacle to developing universal AI-based segmentation models. Addressing the MICCAI BraTS 2025 "Generalizability of Segmentation Methods Across Tumors" (GoAT) challenge, we developed a highly tailored framework within the nnU-Net v2 architecture. This features a deep, six-level residual encoder U-Net with a Focal Loss objective for complex features. Our core contribution is a novel dynamic batching strategy (3→2→1). This approach maximizes GPU memory utilization, enabling high-resolution training of our large-capacity model on a single consumer-grade GPU—obviating the need for multi-GPU compute clusters—while improving training efficiency and promoting generalization. After 5-fold cross-validation on the official training data (n=1,351), our model was evaluated on the blind validation set (n=451). Our solution achieved exceptional mean and median Dice scores of 0.8704 and 0.9367 (WT), 0.8542 and 0.9382 (TC), and 0.7759 and 0.8989 (ET), with a corresponding median 95th percentile Hausdorff Distance of 2.00 mm for the tumor core. These results validate our method's robust generalization across a wide spectrum of tumor morphologies and prove the power of strategic, resource-efficient training innovations in creating a single, clinically-relevant universal model.

Keywords: Multi-domain Generalization · Brain Tumor Segmentation · Brain MRI · Residual U-Net · nnU-Net v2 · Dynamic Batching · BraTS GoAT

S. Bakas et al. (Eds.): MICCAI 2025, LNCS 16376, pp. 489–499, 2026.
https://doi.org/10.1007/978-3-032-16365-3_44

1 Introduction

Brain tumors are not a single disease, but a series of pathological entities with high biological and clinical heterogeneity, with differences across age groups, anatomical locations, and cell origins [20]. These include highly invasive glioblastomas in adults, slowly progressing meningiomas, metastatic lesions from extracranial malignancies, and embryonal tumors such as medulloblastomas, which are common in pediatric populations [13,15,18]. Each type of tumor introduces different radiological characteristics, growth dynamics, and therapeutic plans. Accurate and consistent tumor segmentation is fundamental for neurooncologic management, as it informs diagnosis, guides treatment planning, and contributes critically to prognostic prediction.

Magnetic resonance imaging (MRI) remains the gold standard for the assessment of brain tumors [17]. In clinical practice, multimodal MRI—including native T1-weighted, contrast-enhanced T1-weighted (T1CE), T2-weighted, and fluid-attenuated inversion recovery (FLAIR) sequences—is routinely used to delineate tumor subregions such as the non-enhancing tumor core (NETC), surrounding FLAIR hyperintensity (SNFH), and enhancing tumor tissue (ET) [3,4]. While manual segmentation is widely adopted, it is inherently time-consuming and subject to inter- and intra-observer variability [20]. These limitations are further exacerbated when segmentation must generalize across tumor types and imaging protocols from different institutions.

In the past, most image segmentation models focused on well-classified diseases or groups such as adult gliomas. For example, segmentation models trained for adult gliomas usually have serious segmentation errors when applied to pediatric tumors or metastatic lesions [13,18]. However, in real-world clinical scenarios, medical institutions face gliomas, brain metastases, meningiomas, and pediatric brain tumors during diagnosis and treatment. There are multiple types of tumors. Patients may even come from different regions and ages, and may be diagnosed under different imaging protocols and medical cultures [1,13,15]. All these patients need correct diagnosis, statistical analysis of characteristics, prevalence, age distribution, overall survival, and biological behavior.

This study addresses these challenges by targeting the development of a robust segmentation model capable of performing reliably across multiple tumor types, patient populations, institutions, and imaging protocols [11,12]. As a participant in the MICCAI BraTS 2025 "Generality of Tumor Segmentation Methods" (GoAT) challenge, we propose a framework that seeks not only to optimize segmentation performance but also to enhance its adaptability to real-world clinical diversity. Specifically, we employ SynthStrip to perform robust skull stripping and image enhancement on heterogeneous MRI sequences [9], thereby reducing residual skull artifacts that may affect subsequent segmentation and improving the clarity of the training dataset. Building on nnU-Net v2's auto-configuration pipeline, we develop the `GoAT_ResEncTrainer_XL_Pro`, a deep six-level residual encoder U-Net that uses skip-connection blocks to alleviate gradient vanishing and accelerate convergence [2], enhance hierarchical feature learning for diffuse FLAIR abnormalities and small enhancing tumor cores [8]. To offset the severe class imbalance, we augment the standard Dice loss with Focal Loss to boost sensitivity to under-represented subregions such as enhancing tumor tissue [16]. Finally, we implement a dynamic batch scheduling strategy ($3 \rightarrow 2 \rightarrow 1$) that maximizes GPU memory utilization, enabling high-resolution volume training and further improving the generalization ability across centers and protocols. We believe that when artificial intelligence is designed to reflect the biological heterogeneity of tumors and the clinical complexity of patients, it evolves beyond being a technical instrument—it becomes a bridge toward more equitable, human-centered healthcare.

2 Methods

A core tenet of our methodological approach was to ensure the developed framework remains accessible and readily reproducible. To this end, all model development, training, and inference were conducted on a single workstation equipped with an NVIDIA RTX 5090 GPU, 32GB of VRAM, and 64GB system memory. Crucially, no high-performance computing (HPC) clusters, distributed multi-GPU configurations, or scalable cloud-based resources were required at any stage. This demonstrates that robust, generalizable brain tumor segmentation can be achieved efficiently on widely accessible, off-the-shelf hardware, thereby facilitating cost-effective and reproducible research even in resource-constrained environments.

2.1 Dataset Overview

This study leverages the official BraTS 2025 GoAT training dataset [7]—a uniquely comprehensive, multi-pathology, multi-ethnic, and multi-institutional MRI collection designed to challenge generalizability in brain tumor segmentation. The training cohort consists of 1,351 patients and encompasses 5,404 preoperative MRI scans across four canonical modalities per subject: native T1-weighted (T1), contrast-enhanced T1-weighted (T1CE), T2-weighted (T2), and fluid-attenuated inversion recovery (FLAIR), each accompanied by expert-annotated tumor segmentation masks serving as ground truth. Additionally, an official validation set comprising 451 cases (with withheld annotations) is provided for unbiased model evaluation. The scans have the shape $240 \times 240 \times 155$.

Crucially, this dataset is intentionally heterogeneous, capturing real-world complexity across major neuro-oncological entities and populations. The included pathologies encompass adult gliomas [3–6] (see Fig. 1ae for representative cases), cases from underrepresented sub-Saharan African cohorts (BraTS-SSA) [1] (see Fig. 1fj for representative cases), intracranial meningiomas (BraTS-MEN) [15] (see Fig. 1ko for representative cases), brain metastases (BraTS-MET) [18] (see Fig. 1pt for representative cases), and pediatric brain tumors (BraTS-PED) [13](see Fig. 1uy for representative cases). This design ensures rigorous assessment of algorithmic robustness across imaging domains, anatomical variations, and scanner types.

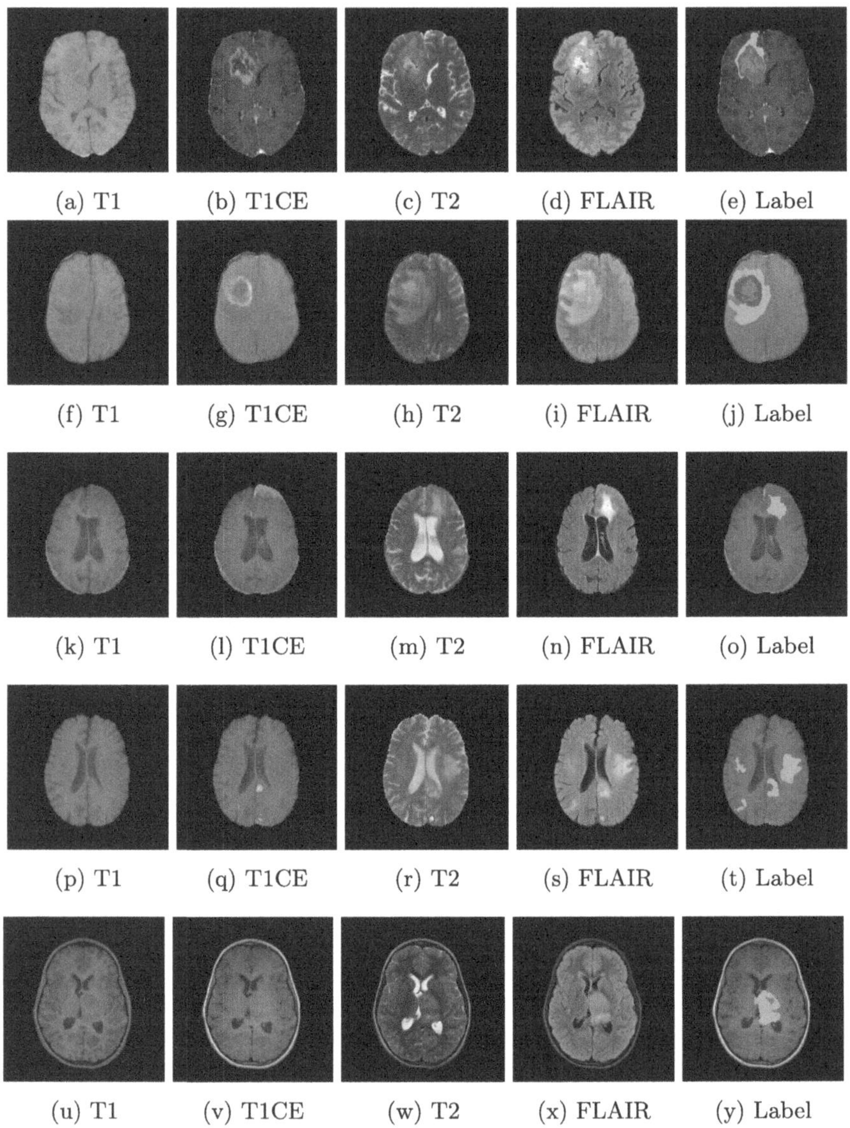

Fig. 1. Representative examples from the five tumor categories in BraTS 2025 GoAT. Each row shows one subject: T1, T1CE, T2, and FLAIR modalities, and segmentation mask on T1CE. Mask color code: red = necrosis (NCR, label 1), green = edema (ED, label 2), blue = enhancing tumor (ET, label 3). (ae) Adult gliomas; (fj) Sub-Saharan African gliomas; (ko) meningiomas; (pt) brain metastases; (uy) pediatric tumors. All data are from official BraTS 2025 training sets [1,3,4,7,13,15,18] (Color figure online).

Segmentation Labels and Definitions. Tumor regions are delineated according to BraTS convention, with voxel-wise ground truth labels as follows:

- **1 (NCR)**: Necrotic (non-enhancing) tumor core—hypointense on T1CE relative to T1.
- **2 (ED)**: Peritumoral edema or infiltrated tissue—typically hyperintense on FLAIR.
- **3 (ET)**: Enhancing tumor—hyperintense on T1CE versus both T1 and normal white matter.
- **0**: Background (non-tumor tissue).

The primary segmentation tasks target three clinically relevant subregions:

1. **Enhancing Tumor (ET):** Label 3.
2. **Tumor Core (TC):** Labels 1 and 3 (NCR + ET).
3. **Whole Tumor (WT):** Labels 1, 2, and 3 (NCR + ED + ET).

These definitions align with clinical radiology and surgical standards, enabling direct translation of segmentation outputs to neuro-oncologic workflows. For clarity, all segmentation masks in Fig. 1 are color-coded as follows: necrotic core in red, edema in green, and enhancing tumor in blue, as per BraTS guidelines.

2.2 Data Preprocessing and Harmonization

A fundamental step in our preprocessing pipeline is aggressive domain harmonization to mitigate variability stemming from multi-site data acquisition. We employed SynthStrip, a state-of-the-art, learning-based skull-stripping tool [9,14], to all 3D MRI volumes. Unlike traditional brain extraction methods, SynthStrip demonstrates robust performance across diverse MRI contrasts and resolutions, making it ideally suited for this multi-domain challenge. By removing all non-brain tissue and enhancing contrast and boundary accuracy, we standardized the input space and enforced that the model learns features intrinsic to the brain and tumor, without being confounded by scanner-specific artifacts or extracranial tissue heterogeneity.

Following skull stripping, all images were resampled to an isotropic resolution of 1 mm^3 and rigidly co-registered, resulting in enhanced anatomical alignment and improved boundary fidelity. Subsequent preprocessing steps followed the nnU-Net v2 ResEncXL default configuration, with intensity normalization (z-scoring) applied independently for each modality of cases, computed over foreground voxels within the brain mask. This comprehensive harmonization pipeline ensures that the model is exposed to standardized, artifact-minimized inputs, facilitating robust cross-domain learning.

2.3 Network Architecture: High-Capacity Residual Encoder U-Net

To address the high complexity and heterogeneity of the Generalist of All Tumors (GoAT) segmentation task, this study uses a high-capacity 3D Residual Encoder

U-Net (ResEncU-Net) architecture [19]. This design decision is based on the trend revealed in recent literature: deep extensions of mature convolutional neural network (CNN) architectures often achieve the best performance, or even surpass the former, compared to exploring new and complex network topologies [11].

Our network uses a six-layer deep encoder-decoder structure, which is designed to obtain a wide receptive field. This feature is crucial for accurately depicting the global context of large tumors and detecting distant multifocal lesions.

In the encoder path, we use ResNet-style residual blocks [8]. Each block consists of two sets of $3\times3\times3$ convolutional layers, instance normalization, and ReLU activation functions, and ends with a skip connection. This residual design aims to alleviate the vanishing gradient problem commonly seen in deep network training, thereby ensuring the trainability of deep structures. The initial number of feature maps of the network is set to 32, and is gradually doubled in six down-sampling stages, eventually reaching 1024 feature channels at the bottleneck of the network.

The symmetrical decoder path uses trilinear upsampling to restore spatial resolution layer by layer. At the same time, by introducing skip connections from the encoder path, high-resolution fine feature information is effectively passed to the decoder. To further enhance the efficiency of gradient propagation throughout the deep network, we follow the standard practice of nnU-Net [11] and introduce a deep supervision mechanism at the intermediate decoding level to ensure that each level can obtain effective learning signals.

2.4 Training Strategy

Our model was developed within the nnU-Net v2 framework [10,11], using a custom trainer, `GoAT_ResEncTrainer_XL_Pro`, to implement our specialized training strategy.

Loss Function. To address class imbalance, particularly for the enhancing tumor subregion, our training objective was a hybrid loss function. We combined the standard Dice and Cross-Entropy (CE) loss with Focal Loss [16], defined as:

$$L_{\text{total}} = L_{\text{DC\_CE}} + 0.5 \cdot L_{\text{Focal}} \quad (1)$$

The Focal Loss component down-weights well-classified examples, forcing the model to focus on harder-to-segment voxels at tumor boundaries.

Dynamic Batch and Patch Strategy. We used a large patch size of $160\times192\times160$ voxels to provide extensive context for the network. To manage GPU memory constraints with this patch size, we introduced a **dynamic batch size schedule**. Training began with a batch size of 3, which was reduced to 2 and then 1 in later epochs. This strategy optimizes training efficiency by allowing for faster learning in early stages while accommodating memory demands later on, without sacrificing the large patch size.

Implementation Details. The model was trained for 1000 epochs using a 5-fold cross-validation scheme on the 1351 training cases. We used the SGD optimizer with Nesterov momentum and a cosine learning rate schedule. Standard nnU-Net data augmentation techniques, including rotation, scaling, elastic deformation, and gamma correction, were applied on-the-fly. All training and inference were conducted on a single host with an NVIDIA RTX 5090 GPU (32GB VRAM), demonstrating the feasibility of our approach on common off-the-shelf hardware.

3 Results

Following a rigorous 5-fold cross validation process, our final model ensemble demonstrated robust and high-fidelity segmentation performance when evaluated on the official BraTS 2025 GoAT blind validation set.

3.1 Quantitative Performance on the Official Validation Set

The quantitative metrics detailed in Table 1 confirm the robust and high-fidelity segmentation capability of our model on the official validation set. Our model demonstrates excellent consistency and high accuracy across the majority of cases, achieving outstanding median Dice scores of 0.9367 (WT), 0.9382 (TC), and a notable 0.8989 for the challenging Enhancing Tumor (ET). This robust performance is further highlighted by the precise boundary delineation, with median 95th percentile Hausdorff Distances reaching an exceptional 2.00 mm for both TC and ET.

While the mean scores are presented for completeness (e.g., 0.8704 for WT Dice), the superior median results are a more robust indicator of the model's practical utility. This discrepancy suggests that a small subset of outlier cases with unique challenges disproportionately influences the mean, whereas the high median values confirm the model's successful and reliable performance on the vast majority of the heterogeneous validation cohort.

Table 1. Detailed quantitative results on the official BraTS 2025 GoAT validation set (n = 451).

Metric	Statistic	Whole Tumor	Tumor Core	Enhancing Tumor
Dice Score	Mean	0.8704	0.8542	0.7759
	Median	0.9367	0.9382	0.8989
	25–75 Quantile	[0.881, 0.964]	[0.869, 0.969]	[0.777, 0.960]
HD95 (mm)	Mean	18.7381	22.2147	29.2360
	Median	2.8284	2.0000	2.0000
	25–75 Quantile	[1.4142, 5.8735]	[1.000, 5.9161]	[1.000, 6.708]
NSD (1mm)	Mean	0.7840	0.7874	0.7786
	Median	0.8484	0.8946	0.9166
	25–75 Quantile	[0.6957, 0.9429]	[0.7089, 0.9763]	[0.7428, 0.9805]

3.2 Qualitative Analysis of Morphological Generalization

To visually demonstrate the model's ability to handle the vast morphological heterogeneity expected in a "generalist" task, Fig. 2 showcases its performance on several distinct tumor presentations from our cross-validation set. As illustrated by the direct comparison with ground truth, the model not only accurately delineates (a) a large, intra-axial mass with irregular, infiltrative margins and a complex necrotic core, but also effectively identifies and segments (b) challenging multifocal, sub-centimeter lesions, demonstrating its detection capabilities. Furthermore, it precisely outlines (c) a solitary, well-circumscribed mass with sharp borders, distinguishing it from adjacent tissues. This demonstrated capacity to handle varied tumor sizes, locations, numbers, and boundary characteristics underscores the model's strong generalization and real-world applicability.

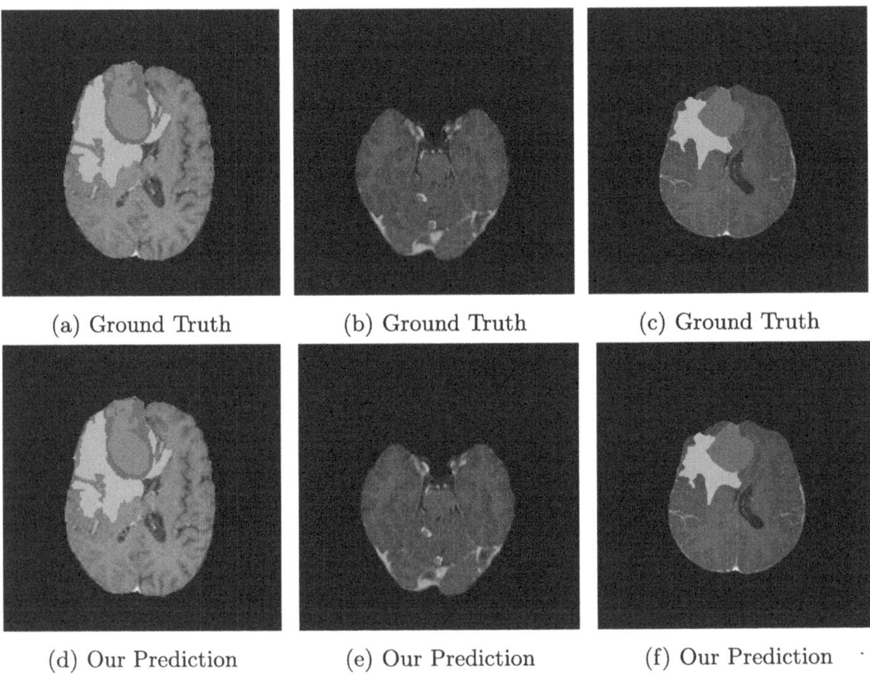

Fig. 2. Qualitative demonstration of the model's generalization across diverse tumor morphologies from the cross-validation set. The top row (a-c) displays the ground truth (GT), and the bottom row (d-f) our model's corresponding predictions. The cases represent three distinct radiological challenges: (a,d) a large, infiltrative intra-axial mass (case: `[BraTS-GoAT-00017]`); (b,e) multifocal, sub-centimeter lesions (case: `[BraTS-GoAT-00683]`); and (c,f) a solitary, well-circumscribed mass (case: `[BraTS-GoAT-02094]`). The model demonstrates high fidelity across these distinct challenges [7]. Image brightness and contrast have been linearly adjusted for display purposes.

3.3 Internal Validation and Model Stability

The model's development was guided by a rigorous 5-fold cross-validation on the training set (n = 1,351). The consistent performance across all folds, with a mean 3-class Dice score of 0.9561 (Table 2), and stable convergence of training and validation losses, confirm the robustness of our training strategy and the absence of significant overfitting.

Table 2. 5-Fold Cross-Validation Performance (VoxelWise) on the Training Set (n = 1351). Values are reported as mean.

Region	DSC
Enhancing Tumor (ET)	0.9386
Tumor Core (TC)	0.9639
Whole Tumor (WT)	0.9657
Average (3-class)	**0.9561**

4 Discussion

In this study, we demonstrated that a single, high-capacity model can achieve robust and generalizable segmentation performance across a highly diverse cohort of brain tumors. Our success builds on three key principles. First, leveraging a deep Residual Encoder U-Net [19] confirms that scaling proven CNN architectures is a powerful strategy for complex, multi-domain tasks, where a large receptive field is critical for handling varied tumor morphologies. Second, to make training this large model with a maximal patch size feasible on standard hardware, we introduced a novel dynamic batch scheduling strategy, a key contribution to improving training efficiency under memory constraints. Finally, aggressive data harmonization using SynthStrip provided a standardized input space, which was crucial for the model's ability to generalize across varied institutional and population-level imaging characteristics.

From a clinical perspective, such a "generalist" model offers substantial workflow advantages over maintaining multiple specialist algorithms. However, our analysis reveals a primary limitation and a clear direction for future work: a performance trade-off between large, infiltrative tumors and the detection of small, sub-centimeter metastatic lesions. Our Dice-centric loss function, while effective for volumetric overlap, deprioritizes tiny foci. Therefore, future work should focus on integrating detection-specific objectives (e.g., Focal loss variants or a dedicated detection branch) or exploring a cascaded detection-then-segmentation approach to improve small lesion recall. Furthermore, incorporating uncertainty estimation will be vital for building clinical trust and ensuring safe deployment. Looking forward, leveraging large-scale, pre-trained foundation models for neuroimaging may be the path toward a truly universal segmentation tool.

5 Conclusion

We presented a universal brain tumor segmentation framework based on a high-capacity ResEnc-UNet with a custom dynamic batching strategy. Our model achieved high-fidelity and robust performance on the diverse BraTS 2025 GoAT validation set. This work demonstrates the feasibility of creating a single, generalist model that can handle significant morphological and domain heterogeneity, representing a practical step towards more integrated and efficient AI tools in clinical neuro-oncology.

Acknowledgements. The authors thank the organizers of the BraTS 2025 Challenge, as well as the numerous institutions and researchers who contributed to the creation and curation of the underlying datasets. We also acknowledge helpful discussions in the challenge forum and support from our institutions high-performance computing center.

References

1. Adewole, M., et al.: The brain tumor segmentation (BraTS) challenge 2023: Glioma segmentation in Sub-Saharan Africa patient population (BraTS-Africa). arXiv preprint arXiv:2305.19369 (2023)
2. Alom, M.Z., Hasan, M., Yakopcic, C., Taha, T.M., Asari, V.K.: Recurrent residual convolutional neural network based on U-Net (R2U-Net) for medical image segmentation. arXiv preprint arXiv:1802.06955 (2018)
3. Baid, U., et al.: The RSNA-ASNR-MICCAI BraTS 2021 benchmark on brain tumor segmentation and radiogenomic classification. arXiv preprint arXiv:2107.02314 (2021)
4. Bakas, S., et al.: Advancing the cancer genome atlas glioma MRI collections with expert segmentation labels and radiomic features. Sci. Data **4**(1), 1–13 (2017)
5. Bakas, S., et al.: Segmentation labels and radiomic features for the pre-operative scans of the TCGA-GBM collection. The Cancer Imaging Archive (2017). https://doi.org/10.7937/K9/TCIA.2017.KLXWJJ1Q
6. Bakas, S., et al.: Segmentation labels and radiomic features for the pre-operative scans of the TCGA-LGG collection. The Cancer Imaging Archive (2017). https://doi.org/10.7937/K9/TCIA.2017.GJQ7R0EF
7. BraTS Challenge Organizers: MICCAI BraTS 2025 GoAT Challenge: Generalizability of Segmentation Methods Across Tumors. https://www.synapse.org/GoAT2025 (2025). Accessed 30 July 2025
8. He, K., Zhang, X., Ren, S., Sun, J.: Deep residual learning for image recognition. In: Proceedings of the IEEE Conference on Computer Vision and Pattern Recognition (CVPR), pp. 770–778 (2016)
9. Hoopes, A., Iglesias, J.E., Dalca, A.V., Fischl, B., Hoffmann, M.: SynthStrip: skull-stripping for any brain image. Neuroimage **260**, 119474 (2022). https://doi.org/10.1016/j.neuroimage.2022.119474
10. Isensee, F., Jaeger, P.F., Kohl, S.A., Petersen, J., Maier-Hein, K.H.: nnU-Net: a self-configuring method for deep learning-based biomedical image segmentation. Nat. Methods **18**(2), 203–211 (2021)

11. Isensee, F., Wald, T., et al.: nnU-Net revisited: a call for rigorous validation in 3D medical image segmentation. In: International Conference on Medical Image Computing and Computer-Assisted Intervention (MICCAI). Springer (2024)
12. Karargyris, A., Umeton, R., Sheller, M.J., et al.: Federated benchmarking of medical artificial intelligence with MedPerf. Nat. Mach. Intell. **5**(8), 799–810 (2023). https://doi.org/10.1038/s42256-023-00652-2
13. Kazerooni, A.F., et al.: BraTS-PEDs: Results of the multi-consortium international pediatric brain tumor segmentation challenge 2023. arXiv preprint arXiv:2404.15009 (2024)
14. Kelley, W.D., Ngo, N., Dalca, A., Fischl, B., Zöllei, L., Hoffmann, M.: Boosting skull-stripping performance for pediatric brain images. In: IEEE International Symposium on Biomedical Imaging (ISBI) (2024)
15. LaBella, D., et al.: The ASNR-MICCAI BraTS 2023 intracranial meningioma segmentation challenge. arXiv preprint arXiv:2305.07642 (2023)
16. Lin, T.Y., Goyal, P., Girshick, R., He, K., Dollár, P.: Focal loss for dense object detection. In: Proceedings of the IEEE International Conference on Computer Vision (ICCV), pp. 2980–2988 (2017)
17. Menze, B.H., et al.: The multimodal brain tumor image segmentation benchmark (BRATS). IEEE Trans. Med. Imaging **34**(10), 1993–2024 (2015)
18. Moawad, A.W., et al.: The BraTS-METS challenge 2023: Brain metastasis segmentation on pre-treatment MRI. arXiv preprint arXiv:2306.00838 (2023)
19. Ronneberger, O., Fischer, P., Brox, T.: U-Net: convolutional networks for biomedical image segmentation. In: International Conference on Medical Image Computing and Computer-Assisted Intervention (MICCAI), pp. 234–241. Springer (2015)
20. Sollmann, N., et al.: A review of deep learning for brain tumor analysis in MRI. NPJ Precis. Oncol. **8**(1), 59 (2024)

Towards Label-Free Brain Tumor Segmentation: Unsupervised Learning with Multimodal MRI

Gerard Comas-Quiles[1](✉), Carles Garcia-Cabrera[2,4], Julia Dietlmeier[3,4], Noel E. O'Connor[3,4], and Ferran Marques[1]

[1] Universitat Politècnica de Catalunya (UPC), Barcelona, Spain
gerard.comas@estudiantat.upc.edu
[2] University College Dublin (UCD), Dublin, Ireland
[3] Dublin City University (DCU), Dublin, Ireland
[4] Insight Research Ireland Center For Data Analytics, Dublin, Ireland

Abstract. Unsupervised anomaly detection (UAD) presents a complementary alternative to supervised learning for brain tumor segmentation in magnetic resonance imaging (MRI), particularly when annotated datasets are limited, costly, or inconsistent. In this work, we propose a novel Multimodal Vision Transformer Autoencoder (MViT-AE) trained exclusively on healthy brain MRIs to detect and localize tumors via reconstruction-based error maps. This unsupervised paradigm enables segmentation without reliance on manual labels, addressing a key scalability bottleneck in neuroimaging workflows. Our method is evaluated in the BraTS-GoAT 2025 Lighthouse dataset, which includes various types of tumors such as gliomas, meningiomas, and pediatric brain tumors. To enhance performance, we introduce a multimodal early-late fusion strategy that leverages complementary information across multiple MRI sequences, and a post-processing pipeline that integrates the Segment Anything Model (SAM) to refine predicted tumor contours. Despite the known challenges of UAD, particularly in detecting small or non-enhancing lesions, our method achieves clinically meaningful tumor localization, with lesion-wise Dice Similarity Coefficient of 0.437 (Whole Tumor), 0.316 (Tumor Core), and 0.350 (Enhancing Tumor) on the test set, and an anomaly Detection Rate of 89.4% on the validation set. These findings highlight the potential of transformer-based unsupervised models to serve as scalable, label-efficient tools for neuro-oncological imaging. The code for this project will be publicly available on GitHub.

Keywords: Autoencoder · Brain Tumor Segmentation · Multimodal · Segment Anything Model · Unsupervised Anomaly Detection · Vision Transformer

1 Introduction

Advancements in medical imaging, particularly magnetic resonance imaging (MRI), have significantly improved the early detection and characterization of

S. Bakas et al. (Eds.): MICCAI 2025, LNCS 16376, pp. 500–511, 2026.
https://doi.org/10.1007/978-3-032-16365-3_45

brain tumors. However, interpreting MRI scans remains a labor-intensive and error-prone process. Studies report that 5–10% of neuroimaging interpretations may overlook critical abnormalities [1,2], underscoring the need for robust and automated diagnostic tools that can support human interpretation.

The Brain Tumor Segmentation (BraTS) Challenge [3,4] has played a central role in advancing brain tumor segmentation techniques, particularly for gliomas. Since its inception in 2012, BraTS has progressively expanded to include additional tumor types and imaging modalities, and to increase clinical relevance. Supervised deep learning methods—especially U-Net architectures [5], 3D CNNs [6], and more recently, transformer-based models [7,8]—have achieved state-of-the-art performance when trained on large, annotated datasets.

Despite these advancements, reliance on manual annotations poses significant limitations in real-world clinical settings. Annotation is not only time-consuming and costly, but also susceptible to inter-observer variability [9], particularly across institutions. These challenges become even more pronounced when dealing with a small number of lesions [10], such as rare tumor types or low-resource environments.

To move beyond models limited to detecting only specific tumor types, the BraTS challenge encouraged research into generalization methods [11]. However, no submissions adopted fully unsupervised learning, underscoring both the technical challenges and the unexplored potential of unsupervised anomaly detection (UAD) in brain tumor segmentation.

In this work, we propose a fully unsupervised brain tumor segmentation pipeline designed for the BraTS Generalizability Across Tumors (GoAT) 2025 challenge. Our method combines a multimodal Vision Transformer Autoencoder (MViT-AE) with a novel postprocessing stage based on the Segment Anything Model (SAM) [12]. The model is trained solely on healthy brain MRIs to learn priors of normal anatomy. During inference, reconstruction errors reveal anomalous regions such as tumors, which are then refined into segmentation masks using morphological operations and SAM-based region proposals.

An overview of the proposed pipeline is shown in Fig. 1, consisting of three stages: multimodal fusion and preprocessing, transformer-based image reconstruction, and SAM-guided postprocessing.

1.1 Related Work

UAD has emerged as a promising strategy for medical image analysis in data-scarce settings. Traditional approaches rely on convolutional autoencoders trained to reconstruct healthy anatomical structures, flagging abnormalities via high reconstruction error [13]. However, these models often suffer from blurry outputs and poor localization.

Variational autoencoders (VAEs) introduced probabilistic modeling to capture latent uncertainty [14], but their reconstructions lack structural detail, limiting segmentation accuracy. Extensions using perceptual losses, adversarial training [15], or memory modules [16] have sought to improve anomaly saliency and boundary sharpness.

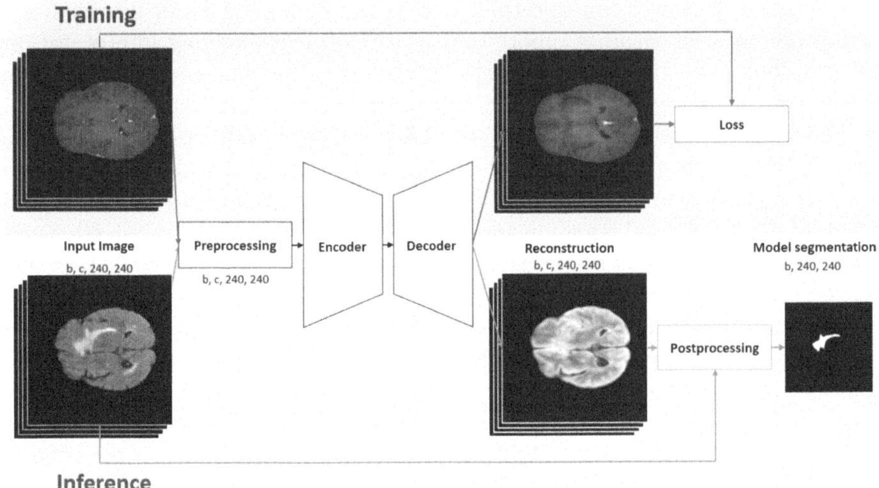

Fig. 1. Overview of the proposed Unsupervised Anomaly Segmentation pipeline, comprising preprocessing, transformer-based reconstruction, and SAM-guided postprocessing. Multimodal MRI slices are used to learn healthy anatomical priors, and reconstruction deviations are used to infer tumor regions.

More recent UAD research has focused on learning disentangled representations through contrastive techniques [17], enabling separation of normal and abnormal features in latent space. These approaches often leverage structural similarity (SSIM) or learned feature distances as anomaly scores.

Despite these efforts, most prior work uses CNN backbones with limited receptive fields, hindering global context modeling. Transformer-based architectures, such as UNETR [7] and TransUNet [8], have demonstrated success in supervised segmentation, but remain largely unexplored in the unsupervised setting.

1.2 Contributions

This paper presents the first fully unsupervised segmentation pipeline evaluated in the BraTS-GoAT setting. Our main contributions include:

- **Multimodal Vision Transformer Autoencoder (MViT-AE):** We introduce a transformer-based autoencoder capable of learning global contextual representations from fused multimodal MRI slices. This addresses the spatial limitations of prior convolutional UAD models and improves reconstruction fidelity.
- **Novel earlyâĂŞlate fusion strategy:** We stack all four MRI modalities as input channels and later, after postprocessing, fuse T1c with T2f to exploit their complementary information, leading to more consistent and robust feature representations.

- **SAM-based postprocessing:** We incorporate SAM into the anomaly detection pipeline to transform coarse reconstruction error maps into high-quality segmentation masks. While semi-supervised SAM extensions (e.g., SemiSAM for heart MRI [18]) have been explored, to the best of our knowledge, this is the first application of SAM in an unsupervised medical segmentation setting.

2 Methods

All experiments were conducted on a workstation equipped with an Intel Core i9-9900K CPU @ 3.80 GHz, 64 GB of RAM, and a NVIDIA GTX 2080 Ti GPU, using the PyTorch framework.

2.1 Data

We used the BraTS-GoAT 2025 dataset, which integrates multiple BraTS challenges to enable evaluation of cross-tumor generalization. The training set includes adult gliomas [19–23], meningiomas [24], and brain metastases [25]. The validation set extends this with additional cohorts, namely gliomas from Sub-Saharan Africa [26] and pediatric brain tumors [27]. The test set composition is not disclosed by the organizers to ensure unbiased evaluation. Each case consists of four mpMRI modalities (T1c, T1n, T2f, T2w) with expert annotations in NIfTI format. The training set consists of 1,352 multiparametric MRI volumes (mpMRI), each containing four modalities (T1c, T1n, T2f, and T2w), with corresponding expert annotations in NIfTI format. Since unsupervised learning requires training on images without anomalies, each volume was split into two pseudo-volumes: one containing slices with anomalies (used for internal validation) and the other containing only healthy brain slices (used for training). This resulted in a training set of 98,354 2D images, each of size 240×240 pixels.

Preprocessing is critical for consistent model learning. MRI intensity values vary widely due to acquisition conditions and lack an absolute physical meaning. We applied z-score normalization on a per-volume basis to standardize intensities while preserving the original distribution, ensuring anomalies remain visible during training.

2.2 Model

Our model, MViT-AE, is based on a 2D Vision Transformer Autoencoder originally designed for unsupervised anomaly detection in industrial images [28]. We retain the ViT encoder, adapting it to handle mpMRI inputs, and use a custom decoder consisting of 6 convolutional layers.

As shown in Fig. 2, each modality is split into 24×24 patches, which are concatenated along the channel dimension, resulting in input vectors of size $24 \times 24 \times 4$. Each patch is flattened into a 576-dimensional vector and projected into a 512-dimensional embedding. Positional embeddings preserve spatial context. The sequence of patch embeddings passes through a Transformer encoder with 6 layers, each having 8 attention heads and a feed-forward network with 1024 hidden units. The encoder output is compressed via a fully connected fusion layer (MLP) into a 512-dimensional latent vector. The decoder reshapes this vector into an $(8, 8, 8)$ feature map and progressively upsamples spatial dimensions while reducing channels to reconstruct all four modalities, producing outputs that match the input size. The model contains approximately 40.7 million parameters.

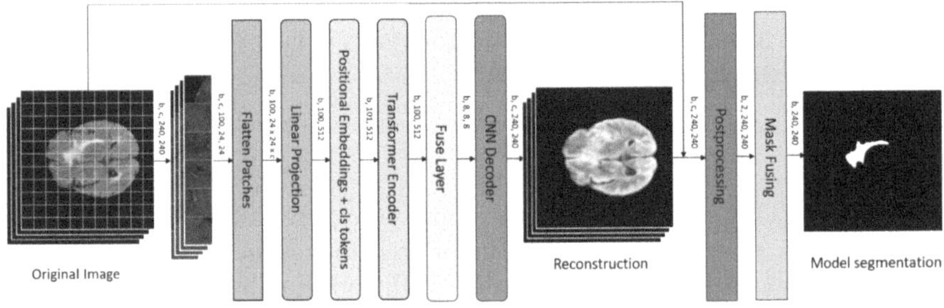

Fig. 2. Overview of the Multimodal ViT-AE (MViT-AE) architecture. The encoder processes multiple input modalities through transformer layers, followed by a fusion layer. The decoder reconstructs each modality, and postprocessing with fusion masking is used to generate the final segmentation.

2.3 Training

We trained the model using the Adam optimizer with a fixed learning rate of 0.0001 and a weight decay of 0.0001, batch size of 32, for 100 epochs. We did not use a learning rate scheduler, data augmentation, or early stopping. The model checkpoint was saved only when the validation loss improved to keep the best-performing version. Future work could focus on hyperparameter tuning to enhance results.

The loss function combines Mean Squared Error (MSE) and Structural Similarity Index Measure (SSIM) losses:

$$L = L_{Rec} + \alpha L_{SSIM},$$

where $L_{SSIM} = 1 - \text{SSIM}(x, \hat{x})$, and $\alpha = 100$ was chosen empirically to balance the contributions of both losses effectively.

Gaussian noise (mean=0, std=0.2) was added during training to improve robustness and encourage the model to learn stable features by simulating subtle variations.

2.4 Postprocessing

Since the model produces reconstructed images rather than direct segmentations, postprocessing is essential for accurate tumor delineation.

We compute residual maps by subtracting the reconstructed images from the originals, using the signed difference to focus on hyperintense, poorly reconstructed areas, which reduces noise compared to absolute differences [13].

The postprocessing steps (Fig. 3) include:

1. **Thresholding**: We set the threshold to the maximum between 20% of the highest residual value and a fixed value of 1.2. This balances adaptability and robustness, and was empirically chosen to optimize validation metrics.
2. **Binarization**: Using Otsu's automatic thresholding method [29], we convert the thresholded residual map into a binary segmentation mask, separating tumor from non-tumor regions.
3. **Removal of small objects**: To reduce false positives caused by small, isolated noise regions, we apply a morphological opening and closing with structure element of size 1.
4. **3D Connected components**: Because tumors typically form contiguous structures in 3D, we identify connected components in the full volume and keep only the largest one, which is most likely the true tumor, discarding smaller irrelevant regions.
5. **Refinement with SAM (Segment Anything Model)**: To further improve segmentation quality, we refine the initial segmentation mask using SAM, a powerful general-purpose segmentation model. SAM is capable of producing high-quality object masks from various prompts such as points, bounding boxes, or coarse masks.

As shown in Fig. 4, applying SAM directly to MRI slices without any guidance results in segmentations that lack medical relevance and fail to accurately capture tumor regions. To address this, we use the initial segmentation mask to generate prompts for SAM:

- We compute a tight bounding box enclosing the predicted tumor region.
- We randomly sample five foreground points from within this region.
- These prompts, consisting of a bounding box and foreground points, are provided to SAM to guide the segmentation.

We accept SAM's refined mask only if it achieves a confidence score above 90%; otherwise, we retry with new points up to three times before falling back to the original mask. This approach leverages SAM's strengths to produce smoother, more accurate boundaries and reduce noise artifacts.

2.5 Mask Fusing

Each MRI modality produces its own reconstruction and residual map. After post-processing each modality independently, T1c-based segmentation identifies

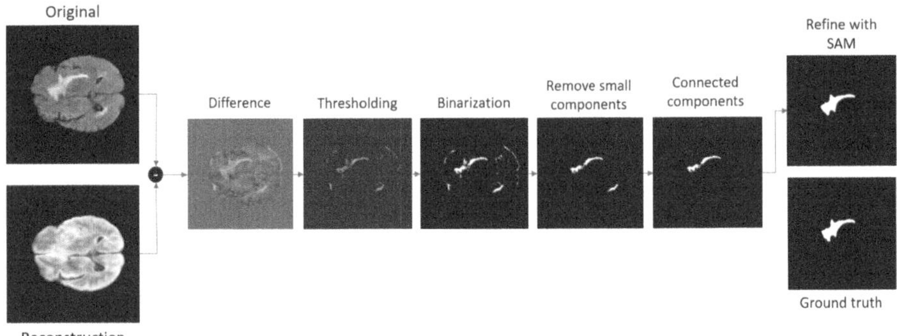

Fig. 3. Postprocessing pipeline: The original and reconstructed images are subtracted to highlight differences. After thresholding and binarization, small irrelevant regions are removed. A 3D connected component algorithm selects the largest region, which is then refined using the Segment Anything Model (SAM) for improved segmentation accuracy.

the Enhancing Tumor (ET), while the difference between T2f and T1c segmentations outlines the Surrounding Non-Enhancing FLAIR Hyperintensity (SNFH) region. Any holes or gaps within the tumor area—regions not classified as either ET or SNFH—are assumed to be Non-Enhancing Tumor (NET). This approach allows us to segment all three main tumor subregions without any manual labels, demonstrating the power of multimodal fusion. To our knowledge, no previous unsupervised method has achieved this level of subregion segmentation.

3 Results

3.1 Quantitative Results

The following quantitative results are based on the validation set from the BraTS-GoAT 2025 challenge, which includes 451 mpMRI volumes. We processed the complete volumes without cropping or patching, but using the same preprocessing as the training dataset.

We evaluated segmentation performance using a lesion-wise Dice Similarity Coefficient (DSC), focusing on five BraTS tumor subregions: ET, NET, SNFH, Tumor Core (ET + NET = TC), and Whole Tumor (TC + SNFH = WT). In addition to DSC, we report the Detection Rate (DR), which measures how often the model detects any part of the tumor. Specifically, DR is computed as the number of cases where the DSC for the WT is greater than zero, divided by the total number of cases.

Table 1 shows the metrics for our model, MViT-AE, both with and without SAM refinement.

Overall, the original MViT-AE model without SAM performed better for most DSC scores. The only exception was the SNFH, where the SAM-refined model scored higher, improving from 0.473 to 0.524.

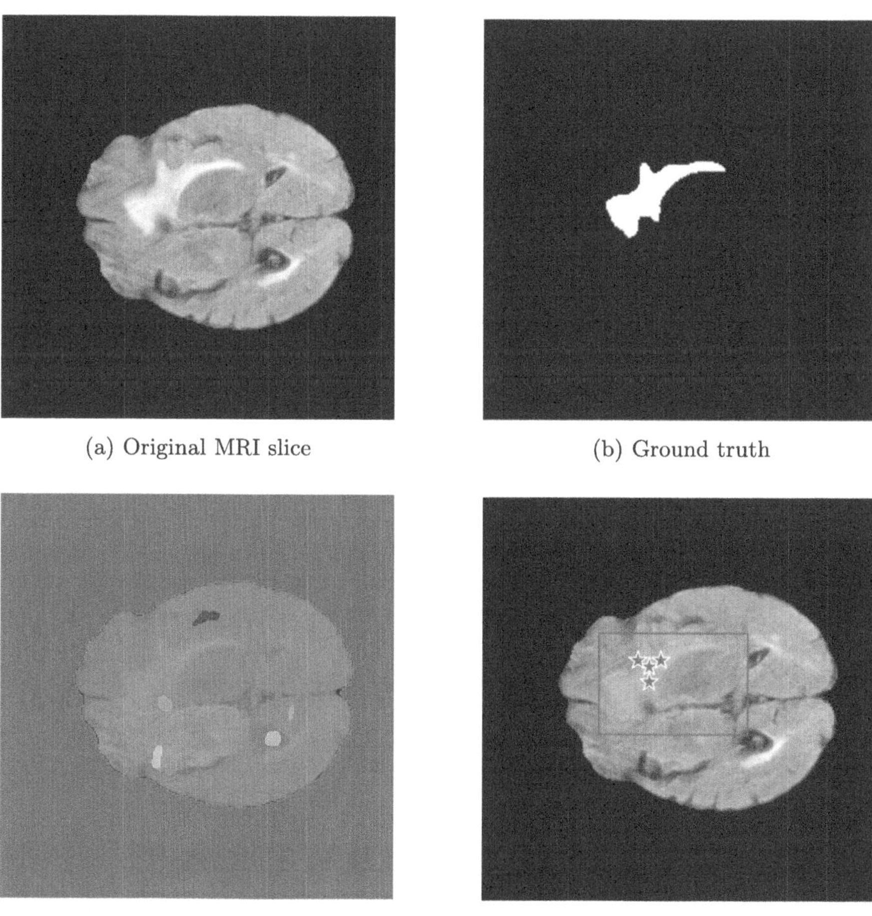

(a) Original MRI slice

(b) Ground truth

(c) Initial SAM segmentation

(d) Prompt SAM segmentation mask

Fig. 4. Comparison of segmentation stages using the Segment Anything Model (SAM). (a) Original MRI slice. (b) Ground truth mask showing the expert-annotated tumor. (c) Initial SAM segmentation without prompts, showing poor accuracy. (d) Refined SAM segmentation using bounding box and point prompts, with clearer tumor boundaries.

Regarding DR, both models show very similar results: 89.4% for MViT-AE and 89.1% for MViT-AE + SAM. This similarity is expected, as the SAM module refines the segmentation mask generated by MViT-AE, but does not introduce new detections i.e. it improves the shape or boundaries of existing masks, but cannot recover tumors missed by the initial model.

These results suggest that while SAM may enhance the segmentation quality in certain regions (e.g., SNFH), it does not consistently improve overall performance and may even degrade it in more localized tumor subregions.

On the independent test set, MViT-AE achieved lesion-wise DSCs of 0.437 (WT), 0.316 (TC), and 0.350 (ET), surpassing validation results and demon-

Table 1. Lesion-wise DSC and DR of MViT-AE With and Without SAM Refinement

Method	DSC ET	DSC NET	DSC SNFH	DSC TC	DSC WT	DR %
MViT-AE	0.289	0.088	0.473	0.279	0.422	89.4
MViT-AE + SAM	0.204	0.082	0.524	0.231	0.371	89.1

strating good generalization to unseen data, despite the undisclosed test set composition.

3.2 Qualitative Results

In this section, we present qualitative examples to better understand how the model leverages the different MRI modalities for tumor detection, and how the SAM optimization helps refine the segmentation.

The results in Fig. 5 highlight the complementary nature of the modalities. In the column corresponding to the T1c-only model, ET (**blue**) core is clearly visible, but SNFH (green) is largely missed. In contrast, the T2f-only model captures SNFH region well, but is less effective at identifying the enhancing part of the tumor. When both modalities are combined, the resulting segmentation benefits from the strengths of each. This fusion results in a more complete and accurate tumor representation.

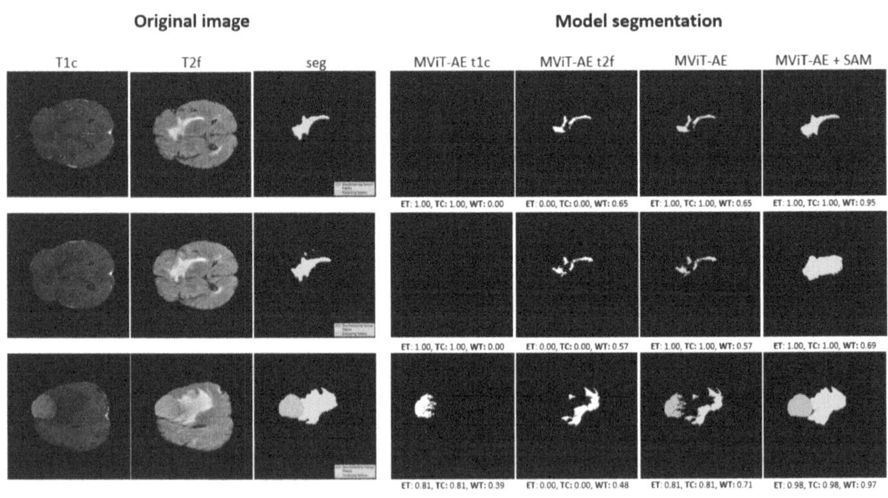

Fig. 5. Qualitative segmentation results for volume 00018 from the BraTS-MEN 2023 dataset. The first three columns show the original input modalities (T1c, T2f) and the ground truth. The following four columns present the outputs of different model branches: MViT-AE with only T1c, only T2f, both combined, and the combination refined using SAM. Each row corresponds to a different slice from the same volume.

Finally, the last column shows the results after applying SAM for post-processing. We observe that the segmentation becomes more anatomically consistent, with smoother boundaries and less pixel-level noise. This refinement significantly improves the visual quality and realism of the predicted masks. However, SAM can occasionally introduce false positives, as seen in the second row, where a part of the brain is mistakenly segmented as tumor.

4 Discussion and Conclusion

We presented an unsupervised brain tumor segmentation pipeline based on MViT-AE, trained exclusively on healthy brain MRI scans. By leveraging reconstruction errors and refining the outputs with SAM, the method localizes tumors without requiring manual annotations.

Our best model achieved a Detection Rate of 89.4%. Most missed cases involved hypointense tumors in T1c, suggesting a need for improved sensitivity to such patterns. While performance remains below state-of-the-art supervised methods, results highlight the promise of unsupervised anomaly detection for this task.

A key limitation is the postprocessing step, which retains only the largest 3D component. This restricts outputs to a single segmentation per volume and negatively impacts lesion-wise metrics when multiple anomalies are present. Another limitation arises from the use of SAM: it refines accurate masks by capturing fine details (e.g., in SNFH regions) but can amplify errors when the initial mask is poor (e.g., in ET regions).

Despite these challenges, the approach reduces reliance on costly labeled datasets and shows potential to generalize across tumor types and imaging protocols. Clinically, it could assist radiologists by flagging suspicious regions, especially in data-scarce settings.

Future work will focus on increasing sensitivity to subtle anomalies, integrating additional imaging sequences, improving computational efficiency, and exploring semi-supervised fine-tuning. Further validation on healthy control datasets and more interpretable outputs will also be essential for clinical translation.

Acknowledgments. We acknowledge the CFIS Mobility Program for the partial funding of this research work, particularly Fundació Privada Mir-Puig, CFIS partners, and donors of the crowdfunding program. This publication has emanated from research conducted with the financial support of Research Ireland under Grant number 12/RC/2289_P2.

References

1. Kim, Y.W., Mansfield, L.T.: Fool me twice: Delayed diagnoses in radiology with emphasis on perpetuated errors. Am. J. Roentgenol., **202**(3), 465–470 (2014). https://doi.org/10.2214/AJR.13.11493. PMID: 24555582

2. Bruno, M.A., Walker, E.A., Abujudeh, H.H.: Understanding and confronting our mistakes: the epidemiology of error in radiology and strategies for error reduction. In: RadioGraphics. vol. 35, no. 6, pp. 1668–1676 (2015). https://doi.org/10.1148/rg.2015150023. PMID: 26466178
3. Menze, B.H., Jakab, A., et al.: The multimodal brain tumor image segmentation benchmark (brats). IEEE Trans. Med. Imaging (2015)
4. Bakas, S., et al.: Advancing the cancer genome atlas glioma MRI collections with expert segmentation labels and radiomic features. Sci. Data (2017)
5. Ronneberger, O., Fischer, P., Brox, T.: U-net: convolutional networks for biomedical image segmentation. MICCAI (2015)
6. Isensee, F., Jaeger, P.F., Kohl, S.A., Petersen, J., Maier-Hein, K.H.: NNU-net: a self-configuring method for deep learning-based biomedical image segmentation. Nat. Methods (2021)
7. Kim, J.W., Khan, A.U., Banerjee, I., et al.: Unetr: transformers for 3d medical image segmentation. CVPR (2022)
8. Chen, J., Lu, Y., Yu, Q., et al.: Transunet: transformers make strong encoders for medical image segmentation. In: MICCAI (2021)
9. de Sutter, S., et al.: Interobserver ground-truth variability limits performance of automated glioblastoma segmentation on [f]fet pet. EJNMMI Phys. **12**, 06 (2025). https://doi.org/10.1186/s40658-025-00767-y
10. van der Loo, I., Bucho, T.M.T., Hanley, J.A., Beets-Tan, R.G., Imholz, A.L., Trebeschi, S.: Measurement variability of radiologists when measuring brain tumors. European J. Radiol. **183**, 111874 (2025). https://doi.org/10.1016/j.ejrad.2024.111874, https://www.sciencedirect.com/science/article/pii/S0720048X24005904
11. Bakas, S., et al.: The 2023 brats challenge: multi-institutional analysis of brain tumor segmentation and generalization. arXiv preprint arXiv:2309.07347 (2023)
12. Kirillov, A., Mintun, E., Ravi, N., et al.: Segment anything. arXiv preprint arXiv:2304.02643 (2023)
13. Baur, C., Denner, S., Wiestler, B., Navab, N., Albarqouni, S.: Autoencoders for unsupervised anomaly segmentation in brain MR images: a comparative study. Med. Image Anal. (2021)
14. Zimmerer, D., Kohl, S.A., Petersen, J., Isensee, F., Maier-Hein, K.H.: Context-encoding variational autoencoder for unsupervised anomaly detection. In: MICCAI (2019)
15. Xi, C., Ender, K.: Unsupervised detection of lesions in brain MRI using constrained adversarial auto-encoders. MedIA (2018)
16. Venkataramanan, S., Peng, K.C., Singh, R.V., Mahalanobis, A.: Attention guided anomaly localization in images (2020). https://arxiv.org/abs/1911.08616
17. Wijanarko, H., Calista, E., Chen, L.F., Chen, Y.S.: Tri-vae: Triplet variational autoencoder for unsupervised anomaly detection in brain tumor MRI. In: 2024 IEEE/CVF Conference on Computer Vision and Pattern Recognition Workshops (CVPRW), pp. 3930–3939 (2024). https://doi.org/10.1109/CVPRW63382.2024.00397
18. Zhang, Y., Yang, J., Liu, Y., Cheng, Y., Qi, Y.: Semisam: enhancing semi-supervised medical image segmentation via SAM-assisted consistency regularization (2024). https://arxiv.org/abs/2312.06316
19. Menze, B., et al.: The multimodal brain tumor image segmentation benchmark (brats). IEEE Trans. Med. Imaging **99**, 12 (2014). https://doi.org/10.1109/TMI.2014.2377694

20. Bakas, S., et al.: Advancing the cancer genome atlas glioma MRI collections with expert segmentation labels and radiomic features. Sci. Data, **4** (2017). https://doi.org/10.1038/sdata.2017.117
21. Bakas, S., Akbari, H., Sotiras, A., Bilello, M., Rozycki, M., Kirby, J., et al.: Segmentation labels and radiomic features for the pre-operative scans of the TCGA-GBM collection. Cancer Imaging Archive (2017)
22. Bakas, S., Akbari, H., Sotiras, A., Bilello, M., Rozycki, M., Kirby, J., et al.: Segmentation labels and radiomic features for the pre-operative scans of the TCGA-LGG collection. Cancer Imaging Archive (2017)
23. Baid, U., et al.: The rsna-asnr-miccai brats 2021 benchmark on brain tumor segmentation and radiogenomic classification (2021). https://arxiv.org/abs/2107.02314
24. LaBella, D., et al.: The ASNR-MICCAI brain tumor segmentation (brats) challenge 2023: intracranial meningioma (2023). https://arxiv.org/abs/2305.07642
25. Moawad, A.W., et al.: The brain tumor segmentation (brats-mets) challenge 2023: brain metastasis segmentation on pre-treatment MRI (2024). https://arxiv.org/abs/2306.00838
26. Adewole, M., et al.: The brain tumor segmentation (brats) challenge 2023: glioma segmentation in sub-saharan africa patient population (brats-africa) (2023). https://arxiv.org/abs/2305.19369
27. Kazerooni, A.F., et al.: The brain tumor segmentation (brats) challenge 2023: Focus on pediatrics (cbtn-connect-dipgr-asnr-miccai brats-peds) (2024). https://arxiv.org/abs/2305.17033
28. Mishra, P., Verk, R., Fornasier, D., Piciarelli, C., Foresti, G.L.: VT-ADL: a vision transformer network for image anomaly detection and localization. In: 2021 IEEE 30th International Symposium on Industrial Electronics (ISIE), pp. 01–06. IEEE (2021). https://doi.org/10.1109/isie45552.2021.9576231
29. Otsu, N.: A threshold selection method from gray-level histograms. IEEE Trans. Syst. Man Cybern. **1**, 62–66 (1979). https://doi.org/10.1109/TSMC.1979.4310076

ADMFNet: Enhancing Cross-Tumor Generalization in Multi-Modal MRI Segmentation

Hongjuan Wang, Yixin Zhang, Jindong Sun(✉), Xinjun An, Liying Zhu, and Chunyao Li

College of Intelligent Equipment, Shandong University of Science and Technology, Taian, China
jdsun@sdust.edu.cn

Abstract. To address the challenge of generalizing brain tumor segmentation across diverse tumor types, the BraTS 2025 Challenge introduced the Generalizability Across Tumors (GoAT) task, focusing on robustness under distribution shifts. In response, we propose ADMFNet (Adaptively Modulated DMF Network), a novel 3D segmentation network designed to enhance cross-distribution performance in multimodal MRI.

ADMFNet features a multi-scale encoder-decoder architecture based on dilated convolutional units (DMFUnit) and incorporates a lightweight Adaptation Module to reduce feature mismatch between encoder and decoder stages, improving cross-modal fusion. The model is trained on the BraTS-GoAT dataset, which includes four MRI modalities: T1n, T1c, T2f, and T2w. Ground truth follows BraTS annotation standards, and training uses class-balanced Generalized Dice Loss.

On the GoAT testing set, ADMFNet achieves Dice scores of 0.696 (WT), 0.744 (TC), and 0.717 (ET), with corresponding NSD (1.0 mm) values of 0.616, 0.708, and 0.732. The model shows excellent performance on clearly defined regions such as edema and radiation cavities (Dice = 1.000), and maintains solid results on challenging areas including non-enhancing tumor cores and cystic components.

Keywords: Brain tumor segmentation · Generalization · Multimodal MRI · Deep learning · BraTS 2025 Challenge

1 Introduction

In recent years, automatic brain tumor segmentation has become a pivotal area in computer-aided diagnosis, personalized treatment planning, and intraoperative navigation. Multimodal MRI-based methods, leveraging MRI's superior soft-tissue contrast, are widely used for tumor detection and assessment. However, the heterogeneity of brain tumors in spatial morphology, histological characteristics, and biological behavior poses challenges to conventional segmentation algorithms, particularly in generalization across patients, tumor types, and imaging devices.

S. Bakas et al. (Eds.): MICCAI 2025, LNCS 16376, pp. 512–523, 2026.
https://doi.org/10.1007/978-3-032-16365-3_46

Deep learning approaches, especially encoder-decoder architectures like U-Net [1], have revolutionized medical image segmentation. Yet, as applications extend to multi-center settings with heterogeneous diseases, generalization and robustness issues emerge. Traditional U-Net models, relying on skip connections for feature fusion, often suffer from semantic discrepancies between shallow and deep features, leading to feature transmission mismatch and degraded performance. To address this, techniques such as channel attention modules [2] and transformation layers [3] have been introduced to optimize cross-layer fusion.

Domain shifts due to variations in imaging devices, acquisition protocols, disease distributions, or patient characteristics further hinder model performance in unseen environments. To tackle this, domain generalization techniques like invariant feature learning [4], adversarial training [5], and meta-learning [6], as well as domain adaptation methods like feature alignment and style transfer [7], have gained traction. For multimodal MRI, methods incorporating feature enhancement and cross-modal consistency constraints [8] show promise in addressing challenges like BraTS.

The BraTS Challenge [9] has standardized evaluation protocols and driven advancements in model generalization. The newly introduced GoAT task in BraTS 2025 emphasizes segmentation under distribution shifts, requiring algorithms to consistently identify tumor subregions across diverse tumor types and imaging protocols, demanding better feature representation and domain adaptation.

To address the scale variability and heterogeneity of brain tumors, multi-scale feature extraction and fusion mechanisms have proven effective. Approaches such as multi-scale convolutions, atrous convolutions, and feature pyramid networks [10] enable models to capture both local details and global context, enhancing segmentation accuracy and adaptability.

Despite the success of encoder-decoder networks on large-scale medical imaging datasets, two critical challenges persist: (1) semantic mismatch between encoder and decoder features, impairing information flow; (2) limited feature adaptation mechanisms for cross-distribution environments, restricting universal representation learning.

To overcome these challenges, we propose ADMFNet (Adaptively Modulated DMF Network), a novel 3D medical image segmentation network. Building on DMFNet's multi-scale feature extraction [11], ADMFNet introduces a lightweight Adaptation Module to mitigate encoder-decoder feature mismatch. Using bottleneck-style channel transformation and nonlinear activation, the module enhances feature consistency and model generalization while maintaining computational efficiency.

ADMFNet was systematically evaluated on the BraTS-GoAT multimodal MRI dataset [12–28]. Results show competitive segmentation performance across major tumor subregions and superior robustness in cross-distribution generalization, providing an effective solution for multimodal medical image segmentation.

2 Method

2.1 Overview

To address the brain tumor segmentation task of the BraTS 2025 dataset, we propose an enhanced 3D deep learning framework—the Adaptively Modulated DMF Network (ADMFNet). This framework integrates robust data preprocessing, a novel network architecture featuring an adaptation module, and a class-balanced loss function, aiming to achieve accurate segmentation of tumor subregions, including necrotic/non-enhancing tumor core, peritumoral edema, and enhancing tumor.The overall pipeline consists of three key components: data preprocessing, network architecture, and loss function design, which are elaborated in the following subsections.

2.2 Data Preprocessing

To enhance the robustness and generalization ability of the segmentation model, we adopt a standardized data preprocessing and augmentation strategy, as illustrated in Fig. 1. The preprocessing includes image normalization, voxel alignment, size normalization, and various data augmentation techniques.

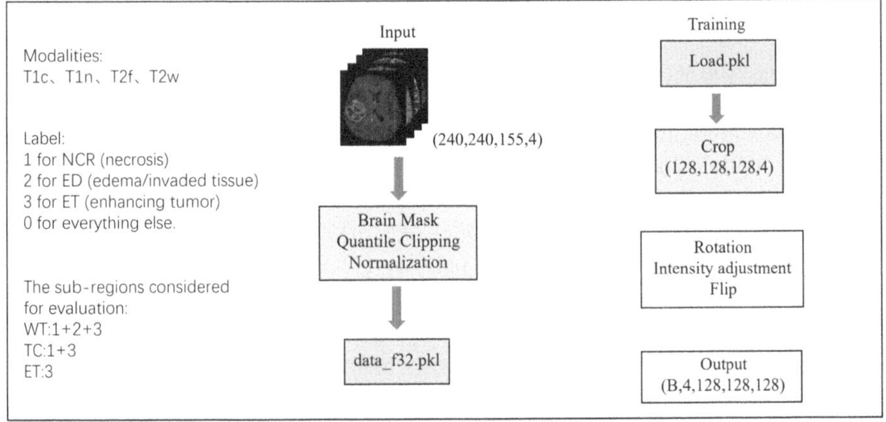

Fig. 1. The preprocessing pipeline of the BraTS-GoAT dataset, including modality alignment, intensity normalization, and data augmentation.

The raw inputs are multimodal brain MRI scans (T1c, T1n, T2f, T2w) provided by the BraTS-GoAT dataset(see Fig. 2). Each modality was clipped to the 0.2–99.8th percentile within the brain mask and then z-score normalized; standard deviation values smaller than 10^{-6} were replaced by 1.0 to ensure stability. The four modalities were stacked into a 4D tensor and stored as `.pkl` files.

During training, the data were randomly cropped into 128^3 patches and augmented with random rotations ($\pm 10°$), intensity perturbations ($\pm 10\%$), and flipping. For inference, volumes were zero-padded to a fixed size before being fed

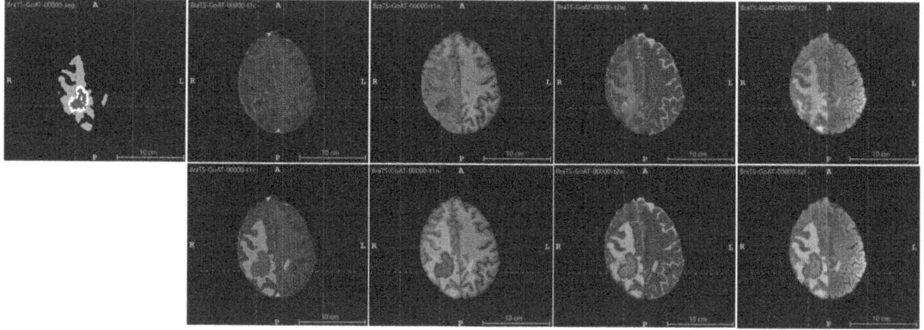

Fig. 2. Examples of multimodal brain MRI scans provided in the BraTS-GoAT dataset, including T1c, T1n, T2f, and T2w sequences.

into the model. All steps were conducted with a fixed random seed (1024) to ensure reproducibility.

During inference, the data are zero-padded to (240, 240, 160, 4) before being passed to the model. All preprocessing steps are conducted under a fixed random seed (1024) to ensure experimental reproducibility.

The label encoding scheme is as follows:

- 1 for necrotic/non-enhancing tumor core (NCR)
- 2 for peritumoral edema (ED)
- 3 for enhancing tumor (ET)

The composite region definitions are:

- WT (Whole Tumor): union of all labeled regions (1, 2, 3)
- TC (Tumor Core): union of ET and NCR (1, 3)
- ET (Enhancing Tumor): label 3 only

2.3 Overall Architecture of ADMFNet

The proposed ADMFNet (Adaptively Modulated DMF Network) is a 3D convolutional neural network built upon the DMFNet backbone. It adopts an encoderâĂŞadaptationâAŞdecoder architecture, as illustrated in Fig. 3.

The model input is a tensor of shape (B, 4, 128, 128, 128), and the output is a softmax-activated segmentation probability map of the same shape (B, 4, 128, 128, 128).The encoder consists of four hierarchical feature extraction stages, each employing stride-2 convolutions followed by stacked DMFUnits to progressively reduce spatial resolution while enhancing semantic abstraction. The feature map size is gradually downsampled from 128Âş to 8Âş, while the number of channels increases from 32 to 384, and is finally compressed to 256 to match the decoder pathway.

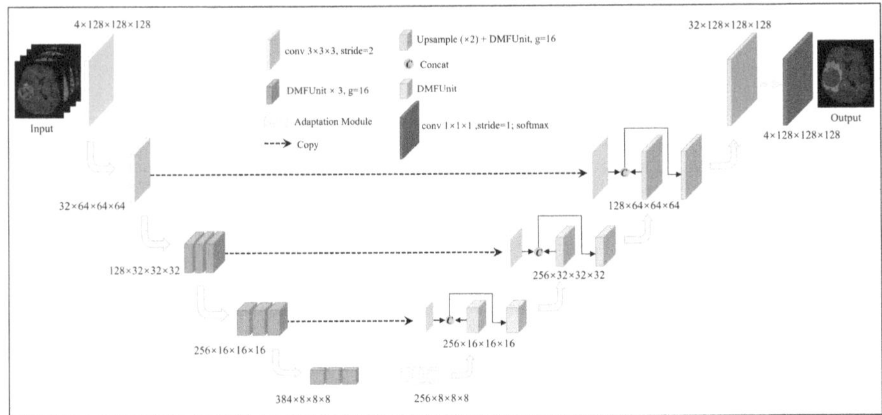

Fig. 3. Overview of the ADMFNet architecture, consisting of a multi-scale encoder, adaptation module, and decoder with skip connections.

Between the encoder and decoder, we insert a lightweight Adaptation Module designed to adjust the channel-wise representation of encoded features. The decoder uses progressive upsampling and skip connections to fuse encoder features, with DMFUnits applied after each fusion to refine the decoded representations. The final output is a semantic segmentation map produced after softmax activation.

2.4 Multi-Scale Feature Extraction Module (DMFUnit)

The Dilated Multi-Fiber Unit (DMFUnit) is the core building block of ADMFNet, designed to efficiently extract multi-scale contextual features while maintaining parameter efficiency [29]. Each DMFUnit first uses two consecutive $1\times1\times1$ convolutions to compress and then restore the channel dimensions of the input features, facilitating efficient feature transformation and information mixing. The transformed features are then processed by three $3\times3\times3$ convolutional layers with different dilation rates (e.g., 1, 2, and 3) to capture contextual information at various spatial scales. Instead of simple parallel branches, the outputs from these dilated convolutions are adaptively fused via learnable weights, allowing the network to dynamically emphasize useful receptive fields for each voxel. A subsequent $3\times3\times1$ convolution further integrates information along the spatial dimension. Finally, a residual connection adds the original input features to the fused output, promoting stable gradient flow and better feature reuse. This design expands the network's receptive field and enables robust multi-scale representation learning, providing a strong foundation for large-volume medical image segmentation tasks.

2.5 Channel Adaptation Module (Adaptation Module)

The Adaptation Module, a key innovation of this work, aims to bridge the semantic gap between the encoder and decoder, mitigating feature distortion during information decoding. Its structure is illustrated in Fig. 4.

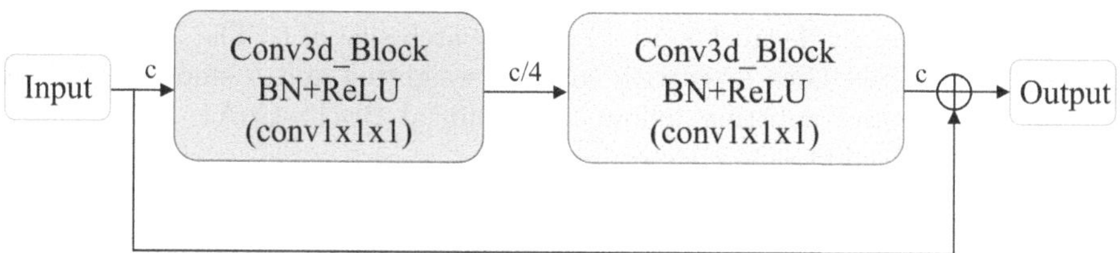

Fig. 4. Detailed structure of the adaptation module. The module employs a bottleneck 1×1×1 convolution with batch normalization (BN) and ReLU activation, followed by a residual connection to facilitate feature alignment.

The module adopts a channel bottleneck architecture composed of two 1×1×1 convolutional layers, with batch normalization and ReLU activation applied between them. The first convolution reduces the channel dimension to 1/4 of the original size, while the second restores it to the original number of channels. Finally, a residual connection adds the module output back to the input feature map to facilitate feature alignment.

This channel remapping mechanism enhances feature reconstruction capability with negligible computational overhead, improving the adaptability of features at the initial stage of decoding.

2.6 Loss Function

To optimize the segmentation performance, we employ the Generalized Dice Loss (GDL) as the primary loss function [30], which specifically addresses the class imbalance in multi-class segmentation tasks. The GDL is defined as:

$$\mathcal{L}_{\mathrm{GDL}} = 1 - 2 \cdot \frac{\sum\limits_{c} w_c \sum\limits_{i} p_{ic} g_{ic}}{\sum\limits_{c} w_c \sum\limits_{i} (p_{ic} + g_{ic}) + \epsilon}, \quad w_c = \frac{1}{(\sum_i g_{ic})^2} \tag{1}$$

where pic and g_{ic} denote the predicted and ground truth labels of voxel i for class c, respectively. The class weight w_c mitigates the imbalance between foreground and background regions, and $\epsilon = e^{-5}$ is a smoothing constant for numerical stability.

The loss function operates on the softmax-activated model outputs. During training, we monitor the Dice scores for each class (NCR, ED, ET) and record the loss curves to assist in convergence analysis.

2.7 Implementation Details

The model was trained for 200 epochs on a single NVIDIA GeForce RTX 4060 Ti GPU (16 GB), with an average runtime of 32 minutes per epoch (≈107 h in total). During inference, processing the entire test dataset consisting of 451 samples took approximately 25 minutes, with GPU memory usage nearing its maximum capacity. We used the Adam optimizer with AMSGrad (initial learning rate 1×10^{-3}, weight decay 1×10^{-5}) and a batch size of 6. The loss function was the Generalized Dice Loss with squared weighting and a smoothing term ($\epsilon = 10^{-5}$). Dataset splitting followed the official BraTS-GoAT patient-level partition without additional cross-validation.

3 Results and Analysis

3.1 Loss Curve and Training Stability

To assess the training stability and convergence of the proposed model, we trained it for 200 epochs on the full training set using a combined Dice and Cross Entropy loss function. The training loss decreased rapidly within the first 10 epochs, indicating swift adaptation to the data distribution. After approximately 50 epochs, the loss curve stabilized between 0.22 and 0.26, demonstrating effective convergence.

The smoothed loss curve closely aligned with the raw loss values, showing minimal fluctuations and confirming the absence of overfitting or instability during training. These results validate the model's robust convergence, providing a reliable basis for subsequent validation and testing phases.

3.2 Validation Performance and Generalization Analysis

We systematically evaluated the proposed model on the 451 cases in the official BraTS-GoAT validation set. The model predictions were submitted to the challenge evaluation server, and the reported quantitative segmentation results for different tumor subregions are summarized in Table 1, demonstrating the model's robust generalization capability.

Segmentation of Major Tumor Regions. The model achieved a Dice score of 0.72 and an NSD (1 mm) of 0.71 for Enhancing Tumor (ET), indicating accurate boundary delineation. The NSD at 0.5 mm was 0.45, suggesting some deviation under stricter boundary evaluation. For Tumor Core (TC), Dice and NSD (1 mm) reached 0.78 and 0.70, respectively, outperforming ET and reflecting robust segmentation of core regions. Whole Tumor (WT) exhibited the highest performance, with Dice = 0.81 and NSD (1 mm) = 0.69, consistent with the relatively lower segmentation difficulty of WT regions.

Table 1. Quantitative evaluation of the model on the BraTS-GoAT validation set.

Region	Dice	NSD (1 mm)
Whole Tumor (WT)	0.805	0.685
Tumor Core (TC)	0.783	0.703
Enhancing Tumor (ET)	0.720	0.711
Edema (ED)	1.000	1.000
Radiation Cavity (RC)	1.000	1.000
NETC	0.607	0.613
Cystic Component	0.634	0.638
SNFH	0.802	0.771

Lesion-wise Analysis. Lesion-wise Dice for ET was 0.68, with NSD (1 mm) of 0.67, closely matching global metrics and indicating sensitivity to small lesions. TC and WT obtained lesion-wise Dice scores of 0.74 and 0.69, respectively. However, WT showed a low NSD (0.5 mm) of 0.31, suggesting room for improvement in fine-grained boundary segmentation.

Segmentation of Other Pathological Regions. Non-Enhancing Tumor Core (NETC) achieved Dice = 0.61 and NSD (1 mm) = 0.61, reflecting moderate performance and the challenge of feature extraction in this region. Peritumoral Edema (ED) and Radiation Cavity (RC) reached perfect scores (Dice = 1.000), likely due to label characteristics or dataset distribution, and should be interpreted with caution. Skull-Nasal Fossa Hyperintensity (SNFH) attained Dice = 0.80 and NSD (1 mm) = 0.77, demonstrating reliable segmentation of complex lesions.

Summary. Overall, the model demonstrated strong Dice performance, particularly for WT and TC regions. NSD evaluation at 0.5 mm highlighted limitations in boundary precision, suggesting that while the model robustly identifies major lesion areas, further refinement is needed for fine-grained boundary alignment.

3.3 Testing Performance and Generalization Evaluation

To further evaluate the model's robustness under distributional shifts, the trained ADMFNet was submitted to the official BraTS-GoAT testing phase. Quantitative results obtained from the challenge server are presented in Table 2, demonstrating consistent segmentation quality across unseen tumor populations.

Performance on Major Tumor Regions. The model achieved Dice scores of 0.717 (ET), 0.744 (TC), and 0.696 (WT), with NSD (1 mm) values of 0.732, 0.708, and 0.616, respectively. The results indicate that ADMFNet maintains robust segmentation quality on the unseen testing data, particularly in the core and enhancing tumor regions.

Table 2. Quantitative evaluation of ADMFNet on the BraTS-GoAT testing set.

Region	Dice	NSD (1 mm)
Whole Tumor (WT)	0.696	0.616
Tumor Core (TC)	0.744	0.708
Enhancing Tumor (ET)	0.717	0.732

Comparison with Validation Phase. Compared with validation results (WT: 0.805 → 0.696; TC: 0.783 → 0.744; ET: 0.720 → 0.717), performance degradation remains within 0.05âĂŞ0.1, suggesting that the model generalizes well under distributional shifts. The Adaptation Module effectively mitigates feature mismatch and enhances domain robustness.

Observations. Despite a moderate drop in boundary accuracy for Whole Tumor, the model demonstrates stable Dice and NSD consistency across tumor subregions. This stability highlights the advantage of the proposed adaptation mechanism in maintaining semantic consistency between encoder and decoder representations even under unseen domain variations.

3.4 Overall Summary of Results

Table 3 summarizes both validation and testing phase results for a comprehensive comparison.

Table 3. Summary comparison between validation and testing results.

Region	Validation		Testing	
	Dice	NSD	Dice	NSD
Whole Tumor (WT)	0.805	0.685	0.696	0.616
Tumor Core (TC)	0.783	0.703	0.744	0.708
Enhancing Tumor (ET)	0.720	0.711	0.717	0.732

The results confirm that ADMFNet exhibits stable and reliable segmentation performance, maintaining competitive accuracy on the unseen testing set. The small metric variation between validation and testing phases further demonstrates its strong generalization capability across tumor types and acquisition domains.

4 Discussion and Conclusion

This study presented ADMFNet, developed for the BraTS 2025 GoAT task, and analyzed both its validation and testing performance.

The validation phase demonstrated that ADMFNet achieved Dice scores of 0.805 (WT), 0.783 (TC), and 0.720 (ET), while the testing phase maintained comparable performance of 0.696, 0.744, and 0.717, respectively. The minor reduction confirms the network's strong generalization across unseen tumor types and imaging protocols.

The Adaptation Module effectively improved feature alignment between encoder and decoder paths, mitigating semantic mismatches and enhancing cross-domain robustness. Meanwhile, the DMFUnit expanded the receptive field through dilated convolutions, improving multi-scale perception and boundary delineation.

Although minor degradation was observed for WT regions under testing conditions, the results indicate that ADMFNet achieves a strong balance between segmentation precision and domain generalization.

Strengths

- Consistent Dice and NSD performance across validation and testing datasets.
- Enhanced feature fusion via Adaptation Module improves cross-domain consistency.
- Robust and interpretable performance under domain shifts.

Limitations and Future Work

- Boundary sensitivity remains limited for large or irregular tumors.
- Future work will explore boundary-aware losses, adaptive data augmentation, and hierarchical attention fusion to further improve segmentation of small or heterogeneous lesions.

Acknowledgements. This work was supported by the Natural Science Foundation of Shandong Province (ZR2019MF003), the National Natural Science Foundation of China (61976126), and the Science, Technology Programme of Tai'an City (2023GX024), the Natural Science Young Foundation of Shandong Province (ZR2025QC700) and it was also supported by the Postgraduate Education Quality Improvement Program of Shandong University of Science and Technology (Yzlts2023069).

Disclosure of Interests. The authors have no competing interests to declare that are relevant to the content of this article.

References

1. Ronneberger, O., Fischer, P., Brox, T.: U-Net: convolutional networks for biomedical image segmentation. In: MICCAI, pp. 234–241 (2015)
2. Woo, S., Park, J., Lee, J.Y., Kweon, I.S.: CBAM: convolutional block attention module. In: ECCV, pp. 3–19 (2018)

3. He, K., Zhang, X., Ren, S., Sun, J.: Deep residual learning for image recognition. In: CVPR, pp. 770–778 (2016)
4. Dou, Q., et al.: Domain generalization via model-agnostic learning of semantic features. In: NeurIPS (2019)
5. Kamnitsas, K., et al.: Unsupervised domain adaptation in brain lesion segmentation with adversarial networks. In: IPMI, pp. 597–609 (2017)
6. Li, D., Yang, Y., Song, Y.Z., Hospedales, T.M.: Learning to generalize: meta-learning for domain generalization. In: AAAI, pp. 3490–3497 (2018)
7. Zhang, Y., Yang, Q.: A survey on multi-task learning. IEEE Trans. Knowl. Data Eng. **34**(12), 5586–5609 (2021)
8. Valvano, G., Leo, A., et al.: Learning cross-modality representations for multimodal brain tumor segmentation. Med. Image Anal. **78**, 102409 (2022)
9. Bakas, S., Reyes, M., et al.: Identifying the best machine learning algorithms for brain tumor segmentation, progression assessment, and overall survival prediction in the BRATS challenge. arXiv preprint arXiv:1811.02629 (2018)
10. Chen, L.C., Papandreou, G., et al.: DeepLab: semantic image segmentation with deep convolutional nets, atrous convolution, and fully connected CRFs. IEEE Trans. Pattern Anal. Mach. Intell. **40**(4), 834–848 (2018)
11. Chen, S., et al.: DMFNet: a CNN for joint segmentation of brain tumor and normal tissue in MRI. Neurocomputing **405**, 112–123 (2020)
12. Karargyris, A., Umeton, R., Sheller, M.J., Aristizabal, A., George, J., Wuest, A., Pati, S., et al.: Federated benchmarking of medical artificial intelligence with MedPerf. Nat. Mach. Intell. **5**, 799–810 (2023). https://doi.org/10.1038/s42256-023-00652-2
13. Bakas, S., et al.: Identifying the best machine learning algorithms for brain tumor segmentation, progression assessment, and overall survival prediction in the BRATS challenge. *arXiv preprint* arXiv:1811.02629 (2018)
14. Baid, U., et al.: The RSNA-ASNR-MICCAI BraTS 2021 benchmark on brain tumor segmentation and radiogenomic classification. arXiv preprint arXiv:2107.02314 (2021)
15. Menze, B.H., et al.: The multimodal brain tumor image segmentation benchmark (BRATS). IEEE Trans. Med. Imaging **34**(10), 1993–2024 (2015). https://doi.org/10.1109/TMI.2014.2377694
16. Bakas, S., et al.: Advancing the cancer genome atlas glioma MRI collections with expert segmentation labels and radiomic features. Sci. Data **4**, 170117 (2017). https://doi.org/10.1038/sdata.2017.117
17. Bakas, S., et al.: Segmentation labels and radiomic features for the pre-operative scans of the TCGA-GBM collection. Cancer Imaging Archive (2017). https://doi.org/10.7937/K9/TCIA.2017.KLXWJJ1Q
18. Bakas, S., et al.: Segmentation labels and radiomic features for the pre-operative scans of the TCGA-LGG collection. Cancer Imaging Archive (2017). https://doi.org/10.7937/K9/TCIA.2017.GJQ7R0EF
19. Baid, U., et al.: The BraTS-GLI challenge on brain tumor segmentation in longitudinal MRI. arXiv preprint arXiv:2405.18368 (2024). https://doi.org/10.48550/arXiv.2405.18368
20. Abdel Khalek, M., et al.: BraTS-Local-Inpainting challenge: brain tumor inpainting using context-aware learning. arXiv preprint arXiv:2305.08992 (2023). https://doi.org/10.48550/arXiv.2305.08992
21. Haque, A., et al.: The brain tumor segmentation challenge on meningioma MRI (BraTS-MEN). arXiv preprint arXiv:2305.07642 (2023). https://doi.org/10.48550/arXiv.2305.07642

22. Haque, A., et al.: Post-treatment meningioma MRI segmentation in the BraTS-MEN-RT Challenge. arXiv preprint arXiv:2405.18383 (2024)
23. Bakas, S., et al.: BraTS-MET: brain metastases segmentation challenge 2023. arXiv preprint arXiv:2306.00838 (2023). https://doi.org/10.48550/arXiv.2306.00838
24. Baid, U., et al.: Brain tumor synthesis with paired and unpaired MR images: the BraSyn challenge. arXiv preprint arXiv:2305.09011 (2023). https://doi.org/10.48550/arXiv.2305.09011
25. Bakas, S., et al.: Pathological verification of brain tumor segmentation (BraTS-Path). arXiv preprint arXiv:2405.10871 (2024)
26. Baheti, B., et al.: BraTS-PED challenge: pediatric brain tumor segmentation from multi-site MRI scans (2023). arXiv preprint arXiv:2305.17033 (2023). https://doi.org/10.48550/arXiv.2305.17033
27. Baheti, B., et al.: BraTS-PED challenge 2024. pediatric brain tumor segmentation. arXiv preprint arXiv:2404.15009 (2024). https://doi.org/10.48550/arXiv.2404.15009
28. Adewole, M., Rudie, J.D., Gbadamosi, A., et al.: The brain tumor segmentation (BraTS) challenge 2023: glioma segmentation in sub-saharan africa patient population (BraTS-Africa). arXiv preprint arXiv:2305.19369 (2023). https://doi.org/10.48550/arXiv.2305.19369
29. Chen, C., Liu, X., Ding, M., Zheng, J., Li, J.: 3D dilated multi-fiber network for real-time brain tumor segmentation in MRI. Neurocomputing **395**, 162–171 (2020)
30. Sudre, C.H., Li, W., Vercauteren, T., Ourselin, S., Jorge Cardoso, M.: Generalised dice overlap as a deep learning loss function for highly unbalanced segmentations. In: Cardoso, M.J., et al., (eds.) DLMIA/ML-CDS -2017. LNCS, vol. 10553, pp. 240–248. Springer, Cham (2017). https://doi.org/10.1007/978-3-319-67558-9_28

Enhancing Brain Tumor Segmentation Generalizability via Pseudo-Labeling and Ratio-Adaptive Postprocessing

To-Liang Hsu, Dang Khoa Nguyen, Pai Lin, Ching-Ting Lin, and Wei-Chun Wang(✉)

Artificial Intelligence and Robotics Innovation Center, China Medical University Hospital, China Medical University, Taichung, Taiwan
017141@tool.caaumed.org.tw

Abstract. The 2025 BraTS Generalizability Across Tumors (GoAT) challenge highlights the need for segmentation models that perform robustly across diverse brain tumor types. We propose a segmentation pipeline that integrates pseudo-label supervised fine-tuning, architectural ensembling, and a novel ratio-adaptive postprocessing strategy. By generating high-quality pseudo-labels from unlabeled cases and fine-tuning multiple nnUNet variants, we enhance model generalization, particularly for whole tumor segmentation. Our ensemble of heterogeneous architectures—including ResNetEncoder variants and U-MambaBot—further improves performance across all tumor subregions. To refine predictions, we introduce a ratio-adaptive thresholding scheme that dynamically adjusts postprocessing cutoffs based on predicted tumor volume, achieving a better balance between precision and recall. Together, these strategies yield strong lesion-wise Dice scores across tumor compartments on the validation set, demonstrating effective tumor-type-agnostic segmentation. Our final test-phase submission achieved lesion-wise Dice scores of 0.828 (WT), 0.827 (TC), and 0.800 (ET), co-ranking first place in the BraTS 2025 Lighthouse GoAT Challenge. We also explore a multitask anatomical segmentation approach as a potential future direction.

Keywords: Brain tumor segmentation · Pseudo-labeling · nnU-Net · UMambaBot · Postprocessing

1 Introduction

The Brain Tumor Segmentation (BraTS) challenge has long focused on creating benchmark datasets and evaluation protocols for segmenting adult brain gliomas [1]. In 2025, the BraTS Generalizability Across Tumors (GoAT) challenge expands this mission by unifying datasets across diverse tumor types, including gliomas [2–7], meningiomas [8], metastases [9], and pediatric brain

T.-L. Hsu and D. K. Nguyen—Equal contribution.

S. Bakas et al. (Eds.): MICCAI 2025, LNCS 16376, pp. 524–537, 2026.
https://doi.org/10.1007/978-3-032-16365-3_47

tumors [10,11]. This expansion reflects a shift toward algorithmic generalization, where the goal is no longer to optimize for a single tumor type, but to develop models that perform robustly across heterogeneous, previously unseen tumor types.

The GoAT task emphasizes type-agnostic segmentation of tumor subregions—enhancing tumor (ET), tumor core (TC), and whole tumor (WT)—using the standard four MRI modalities (T1, T1Gd, T2, FLAIR). While the label schema is consistent across all datasets, the presence, appearance, and frequency of subregions vary significantly between tumor types. This introduces challenges such as inconsistent lesion appearance and domain shifts due to differing patient demographics and imaging protocols.

To address the generalization challenges posed by the GoAT task, we propose a robust segmentation pipeline based on three key components. First, we adopt a pseudo-labeling strategy to incorporate unlabeled training data and improve model generalization. Second, we ensemble diverse model architectures, including nnUNet ResEnc variants and U-MambaBot, to boost robustness. Finally, we introduce a novel ratio-adaptive postprocessing strategy that dynamically filters predictions based on tumor volume. We also briefly explore multitask anatomical supervision via TumorSurfer, though its tumor segmentation performance was ultimately limited.

2 Methods

2.1 Dataset

GoAT Dataset. The provided dataset includes 1,351 labeled and 1,138 unlabeled pre-operative MRI cases. According to the organizers, Meningioma and Metastases are more prevalent in the unlabeled set, while the labeled set contains relatively fewer cases of these subtypes.

Pseudo-Labels. We hypothesize that labeled training data may not fully capture the diversity of brain lesion types, and there is a likely tumor distribution shift between labeled training data and validation or hidden test data. Thus, incorporating both labeled and unlabeled training data could enhance model generalizability across various brain tumors. Li et al. [12] demonstrated that supervised pretraining generally outperforms self-supervised methods in medical imaging tasks. Motivated by this, we adopt a pseudo-labeling strategy to convert unlabeled data into additional supervision, rather than relying on self-supervised representation learning.

The pseudo-label generation process involved three steps. First, we trained three nnU-Net ResEnc variants (M, L, XL) on labeled training data. These models were then ensembled by averaging their softmax predictions, yielding stable performance on the validation set (lesion-wise WT Dice 0.81, TC Dice 0.82). Second, we applied conservative postprocessing to the ensemble predictions: only connected components smaller than 10 voxels were removed. This choice prioritizes sensitivity, as false positives can be further suppressed downstream, whereas false negatives cannot be recovered once removed. Third, the refined pseudo-labels were combined with the original labeled set, forming a mixed training dataset of 2,489 cases. Validation data was neither used for generating pseudo-labels nor included in the training process.

2.2 Preprocessing

All MRI scans were preprocessed using nnU-Net v2's built-in pipeline. Specifically, images were resampled to a common voxel spacing, cropped to foreground regions, and normalized via per-volume z-score of non-zero voxels.

2.3 Models

nnUNet Baseline. As our primary baseline, we adopted the vanilla nnU-Net v2 architecture (3D full resolution), following its default configuration without modifications to architecture, preprocessing, or training schedules. nnU-Net, introduced by Isensee et al. [13,14], is a self-configuring deep learning framework for biomedical image segmentation. It automatically adapts model depth, patch size, preprocessing, and augmentation strategies to the input dataset, removing the need for manual tuning. This standardized and reproducible setup has achieved state-of-the-art results across a wide range of medical imaging benchmarks and serves as a strong baseline for the BraTS GoAT task.

nnUNet ResNet Encoder Variants. We explored nnUNet ResEnc variants (M, L, XL), which incorporate ResNet-style residual connections in the encoder with increasing model sizes (Medium, Large, Extra Large) to improve feature extraction and segmentation performance, as shown by Isensee et al. [15].

Semi-supervised Learning with Mean Teacher (MT). To improve the generalizability of segmentation models across tumor subregions and characteristics, we utilize unlabeled training data and adapt the uncertainty-aware self-ensembling mean teacher (UA-MT) framework proposed by Yu et al. [16] for semi-supervised 3D left atrium segmentation. This method leverages both labeled and unlabeled MRI data to enhance segmentation performance. The framework includes a student model and a teacher model. The student model is trained by minimizing a segmentation loss on labeled data and a consistency loss, ensuring predictions for the same input under different perturbations align with the teacher model's targets. The teacher model generates these targets and estimates their uncertainty, enabling the student to learn from reliable predictions. The uncertainty-guided consistency loss enhances the student model's robustness and accuracy, effectively utilizing unlabeled data for brain tumor segmentation. We made two modifications to the original framework. First, to reduce the computational cost of uncertainty estimation, which practically required T = 3 stochastic forward passes per batch, we adopted the single-forward-pass uncertainty method proposed by Assefa et al. [17]. Second, we enabled the student model to learn from additional pseudo-labels. Only the student model is used during inference.

U-Mamba. U-Mamba architecture networks using hybrid CNN-SSM blocks, provide two implementation including U-MambaEnc with U-Mamba block used in all encoder blocks, another variant is U-MambaBot with a single Mamba-based SSM block at the bottleneck for capturing long-range dependencies in MRI images and the rest with plain Residual convolutional blocks for local feature extraction. We found that training U-MambaBot is more efficient than that for U-MambaEnc, so U-MambaBot is selected, the network leverages nnU-Net's self-configuring default plan version and training followed the default nnU-Net v2 framework on 3D full resolution data with the following configuration: patch size of (128 x 160 x 112), batch size of 2, and inference with test-time augmentation by default. U-MambaBot demonstrated superior dice and boundary accuracy compared to leading CNN and Transformer segmentation models in [18]

TumorSurfer. Inspired by prior work on anatomical priors and context-aware segmentation [19–21], we explored a multitask learning approach, **TumorSurfer**, that simultaneously predicts anatomical structures and tumor subregions. While standard nnU-Net treats the background as a single undifferentiated class, TumorSurfer explicitly predicts both tumor subregions and anatomical regions (e.g., cortex, ventricles, brainstem). This encourages the model to leverage structural priors from healthy tissue and refine tumornon-tumor boundaries. We did not use the unlabeled dataset in this setting.

To provide anatomical supervision, we used FastSurfer [22] to segment 1,351 BraTS cases. However, FastSurfer performed poorly in pathological regions, and only 709 cases (52.5%) passed quality control. We trained a separate nnU-Net model, **SimpleSurfer**, on these high-quality cases using all four MRI modalities and consolidated FastSurfer's 95 fine-grained labels into 11 anatomically meaningful classes. For the remaining 642 cases with poor-quality segmentations, we re-generated anatomical pseudo-labels using SimpleSurfer. Figure 1 illustrates the segmentation differences.

TumorSurfer employs a ResNetEnc-L-based architecture within the nnU-Net framework and was trained on merged labels combining anatomical pseudo-labels and tumor ground truth, with priority given to tumor labels in overlapping regions. To address severe class imbalance, we adopted patch oversampling on tumor-positive voxels and inverse-volume loss weighting, preventing large anatomical classes such as white matter or cortex from dominating training. This design allows TumorSurfer to jointly learn anatomical priors and tumor subregions within a unified multitask framework.

2.4 Training

Optimizer and Schedule. We first trained three nnU-Net ResEnc variants (M, L, XL) on labeled training data only, using the default nnU-Net v2 configuration: 1000 epochs, an initial learning rate of 1e-2, and the SGD optimizer with Nesterov momentum. These models were trained from scratch. For fine-tuning on the mixed dataset (labeled + pseudo-labeled), ResEnc-L and ResEnc-XL were

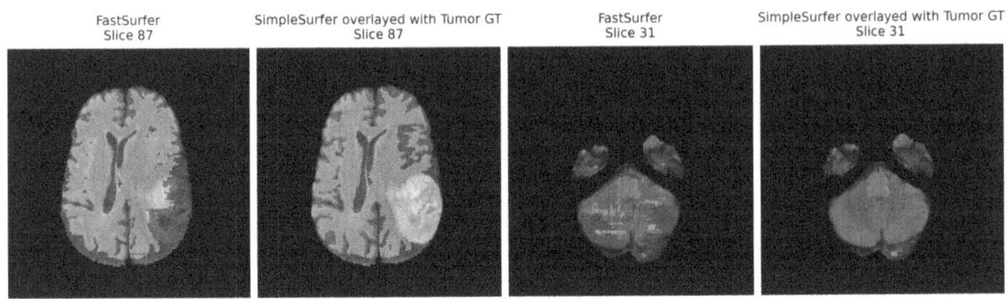

Fig. 1. Comparison between FastSurfer and SimpleSurfer anatomical segmentation on training case GoAT-00024. FastSurfer outputs appear conservative in cortical regions and exhibit noisy labeling in the cerebellum. SimpleSurfer shows more complete segmentation of both cortex and cerebellum, with clearer delineation of structures such as the insula. Tumor ground truth is overlaid on the SimpleSurfer output to illustrate the composite label used for TumorSurfer training.

trained for 300 epochs with a learning rate of 2e-4, while ResEnc-M was retrained for 1000 epochs from its labeled-only checkpoint with a learning rate of 3e-3. U-MambaBot was trained from scratch on the mixed dataset using nnU-Net defaults.

Loss Functions. For all fine-tuned models, we employed the DiceTopKFocal loss [23], a composite of Dice, Top-K, and Focal losses, to better handle hard positive tumor subregions.

Data Augmentation. Unless otherwise noted, all models used nnU-Net v2's default on-the-fly augmentation pipeline. This includes random rotations, scaling factors, and mirroring along all spatial axes. No custom augmentations were introduced beyond nnU-Net defaults.

Checkpoint Selection. Following nnU-Net v2's default protocol, model checkpoints were selected based on the best validation Dice score, with exponential moving average (EMA) weights used for evaluation rather than raw last-epoch parameters.

Hardware. All models were trained using PyTorch on a single NVIDIA V100 GPU (32GB).

2.5 Test-Time Augmentation and Ensembling

During inference, we applied nnU-Net v2's default test-time augmentation (TTA) strategy, which generates 8 variants of each scan by mirroring along the three spatial axes. Model predictions from all augmented inputs were aggregated by averaging softmax probabilities voxel-wise. For ensembling, we combined outputs from multiple models with diverse architectures in the same way—averaging their softmax maps—to smooth over individual model errors and enhance robustness across tumor types. Unless otherwise specified, all reported experiments used this fixed combination of 8-way TTA and softmax-averaged ensembling. For the final Docker submission, however, TTA was disabled to reduce inference time, while ensembling across models was retained.

2.6 Postprocessing

Well-designed postprocessing strategies have demonstrated measurable gains in segmentation accuracy in past BraTS challenges. However, compared to single-tumor type challenges, GoAT emphasizes generalization across all types of tumors without providing tumor type annotations. This constraint complicates the design of a robust, type-agnostic postprocessing pipeline.

Fixed Thresholding. Traditional threshold-based methods eliminate or relabel components whose voxel volume falls below a predefined cutoff. For instance, Zeineldin et al. [24] proposed relabeling small enhancing tumor (ET) components as non-enhancing tumor core (NETC). Ferreira et al. [25] applied fixed thresholds of 250 voxels for whole tumor (WT), 150 for tumor core (TC), and 100 for ET. Capellán-Martín et al. [26] introduced tumor-type-specific cutoffs for pediatric, meningioma, and metastasis tumors (130, 110, and 15 voxels, respectively).

Ratio-Adaptive Thresholding. To overcome the rigidity of fixed thresholds and maintain tumor-type agnosticism, we propose a ratio-adaptive thresholding strategy. This method dynamically adjusts filtering thresholds based on the predicted tumor volume, enabling more context-aware refinement.

First, we computed the average predicted volume of WT components in each case, excluding those smaller than 10 voxels to avoid noise. Next, thresholds are defined as:

$$\mathrm{ET}_{\mathrm{thresh}} = \min(0.0005 \times \text{avg predicted WT volume}, 100)$$

$$\mathrm{WT}_{\mathrm{thresh}} = \max\left(\min(0.005 \times \text{avg predicted WT volume}, 250), 10\right)$$

These thresholds blend prior fixed rules with adaptive scaling. The upper bounds (100 for ET, 250 for WT) are informed by previous literature [25], while the lower bound of 10 voxels ensures minimal noise removal.

3 Results

All reported results are based on the BraTS GoAT official evaluation platform, which ensures consistency across submissions. The primary metric is lesion-wise Dice, which differs from conventional Dice in that it evaluates connected components independently, thereby penalizing false positives and false negatives more strongly. False positive and false negative lesion counts are also reported by the platform on a per-case basis and aggregated across the validation set. Unless otherwise specified, reported scores represent averages over all cases within each subregion (ET, NETC, SNFH, TC, WT).

We report lesion-wise Dice scores on the hold-out validation set for single models and model ensembles in Tables 1 and 2. To compare postprocessing strategies, detailed results are shown in Table 3, and the final postprocessed ensemble scores are presented in Table 4. Due to submission quota constraints and the need to prioritize promising configurations, not all models or ensemble variants were exhaustively evaluated. Our analysis focuses on representative settings that demonstrated strong internal performance. Finally, the test-phase evaluation provded by the BraTS organizers is reported in Table 5.

3.1 Individual Model Results

In Table 1, among models trained solely on labeled data (nnUNet Baseline, TumorSurfer, ResEncM), ResEncM achieved the highest Dice scores in most subregions. For models trained with additional pseudo-labeled data (ResEncXL, ResEncXL MT, UMambaBot), ResEncXL led in ET (0.730), while UMambaBot outperformed others in SNFH (0.780) and WT (0.816).

TumorSurfer achieved high anatomical accuracy during training, with Dice scores exceeding 0.9 for most structures— Cerebral white matters (0.925), ventricles (0.969), brainstem (0.972), cerebellum (0.977), and cortex (0.900). However, due to the lack of anatomical ground truth in BraTS, external validation remains limited. Despite its strong anatomical capability, TumorSurfer underperformed in tumor segmentation compared to the nnUNet baseline. Figure 2 illustrates TumorSurfer's predicted anatomy and tumor outputs.

3.2 Model Ensemble Results

In Table 2, BaselineEnsemble—comprising three nnUNet models with ResNetEnc M, L, and XL encoders—performed comparably to FinetunedEnsemble, which included two fine-tuned models (ResEnc L and XL) trained with pseudo-labeled data. Merging these into a 5-model ensemble (601 + 603) led to consistent improvements across most tumor subregions. Building on this strong baseline, we explored additional ensemble configurations. Adding ResEncXL MT (a Mean Teacherbased model) resulted in slightly lower performance in ET and TC, whereas replacing it with a pseudo-labeled ResEnc M model led to modest gains across all core subregions, forming our 6-model ensemble. Although this process was not a systematic search, it guided us toward an effective composition. The final 7-model ensemble—further expanded with UMambaBot—achieved the best overall Dice scores across tumor types.

3.3 Postprocessing Results

Table 3 compare the three postprocessing strategies defined in Sect. 2.6. For the fixed-threshold baseline, we adopted the approach of Ferreira et al. [25]. In contrast, our ratio-adaptive methods dynamically adjust thresholds based on predicted tumor volume, with variants that either relabel or discard small ET components. Among these, the discard-based strategy yielded the best lesion-wise Dice scores, particularly improving ET while preserving other subregions. As shown in Table 4, postprocessing consistently improved ensemble performance across all settings, with the 7-model ensemble achieving the strongest overall results.

3.4 Test-Phase Evaluation Results

Following the validation phase, our final 7-model ensemble with ratio-adaptive postprocessing was evaluated on the BraTS 2025 GoAT test set by the official organizers. As summarized in Table 5, our model achieved mean lesion-wise Dice scores of 0.800 (ET), 0.827 (TC), and 0.828 (WT). These results placed our solution among the **co-first-place winners** in the BraTS 2025 Lighthouse Challenge, demonstrating strong generalization across heterogeneous tumor types (Table 5).

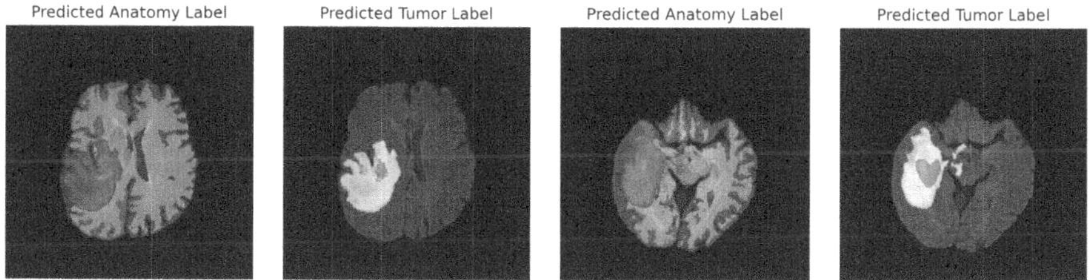

Fig. 2. TumorSurfer Prediction of Anatomical Labels and Tumor Labels on validation set case GoAT-02491.

4 Discussion

The results from Tables 1, 2, and 4 highlight several key factors contributing to improved performance on the validation set for lesion-wise Dice scores in brain tumor segmentation. Below, we discuss the impact of pseudo-labels, ensemble strategies with diverse model architectures, and adaptive post-processing, alongside future improvement directions.

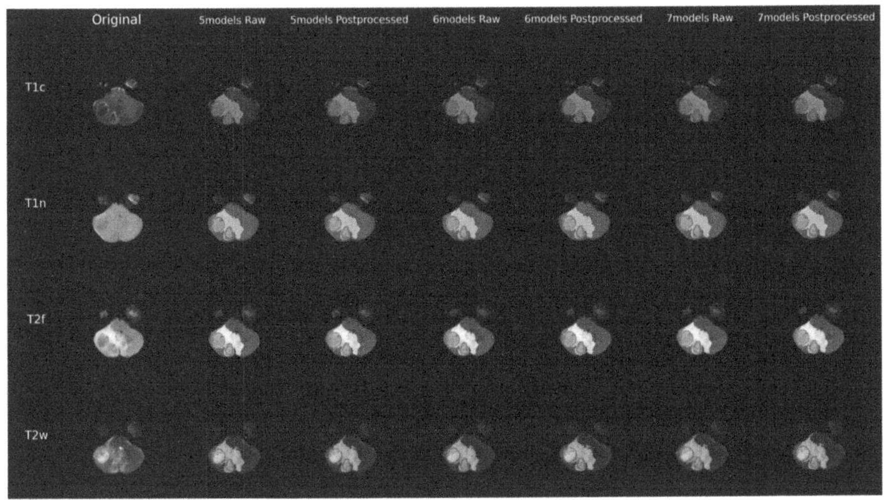

Fig. 3. Sample outputs of different ensembles on validation set case GoAT-02586.

Table 1. Lesion-wise Dice scores of single models before postprocessing. Models marked "Yes" in the *+Pseudo-Labeled Data* column were trained using additional unlabeled data with pseudo-labels. Best scores per column are bolded.

Model	+Pseudo-Labeled	ET	NETC	SNFH	TC	WT
nnUNet Baseline	No	0.725	0.656	0.776	0.807	0.793
TumorSurfer	No	0.681	0.635	0.741	0.765	0.713
ResEncM	No	0.728	**0.668**	**0.780**	**0.820**	0.791
ResEncXL	Yes	**0.730**	0.652	0.774	0.817	0.801
ResEncXL MT	Yes	0.724	0.661	0.778	0.811	0.802
UMambaBot	Yes	0.722	0.657	**0.780**	0.818	**0.816**

Table 2. Lesion-wise Dice scores of ensemble models before postprocessing. Best scores per column are bolded. BaselineEnsemble trained nnUNets with different ResNetEncoder size. FinetunedEnsemble trained nnUNets finetuned with pseudo-labeled data.

Model	ET	NETC	SNFH	TC	WT
BaselineEnsemble (ResEnc M, L, XL)	0.740	0.655	0.782	0.817	0.807
FinetunedEnsemble (ResEnc L, XL)	0.737	0.656	0.777	0.819	0.809
5 models ensemble (Baseline + Finetuned)	0.742	0.658	0.780	0.823	0.810
5 models + MT	0.739	0.658	**0.783**	0.820	0.811
6 models (5 models + Finetuned ResEnc M)	0.740	0.658	**0.783**	0.821	0.813
7 models (6 models + UMamba)	**0.745**	**0.662**	0.782	**0.824**	**0.816**

Table 3. Lesion-wise Dice scores, false positives (FP), and false negatives (FN) for ET, TC, and WT under different postprocessing strategies.

Method	ET			TC			WT		
	Dice	FP	FN	Dice	FP	FN	Dice	FP	FN
5 models ensemble (Raw)	0.742	66	**62**	0.823	17	**65**	0.810	54	**66**
Fixed Thresholding	0.746	**7**	88	0.816	**3**	87	0.824	**16**	82
Ratio-Adapt. (ET→NETC)	0.751	17	68	0.822	15	68	0.827	31	71
Ratio-Adapt. (ET→Discard)	**0.751**	17	68	**0.824**	10	68	**0.827**	31	71

Table 4. Postprocessed results for ensemble models using 5, 6, and 7 models. Postprocessing consistently improves performance across most tumor subregions.

Model	ET	NETC	SNFH	TC	WT
5models Raw	0.742	0.658	0.780	0.823	0.810
5models Postprocessed	0.751	0.658	**0.789**	0.824	0.827
6models Raw	0.740	0.658	0.783	0.821	0.813
6models Postprocessed	0.752	0.658	**0.789**	0.824	0.828
7models Raw	0.745	**0.662**	0.782	0.824	0.816
7models Postprocessed	**0.756**	**0.662**	0.788	**0.827**	**0.831**

Table 5. Final test-phase results on the BraTS 2025 GoAT Challenge test set. Lesion-wise Dice and NSD@1 mm (Normalized Surface Dice at 1 mm tolerance) are reported as mean values across all cases.

Metric	ET	TC	WT
Lesion-wise Dice	**0.800**	**0.827**	**0.828**
Lesion-wise NSD @ 1 mm	**0.826**	**0.801**	**0.763**

4.1 Pseudo-Label Supervised Training

As shown in Table 1, incorporating pseudo-labeled training data led to consistent improvements in whole tumor (WT) segmentation, both in individual models (e.g., ResEncXL, UMambaBot) and ensemble settings. While the benefits across other subregions were mixed, the added data appears to improve generalization by exposing models to greater tumor variability. This suggests that pseudo-labels are especially useful for learning coarse tumor extents and enriching ensemble diversity, even if their impact on finer subregion boundaries remains limited.

4.2 Ensemble with Diverse Model Architectures:

Table 2 demonstrates the strength of ensemble strategies combining models with varied architectures, such as ResNetEncoder sizes (M, L, XL) and UMambaBot. The 7-model ensemble, which included diverse architectures and additional pseudo-labeled training data, achieved the highest performance across all tumor subregions. This improvement can be attributed to diversity in feature extraction and modeling approaches that mitigated individual model weaknesses. By combining ResNetEncoder models with U-MambaBot, the 7-model ensemble integrates local feature extraction via convolutions with long-range context modeling via SSMs, yielding improved segmentation performance.

4.3 Postprocessing

The proposed ratio-adaptive thresholding strategy outperformed both the raw and fixed-threshold baselines by achieving a better balance between precision and recall, particularly for Enhancing Tumor (ET) and Whole Tumor (WT).

As shown in Table 3, the fixed-threshold method achieved the lowest ET false positive count (reducing it from 66 to 7), but at the cost of a substantial increase in false negatives (from 62 to 88), often suppressing small but valid lesions—especially in metastases cases.

In contrast, the ratio-adaptive method reduced ET false positives to 17 while limiting false negatives to 68, offering a more balanced trade-off. By scaling thresholds based on predicted WT volume, the method adapts to case-specific tumor size and improves generalization across diverse tumor types—a crucial requirement in the GoAT task.

We also tested reassigning small ET components to NETC, as suggested in prior work, but this degraded TC Dice and increased TC false positives. As a result, we adopted the discard strategy, which better preserves tumor subregion integrity without introducing ambiguous label transitions.

4.4 Future Improvements

While pseudo-label fine-tuning proved effective, our attempt to incorporate semi-supervised learning via the Mean Teacher framework underperformed on the validation set and was excluded from the final ensemble. This may be due to suboptimal training configurations and the instability of Mean Teacher models under noisy pseudo-labels.

We also observed weaker tumor segmentation in our multitask model, TumorSurfer (Table 1), despite its strong anatomical performance. We attribute this to three factors: (1) capacity dilution from sharing features between 13 anatomical classes and tumor subregions; (2) voxel imbalance favoring dominant structures like white matter and cortex, even with inverse-volume weighting; and (3) sharp label boundaries introduced during tumoranatomy overlap resolution, which may have hindered margin learning.

Nevertheless, TumorSurfer achieved Dice scores above 0.9 on major anatomical structures, suggesting meaningful priors were learned. Future work may explore decoupling anatomical and tumor pathways—e.g., guiding tumor post-processing with pre-trained anatomical segmenters or applying anatomy-aware attention during decoding.

Acknowledgements. We would like to thank Ting-Yu Lai for her help during the early setup of the experiments.

References

1. Karargyris, A., et al.: Federated benchmarking of medical artificial intelligence with MedPerf. Nat. Mach. Intell. **5**, 799–810 (2023). https://doi.org/10.1038/s42256-023-00652-2
2. Baid, U., Rane, S.M., Talbar, S.N., et al.: The RSNA-ASNR-MICCAI BraTS 2021 Benchmark on Brain Tumor Segmentation and Radiogenomic Classification. arXiv preprint arXiv:2107.02314 (2021)
3. Menze, B.H., et al.: The multimodal brain tumor image segmentation benchmark (BRATS). IEEE Trans. Med. Imaging **34**(10), 1993–2024 (2015). https://doi.org/10.1109/TMI.2014.2377694
4. Bakas, S., et al.: Advancing the cancer genome atlas glioma MRI collections with expert segmentation labels and radiomic features. Sci. Data **4**, 170117 (2017). https://doi.org/10.1038/sdata.2017.117
5. Adewole, M., Rudie, J.D., Gbadamosi, A., et al.: The brain tumor segmentation (BraTS) challenge 2023: glioma segmentation in sub-Saharan Africa patient population (BraTS-Africa). arXiv preprint arXiv:2305.19369 (2023). https://doi.org/10.48550/arXiv.2305.19369
6. Bakas, S., Akbari, H., Sotiras, A., Bilello, M., Rozycki, M., Kirby, J., et al.: Segmentation labels and radiomic features for the pre-operative scans of the TCGA-GBM collection. Cancer Imaging Archive (2017). https://doi.org/10.7937/K9/TCIA.2017.KLXWJJ1Q
7. Bakas, S., Akbari, H., Sotiras, A., Bilello, M., Rozycki, M., Kirby, J., et al.: Segmentation labels and radiomic features for the pre-operative scans of the TCGA-LGG collection. Cancer Imaging Archive (2017). https://doi.org/10.7937/K9/TCIA.2017.GJQ7R0EF
8. LaBella, D., et al.: The ASNR-MICCAI brain tumor segmentation (BraTS) challenge 2023: intracranial meningioma. arXiv preprint arXiv:2305.07642 (2023). https://doi.org/10.48550/arXiv.2305.07642

9. Moawad, A.W., et al.: The brain tumor segmentation (BraTS-METS) challenge 2023: brain metastasis segmentation on pre-treatment MRI. arXiv preprint arXiv:2306.00838 (2023). https://doi.org/10.48550/arXiv.2306.00838
10. Kazerooni, A.F., et al.: The brain tumor segmentation (BraTS) challenge 2023: focus on pediatrics (CBTN-CONNECT-DIPGR-ASNR-MICCAI BraTS-PEDs). arXiv preprint arXiv:2305.17033 (2023). https://doi.org/10.48550/arXiv.2305.17033
11. Kazerooni, A.F., et al.: The brain tumor segmentation in pediatrics (BraTS-PEDs) challenge: focus on pediatrics (CBTN-CONNECT-DIPGR-ASNR-MICCAI BraTS-PEDs). arXiv preprint arXiv:2404.15009 (2024). https://doi.org/10.48550/arXiv.2404.15009
12. Li, W., Yuille, A., Zhou, Z.: How well do supervised 3D models transfer to medical imaging tasks? arXiv preprint arXiv:2501.11253 (2025). https://doi.org/10.48550/arXiv.2501.11253
13. Isensee, F., Jaeger, P.F., Kohl, S.A.A., Petersen, J., Maier-Hein, K.H.: nnU-Net: a self-configuring method for deep learning-based biomedical image segmentation. Nature Methods **18**, 203–211 (2021). https://doi.org/10.1038/s41592-020-01008-z
14. Isensee, F., Ulrich, C., Wald, T., Maier-Hein, K.H.: Extending NNU-Net is all you need. In: Deserno, T.M., Handels, H., Maier, A., Maier-Hein, K., Palm, C., Tolxdorff, T. (eds.) Bildverarbeitung für die Medizin 2023, Informatik aktuell, pp. 33–38. Springer Vieweg, Wiesbaden (2023). https://doi.org/10.1007/978-3-658-41657-7_7
15. Isensee, F., et al.: nnU-Net revisited: A call for rigorous validation in 3D medical image segmentation. In: Proceeding MICCAI, pp. 488–498. Springer (2024)
16. Yu, L., Wang, S., Li, X., Fu, C.-W., Heng, P.-A.: Uncertainty-aware self-ensembling model for semi-supervised 3D left atrium segmentation. In: Proceeding MICCAI, pp. 605–613. Springer (2019)
17. Assefa, M., Naseer, M., Ganapathi, I.I., Ali, S.S., Seghier, M.L., Werghi, N.: DyCON: dynamic uncertainty-aware consistency and contrastive learning for semi-supervised medical image segmentation. In: *Proc. CVPR*, pp. 30850–30860 (2025)
18. Ma, J., Li, F., Wang, B.: U-Mamba: Enhancing long-range dependency for biomedical image segmentation. arXiv preprint arXiv:2401.04722 (2024). https://doi.org/10.48550/arXiv.2401.04722
19. Tampu, I.E., Haj-Hosseini, N., Eklund, A.: Does anatomical contextual information improve 3D U-Net-based brain tumor segmentation? Diagnostics**11**(7), 1159 (2021). https://doi.org/10.3390/diagnostics11071159
20. Mathai, T.S., Liu, B., Summers, R.M.: Segmentation of mediastinal lymph nodes in CT with anatomical priors. Int. J. Comput. Assist. Radiol. Surg. **19**(8), 1537–1544 (2024). https://doi.org/10.1007/s11548-024-03165-4
21. Huang, H., et al.: A deep multi-task learning framework for brain tumor segmentation. Front. Oncol. **11**, 690244 (2021). https://doi.org/10.3389/fonc.2021.690244
22. Henschel, L., Conjeti, S., Estrada, S., Diers, K., Fischl, B., Reuter, M.: FastSurfer – A fast and accurate deep learning-based neuroimaging pipeline. NeuroImage **219**, 117012 (2020). https://doi.org/10.1016/j.neuroimage.2020.117012
23. Ma, J., et al.: Loss Odyssey in Medical Image Segmentation. Med. Image Anal. **71**, 102035 (2021). https://doi.org/10.1016/j.media.2021.102035
24. Zeineldin, R.A., Karar, M.E., Burgert, O., Mathis-Ullrich, F.: Multimodal CNN networks for brain tumor segmentation in MRI: a BraTS 2022 challenge solution. In: Bakas, S., Reyes, M., Rieke, N., Menze, B.H., Baust, M. (eds.) Brainlesion: Glioma, Multiple Sclerosis, Stroke and Traumatic Brain Injuries. BrainLes 2022,

LNCS, vol. 13769, pp. 140–151. Springer, Cham (2023). https://doi.org/10.1007/978-3-031-33842-7_11

25. Ferreira, A., et al.: How we won BraTS 2023 Adult Glioma challenge? Just faking it! Enhanced synthetic data augmentation and model ensemble for brain tumour segmentation. arXiv preprint arXiv:2402.17317 (2024). https://arxiv.org/abs/2402.17317
26. Capellán-Martín, D., et al.: Model ensemble for brain tumor segmentation in magnetic resonance imaging. In: Brain Tumor Segmentation, and Cross-Modality Domain Adaptation for Medical Image Segmentation: MICCAI Challenges, BraTS 2023 and CrossMoDA 2023, LNCS, vol. 14465, pp. 221–232. Springer, Cham (2023). https://doi.org/10.1007/978-3-031-76163-8_20

Ensemble-Based Generalization for Brain Tumor Segmentation Using NnU-Net Variants and Swin UNETR

Vaidehi Satushe[1(✉)], Madhav Arora[2], Vibha Vyas[1], and Shilpa Metkar[1]

[1] COEP Technological University, Pune, India
vaidehisatushe@gmail.com, {vsv.extc,metkars.extc}@coeptech.ac.in
[2] Netaji Subhas University of Technology, New Delhi, India
eragon.cube@outlook.com

Abstract. We employed an ensemble technique for the BraTS Generalizability Across Tumors (BraTS-GoAT) task of the BraTS-Lighthouse 2025 Challenge, where it performed well on the unseen test validation dataset. To enhance models' segmentation capabilities, we applied specific preprocessing techniques tailored to BraTS, focused on training different tumor regions, and made several minor adjustments to the pipeline. We also used the BraTS ranking criteria to identify the nnU-Net variant that met the challenge's requirements most effectively. Our results for the whole tumor, tumor core, and enhanced tumor were Dice similarity coefficients of 0.84, 0.87, and 0.90 and HD95 values of 3.39, 3.12, and 2.64, respectively.

Keywords: nnU-Net · Medical Image Segmentation · Brain Tumor Segmentation · SwinU-Net

1 Introduction

Brain tumor segmentation is a highly challenging problem in medical imaging. Precise tumor delineation is essential, as it enhances treatment quality by aiding in monitoring therapy responses, planning treatments, and making diagnoses [15]. Detailed segmentation and analysis of tumor subregions can identify new imaging biomarkers, leading to more accurate disease classification [11] and improved predictions of treatment outcomes [10]. The Segmentation Challenge [5,14] offers the most extensive publicly available annotated dataset, serving as a leading benchmark for evaluating and comparing segmentation techniques.

The BraTS 2025 dataset features 1,351 subjects data with reference annotations to train and 451 unannotated subjects data to validate. Models can be evaluated and compared through an online evaluation tool. Our primary focus

V. Satushe and M. Arora—Equal contribution.

S. Bakas et al. (Eds.): MICCAI 2025, LNCS 16376, pp. 538–548, 2026.
https://doi.org/10.1007/978-3-032-16365-3_48

will be on the Generalizability Across Tumors Challenge, though BraTS 2025 also includes other related competitions.

Recent high-performing entries in the BraTS challenge have predominantly utilized deep neural networks [9]. Enhancements to this model include densely connected layers [7], attention mechanisms, and residual connections [1,6,16], which have all been applied to improve brain tumor segmentation. Noteworthy submissions from 2018 [2] and 2019 [11] incorporated a second decoder for auxiliary tasks, extending the encoder-decoder framework to enhance regularization.

Training approaches are adapted to address challenges unique to brain tumor segmentation, such as class imbalance, often using specialized loss functions like focal loss and Dice loss [2]. The BraTS evaluation criteria focus on overlapping regions of the whole tumor, tumor core, and enhanced tumor [5]. Employing all three class labels can boost performance, and effectively managing data ambiguity has been shown to improve results.

The advanced brain tumor segmentation techniques previously mentioned [8] are highly specialized and have been developed through rigorous trial and error. Recently, we introduced an ensemble technique, an advanced segmentation framework that automatically creates pipelines for various biological datasets. nnU-Net has shown its capability by achieving top performance across most of the 25 datasets it has been tested on [12]. In the upcoming discussion, we will analyse the effectiveness of ensemble models for segmenting and exploring their potential as a foundational framework for developing new segmentation models.

2 Dataset Specification

This study utilises the official BraTS 2025 GoAT training dataset [13], a uniquely comprehensive MRI collection encompassing multiple pathologies, ethnicities, and institutions, specifically designed to test the generalizability of brain tumor segmentation methods. Among these, 1,351 scans are annotated with segmentation labels for training purposes with an additional 1,138 unlabelled data, while a set of 451 scans are reserved for public leaderboard validation. An additional test set is also curated, but its details are kept hidden from the participants.

Each patient case includes four types of MRI contrasts: pre-contrast native T1-weighted (T1N), contrast-enhanced T1-weighted (T1C), T2-weighted (T2W), and T2-weighted Fluid Attenuated Inversion Recovery (T2-FLAIR or T2F). Each scan has been meticulously annotated by up to four raters and reviewed by expert neuroradiologists. The key annotated regions are the ET (enhancing tumor), NCR (necrosis), and ED (edema/invaded tissue).

For preprocessing, the MRI scans underwent skull stripping, co-registration to a standard anatomical template, and interpolation to an isotropic resolution of $1mm^3$. The dimensions of the images and labels are $240 \times 240 \times 155$. An example slice for each contrast type with its segmentation is illustrated in Fig. 1.

Before being input into the network, additional processing was applied to exclude zero-voxel regions, thus reducing computational requirements. To address the qualitative nature of MR image intensities, voxel intensities were

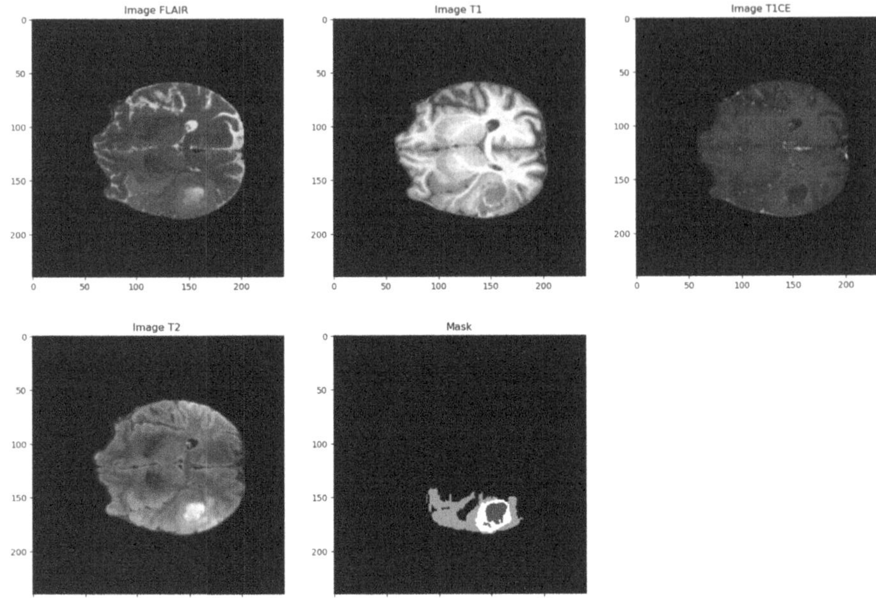

Fig. 1. Example of an axial slice from a single patient.

normalized based on their mean and standard deviation [4]. An axial slice from a single patient displaying FLAIR contrast for the three tumor sub-regions superimposed with three sub-regions of the tumor part on the T1 image as shown in Fig. 2.

3 Methods

3.1 Nn-UNet Baseline

Our methodology leverages an ensemble model, an advanced, cascaded framework designed for configuring segmentation techniques. For in-depth details on nnU-Net, please refer to [16]. Initially, we deploy nnU-Net in its standard form to set a baseline before applying any modifications. Here is an overview of the design choices implemented in nnU-Net:

nnU-Net normalizes brain voxels by adjusting for the standard deviation and subtracting the mean, while keeping non-brain voxels at zero. The architecture, shown in Fig. 1, features an encoder and decoder connected through skip links, echoing the structure of the 3D U-Net [9]. nnU-Net maintains a straightforward design, avoiding complex architectural changes and relying on basic convolution operations.

SwinUNETR is a Vision Transformer-based hierarchical model for localized self-attention with shifted windows. For each task, we trained a 3D SwinUNETR model with five-fold cross validation.

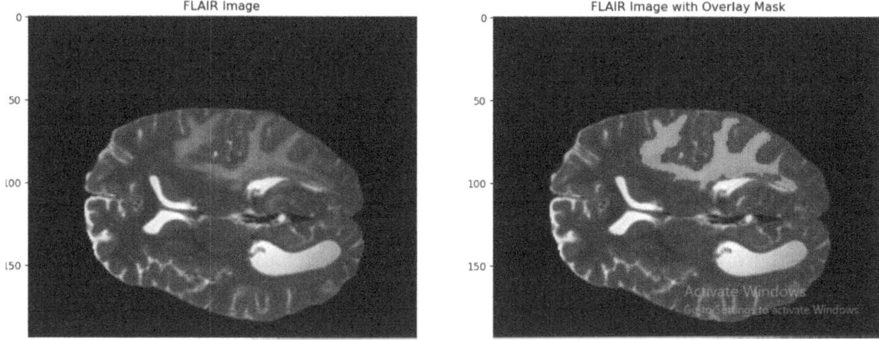

Fig. 2. Example of an axial slice from a single patient displaying FLAIR contrast for the three tumor sub-regions superimposed with three sub-regions of tumor part on the T1 image.

Modified nnU-Net: we modified the architecture of last year's winner's nnU-Net with multiple components. Because of how straightforward nnU-Net is to adapt to new datasets and the fact that the entire code and models has been open-sourced, nnU-Net makes a fantastic baseline for further experimentation. we used group normalization instead of batch normalization, used an asymmetrically large en- Extending nn-UNet for brain tumor segmentation 3 coder for the U-Net, and axial attention in the decoder.

For the BraTS 2025 dataset, nnU-Net processes input patches of size $128 \times 128 \times 128$. Downsampling is accomplished with strided convolutions, while upsampling is managed through transposed convolutions. The feature maps in both the encoder and decoder are designed to be consistent, except at the two lowest resolutions in the decoder, where auxiliary outputs are used for deep supervision.

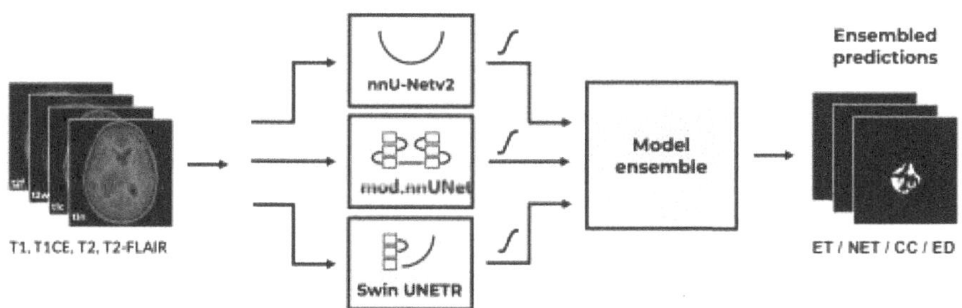

Fig. 3. Proposed Method: Outputs are produced by employing three cutting-edge deep learning models that are utilised in conjunction with ensemble techniques.

3.2 BraTS-Specific Modifications

We employ nnU-Net as a core framework for developing new methodologies and establishing a consistent baseline for segmentation. To highlight its adaptability, we integrate BraTS-specific improvements into the nnU-Net setup.

The training labels cover areas like"Edema", "non-enhancing tumor and necrosis", and "enhancing tumor". However, for evaluation, we focus on three overlapping segments: the tumor core (including non-enhancing tumor, necrosis, and enhancing tumor), the enhancing tumor, and the overall tumor (which encompasses all three categories). Previous studies [3] have shown that directly addressing these combined regions, rather than individual classes, enhances performance in BraTS evaluations.

To implement this, we modify the optimization target to focus on these tumor subregions and replace the softmax function with a sigmoid activation in our network architecture. We also switch to binary cross-entropy loss to optimize each region separately, instead of using traditional cross-entropy.

3.3 Nn-UNet Modifications

As the BraTS dataset has expanded, managing batch size in nnU-Net has become crucial. Using a smaller batch size can result in noisier gradients and limit the model's ability to fit the training data effectively, potentially reducing overfitting. With larger datasets, increasing the batch size can be advantageous if balanced with the bias-variance trade-off. To enhance model performance, we have increased the batch size from 2 to 5 in the nnU-Net configuration.

The conventional method for calculating Dice loss involves assessing each minibatch sample individually before averaging. This approach can produce large gradients from minor errors, especially when labeled voxels are scarce, impacting training updates significantly. These large gradients aim to correct inaccuracies in model predictions.

However, if the model's predictions are accurate but the reference segmentations are not, these large gradients may not be helpful. To address this, we compute Dice loss differently: instead of evaluating each sample separately, we consider each sample in the batch as part of a larger aggregate, a technique known as batch Dice [14]. This method helps balance the influence of samples with few annotated voxels by incorporating them with other samples in the batch.

3.4 Mathematical Model of Advanced NnU-Net

The advanced nnU-Net model for brain tumor segmentation incorporates several key components: residual blocks, attention mechanisms, and Hausdorff distance (HD) loss. Here's a detailed breakdown of its mathematical framework:

Residual Blocks. Residual blocks are integral to capturing complex spatial features within the network. They are mathematically defined as follows:

$$H(x) = F(x) + x \tag{1}$$

In this equation: x is the input to the residual block. $F(x)$ represents the residual function that the network learns. $H(x)$ is the output of the residual block.

Attention Mechanisms Attention mechanisms in nnU-Net help highlight important regions of the image for more accurate segmentation.

Hausdorff Distance (HD) Loss. To enhance boundary precision in segmentation tasks, nnU-Net uses Hausdorff distance as part of its loss function. These components work together to refine the segmentation process, improving both feature extraction and boundary delineation in the advanced nnU-Net model.

By integrating these components, nnU-Net achieves a more precise and effective segmentation process, improving the model's ability to accurately identify and delineate brain tumors. Each element plays a role in refining the overall performance and accuracy of the segmentation outcomes.

4 Results

This section provides a detailed assessment of the enhanced nnU-Net, comparing its performance both quantitatively and qualitatively against the baseline nnU-Net, including insights from an ablation study.

The segmentation metrics for the whole tumor, tumor core, and enhancing tumor show Dice similarity coefficients of 0.84, 0.87, and 0.90 and HD95 values of 3.39, 3.12, and 2.64 respectively. The higher Dice scores indicate a significant improvement in segmentation accuracy, suggesting a closer alignment between the predicted segmentations and the true ground truth. A lower HD95 value suggests that a greater portion of the segmented boundary aligns closer to the actual boundary, indicating improved segmentation accuracy.

Our results clearly demonstrate that architectural enhancements and normalization strategies significantly uplift segmentation quality. Notably, the Modified nnUNet, which incorporates Group Normalization and custom loss functions, outperforms both baseline nnUNet and Swin-UNet in terms of both region overlap (Dice) and boundary precision (HD95). Achieving an average Dice of approximately 0.86 and the lowest average HD95 (2.64 mm), our model surpasses standard nnUNet (Dice 0.85, HD95 3.28 mm) and Swin-UNet (Dice 0.86, HD95 2.93 mm). These figures indicate more accurate delineation of tumor regions and tighter segmentation boundaries.

The superiority of GroupNorm over BatchNorm in small-batch 3D medical imaging is well-established. Since GroupNorm's normalization is independent of batch size, it yields more reliable convergence and improved accuracy in limited memory environments.

In summary, our modified approach, which integrates GroupNorm and Transformer-inspired architecture refinements, leads to a robust model that excels in both region overlap and boundary metrics.

Overall, the ensemble model demonstrates better performance through superior Dice and HD95 scores, leading to more accurate segmentation and more precisely defined tumor boundaries (Fig. 1 and 2) (Table 1, 2 and 3).

Table 1. Dice and HD95 metrics for different model variants

Model	Dice				HD95 (mm)			
	WT	TC	ET	Avg	WT	TC	ET	Avg
nnUNet	0.81	0.84	0.87	0.84	3.71	3.34	2.81	3.29
Swin-Unet	0.84	0.86	0.89	0.87	3.34	2.94	2.54	2.95
Modified nnUNet	0.85	0.87	0.88	0.86	3.15	2.80	2.32	2.75

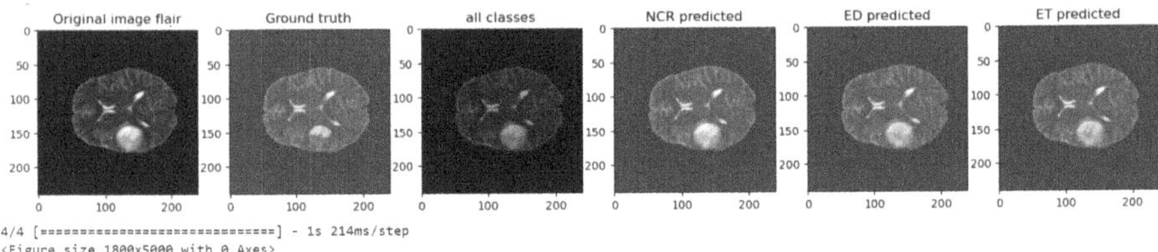

Fig. 4. Qualitative outcome of the suggested framework.

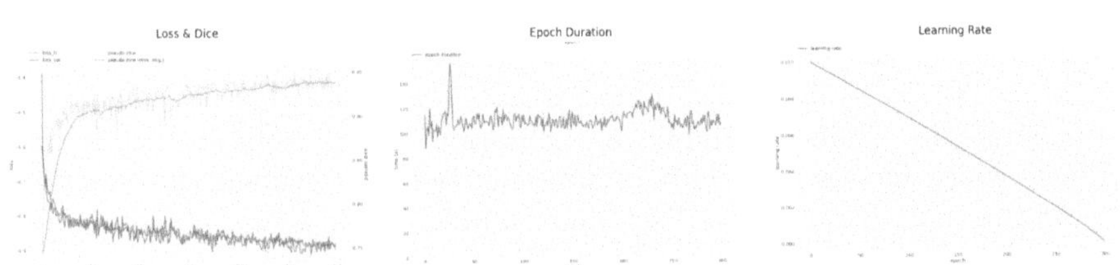

Fig. 5. Training progress over 300 epochs: (top) training/validation loss (blue/red) and pseudo-Dice score (dotted/raw, solid/moving average), (middle) epoch duration per iteration, and (bottom) learning rate schedule. (Color figure online)

Table 2. Training Metrics Over 300 Epochs

Metric	Epoch 0âĂŞ1	Epoch 150	Epoch 300
Training Loss (loss_tr)	0.40	0.85	0.89
Validation Loss (loss_val)	0.60	0.85	0.90
Pseudo Dice (raw)	0.75	0.92	0.94
Pseudo Dice (smoothed)	0.78	0.93	0.945
Epoch Duration (s)	110âĂŞ120	110âĂŞ120	110âĂŞ120
Learning Rate	0.010	0.0045	0.0001

4.1 Qualitative Results

Figure 3 compares the baseline and advanced nnU-Net segmentations using sample instances from the dataset. The comparison highlights how incorporating the attention gate and HD loss improves segmentation accuracy, resulting in the advanced nnU-Net achieving more precise tumor segmentations with fewer false positives. Figure 6 shows that the segmentations results proved excellent value here. In both tasks, the model has apparent capture of the core and peripheral regions of the brain tumor, maintaining the intricate structures and boundaries shown in the ground-truth masks. The error maps show relatively isolated and tiny error spots, mostly close to the boundaries, indicating that most of the errors are rather some mis-classifications and not radical mis-segmentations. Case 2 shows the boundaries differences slightly more evident, but the edges are still trapped to some regions and not numerous. In aggregate, the model continually produces accurate estimates with clear contouring of tumor volumes. Altogether, the results demonstrate a stable and precise model with only a couple of margins for improvement.

Table 3. BraTS GoAT 2025 Challenge âĂŞ Summary of Lesion-wise Dice and NSD Scores.

Metric	ET (Dice)	TC (Dice)	WT (Dice)	ET (NSD)	TC (NSD)	WT (NSD)
Mean	0.7858	0.8135	0.8185	0.8049	0.7839	0.7518
Std	0.2821	0.2878	0.2540	0.2813	0.2882	0.2591

4.2 Testing Phase Results on Unseen Test Data

5 Discussion

This document details our approach for the BraTS 2025 competition. We have refined the nn-UNet structure by employing a larger network, substituting

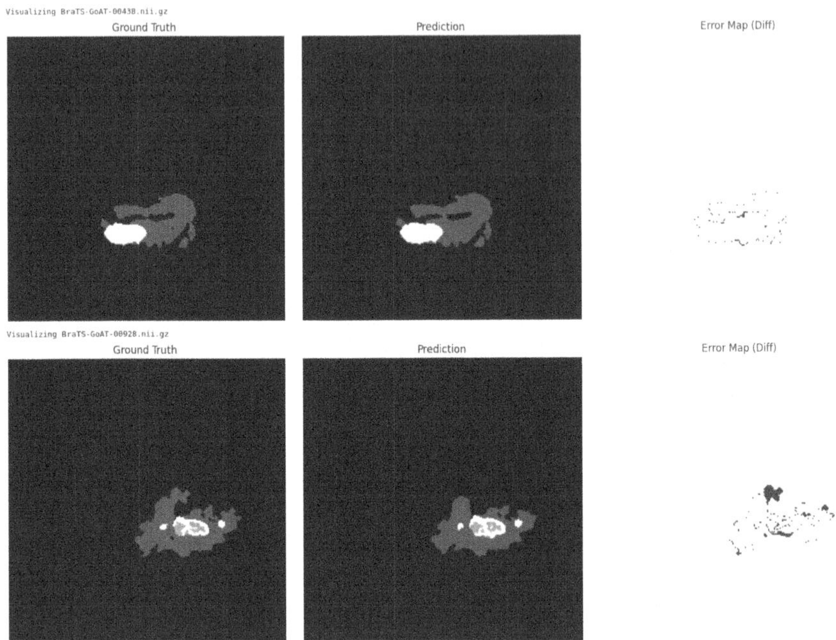

Fig. 6. Predicted vs Groundtruth image.

group normalization for batch normalization, and integrating an axial attention decoder. These adjustments provide a modest improvement over the original nn-UNet.

The nn-UNet framework remains a central element of our strategy due to its flexibility, stability, and ease of implementation. We were able to quickly develop a solid foundation with minimal adjustments.

When modifying 3D data, it is important to account for GPU RAM availability to ensure efficient and smooth training. The larger U-Net and axial attention decoder proposed can significantly increase memory usage, even with modest RAM capacity. Proper calibration is essential to manage memory consumption, as small changes can lead to substantial increases. Group normalization helps address this issue by allowing for smaller batch sizes without significantly impacting performance.

6 Conclusion

The combination of nnU-net, Swin UNETR and Modified nnU-net ensemble prediction led to superior segmentation accuracy for all tumor types. In this work, we looked into ensembling techniques that make the best use of the generalizability of deep learning models and approaches between a wide range of data distributions and tasks. We also qualify the success of our approach in the challenge ranking positions over unseen test cases, where we were ranked first in the GoAT task.

Acknowledgements. The authors would like to thank Dr Nilesh Kurwale, Neurosurgeon, Dinanath Mangeshkar Hospital, Pune, India, for explaining the medical concepts.

References

1. Adewole, M., et al.: The brain tumor segmentation (brats) challenge 2023: glioma segmentation in sub-Saharan Africa patient population (brats-Africa). arXiv preprint (2023). https://arxiv.org/abs/2305.19369
2. Banan-Khojasteh, S.M., Balafar, M.A.: Automatic brain tumor segmentation in multimodal MRI images using deep learning. In: Applied Artificial Intelligence: A Biomedical Perspective (2023). https://doi.org/10.1201/9781003324430-7
3. Bhardawaj, F., Jain, S.: Cad system design for two-class brain tumor classification using transfer learning. Current Cancer Therapy Rev. **20**(2) (2023). https://doi.org/10.2174/1573394719666230816091316
4. Chauhan, A.S., Singh, J., Kumar, S., Saxena, N., Gupta, M., Verma, P.: Design and assessment of improved convolutional neural network based brain tumor segmentation and classification system. J. Integrated Sci. Technol. **12**(4) (2024). https://doi.org/10.62110/sciencein.jist.2024.v12.793
5. Hou, Q., Peng, Y., Wang, Z., Wang, J., Jiang, J.: Mfd-net: Modality fusion diffractive network for segmentation of multimodal brain tumor image. IEEE J. Biomed. Health Inform. **27**(12), 5958–5969 (2023). https://doi.org/10.1109/JBHI.2023.3318640
6. Imtiaz, R., Mirza, M.W., Siddiq, A., Farooq-I-Azam, M., Khan, I.R., Rahardja, S.: Brain tumor segmentation from MR images using customized u-net for a smaller dataset. In: BioCAS 2023 - IEEE Biomedical Circuits and Systems Conference (2023). https://doi.org/10.1109/BioCAS58349.2023.10389092
7. Jiang, Y., Zhang, Y., Lin, X., Dong, J., Cheng, T., Liang, J.: Swinbts: A method for 3D multimodal brain tumor segmentation using swin transformer. Brain Sci. **12**(6) (2022). https://doi.org/10.3390/brainsci12060797
8. Kim, B.H., et al.: Validation of MRI-based models to predict MGMT promoter methylation in gliomas: Brats 2021 radiogenomics challenge. Cancers **14**(19) (2022). https://doi.org/10.3390/cancers14194827
9. Lee, S., Lee, M.: Metaswin: a unified meta vision transformer model for medical image segmentation. PeerJ Computer Science **10** (2024). https://doi.org/10.7717/peerj-cs.1762
10. Liu, P., Dou, Q., Wang, Q., Heng, P.A.: An encoder-decoder neural network with 3D squeeze-and-excitation and deep supervision for brain tumor segmentation. IEEE Access **8**, 34029–34037 (2020). https://doi.org/10.1109/ACCESS.2020.2973707
11. Liu, Y., Zhang, Z., Yue, J., Guo, W.: Scanext: Enhancing 3d medical image segmentation with dual attention network and depth-wise convolution. Heliyon **10**(5) (2024). https://doi.org/10.1016/j.heliyon.2024.e26775

12. Mehta, R., et al.: Qu-brats: Miccai brats 2020 challenge on quantifying uncertainty in brain tumor segmentation – analysis of ranking scores and benchmarking results. Mach. Learn. Biomed. Imaging **1** (2022). https://doi.org/10.59275/j.melba.2022-354b
13. Organizers, B.C.: Miccai brats 2025 goat challenge: Generalizability of segmentation methods across tumors (2025). Accessed: 30-07-2025
14. Singh, S., Garg, V., Loganathan, S.: Brain tumor segmentation using 3D unet. Int. J. Multidisc. Res. (IJFMR) **5**(6) (2023). https://doi.org/10.36948/ijfmr.2023.v05i06.8815
15. Sridhar, S.R.: Automated brain tumor detection using ideal shallow neural network with artificial jellyfish optimization. Current Med. Imaging **20**, 1–15 (2024). https://doi.org/10.2174/1573405620666230731120924
16. Tixier, F., Jaouen, V., Hognon, C., Gallinato, O., Colin, T., Visvikis, D.: Evaluation of conventional and deep learning based image harmonization methods in radiomics studies. Phy. Med. Biol. **66**(24) (2021). https://doi.org/10.1088/1361-6560/ac39e5

Author Index

S. Bakas et al. (Eds.): MICCAI 2025, LNCS 16376, pp. 549–552, 2026.
https://doi.org/10.1007/978-3-032-16365-3

The manufacturer's authorised representative in the EU is Springer Nature Customer Service Centre GmbH, Europaplatz 3, 69115 Heidelberg, Germany. If you have any concerns regarding our products, please contact ProductSafety@springernature.com

Printed and bound by CPI Group (UK) Ltd, Croydon, CR0 4YY
07/07/2026
02160917-0018